FLAVIVIRUS ENCEPHALITIS

Edited by **Daniel Růžek**

Flavivirus Encephalitis
Edited by Daniel Růžek

Published by InTech
Janeza Trdine 9, 51000 Rijeka, Croatia

Publishing Process Manager Masa Vidovic

Technical Editor Teodora Smiljanic

Cover Designer InTech Design Team

Additional hard copies can be obtained from orders@intechopen.com

Flavivirus Encephalitis, Edited by Daniel Růžek
p. cm.
ISBN 978-953-307-669-0

For EU product safety concerns:
IN TECH d.o.o., Prolaz Marije Krucifikse Kozulić 3, 51000 Rijeka, Croatia,
info@intechopen.com or visit our website at intechopen.com.

Meet the editor

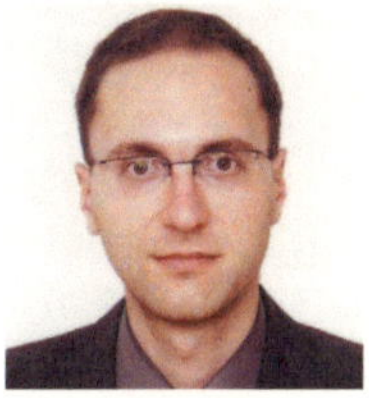

Dr. Daniel Růžek is a research scientist at the Institute of Parasitology, Academy of Sciences of the Czech Republic, and assistant professor at the Department of Medical Biology, Faculty of Science, University of South Bohemia. He received his Ph.D. in the field of molecular and cellular biology and genetics from the Academy of Sciences of the Czech Republic and University of South Bohemia. He had postdoctoral training at the Department of Virology and Immunology, Texas Biomedical Research Institute (formerly Southwest Foundation for Biomedical Research), San Antonio, USA. His primary field is virology with research emphasis on vector-borne viruses, especially tick-borne encephalitis virus, Omsk hemorrhagic fever virus, dengue virus, and West Nile virus. He is a recipient of several scientific awards through various organizations, e.g., in 2009 he was awarded with a prestigious international Sinnecker-Kunz Award for young researchers in the field of tick-borne diseases.

Contents

Preface

Encephalitis in humans is of public health concern worldwide because of its high morbidity and mortality. The disease can be characterized as an inflammatory process in the brain parenchyma associated with clinical evidence of brain dysfunction. There are several causes leading to the development of encephalitis, which includes non-infective processes and microbial infections. Infectious encephalitis can be caused by bacterial or protozoal infestation, but viruses are the most common causative agents. Herpes simplex virus type 1, varicella-zoster virus, Epstein-Barr virus, the mumps virus, the measles virus, or enteroviruses belong to the most important.

The genus Flavivirus represents a diverse group of viruses. Most of them are transmitted by mosquitoes or ticks. Flaviviruses cause flu-like diseases, fever, or hemorrhagic fever, but several members of this group also represent important causative agents of encephalitis. These include the West Nile virus occurring in large areas of the world, the tick-borne encephalitis virus prevalent across Eurasia, Japanese encephalitis in Asia, Murray Valley encephalitis in Australia, New Guinea, and New Zealand, and St. Louis encephalitis virus in the United States.

The book *Flavivirus Encephalitis* provides the most recent information about selected aspects associated with encephalitic flaviviruses. The book contains chapters that cover a wide spectrum of subjects including flavivirus biology, virus-host interactions, the role of vectors in disease epidemiology, neurological dengue, and West Nile encephalitis. Special attention is paid to tick-borne encephalitis and Japanese encephalitis viruses. Leading experts from several countries all over the world have written chapters for this impressive collection. The multi-authored characteristic of this volume offers a wide spectrum of knowledge and experience, as the authors are specialists in different fields and express diverse approaches and concepts. The book uniquely combines up-to-date reviews with cutting-edge original research data. Hence, it provides a good source of information for students, medical professionals, as well as experts in the field of viral neuroinfections, and all others interested in this topic.

I would like to acknowledge sincerely all contributing authors for their time and effort in preparing the various chapters and their excellent work. Also I would like to thank Masa Vidovic from InTech Open Access Publisher for her excellent technical support during the realization process of this book. Last but not least, I would like to acknowledge the Czech Science Foundation (projects No. P302/10/P438, and No. P502/11/2116) for financial support.

Dr. Daniel Růžek
Academy of Sciences of the Czech Republic
Institute of Parasitology

and

University of South Bohemia
Faculty of Science
Department of Medical Biology
České Budějovice,
Czech Republic

Part 1

Encephalitic Flaviviruses - General Concepts, Dengue, West Nile

1

Encephalitic Flaviviruses

Duncan R. Smith
Institute of Molecular Biosciences and Center for Emerging and Neglected Infectious Diseases, Mahidol University
Thailand

1. Introduction

As defined by the Infectious Diseases Society of America, encephalitis is "the presence of an inflammatory process of the brain associated with clinical evidence of neurologic dysfunction"(Tunkel et al., 2008). In the absence of appropriate data, it is difficult to estimate the worldwide incidence of encephalitis, but in Southeast Asia Japanese encephalitis virus infections alone causes some 30,000 to 50,000 cases of encephalitis annually (Misra & Kalita, 2010; Tsai, 2000) and causes of encephalitis include, but are not limited to, bacterial, viral, fungal and parasite infections as well as autoimmune and post infectious encephalitis where the encephalitis follows a usually mild viral infection or vaccine immunization and results from an inappropriate immune response. More than one hundred different infectious agents have been known to cause encephalitis, and while bacteria such as *Mycobacterium tuberculosis* (TB) and *Bartonella henselae* (the agent that causes cat scratch disease) are significant causes of encephalitis, viral infections are responsible for the majority of cases of infectious encephalitis. Viruses that can cause encephalitis include rabies virus, herpes simplex virus, enteroviruses including polioviruses, coxsackieviruses, echoviruses and a number of arboviruses (arthropod-borne viruses).

	Primary vector species	Probable natural reservoir	Human disease	Encephalitis
Mammalian tick-borne virus group				
Gadgets Gully virus	Ixodes	Birds	No reports to date	
Kyasanur Forest disease virus	Ixodes, Haemophysalis	Monkeys, small mammals	Yes	No
Langat virus	Ixodes, Haemaphysalis	Forest rats	Yes	Possible
Louping ill virus	Ixodes	Sheep, deer, birds	Yes	Yes
Omsk hemorrhagic fever virus	Dermacentor	Mammals, rodents	Yes	No
Powassan virus	Ixodes, Dermacentor, Haemaphysalis	Rodents, mustelids, lagomorphs	Yes	Yes
Royal Farm virus	Argas	Rodents	No reports todate	
Tick-borne encephalitis virus	Ixodes	Rodents	Yes	Yes
Seabird tick-borne virus group				
Kadam virus	Rhipicephalus	Cloven hooved mammals, rodents	No reports to date	
Meaban virus	Ornithodores	Seabirds	No reports to date	
Saumarez Reef virus	Ixodes	Seabirds	No reports to date	
Tyuleniy virus	Ixodes	Seabirds	No reports to date	

Table 1. Tick-borne flavivirus species

There are over 500 known arboviruses, which predominantly belong to the *Togaviridae, Bunyaviridae, Rhabdoviridae, Reoviridae* and *Flaviviridae* families, and viruses that cause encephalitis in humans belong to all of these families. Encephalitis causing *Togaviridae* belong to the *Alphavirus* genus and include Ross River, Chikungunya and Western-, Eastern- and Venezuelan equine encephalitis viruses, while encephalitis causing viruses in the family *Bunyaviridae* belong to the *Nairovirus* (Crimean-Congo hemorrhagic fever virus), *Phlebovirus* (Rift Valley fever virus) and *Orthobunyavirus* (La Crosse virus) genera. Chandipura virus (family *Rhabdoviridae*, genus *Vesiculovirus*) has been associated with encephalitis, although there remains little further information. The family *reoviridae* contains 12 genera (*Orthoreovirus, Orbivirus, Rotavirus, Coltivirus, Aquareovirus, Cypovirus, Fijivirus, Phytoreovirus, Oryzavirus, Mycoreovirus, Seadornavirus and Idnoreovirus*) at least two of which contain arboviruses associated with encephalitis, namely the genera *Coltivirus* (Colorado Tick fever virus) and *Seadornavirus* (Banna virus). The family *Flaviviridae* contains only three genera (*Hepacivirus, Pestivirus and Flavivirus*) but the *Flavivirus* genus contains some of the most widespread and important arboviruses as well as the most important and widespread viruses associated with encephalitis.

	Primary vector species	Probable natural reservoir	Human disease	Encephalitis
Aroa virus group				
Aroa virus	Not known	Rodents	No reports to date	
Dengue virus group				
Dengue virus	Aedes	Primates	Yes	Occasional
Kedougou virus	Aedes	Primates (?)	No reports to date	
Japanese encephalitis group				
Cacipacore virus	Culex	Birds (?)	No reports to date	
Koutango virus	Culex	Rodents (?)	Yes	No
Japanese encephalitis virus	Culex	Migrating birds, domestic fowl, pigs	Yes	Yes
Murray Valley encephalitis virus	Culex	Birds, feral pigs (?)	Yes	Yes
St. Louis encephalitis virus	Culex	Birds	Yes	Yes
Usutu virus	Culex	Rodents, birds	Yes	No
West Nile virus	Culex	Birds of family Corvidae, passerines	Yes	Yes
Yaounde virus	Culex	Birds (?)	No reports to date	
Kokobera virus group				
Kokobera virus	Culex	Macropods, Marsuplials	Yes	No
Ntaya virus group				
Bagaza virus	Culex	Birds	Yes	Possible
Ilheus virus	Psorophora, Aedes	Birds	Yes	Possible
Israel turkey meningoencephalomyelitis virus	Not known	Birds	No reports to date	
Ntaya virus	Aedes (?) Culex (?)	Not known	Yes	No
Tembusu virus	Culex	Birds	No reports to date	
Spondweni virus group				
Zika virus	Aedes	Primates	Yes	No
Yellow fever virus group				
Banzi virus	Culex	Rodents	Yes	No
Bouboui virus	Anopheles	Primates	No reports to date	
Edge Hill virus	Aedes	Wallabies, bandicoots	Possible	No
Jugra virus	Aedes	Bats	No reports to date	
Saboya virus	Phlebotomines	Rodents	No reports to date	
Sepik virus	Ficalbia	Sheep (?) Humans (?)	Possible	No
Uganda S virus	Aedes	Birds, Rodents (?)	No reports to date	
Wesselsbron virus	Aedes	Ruminants (Artiodactyla)	Yes	Possible
Yellow fever virus	Aedes	Primates	Yes	No

Table 2. Mosquito-borne flavivirus species

A total of 53 species of flaviviruses are listed in the latest version of the International Committee on Taxonomy of Viruses Master species list version 9 (ICTV, 2011). A further 23 viruses are considered to be strains belonging to the 53 species, while another two viruses (Cell fusing agent virus and Tamana bat virus) are considered tentative species in the genus (ICTV, 2011). The genus *Flavivirus* is divided into three clusters, the mosquito-borne cluster, the tick-borne cluster and the "no known arthropod vector" cluster. All flaviviruses of human importance belong to the mosquito-borne or tick-borne clusters. While flaviviruses that cause human disease are found in the "no known arthropod vector" cluster, these have not yet been responsible for significant outbreaks of human disease. Classification of flaviviruses was originally based upon classical studies using cross-neutralization tests, with viruses that induce cross reacting antibodies being placed into the same "serogroup". In recent times however grouping of flaviviruses has been predominantly based upon genetic analysis with viruses being placed into groups based upon sequence analysis. For the majority of flaviviruses, these groupings are synonymous, although some differences do occur. For example the Cacipacoré virus which was originally considered an ungrouped flavivirus based on cross neutralization tests is now considered part of the Japanese encephalitis group based upon sequence data and phylogenic analysis.

The tick-borne cluster of flavivirus is commonly divided into the mammalian tick-borne virus group and the seabird tick-borne virus group (see Table 1), while the mosquito -borne flaviviruses are commonly segregated into 7 groups (See Table 2). The no known arthropod vector group currently consists of 12 virus species, divided into 3 groups (See Table 3).

	Primary vector species	Probable natural reservoir	Human disease	Encephalitis
Entebbe virus group				
Entebbe bat virus	Unknown	Bats	No reports to date	
Yokose virus	Unknown	Bats	No reports to date	
Modoc virus group				
Apoi virus	Unknown	Rodents	Possible	
Cowbone Ridge virus	Unknown	Rodents	No reports to date	
Jutiapa virus	Unknown	Rodents (?)	No reports to date	
Modoc virus	Unknown	Rodents (?)	Possible	Possible
Sal Vieja virus	Unknown	Rodents	No reports to date	
San Perlita virus	Unknown	Rodents	No reports to date	
Rio Bravo virus group				
Bukalasa bat virus	Unknown	Bats	No reports to date	
Carey Island virus	Unknown	Bats	No reports to date	
Dakar bat virus	Unknown	Bats	No reports to date	
Montana myotis leukoencephalitis virus	Unknown	Bats	No reports to date	
Phnom Penh bat virus	Unknown	Bats	No reports to date	
Rio Bravo virus	Unknown	Bats	Possible	No

Table 3. No known arthropod vector flavivirus species

As with all arboviruses, arboviral flaviviruses are maintained in natural cycles in which they multiply in a blood sucking arthropod such as a mosquito or tick and are then transmitted to a vertebrate host via the saliva when the insect takes a blood meal. Replication of the virus in the vertebrate host causes viremia of a sufficient level to allow infection of a naïve mosquito as it feeds. When infected, the arthropod becomes infected for life while in contrast the vertebrate host normally undergoes an acute but normally self limiting infection. In natural transmission cycles neither the arthropod vector nor the vertebrate suffer significant consequences of the infection. With the exception of urban cycles of yellow fever and dengue fever viruses, humans are not the principal amplifying host and infection in humans occurs when the vector feeds on humans as an alternate to its normal vertebrate host. In these cases infection is normally a dead end for virus transmission as the disease is usually of a low titer viremia, although the consequences may be significant for the human host. The "no known arthropod vector group" of flaviviruses remains poorly understood. They are predominantly associated with either rodents or bats, and the ecology of their transmission remains largely undefined. There are scattered reports of possible infections of humans, usually by direct infection, although there is little confirmatory evidence linking the pathogen with the disease. These viruses are however of significant interest given their potential for emerging into the human population.

2. The encephalitic flaviviruses

2.1 Epidemiology

2.1.1 The Japanese encephalitis group.

The Japanese encephalitis group of the mosquito-borne flavivirus cluster consists of 8 virus species (Table 2) of which 4 viruses (Japanese encephalitis virus, Murray Valley encephalitis virus, St. Louis encephalitis virus and West Nile virus) have been consistently associated with encephalitis in cases of human infection.

2.1.1.1 Japanese encephalitis virus

Japanese encephalitis is one of the most important encephalitic diseases worldwide, resulting in some 35,000 to 50,000 deaths annually (Misra & Kalita, 2010; Tsai, 2000). Humans can become infected as a consequence of the bite of an infected mosquito, although evidence suggests that humans are not a natural host, but rather a dead-end host for Japanese encephalitis virus infection (Rosen, 1986). Naturally Japanese encephalitis virus is transmitted in an enzootic cycle among birds, particularly ardeid wading birds, and mosquitoes, principally *Culex tritaeniorhynchus* (Halstead & Jacobson, 2003) and *Culex quinquefasciatus*. The geographic distribution of Japanese encephalitis virus is mainly in the Asian region including India, China, and all of South-East Asia, although outbreaks have also been reported in Australia. Pigs have become an important host for maintaining, amplifying and spreading Japanese encephalitis virus as they undergo a long lasting viremia upon infection and are a preferred feeding source for *Culex tritaeniorhynchus*. The commercial pig farm industry both provides a source of susceptible animals in endemic areas, as well as potentially spreading the disease through the transport of infected animals. In Southeast Asian countries Japanese encephalitis virus is the leading reported cause of acute encephalitis in children, accounting for approximately 40% of cases (Solomon et al., 2002; Srey et al., 2002).

2.1.1.2 Murray Valley encephalitis virus

Murray Valley encephalitis virus (sometimes called Australian encephalitis) is spread primarily by *Culex annulirostris*, and is believed to be endemic only in Australia and Papua New Guinea. Since the last major outbreak in Australia in 1974, which infected nearly 60 patients, only sporadic outbreaks have been recorded.

2.1.1.3 St. Louis encephalitis virus

St. Louis encephalitis virus is distributed over much of the Americas, and is found in Canada (Ontario), the United States (especially in western states and in the southeast), Trinidad, Jamaica, Panama, Brazil, and Argentina. In North America approximately 25-50 individuals are symptomatically infected each year and significant outbreaks affecting up to

800 people per 100,000 occur every 5 to 15 years in the Americas. The last major epidemic recorded was in 1990 in Florida which resulted in 11 deaths. Passeriforme and Columbiforme birds are believed to be the major reservoir species, and transmission is by *Culex* spp mosquitoes.

2.1.1.4 West Nile virus

West Nile virus is the most wide spread flavivirus with a worldwide distribution including Africa, Asia, Europe, and North America (Bakonyi et al., 2005). West Nile virus is naturally maintained in a cycle between bird feeding mosquitoes and wild animals, mainly birds. The natural cycle primarily involves the *Culex* species of mosquitoes in particular *Culex pipiens, Culex quinquefasciatus* and *Culex restuans* which are the most important West Nile virus vectors. A broad range of mammalian species are found to be susceptible to natural infection with West Nile virus following infectious mosquito bite(s) and includes humans, horses, cats, rabbits, skunks, squirrels, chipmunks, and two species of bats (Marfin et al., 2001). Although initially West Nile virus was considered to have a minor human health impact, West Nile virus epidemics have become widely distributed causing several hundreds of reported cases in Romania in 1996 (Tsai et al., 1998), Russia in 1999 (Platonov et al., 2001), and Israel in 2000 (Chowers et al., 2001). West Nile virus has also been a significant cause of human illness in the United States. By the end of 2002, West Nile virus activity had been identified in 44 states and the District of Columbia resulting in reports of over 4,000 human cases of West Nile disease (including several thousand cases of meningoencephalitis cases and almost 300 deaths). Reported deaths were also recorded for wild animals including 16,741 dead birds and 14,571 equine cases (Centers for Disease Control and Prevention (CDC), 2003). Phylogenetic analyses have shown 2 distinct lineages of West Nile virus strains which were isolated in different geographic regions: I and II (Berthet et al., 1997; Lanciotti et al., 1999; Savage et al., 1999). Lineage I has a wide distribution including Africa, Asia, Europe, and North America and is associated with all the outbreaks of human and equine diseases. Lineage II is restricted to endemic enzootic infections in Africa and has not been associated with human encephalitis (Berthet et al., 1997).

2.1.2 The tick-borne encephalitis group

The tick-borne encephalitis group consists of two main subgroups (the mammalian tick-borne virus group and the seabird tick-borne virus group), with human pathogens being limited to the mammalian tick-borne group (Table 1). Three virus species within this group have a consistent association with encephalitis, namely Louping ill virus, Powassan virus and Tick-borne encephalitis virus. The position of the Kadam virus within the seabird tick-borne cluster remains somewhat controversial, but this virus has not been associated with significant levels of human infection nor encephalitis, and as such is not discussed further in this article. Similarly Langat virus is naturally attenuated and does not seem to be associated with human disease under natural conditions. While there are reports of Langat associated encephalitis in humans, these have occurred solely in large scale vaccination trials attempting to use Langat virus to protect against Tick-borne encephalitis virus infection in Russia.

2.1.2.1 Louping ill virus

Louping ill virus occurs mainly in the British Isles, where sheep are the most important reservoir host for this virus, but amplification can also occur in grouse and mountain hares which have been implicated as maintenance hosts via non-viremic transmission between cofeeding ticks. The principal vector for transmission is the tick *Ixodes ricinus*, although other species of tick including *Rhipicephalus appendiculatus*, *Ixodes persulcatus* and *Haemaphysalis anatolicum* are capable of transmitting the virus. Louping ill virus produces a symptomatic disease in sheep which may have a neurological component including encephalitis. Fewer than 100 cases of Louping ill infection of humans have been reported in the British Isles, most commonly in agricultural workers, although a number of cases of laboratory based infection have been reported. While direct tick transmission to humans is a possibility, there are few reliable reports of transmission by this route, and infection may arise predominantly through contact with sick animals or infected tissues or fluids.

2.1.2.2 Powassan virus

Only between 20 and 50 cases of human Powassan virus infection have been reported since the first identified case of a boy who died from infection with the virus in Powassan, Ontario in 1958. The virus is widely distributed in North America in both Canada and in the United States, and reports have identified Powassan virus in locations in southeastern Siberia. The virus is maintained in transmission cycles that include several species of small wild mammals including the woodchuck (*Marmota monax*), squirrels, chipmunks and deer mice and several species of *Ixodes* ticks. In eastern and central Canada, the transmission cycle between the woodchuck and the tick *Ixodes cookei* may be of particular importance.

2.1.2.3 Tick-borne encephalitis virus

Tick-borne encephalitis virus is one of the most important tick-borne flaviviruses causing a serious acute central nervous system infection and the distribution of this disease stretches from seven countries in northern Asia to central Asia and 25 Western European countries (Charrel et al., 2004). Naturally, Tick-borne encephalitis virus is maintained in a cycle involving ticks and wild vertebrate hosts. While several different species of tick have been found to be biologically competent to transmit Tick-borne encephalitis virus in the laboratory, in nature, because of specific ecological limiting factors, only *Ixodes ricinus* in Europe, and *Ixodes persulcatus* and *Haemaphysalis concinna* in Russia, appear to play a significant role in the virus maintenance (Labuda & Randolph, 1999). There are three subtypes of Tick-borne encephalitis virus, the European (also known as Central European encephalitis virus), Siberian (also known as west-Siberian encephalitis virus) and Far-eastern (also known as Russian Spring/Summer encephalitis virus), in which the degrees of virulence are different (Mansfield et al., 2009). Transmission of Tick-borne encephalitis virus through raw milk or cheese from goats, sheep and cows was previously responsible for 10 to 20% of cases of Tick-borne encephalitis virus transmission in central Europe.

2.2 Pathogenesis and clinical features

All of the encephalitic flaviviruses have several features in common and they all raise a significant immune response. The initial response is generally a non-specific innate response that occurs within the first few days after infection, and pathogen specific humoral (antibody) and cell mediated immunity begin four to seven days after infection. The antibody response raised is frequently extremely broad and cross reactive with other flaviviruses and generates lifelong immunity towards the homotypic virus as well as potentially partial protection against other flaviviruses. With each of the encephalitic flaviviruses, symptomatic infections are greatly outnumbered by asymptomatic infections, and symptomatic infections generally generate a broad spectrum of responses in patients ranging from a mild disease typically characterized by fever and headache to severe encephalitis or meningitis leading often to coma and death. The broad range of responses to the infecting pathogen suggests a complex interplay between host and viral factors that remains largely unexplained. Where encephalitis is a component of the disease pathology, long term neurological deficit is common. The underlying mechanism by which some flaviviruses, but not others, cause encephalitis is still the subject of considerable investigation. Where flavivirus infection does lead to encephalitis, the mechanism by which the virus crosses the blood brain barrier remains to be fully elucidated, and several mechanisms have been proposed. Studies of neurotropism in a hamster model of St. Louis encephalitis virus infection have shown the importance of axonal transport through olfactory neurons (Monath et al., 1983), thus evading the blood brain barrier. However, postmortem studies on patients who died from Japanese encephalitis virus infection showed diffuse infection throughout the brain, indicating a hematogenous route of entry (Desai et al., 1995; Johnson et al., 1985). Infection of parenchyma may therefore result from either simple diffusion from vascular endothelial cells at sites where the integrity of the blood brain barrier has been compromised due to trauma, or through replication of the virus in the endothelial cells of brain capillaries, and release of the virus into the brain. Alternatively, some evidence has suggested a role for overproduction of inflammatory cytokines as a consequence of activation of the Toll-like receptor (TLR) 3 as causative in weakening the blood brain barrier in West Nile virus infections (Wang et al., 2004). However, a simple increase in permeability of the blood brain barrier seems not to be the primary determinant of lethality in animal model systems (Morrey et al., 2008), suggesting that additional factors need to be elucidated. Whether all encephalitic flaviviruses use the same mechanism, or indeed whether a specific virus utilizes several pathways remains to be determined.

2.2.1 The Japanese encephalitis virus group

2.2.1.1 Japanese encephalitis virus

Population based studies in areas with endemic Japanese encephalitis have estimated the ratio of overt: inapparent Japanese encephalitis virus infections as approximately 1:250 (Gajanana et al., 1995). Where symptomatic infection occurs, symptoms start some five to 15 days after infection. Mild infections are generally characterized by a fever and headaches while more severe disease is characterized by nausea and vomiting, neck stiffness, stupor, disorientation, convulsions and paralysis. While a proportion of patients make a rapid and spontaneous recovery, up to 30% of patients admitted to hospital with Japanese encephalitis die. For non-fatal cases of Japanese encephalitis, approximately 50% of the survivors suffer from severe neurological sequelae, and even those who have been classed as having "good recovery" have evidence of neurological damage (Kumar et al., 1993; Solomon et al., 2000). There is some evidence that Japanese encephalitis virus may establish a latent infection in some patients that can lead to recurrence of symptoms many months later (Sharma et al., 1991).

2.2.1.2 Murray Valley encephalitis virus

Serological surveys suggest that only 1 in 1000 infections with Murray Valley Encephalitis virus result in a symptomatic disease. Where a symptomatic infection does occur, symptoms arise some one to four weeks after exposure to the virus and may include headache, nausea, vomiting, myalgia and a rash. In a proportion of symptomatic cases lethargy, confusion, convulsions and fits may occur indicative of neurological involvement and coma and death may follow. Up to 25% of cases of symptomatic Murray Valley encephalitis infection are fatal, and survivors may show long term neurological deficits.

2.2.1.3 St. Louis encephalitis virus

As with other flavivirus infections, infections with St. Louis encephalitis virus are generally asymptomatic, with an inapparent: apparent infection ratios of between 16:1 and 425:1. The incubation period between infection and the onset of symptoms is believed to be 21 days, and symptomatic infection usually results in a mild disease characterized by headache, tiredness and dizziness, sometimes with nausea and vomiting. Severe disease with neurologic involvement including encephalitis or aseptic meningitis is rare, and more commonly found in older adults. Long term disability and death can occur, and the disease is fatal in up to 10% of patients.

2.2.1.4 West Nile virus

Most infections with West Nile virus are asymptomatic and symptomatic West Nile fever occurs in only 20-30% of cases of infection. West Nile fever is a flu-like illness which develops 3 - 14 days post infection and is characterized by fever, headache, back pain, fatigue, arthralgia and myalgia (Hayes et al., 2005) with symptoms sometimes persisting for several weeks. A maculopapular rash occurs in about 50% of cases. Neurological involvement occurs in less than 1% of infections, and is characterized by encephalitis in 60% of cases, and meningitis in 40% of cases. Neurological involvement can result in long term cognitive and neurological deficits.

2.2.2 The tick-borne encephalitis group

2.2.2.1 Louping ill virus

Given the small number of cases of Louping ill virus infection recorded, accurate clinical data is somewhat scarce. A four to seven day incubation period is believed to occur after infection before the onset of symptoms. Evidence suggests that the disease evinces with a mild fever, headache and tiredness which may be mistaken for flu, and serological studies in abattoir workers suggest a greater degree of exposure to the virus than symptomatic cases would suggest. In some infections the mild symptoms maybe the only pathological expression of the disease, however, in other infections after an apparent remission period of approximately one week, the fever recurs together with neurologic complications which can include meningoencephalitis or paralytic poliomyelitis. Even with the severe form of Louping ill virus infection, death is rare, and although convalescence maybe prolonged, there are no apparent long term neurological deficits.

2.2.2.2 Powassan virus

While an extremely limited number of cases of infection with Powassan virus have been recorded, serological evidence suggests that large numbers of people have been exposed to the virus. Serological surveys in Ontario between 1959 and 1961 suggested an average yearly exposure of approximately 2% of the population, suggesting that symptomatic infections with Powassan virus are significantly outnumbered by asymptomatic infections. Where symptomatic infection occurs, an estimated 8 to 34 days after infection, early symptoms include headache, lethargy and disorientation, while in the later progression of the disease, encephalopathy is extremely common. The case fatality rate for Powassan virus infection is believed to be 10 to 15%, but severe, long term neurological sequelae are present in up to 50% of the survivors (Ebel, 2010; Gholam et al., 1999).

2.2.2.3 Tick-borne encephalitis virus

An estimated 90% of cases of infection with Tick-borne encephalitis virus are believed to be asymptomatic or to result in a non-specific illness. Symptomatic disease, which may last from two to four days is characterized by a non-specific flu like disease with fever, headache, myalgia and vomiting and occurs after an incubation period of one to two weeks, although the range of onset of symptoms extends between two days and one month. Reports suggest infection through raw milk and milk products may lead to a faster onset of symptoms. In approximately one third of cases the disease presents as a biphasic disease and after an approximately one week (range 1 to 20 days) asymptomatic period the second phase of the disease occurs. The second phase of the disease is heralded by the onset of a high fever coupled with central nervous system involvement and involves symptoms of meningitis (fever, headache, stiff neck) or encephalitis (drowsiness, confusion, sensory disturbances, paralysis) or meningoencephalitis. Encephalitis is more commonly found in adults over the age of 40, while children are more likely to experience meningitis. Infection with Tick-borne encephalitis virus may result in mortality or long-term neurological sequelae in 35–58% of patients. The fatality rate associated with clinical infection is 0.5–20% (World Health Organization, 2006), although the Far Eastern subtype is generally associated with a higher mortality rate (5 to 20% fatality rate) than the European subtype (1 -2%). As with Japanese encephalitis virus, some data suggests that the Tick-borne encephalitis virus may be able to establish latent infections leading to the recurrence of symptoms after a long remission period (Ogawa et al., 1973).

2.3 Flavivirus life cycle

Flaviviruses are spherical viruses some 40-60nm in diameter consisting of three structural proteins, Envelope (E), Membrane (M) and Capsid (C) and a single stranded (+) sense RNA molecule of approximately 11kb. The RNA contains both 5′ and 3′ untranslated regions and is usually not polyadenylated (although some strains of tick-borne encephalitis may contain a poly(A) tract) and encodes the three structural proteins (C, E and pre-M), as well as seven non-structural proteins (NS1, NS2A, NS2B, NS3, NS4A, NS4B and NS5) and is translated as a single open reading frame and processed by host and virally encoded proteases (Henchal & Putnak, 1990; Perera & Kuhn, 2008). The viruses contain a significant amount of lipid (15-20% by weight) that is similar in content to the host cell membranes (Russell et al., 1980).

Flaviviruses predominantly enter into both insect and mammalian cells through endocytosis into clathrin coated pits following binding to a specific receptor or receptors. While clathrin mediated endocytosis has been clearly established for a number of different flaviviruses through studies using biochemical and genetic characterization methods in a wide range of cell types, characterization of the receptor or receptor complexes used in the initial binding remains much more poorly characterized, and evidence suggests that virus entry may be cell type specific. However, it is clear that it is an interaction between the flavivirus envelope (E) glycoprotein that mediates the interaction of the virus with the host cell and the flavivirus E glycoprotein is believed to contain the components responsible for several important viral functions including target cells binding, induction of protective immunity, mediation of membrane fusion and virus assembly (Chang, 1997; Heinz, 1990; Kimura & Ohyama, 1988; Klasse et al., 1998). The E protein is highly conserved amongst all flaviviruses and shares common features. Conservation of cysteine residues and similar hydrophobicity profiles suggest a common folded structure of the E protein for all flaviviruses. Recently high resolution flavivirus E protein crystal structures of dengue virus serotype 2 (Modis et al., 2003) and tick-borne encephalitis (Rey et al., 1995) have shown their close relationship in overall dimeric structure, protein folding and a similar set of six disulfide bonds (Modis et al., 2003; Rey et al., 1995). The approximately 55 to 60kDa E protein contains 494 to 501 amino acids folded into three distinct structural and functional domains; domains I, II and III which correlate well with the previously defined antigenic domains C, A, and B. (Chang, 1997; Heinz et al., 1983; Roehrig et al., 1983). Domain I and III (C and B) contain predominately subcomplex- and type-specific epitopes, whereas domain II (A) the dimerization domain, contains broadly flavivirus-cross-reactive epitopes and also subtype-specific epitopes (Mandl et al., 1989). The flavivirus domain III has been shown to participate in virus attachment through its interaction with a cellular receptor (Chu et al., 2005; Crill & Roehrig, 2001; Hung et al., 2004; Hurrelbrink & McMinn, 2001; Volk et al., 2004). The participation of domain III in cell entry appears to involve the presence of a putative receptor binding loop (Modis et al., 2003) and a heparan sulphate binding site (Chen et al., 1997; Mandl et al., 1989; Twiddy et al., 2002; Wu et al., 2004) including the membrane fusion peptides (Allison et al., 2001). Apparently the flavivirus E glycoprotein is a crucial determinant of the host range, tissue tropism, and virulence of the virus (Crill & Chang, 2004; Mandl, 2005). After virus entry into the target cell, the acid environment of the endosome vesicle triggers conformational changes in the virions and fusion of viral and cell membranes and particle disassembly occur (Dimitrov, 2004; Marsh, 1984).

The non-structural proteins then initiate the replication of the viral genome in close association with the ER, and the newly synthesized RNA is packaged by the C protein forming a nucleocapsid complex. The nucleocapsids bud from the ER and become enveloped by a lipid membrane carrying with it associated envelope (E) and the pre-membrane (prM) proteins which have formed initially into prM/E heterodimers and subsequently these heterodimers associate into trimers (Kuhn et al., 2002; Perera & Kuhn, 2008). The newly assembled particle is in an immature form, in which the prM/E heterodimers project from the surface as 60 trimeric spikes and has a diameter of approximately 600 Angstroms (Li et al., 2008; Yu et al., 2009). After budding from the ER, the immature viruses transit the secretory pathway, where the prM protein is cleaved by the cellular furin protease after a major conformational change induced by the acidic environment of the trans-Golgi network resulting in exposure of a furin cleavage site (Li et al., 2008; Yu et al., 2009). In the slightly acidic pH of the trans-Golgi network the cleaved "pr" domain of the prM protein remains in association with the essentially mature virus particle, preventing premature membrane fusion inside the cell. Exposure to a neutral pH upon virion exposure to the extracellular milieu induces dissociation of the "pr" peptide from the now mature virion (Yu et al., 2009).

2.4 Current and future vaccine development

The development of vaccines to protect against infections by members of the flavivirus genus has been extremely uneven. It is of note that the vaccine against the prototype flavivirus, Yellow fever virus, the causative agent of yellow fever, is one of the most successful live attenuated vaccines, with the currently used YF-17D derivatives capable of inducing a protective level of neutralizing antibodies in 99% of recipients within 30 days from a single dose (Monath, 2001). In contrast, the effort to develop an effective live attenuated vaccine or vaccines against dengue virus remain incomplete, despite more than

60 years of investigation since the pioneering studies of Sabin and Schlesinger (Sabin & Schlesinger, 1945). For the flaviviruses that are associated with encephalitis, the picture is somewhat more promising.

2.4.1 Japanese encephalitis virus

For the most significant flavivirus causing encephalitis, Japanese encephalitis virus, vaccines have been available since the 1950s. The original vaccine widely distributed in much of Asia was a formalin inactivated whole virus formulation grown in mouse brain using either the Nakayama or Beijing-1 strains (Halstead & Thomas, 2010). Despite acceptable protection levels after one, two or three vaccination doses and a significant decrease in the number of cases of Japanese encephalitis in countries where the vaccine was widely used (Solomon, 2004; Solomon et al., 2000), possibly unfounded concerns as to adverse reactogenicity of this formulation (Halstead & Thomas, 2010) led to discontinuation of production of this vaccine. The mouse brain produced vaccine was developed in Japan and used in much of Asia for indigenous populations as well as used for vaccination of travelers to endemic areas. China however developed its own, cell culture produced, whole virus inactivated vaccine for Japanese encephalitis based on culture of the P-3 or Beijing-3 strain of Japanese encephalitis in primary hamster kidney (PHK) cells, which was later superseded by the production of a live attenuated vaccine, SA14-14-2. This vaccine has been reported to induce excellent, long lived protection after a single dose administration and is currently distributed in China and several other Asian countries. The SA14-14-2 vaccine strain was the starting point for development of a further, whole virus formalin inactivated vaccine IXARO (IC51) developed originally by the Walter Reed Army Institute of Research. This vaccine is produced in Vero (African green monkey kidney) cells and induces high levels of protection after two or three doses. It is expected that this vaccine will be widely distributed (Halstead & Thomas, 2010). One further Japanese encephalitis vaccine candidate is currently on the brink of being widely marketed and distributed. This vaccine, the so called IMOJEV (JE-CV and previously called ChimeriVax-JE) vaccine is a live attenuated recombinant vaccine based upon the exceedingly well characterized YF-17D backbone, with the prM and E coding sequences from Japanese encephalitis virus replacing the equivalent YF-17D sequences. This vaccine offers levels of protection apparently equivalent or greater than other existing vaccines with a single dose administration generating protective antibody levels in 95% (children) or 99% (adults) of recipients by 1 month post-administration (Halstead & Thomas, 2010). Overall, with three effective and apparently safe vaccines either being distributed or in the process of being distributed, the outlook for control of Japanese encephalitis is promising.

2.4.2 West Nile virus

There is currently no licensed vaccine to protect against West Nile virus infection for use in humans although five vaccines are available for vaccination of horses. Two of these vaccines, the West Nile-Innovator™ (Fort Dodge Animal Health) and the Boehringer-Ingelheim Vetera™ vaccine consist of whole inactivated virus. In both cases the vaccine is derived from an equine isolate of West Nile virus. The third vaccine available (Prevenile™, Intervet/Schering-Plough Animal Health) is a chimeric vaccine using the Yellow fever vaccine YF-17D backbone and the pre-membrane and envelope proteins of West Nile virus, although a recall notice is currently in effect on this vaccine due to reports of adverse reactions (http://www.prevenile.com/PDF/PreveNile%20Letter.pdf; accessed 17/02/2011). The fourth horse vaccine for West Nile virus (Recombitek™, Merial) is a recombinant canarypox vector containing the pre-membrane and envelope proteins of West Nile virus, while the fifth vaccine (West Nile- Innovator® DNA, Fort Dodge Animal Health) is a DNA vaccine encoding the West Nile virus prM and E proteins.

Perhaps unsurprisingly, development of a human vaccine largely follows from the progress made with equine vaccines. A phase II trial of a chimeric YF-17D backbone with the West Nile pre-membrane and envelope proteins has been undertaken (Biedenbender et al., 2011). This vaccine largely follows the equine Prevenile vaccine strategy, but includes three mutations in the E protein predicted to reduce neurovirulence, and results from the Phase II study suggest that the construct is highly immunogenic and well tolerated (Biedenbender et al., 2011). Similarly, a Phase I trial of DNA vaccine encoding the pre-membrane and envelope proteins of the NY99 strain of West Nile virus was completed in 2007 (Martin et al., 2007).

Other potential vaccine candidates include a live attenuated Schwarz strain of measles virus expressing the secreted form of E protein from a virulent strain of West Nile virus (Despres et al., 2005), a live attenuated WNV/Dengue 4 virus chimera (Pletnev et al., 2003), RepliVax WN, a defective pseudoinfectious West Nile virus lacking a functional capsid gene (Mason et al., 2006; Widman et al., 2008; Yamshchikov et al., 2004), an attenuated West Nile prototype virus (Yamshchikov et al., 2004) and a plasmid DNA vaccine containing the infectious full-length RNA genome of Kunjin (KUN) virus (Hall et al., 2003), a subtype of West Nile virus. In addition subunit vaccines including a bacterially expressed domain III of West Nile virus E protein (Chu et al., 2007; Martina et al., 2008) and a recombinant truncated E (trE) and NS1 protein construct expressed in *Drosophila* S2 cells (Lieberman et al., 2007; Watts et al., 2007) are under investigation.

As with Japanese encephalitis virus, the prospect for a human vaccine for West Nile virus infections is promising, with the leading candidates at various stages of clinical trials as well as a number of promising candidates still at the early developmental stage.

2.4.3 Murray Valley encephalitis virus

There is currently no vaccine to protect against infection with Murray Valley encephalitis, and given the limited distribution and low incidence of cases, it is possible that a specific commercial vaccine against Murray Valley encephalitis will not be developed. However, animal studies have suggested that immunization with a live chimeric anti-Japanese encephalitis vaccine (ChimeriVax-JE) may provide protection against the closely related Murray Valley encephalitis virus (Lobigs et al., 2009). However, preliminary animal based studies using Murray Valley encephalitis recombinant subviral particles (Kroeger & McMinn, 2002) or E and NS1 proteins expressed in a recombinant vaccinia virus (Hall et al., 1996) have been undertaken which may possibly lead to the development of a specific Murray Valley encephalitis vaccine.

2.4.4 St. Louis encephalitis virus

There is currently no commercially licensed vaccine to protect against infection with St. Louis encephalitis virus. The development of possible vaccines follows closely the development of West Nile virus vaccines. Potential vaccine constructs evaluated at least in animal studies include chimeric yellow fever/ St. Louis encephalitis virus constructs consisting of the well characterized yellow fever vaccine strain YF-17D backbone with the pre-membrane and envelope coding sequences of a virulent (MSI-7) or an attenuated

(CorAn9124) strain of St. Louis encephalitis virus (Pugachev et al., 2004) and a chimeric dengue serotype 4/ St. Louis encephalitis virus construct consisting of the dengue serotype 4 backbone and the pre-membrane and envelope coding sequences of Hubbard strain of St. Louis encephalitis virus (Blaney et al., 2008). In addition a prime/boost strategy using sequential immunization with a vaccinia virus expressing St. Louis encephalitis virus pre-membrane and envelope proteins followed by purified recombinant envelope protein (Venugopal et al., 1995) and a DNA vaccine candidate based upon expression of the St. Louis encephalitis virus pre-membrane and envelope proteins under control of the cytomegalovirus immediate-early promoter have been investigated in mice (Phillpotts et al., 1996).

2.4.5 Louping ill virus

Probably as a reflection of the extremely low incidence of Louping ill virus infections in humans, little vaccine development has taken place, although a vaccine for sheep has been in use in the United Kingdom since before 1935. The original vaccine was prepared from formalin inactivated virus grown in sheep brains, but this practice was halted when causal evidence of a link with spread of the sheep prion disease Scrapie was uncovered (Nathanson, 2007). The current sheep vaccine is made by formalin inactivation of virus grown in cultured cells. At this point it seems unlikely that a human vaccine will be developed.

2.4.6 Powassan virus

There is currently no vaccine to protect against infection with Powassan virus, and given the extremely small number of cases reported so far, it is somewhat unlikely that a concerted vaccine development program will be initiated, in the absence of a significant increase in the number of cases. It is possible that some degree of protection against Powassan virus infection may be induced by immunization with a vaccine developed against a different member of the tick-borne encephalitis group, but this remains speculative at the moment.

2.4.7 Tick-borne encephalitis virus

There are currently two vaccines available for prophylactic protection against Tick-borne encephalitis virus infections. These vaccines, FSME-Immun (Baxter, Austria) and Encepur (Novartis, Germany) are both formalin inactivated whole virus produced in primary chicken embryo fibroblasts and are distributed in adult and child formulations. FSME-Immun is derived from the Austrian Neudorfl strain, while Encepur is derived from the German K23 isolate. Both vaccines protect against all three subtypes (European, far-Eastern and Siberian) of Tick-borne encephalitis virus and are able to be administered in conventional and rapid immunization schedules, although evidence suggests that the conventional schedules offer better protection. Both vaccines have undergone considerable formulation changes since their original introduction as a consequence of adverse immunization events and as both viruses are manufactured using chicken eggs, the possibility of hypersensitivity reactions remains. Two further vaccines are available or undergoing trials in Russia, the KKhv and IPVE vaccines (Demicheli et al., 2009) but there are few if any reports in the English language literature about these formulations. Overall, vaccination coverage rates vary dramatically among Tick-borne encephalitis virus endemic countries, but where effective vaccination programs are in place as in Austria, a significant reduction in Tick-borne encephalitis virus incidence has been observed (Petri et al., 2010). However, significant numbers of hospitalizations still occur in endemic countries, despite the availability of vaccines which probably results from the high cost of the vaccines as well as the requirement for multiple booster shots to maintain effective protection (Widman et al., 2008). Several studies have attempted to use the naturally attenuated Langat virus as the basis of a vaccine against Tick-borne encephalitis virus infection. These include large scale (more than 600,000 individuals) testing in the former USSR of the Yelantsev strain of Langat virus but due to an unacceptably high incidence of vaccine associated complications, this approach was discontinued. However, a Langat/Dengue 4 chimeric live vaccine which replaces the dengue serotype 4 pre-membrane and envelope proteins with the corresponding sequences from the Langat virus TP21 strain is currently under development (Pripuzova et al., 2009). Other potential live attenuated virus vaccine candidates include a recombinant vaccinia virus expressing the tick-borne virus non-structural NS1 protein (Aleshin et al., 2005), a vaccinia virus vector carrying the tick-borne encephalitis virus prM/E sequences (Holzer et al., 1999) and a self-replicating noninfectious Tick-borne encephalitis virus RNA vaccine based upon the Neudoerfl tick-borne encephalitis strain, but containing a large deletion of the sequences coding for the capsid protein (Aberle et al., 2005). Potential nucleic acid based (Aberle et al., 1999; Schmaljohn et al., 1997) and subunit vaccines are also at an early stage of development.

2.5 Therapeutic agents

Current treatment for all flavivirus infections is primarily supportive and orientated towards alleviating symptoms and there are no specific antivirals marketed to combat flaviviral infections. Small scale trials of existing antiviral agents such as ribavirin (Chowers et al., 2001) and interferon-α (Solomon et al., 2003) have proved disappointing. There are however a large number of compounds currently in the developmental pipeline targeted against a number of different processes in the flavivirus life cycle. In addition, therapeutic immunoglobulins have shown some promise in animal model systems of West Nile virus infection (Ben-Nathan et al., 2003; Oliphant et al., 2005). Current drug compound discovery primarily centers on inhibition of virus entry, replication and translation, polyprotein processing, virus assembly and cellular host proteins, and while drug development primarily focuses on a specific flavivirus, the hope is that a broad spectrum anti-flaviviral compound will be discovered. However, the apparent lack of efficacy of ribavirin and interferon-α, towards West Nile virus, while these are effective treatments for infections with Hepatitis C virus which is a closely related member of the family *Flaviviridae* (genus *Hepacivirus*), suggests that this may be an unrealistic objective.
Potential entry inhibitors being evaluated include sulfated glycosaminoglycans, sulfated galactomannans and quinazolines which either directly interact with the virus to prevent binding to the cell, or interfere with the process of membrane fusion leaving the virus trapped at the cell surface. However, the wide sequence diversity of the flavivirus E protein suggests that these molecules may have a narrowly defined application. In addition, a significant amount of research has suggested that even a single flavivirus may use multiple proteins to enter into cells, and that these proteins may differ between different cell types. Of even greater concern are the several studies that imply multiple mechanisms of entry for some flaviviruses, in addition to endocytosis into clathrin coated pits (Acosta et al., 2009; Suksanpaisan et al., 2009), all of which may serve to make the initial host cell: virus interaction a less than desirable target.
Significant attention has focused therefore on the flaviviral proteins with enzymatic activity, namely the NS3 and NS5 proteins. The NS3 protein has both protease and helicase activities,

while the NS5 protein has methyltransferase and RNA-dependent RNA polymerase activities. These proteins, from several different flaviviruses, have been cloned either as a complete functional unit of or as a sub-domain expressing a single activity in a number of reporter systems, and adapted to high throughput screening assays, allowing the assay of many thousands of potential compounds. There are several recent comprehensive reviews on the progress of anti-flavivirus drug development (Bollati et al., 2010; Noble et al., 2010; Parkinson & Pryde, 2010; Pastorino et al., 2010; Paula et al., 2009).

3. Conclusions

The genus flavivirus contains some of the most important vector-borne human pathogens, which are widely distributed around the world. Several flaviviruses including some of the most important encephalitis causing viruses such as Japanese encephalitis virus, West Nile virus and Tick-borne encephalitis virus (both European and Far-Eastern) are considered to be emerging infectious diseases in that they have recently shown an increase in "incidence, impact or geographic range" (Jones et al., 2008). Increases in the geographic range of a vector borne disease may follow the natural expansion of a host species into new geographical locations, or, possibly sudden importation as a result of human activity (Pfeffer & Dobler, 2010). However, the sudden and explosive epidemic of chikungunya virus (a member of the family *Togaviridae*, genus *Alphavirus*) infections in the Indian Ocean Islands, India and much of Southeast Asia (Staples et al., 2009) occurred largely as a result of the adaptation of the chikungunya virus to transmission by a new host (*Aedes albopictus* instead of *Aedes aegypti*) and spread internationally by infected humans. This was clearly illustrated by the outbreak of chikungunya fever in Italy in 2007, where the disease was imported by an infected but presumably pre-symptomatic traveler from India and the virus became established in the local *Aedes albopictus* population. As such, there are several potential mechanisms by which vector borne diseases may become established in new areas, exposing new populations to the hazards of these diseases.

Total eradication of the encephalitic flaviviruses seems highly unlikely. While it was possible to eliminate the Smallpox virus from nature, this virus was spread through direct contact with an infected person or with contaminated fluids or objects, and there is no natural reservoir for this virus apart from the human population. With flaviviruses, numerous natural host reservoirs exist in the wild, and transovarial transmission of both tick-borne and mosquito borne flaviviruses has been documented. Given the inability to eradicate these diseases from the wild, efforts to control these diseases and their transmission are focused on vector control policies as well as on prevention and cure of the disease where human infection does occur. Immunization clearly offers the best solution to prevention of these diseases in humans, and as has been seen in the previous section, effective vaccines for Japanese encephalitis and tick-borne encephalitis are already available, while vaccines for the remaining encephalitis causing diseases (with a few exceptions) are generally well advanced. As such research in vaccine development will be essentially focused on improvement, both with regards to lowering the incidence of adverse events, as well as reducing the cost of the vaccines. With effective vaccines, the critical issue is one of cost. Both tick- and mosquito borne encephalitic flaviviruses are common in the developing nations of the world, and the main mission will be to make the vaccines affordable for people in resource poor countries, and ensure the vaccine is delivered to susceptible population groups. This will also entail careful integration of the new vaccines with existing immunization programs.

To date, drug development somewhat lags behind vaccine development and there are currently no specific anti-flaviviral drugs available, nor any drugs specifically designed to combat the consequences of encephalitic manifestations of the disease. However, the advent of new technologies has provided a significant boost to drug development programs although it remains to be seen whether this will genuinely result in new therapies and whether these potential drugs will be broad spectrum or specific to a particular virus species. This research however remains of vital importance. While vaccine programs are ideal for long-term disease control, vaccine development for flaviviruses takes years or decades for a safe, effective and cheap vaccine to be produced. In the event of a massive explosion of a previously unregarded flaviviral disease, a broad spectrum anti-flaviviral agent may be the only practical solution to reduce high levels of morbidity and mortality.

4. Acknowledgement

The author gratefully acknowledges the Office of the Higher Education Commission and Mahidol University under the National Research Universities Initiative, The Thailand Research Fund and The National Center for Genetic Engineering and Biotechnology, National Science and Technology Development Agency for support of his studies on the pathogenesis of arboviruses.

5. References

Aberle, J. H., Aberle S. W., Allison S. L., Stiasny K., Ecker M., Mandl C. W., Berger R., Heinz F. X. (1999). A DNA immunization model study with constructs expressing the tick-borne encephalitis virus envelope protein E in different physical forms. *J Immunol* 163(12):6756-6761.

Aberle, J. H., Aberle S. W., Kofler R. M., Mandl C. W. (2005). Humoral and cellular immune response to RNA immunization with flavivirus replicons derived from tick-borne encephalitis virus. *J Virol* 79(24):15107-15113.

Acosta, E. G., Castilla V., Damonte E. B. (2009). Alternative infectious entry pathways for dengue virus serotypes into mammalian cells. *Cell Microbiol* 11(10):1533-1549.

Aleshin, S. E., Timofeev A. V., Khoretonenko M. V., Zakharova L. G., Pashvykina G. V., Stephenson J. R., Shneider A. M., Altstein A. D. (2005). Combined prime-boost vaccination against tick-borne encephalitis (TBE) using a recombinant vaccinia virus and a bacterial plasmid both expressing TBE virus non-structural NS1 protein. *BMC Microbiol* 5:45.

Allison, S. L., Schalich J., Stiasny K., Mandl C. W., Heinz F. X. (2001). Mutational evidence for an internal fusion peptide in flavivirus envelope protein E. *J Virol* 75(9):4268-4275.

Bakonyi, T., Hubalek Z., Rudolf I., Nowotny N. (2005). Novel flavivirus or new lineage of West Nile virus, central Europe. *Emerg Infect Dis* 11(2):225-231.

Ben-Nathan, D., Lustig S., Tam G., Robinzon S., Segal S., Rager-Zisman B. (2003). Prophylactic and therapeutic efficacy of human intravenous immunoglobulin in treating West Nile virus infection in mice. *J Infect Dis* 188(1):5-12.

Berthet, F. X., Zeller H. G., Drouet M. T., Rauzier J., Digoutte J. P., Deubel V. (1997). Extensive nucleotide changes and deletions within the envelope glycoprotein gene of Euro-African West Nile viruses. *J Gen Virol* 78 (Pt 9):2293-2297.

Biedenbender, R., Bevilacqua J., Gregg A. M., Watson M., Dayan G. (2011). Phase II, randomized, double-blind, placebo-controlled, multicenter study to investigate the immunogenicity and safety of a West Nile virus vaccine in healthy adults. *J Infect Dis* 203(1):75-84.

Blaney, J. E., Jr., Speicher J., Hanson C. T., Sathe N. S., Whitehead S. S., Murphy B. R., Pletnev A. G. (2008). Evaluation of St. Louis encephalitis virus/dengue virus type 4 antigenic chimeric viruses in mice and rhesus monkeys. *Vaccine* 26(33):4150-4159.

Bollati, M., Alvarez K., Assenberg R., Baronti C., Canard B., Cook S., Coutard B., Decroly E., de Lamballerie X., Gould E. A., Grard G., Grimes J. M., Hilgenfeld R., Jansson A. M., Malet H., Mancini E. J., Mastrangelo E., Mattevi A., Milani M., Moureau G., Neyts J., Owens R. J., Ren J., Selisko B., Speroni S., Steuber H., Stuart D. I., Unge T., Bolognesi M. (2010). Structure and functionality in flavivirus NS-proteins: perspectives for drug design. *Antiviral Res* 87(2):125-148.

Centers for Disease Control and Prevention (CDC). (2003). Epidemic/epizootic West Nile virus in the United States: guidelines for surveillance, prevention, and control. *www.cdc.gov/NCIDOD/D VBID/WESTNILE/resources/wnv-guidelines-apr-2001.pdf.*

Chang, G. J. 1997. Molecular biology of dengue viruses. Gluber, D., Kuno G., editor. New York: CAB International. 175-198 p.

Charrel, R. N., Attoui H., Butenko A. M., Clegg J. C., Deubel V., Frolova T. V., Gould E. A., Gritsun T. S., Heinz F. X., Labuda M., Lashkevich V. A., Loktev V., Lundkvist A., Lvov D. V., Mandl C. W., Niedrig M., Papa A., Petrov V. S., Plyusnin A., Randolph S., Suss J., Zlobin V. I., de Lamballerie X. (2004). Tick-borne virus diseases of human interest in Europe. *Clin Microbiol Infect* 10(12):1040-1055.

Chen, Y., Maguire T., Hileman R. E., Fromm J. R., Esko J. D., Linhardt R. J., Marks R. M. (1997). Dengue virus infectivity depends on envelope protein binding to target cell heparan sulfate. *Nat Med* 3(8):866-871.

Chowers, M. Y., Lang R., Nassar F., Ben-David D., Giladi M., Rubinshtein E., Itzhaki A., Mishal J., Siegman-Igra Y., Kitzes R., Pick N., Landau Z., Wolf D., Bin H., Mendelson E., Pitlik S. D., Weinberger M. (2001). Clinical characteristics of the West Nile fever outbreak, Israel, 2000. *Emerg Infect Dis* 7(4):675-678.

Chu, J. H., Chiang C. C., Ng M. L. (2007). Immunization of flavivirus West Nile recombinant envelope domain III protein induced specific immune response and protection against West Nile virus infection. *J Immunol* 178(5):2699-2705.

Chu, J. J., Rajamanonmani R., Li J., Bhuvanakantham R., Lescar J., Ng M. L. (2005). Inhibition of West Nile virus entry by using a recombinant domain III from the envelope glycoprotein. *J Gen Virol* 86(Pt 2):405-412.

Crill, W. D., Chang G. J. (2004). Localization and characterization of flavivirus envelope glycoprotein cross-reactive epitopes. *J Virol* 78(24):13975-13986.

Crill, W. D., Roehrig J. T. (2001). Monoclonal antibodies that bind to domain III of dengue virus E glycoprotein are the most efficient blockers of virus adsorption to Vero cells. *J Virol* 75(16):7769-7773.

Demicheli, V., Debalini M. G., Rivetti A. (2009). Vaccines for preventing tick-borne encephalitis. *Cochrane Database Syst Rev*(1):CD000977.

Desai, A., Shankar S. K., Ravi V., Chandramuki A., Gourie-Devi M. (1995). Japanese encephalitis virus antigen in the human brain and its topographic distribution. *Acta Neuropathol* 89(4):368-373.

Despres, P., Combredet C., Frenkiel M. P., Lorin C., Brahic M., Tangy F. (2005). Live measles vaccine expressing the secreted form of the West Nile virus envelope glycoprotein protects against West Nile virus encephalitis. *J Infect Dis* 191(2):207-214.

Dimitrov, D. S. (2004). Virus entry: molecular mechanisms and biomedical applications. *Nat Rev Microbiol* 2(2):109-122.
Ebel, G. D. (2010). Update on Powassan virus: emergence of a North American tick-borne flavivirus. *Annu Rev Entomol* 55:95-110.
Gajanana, A., Thenmozhi V., Samuel P. P., Reuben R. (1995). A community-based study of subclinical flavivirus infections in children in an area of Tamil Nadu, India, where Japanese encephalitis is endemic. *Bull World Health Organ* 73(2):237-244.
Gholam, B. I., Puksa S., Provias J. P. (1999). Powassan encephalitis: a case report with neuropathology and literature review. *CMAJ* 161(11):1419-1422.
Hall, R. A., Brand T. N., Lobigs M., Sangster M. Y., Howard M. J., Mackenzie J. S. (1996). Protective immune responses to the E and NS1 proteins of Murray Valley encephalitis virus in hybrids of flavivirus-resistant mice. *J Gen Virol* 77 (Pt 6):1287-1294.
Hall, R. A., Nisbet D. J., Pham K. B., Pyke A. T., Smith G. A., Khromykh A. A. (2003). DNA vaccine coding for the full-length infectious Kunjin virus RNA protects mice against the New York strain of West Nile virus. *Proc Natl Acad Sci U S A* 100(18):10460-10464.
Halstead, S. B., Jacobson J. (2003). Japanese encephalitis. *Adv Virus Res* 61:103-138.
Halstead, S. B., Thomas S. J. (2010). New vaccines for Japanese encephalitis. *Curr Infect Dis Rep* 12(3):174-180.
Hayes, E. B., Sejvar J. J., Zaki S. R., Lanciotti R. S., Bode A. V., Campbell G. L. (2005). Virology, pathology, and clinical manifestations of West Nile virus disease. *Emerg Infect Dis* 11(8):1174-1179.
Heinz, F. X., Berger R., Tuma W., Kunz C. (1983). A topological and functional model of epitopes on the structural glycoprotein of tick-borne encephalitis virus defined by monoclonal antibodies. *Virology* 126(2):525-537.
Heinz, F. X., Roehring, J.T. 1990. Flaviviruses. vanRegen-Mortel, M. H. V., Neurath, A.R., editor. Amsterdam: Elsevier Science. 289-305 p.
Henchal, E. A., Putnak J. R. (1990). The dengue viruses. *Clin Microbiol Rev* 3(4):376-396.
Holzer, G. W., Remp G., Antoine G., Pfleiderer M., Enzersberger O. M., Emsenhuber W., Hammerle T., Gruber F., Urban C., Falkner F. G., Dorner F. (1999). Highly efficient induction of protective immunity by a vaccinia virus vector defective in late gene expression. *J Virol* 73(6):4536-4542.
Hung, J. J., Hsieh M. T., Young M. J., Kao C. L., King C. C., Chang W. (2004). An external loop region of domain III of dengue virus type 2 envelope protein is involved in serotype-specific binding to mosquito but not mammalian cells. *J Virol* 78(1):378-388.
Hurrelbrink, R. J., McMinn P. C. (2001). Attenuation of Murray Valley encephalitis virus by site-directed mutagenesis of the hinge and putative receptor-binding regions of the envelope protein. *J Virol* 75(16):7692-7702.
ICTV. (2011). ICTV Master Species List 2009 - Version 9. Date of Access: 12 February 2011, http://ictvonline.org/index.asp
Johnson, R. T., Burke D. S., Elwell M., Leake C. J., Nisalak A., Hoke C. H., Lorsomrudee W. (1985). Japanese encephalitis: immunocytochemical studies of viral antigen and inflammatory cells in fatal cases. *Ann Neurol* 18(5):567-573.
Jones, K. E., Patel N. G., Levy M. A., Storeygard A., Balk D., Gittleman J. L., Daszak P. (2008). Global trends in emerging infectious diseases. *Nature* 451(7181):990-993.
Kimura, T., Ohyama A. (1988). Association between the pH-dependent conformational change of West Nile flavivirus E protein and virus-mediated membrane fusion. *J Gen Virol* 69 (Pt 6):1247-1254.

Klasse, P. J., Bron R., Marsh M. (1998). Mechanisms of enveloped virus entry into animal cells. *Adv Drug Deliv Rev* 34(1):65-91.

Kroeger, M. A., McMinn P. C. (2002). Murray Valley encephalitis virus recombinant subviral particles protect mice from lethal challenge with virulent wild-type virus. *Arch Virol* 147(6):1155-1172.

Kuhn, R. J., Zhang W., Rossmann M. G., Pletnev S. V., Corver J., Lenches E., Jones C. T., Mukhopadhyay S., Chipman P. R., Strauss E. G., Baker T. S., Strauss J. H. (2002). Structure of Dengue Virus: Implications for Flavivirus Organization, Maturation, and Fusion. *Cell* 108(5):717-725.

Kumar, R., Mathur A., Singh K. B., Sitholey P., Prasad M., Shukla R., Agarwal S. P., Arockiasamy J. (1993). Clinical sequelae of Japanese encephalitis in children. *Indian J Med Res* 97:9-13.

Labuda, M., Randolph S. E. (1999). Survival strategy of tick-borne encephalitis virus: cellular basis and environmental determinants. *Zentralbl Bakteriol* 289(5-7):513-524.

Lanciotti, R. S., Roehrig J. T., Deubel V., Smith J., Parker M., Steele K., Crise B., Volpe K. E., Crabtree M. B., Scherret J. H., Hall R. A., MacKenzie J. S., Cropp C. B., Panigrahy B., Ostlund E., Schmitt B., Malkinson M., Banet C., Weissman J., Komar N., Savage H. M., Stone W., McNamara T., Gubler D. J. (1999). Origin of the West Nile virus responsible for an outbreak of encephalitis in the northeastern United States. *Science* 286(5448):2333-2337.

Li, L., Lok S. M., Yu I. M., Zhang Y., Kuhn R. J., Chen J., Rossmann M. G. (2008). The flavivirus precursor membrane-envelope protein complex: structure and maturation. *Science* 319(5871):1830-1834.

Lieberman, M. M., Clements D. E., Ogata S., Wang G., Corpuz G., Wong T., Martyak T., Gilson L., Coller B. A., Leung J., Watts D. M., Tesh R. B., Siirin M., Travassos da Rosa A., Humphreys T., Weeks-Levy C. (2007). Preparation and immunogenic properties of a recombinant West Nile subunit vaccine. *Vaccine* 25(3):414-423.

Lobigs, M., Larena M., Alsharifi M., Lee E., Pavy M. (2009). Live chimeric and inactivated Japanese encephalitis virus vaccines differ in their cross-protective values against Murray Valley encephalitis virus. *J Virol* 83(6):2436-2445.

Mandl, C. W. (2005). Steps of the tick-borne encephalitis virus replication cycle that affect neuropathogenesis. *Virus Res* 111(2):161-174.

Mandl, C. W., Guirakhoo F., Holzmann H., Heinz F. X., Kunz C. (1989). Antigenic structure of the flavivirus envelope protein E at the molecular level, using tick-borne encephalitis virus as a model. *J Virol* 63(2):564-571.

Mansfield, K. L., Johnson N., Phipps L. P., Stephenson J. R., Fooks A. R., Solomon T. (2009). Tick-borne encephalitis virus - a review of an emerging zoonosis. *J Gen Virol* 90(Pt 8):1781-1794.

Marfin, A. A., Petersen L. R., Eidson M., Miller J., Hadler J., Farello C., Werner B., Campbell G. L., Layton M., Smith P., Bresnitz E., Cartter M., Scaletta J., Obiri G., Bunning M., Craven R. C., Roehrig J. T., Julian K. G., Hinten S. R., Gubler D. J. (2001). Widespread West Nile virus activity, eastern United States, 2000. *Emerg Infect Dis* 7(4):730-735.

Marsh, M. (1984). The entry of enveloped viruses into cells by endocytosis. *Biochem J* 218:1-10.

Martin, J. E., Pierson T. C., Hubka S., Rucker S., Gordon I. J., Enama M. E., Andrews C. A., Xu Q., Davis B. S., Nason M., Fay M., Koup R. A., Roederer M., Bailer R. T., Gomez P. L., Mascola J. R., Chang G. J., Nabel G. J., Graham B. S. (2007). A West Nile virus DNA vaccine induces neutralizing antibody in healthy adults during a phase 1 clinical trial. *J Infect Dis* 196(12):1732-1740.

Martina, B. E., Koraka P., van den Doel P., van Amerongen G., Rimmelzwaan G. F., Osterhaus A. D. (2008). Immunization with West Nile virus envelope domain III protects mice against lethal infection with homologous and heterologous virus. *Vaccine* 26(2):153-157.

Mason, P. W., Shustov A. V., Frolov I. (2006). Production and characterization of vaccines based on flaviviruses defective in replication. *Virology* 351(2):432-443.

Misra, U. K., Kalita J. (2010). Overview: Japanese encephalitis. *Prog Neurobiol* 91(2):108-120.

Modis, Y., Ogata S., Clements D., Harrison S. C. (2003). A ligand-binding pocket in the dengue virus envelope glycoprotein. *Proc Natl Acad Sci U S A* 100(12):6986-6991.

Monath, T. P. (2001). Yellow fever: an update. *Lancet Infect Dis* 1(1):11-20.

Monath, T. P., Cropp C. B., Harrison A. K. (1983). Mode of entry of a neurotropic arbovirus into the central nervous system. Reinvestigation of an old controversy. *Lab Invest* 48(4):399-410.

Morrey, J. D., Olsen A. L., Siddharthan V., Motter N. E., Wang H., Taro B. S., Chen D., Ruffner D., Hall J. O. (2008). Increased blood-brain barrier permeability is not a primary determinant for lethality of West Nile virus infection in rodents. *J Gen Virol* 89(Pt 2):467-473.

Nathanson, N. 2007. Epidemiology. In: Knipe, D. M., Howley P. M., editors. Field's virology: Lippincott Williams & Wilkins. p 423-446.

Noble, C. G., Chen Y. L., Dong H., Gu F., Lim S. P., Schul W., Wang Q. Y., Shi P. Y. (2010). Strategies for development of Dengue virus inhibitors. *Antiviral Res* 85(3):450-462.

Ogawa, M., Okubo H., Tsuji Y., Yasui N., Someda K. (1973). Chronic progressive encephalitis occurring 13 years after Russian spring-summer encephalitis. *J Neurol Sci* 19(3):363-373.

Oliphant, T., Engle M., Nybakken G. E., Doane C., Johnson S., Huang L., Gorlatov S., Mehlhop E., Marri A., Chung K. M., Ebel G. D., Kramer L. D., Fremont D. H., Diamond M. S. (2005). Development of a humanized monoclonal antibody with therapeutic potential against West Nile virus. *Nat Med* 11(5):522-530.

Parkinson, T., Pryde D. C. (2010). Small molecule drug discovery for Dengue and West Nile viruses: Applying experience from hepatitis C virus. *Future Medicinal Chemistry* 2(7):1181-1203.

Pastorino, B., Nougairede A., Wurtz N., Gould E., de Lamballerie X. (2010). Role of host cell factors in flavivirus infection: Implications for pathogenesis and development of antiviral drugs. *Antiviral Res* 87(3):281-294.

Paula, T., Pablo R., Eugenia V., Pablo B., Sabino P., Jose M., Antonio M., Dolores H. M., Pablo L., Javier G. S., Vincente S. (2009). New drug targets for hepatitis C and other Flaviviridae viruses. *Infect Disord Drug Targets* 9(2):133-147.

Perera, R., Kuhn R. J. (2008). Structural proteomics of dengue virus. *Curr Opin Microbiol* 11(4):369-377.

Petri, E., Gniel D., Zent O. (2010). Tick-borne encephalitis (TBE) trends in epidemiology and current and future management. *Travel Med Infect Dis* 8(4):233-245.

Pfeffer, M., Dobler G. (2010). Emergence of zoonotic arboviruses by animal trade and migration. *Parasit Vectors* 3(1):35.

Phillpotts, R. J., Venugopal K., Brooks T. (1996). Immunisation with DNA polynucleotides protects mice against lethal challenge with St. Louis encephalitis virus. *Arch Virol* 141(3-4):743-749.

Platonov, A. E., Shipulin G. A., Shipulina O. Y., Tyutyunnik E. N., Frolochkina T. I., Lanciotti R. S., Yazyshina S., Platonova O. V., Obukhov I. L., Zhukov A. N., Vengerov Y. Y., Pokrovskii V. I. (2001). Outbreak of West Nile virus infection, Volgograd Region, Russia, 1999. *Emerg Infect Dis* 7(1):128-132.

Pletnev, A. G., Claire M. S., Elkins R., Speicher J., Murphy B. R., Chanock R. M. (2003). Molecularly engineered live-attenuated chimeric West Nile/dengue virus vaccines protect rhesus monkeys from West Nile virus. *Virology* 314(1):190-195.

Pripuzova, N. S., Tereshkina N. V., Gmyl L. V., Dzhivanyan T. I., Rumyantsev A. A., Romanova L., Mustafina A. N., Lashkevich V. A., Karganova G. G. (2009). Safety evaluation of chimeric Langat/Dengue 4 flavivirus, a live vaccine candidate against tick-borne encephalitis. *J Med Virol* 81(10):1777-1785.

Pugachev, K. V., Guirakhoo F., Mitchell F., Ocran S. W., Parsons M., Johnson B. W., Kosoy O. L., Lanciotti R. S., Roehrig J. T., Trent D. W., Monath T. P. (2004). Construction of yellow fever/St. Louis encephalitis chimeric virus and the use of chimeras as a diagnostic tool. *Am J Trop Med Hyg* 71(5):639-645.

Rey, F. A., Heinz F. X., Mandl C., Kunz C., Harrison S. C. (1995). The envelope glycoprotein from tick-borne encephalitis virus at 2 A resolution. *Nature* 375(6529):291-298.

Roehrig, J. T., Mathews J. H., Trent D. W. (1983). Identification of epitopes on the E glycoprotein of Saint Louis encephalitis virus using monoclonal antibodies. *Virology* 128(1):118-126.

Rosen, L. (1986). The natural history of Japanese encephalitis virus. *Annu Rev Microbiol* 40:395-414.

Russell, P. K., Brandt W. E., Dalrymple J. M., editors. 1980. Chemical and antigenic structure of flaviviruses. New York: Academic Press. 503-529 p.

Sabin, A. B., Schlesinger R. W. (1945). Production of Immunity to Dengue with Virus Modified by Propagation in Mice. *Science* 101(2634):640-642.

Savage, H. M., Ceianu C., Nicolescu G., Karabatsos N., Lanciotti R., Vladimirescu A., Laiv L., Ungureanu A., Romanca C., Tsai T. F. (1999). Entomologic and avian investigations of an epidemic of West Nile fever in Romania in 1996, with serologic and molecular characterization of a virus isolate from mosquitoes. *Am J Trop Med Hyg* 61(4):600-611.

Schmaljohn, C., Vanderzanden L., Bray M., Custer D., Meyer B., Li D., Rossi C., Fuller D., Fuller J., Haynes J., Huggins J. (1997). Naked DNA vaccines expressing the prM and E genes of Russian spring summer encephalitis virus and Central European encephalitis virus protect mice from homologous and heterologous challenge. *J Virol* 71(12):9563-9569.

Sharma, S., Mathur A., Prakash V., Kulshreshtha R., Kumar R., Chaturvedi U. C. (1991). Japanese encephalitis virus latency in peripheral blood lymphocytes and recurrence of infection in children. *Clin Exp Immunol* 85(1):85-89.

Solomon, T. (2004). Flavivirus encephalitis. *N Engl J Med* 351(4):370-378.

Solomon, T., Dung N. M., Kneen R., Gainsborough M., Vaughn D. W., Khanh V. T. (2000). Japanese encephalitis. *J Neurol Neurosurg Psychiatry* 68(4):405-415.

Solomon, T., Dung N. M., Kneen R., Thao le T. T., Gainsborough M., Nisalak A., Day N. P., Kirkham F. J., Vaughn D. W., Smith S., White N. J. (2002). Seizures and raised intracranial pressure in Vietnamese patients with Japanese encephalitis. *Brain* 125(Pt 5):1084-1093.

Solomon, T., Dung N. M., Wills B., Kneen R., Gainsborough M., Diet T. V., Thuy T. T., Loan H. T., Khanh V. C., Vaughn D. W., White N. J., Farrar J. J. (2003). Interferon alfa-2a in Japanese encephalitis: a randomised double-blind placebo-controlled trial. *Lancet* 361(9360):821-826.

Srey, V. H., Sadones H., Ong S., Mam M., Yim C., Sor S., Grosjean P., Reynes J. M. (2002). Etiology of encephalitis syndrome among hospitalized children and adults in Takeo, Cambodia, 1999-2000. *Am J Trop Med Hyg* 66(2):200-207.

Staples, J. E., Breiman R. F., Powers A. M. (2009). Chikungunya fever: an epidemiological review of a re-emerging infectious disease. *Clin Infect Dis* 49(6):942-948.

Suksanpaisan, L., Susantad T., Smith D. R. (2009). Characterization of dengue virus entry into HepG2 cells. *J Biomed Sci* 16:17.

Tsai, T., Popovici F., Cernescu C., Campbell G., Nedelcu N. (1998). West Nile encephalitis epidemic in southeastern Romania. *Lancet* 352:767-771.

Tsai, T. F. (2000). New initiatives for the control of Japanese encephalitis by vaccination: minutes of a WHO/CVI meeting, Bangkok, Thailand, 13-15 October 1998. *Vaccine* 18 Suppl 2:1-25.

Tunkel, A. R., Glaser C. A., Bloch K. C., Sejvar J. J., Marra C. M., Roos K. L., Hartman B. J., Kaplan S. L., Scheld W. M., Whitley R. J. (2008). The management of encephalitis: clinical practice guidelines by the Infectious Diseases Society of America. *Clin Infect Dis* 47(3):303-327.

Twiddy, S. S., Woelk C. H., Holmes E. C. (2002). Phylogenetic evidence for adaptive evolution of dengue viruses in nature. *J Gen Virol* 83(Pt 7):1679-1689.

Venugopal, K., Jiang W. R., Gould E. A. (1995). Immunity to St. Louis encephalitis virus by sequential immunization with recombinant vaccinia and baculovirus derived PrM/E proteins. *Vaccine* 13(11):1000-1005.

Volk, D. E., Beasley D. W., Kallick D. A., Holbrook M. R., Barrett A. D., Gorenstein D. G. (2004). Solution structure and antibody binding studies of the envelope protein domain III from the New York strain of West Nile virus. *J Biol Chem* 279(37):38755-38761.

Wang, T., Town T., Alexopoulou L., Anderson J. F., Fikrig E., Flavell R. A. (2004). Toll-like receptor 3 mediates West Nile virus entry into the brain causing lethal encephalitis. *Nat Med* 10(12):1366-1373.

Watts, D. M., Tesh R. B., Siirin M., Rosa A. T., Newman P. C., Clements D. E., Ogata S., Coller B. A., Weeks-Levy C., Lieberman M. M. (2007). Efficacy and durability of a recombinant subunit West Nile vaccine candidate in protecting hamsters from West Nile encephalitis. *Vaccine* 25(15):2913-2918.

Widman, D. G., Frolov I., Mason P. W. (2008). Third-generation flavivirus vaccines based on single-cycle, encapsidation-defective viruses. *Adv Virus Res* 72:77-126.

World Health Organization. (2006). Vector-Borne Viral Infections Tick-borne encephalitis. *http://www.who.int/vaccine_research/diseases/vector/en/print.html.*

Wu, S. C., Chiang J. R., Lin C. W. (2004). Novel cell adhesive glycosaminoglycan-binding proteins of Japanese encephalitis virus. *Biomacromolecules* 5(6):2160-2164.

Yamshchikov, G., Borisevich V., Seregin A., Chaporgina E., Mishina M., Mishin V., Kwok C. W., Yamshchikov V. (2004). An attenuated West Nile prototype virus is highly immunogenic and protects against the deadly NY99 strain: a candidate for live WN vaccine development. *Virology* 330(1):304-312.

Yu, I. M., Holdaway H. A., Chipman P. R., Kuhn R. J., Rossmann M. G., Chen J. (2009). Association of the pr peptides with dengue virus at acidic pH blocks membrane fusion. *J Virol* 83(23):12101-12107.

2

The Immunopathogenesis of Neurotropic Flavivirus Infection

King NJC et al.*
University of Sydney
Australia

1. Introduction

The flavivirus genus in the *Flaviviridae* family comprises over 70 species, most of which are tick- or mosquito-borne. They are single-stranded, plus-sense RNA viruses, responsible for significant human and animal morbidity and mortality on all inhabited continents. Medically important viscerotropic flaviviruses include dengue, found equatorially across the world, and the prototypic yellow fever virus, found in Africa and South America. Neurotropic members include tick-borne encephalitis virus (TBEV) in Europe, West Nile virus (WNV) in Africa, parts of Europe and the Indian subcontinent, as well as the USA, St Louis encephalitis virus in the USA, and Japanese encephalitis (JEV) and Murray Valley encephalitis (MVE) viruses in Australasia. Many of these have a history of emergence and re-emergence; indeed, following a novel outbreak in 1999 in New York (Lanciotti et al., 1999; CDC, 2010), WNV spread virtually throughout the Americas in less than 10 years and is the most common cause of meningoencephalitis in North America. WNV is now perhaps the most widely spread of all flaviviruses and may comprise 4 or more lineages, based on isolate homologies (C.G. Hayes, 2001; Bakonyi et al., 2005; Vazquez et al., 2010), with Lineage I and II well-defined and of obvious clinical importance in animals and humans (E.B. Hayes et al., 2005; Venter et al., 2009). WNV was first isolated in 1937 in the West Nile region of Uganda (Smithburn et al., 1940). It is a member of the Japanese encephalitis serogroup, together with JEV, Murray Valley and Saint Louis encephalitis viruses (Poidinger et al., 1996). These viruses are usually propagated in a zoonotic cycle between mosquitoes and amplifying hosts, particularly birds (or pigs in the case of JEV), with humans being incidental, since they may not develop high enough virus titres to infect arthropod vectors (C.G. Hayes, 2001). Rare cases of human-to-human WNV transmission have been documented via organ transplants and blood transfusion, as well as vertical transmission to the foetus *in utero* (Iwamoto et al., 2003; Lindsey et al., 2009). Although less than one percent of WNV infections develop neuroinvasive disease, in some 60% of patients presenting with central nervous system (CNS) symptoms denoting neuroinvasive disease, life-threatening encephalitis supervenes (Samuel & Diamond, 2009). The young,

* van Vreden C, Terry RL, Getts DR, Yeung AWS, Teague-Getts M, Davison AM, Deffrasnes C. and Munoz-Erazo L
University of Sydney, Australia

immunocompromised and elderly are at highest risk of developing encephalitis (Weiss et al., 2001; Guarner et al., 2004; Lindsey et al., 2009). Climate change, geographic factors and international travel, as well as local factors, such as mosquito rates and land clearing (E.A. Gould & Higgs, 2009) are cited as influencing the spread and prevalence of arbovirus infections across the globe. Despite considerable effort, the only successful live attenuated vaccine for neurotropic flaviviruses is for JEV (X. Liu et al., 2011), although considerable success has been achieved with a killed vaccine for TBEV (Barrett et al., 2003; Heinz et al., 2007). Treatment for all flavivirus encephalitides remains palliative. Indeed, one of the cardinal features of flavivirus infection complicating treatment approaches is immunopathology, evident in human cases and demonstrable in various animal models. In this review, we analyse the principal elements involved in the immunopathogenesis of flavivirus disease, with a view to novel constructive approaches to disease intervention.

2. Local flavivirus infection - responses of infected cells

Live WNV infection of various cell types leads to an upregulation of various cellular adhesion molecules, either directly or co-modulated by cytokines (Shen et al., 1995b; Shen et al., 1997; Arnold et al., 2004). These molecules include major histocompatibility complex (MHC) class I and II, intracellular adhesion molecule-1 (ICAM-1), vascular cellular adhesion molecule-1 (VCAM-1) and E-selectin (King & Kesson, 1988; Argall et al., 1991; Shen et al., 1997; Verma et al., 2009). The increase in MHC-I in mouse embryonic fibroblasts is independent of tumour necrosis factor (TNF) (Cheng et al., 2004b), although many cell types produce it in response to infection. In both mouse embryonic fibroblasts and human skin fibroblasts it can be induced by type I interferon (IFN)-dependent and -independent pathways (King & Kesson, 1988; Kesson & King, 2001; Cheng et al., 2004a), with the IFN-independent pathway relying on the activation of the transcription factor nuclear factor-κB (Kesson & King, 2001). This seemingly paradoxical increase in immune recognition molecule expression may enable evasion of early NK responses *in vivo* (Lobigs et al., 2003).

3. Earliest local changes in dermis and draining lymph nodes

Flaviviruses, transmitted by the bite of an infected mosquito, are injected with saliva during feeding. While several structural cell types are likely to come into contact with injected virus, the first leukocyte subset that virus is likely to encounter is the Langerhans cell (LC). LC are dendritic cells (DC) in the epidermis replenished by myeloid precursors in the bone marrow (BM) (Steinman, 1991; Merad et al., 2002). Following cutaneous inoculation, virus may infect LC, which increases cell surface expression of MHC-I, MHC-II, adhesion molecules, as well as costimulatory molecules, such as CD80, differentiating into a migratory phenotype in the process (Johnston et al., 1996). LC migrate to draining lymph nodes (DLN) in an accelerated manner in response to live virus, due to the induced soluble factor milieu (Johnston et al., 2000). *In vivo* experiments in mice show that the cytokine IL-1β is crucial for the emigration of LC from the epidermis to DLN (Byrne et al., 2001). It is presumed that these DC pass antigen to CD8α$^+$ DC in the DLN, since LC alone evidently do not initiate antiviral immune responses (Allan et al., 2003; Kissenpfennig et al., 2005; Hildner et al., 2008), but direct evidence of WNV antigen transfer has yet to be shown. While mosquito saliva may skew adaptive responses towards a more Th2-like response profile

(Schneider et al., 2007; Schneider et al., 2010), it is still unclear how its early presence influences disease outcome, since WNV infection in the genetic absence of IFN-γ still results in the generation of neutralising immunity (King et al., 2003). Arrival of virus in the DLN is accompanied by significant induction of CCL2 expression there that recruits monocyte-derived macrophages (MDM) from the bone marrow. The bone marrow undergoes a significant myeloid response to infection, releasing monocytes with a qualitatively different phenotype from the homeostatic state. Monocytes rapidly become TipDC (producing TNF and nitric oxide) in the DLN and likely contribute to the initiation of type 1 immune responses by inducing more IFN-γ from responding T cells than other DC subtypes in the DLN (Davison & King, 2011). Since flaviviruses significantly upregulate MHC expression on infected cells (King & Kesson, 1988; Shen et al., 1997), it is of interest how this influences the outcomes of innate immune interactions, such as with NK cells, and/or bears on the ultimate affinities of later adaptive cytotoxic T cell responses, reviewed in detail elsewhere (King & Kesson, 2003; Lobigs et al., 2003; King et al., 2009).

At the same time, at the dermal site of infection, CCL2, produced by infected cells, also recruits considerable numbers of MDM, which surround the infected focus, becoming DC within 24h of arrival. While it would appear that the DLN and dermis, by both producing CCL2, compete for MDM from the bone marrow, it seems likely that a subtly different cytokine milieu at each site selects for specific MDM subsets. This is suggested by adoptive transfer studies of flow cytometrically-sorted BM-derived monocyte subsets during infection. Thus, although similar numbers of inflammatory (Ly6C^{hi}) monocytes migrated to each site, 5-fold more Ly6C^{lo} monocytes migrated to the DLN than Ly6C^{hi}, while some 2-fold more Ly6C^{hi} monocytes migrated to the focus of infection in the skin than Ly6C^{lo} monocytes. Perhaps consonant with these proportions, immigrant Ly6C^{lo} monocytes in the DLN were 3-fold more likely to become DC, while in the dermis, immigrant Ly6C^{hi} cells were 2-fold more likely to become DC. This suggests that other chemokines may differentially contribute to the recruitment of these cells to the relevant site, but more importantly, it suggests that relevant precursors to specific cells are already ordained before they reach their target site, rather than necessarily being randomly and non-specifically recruited (*e.g.*, by CCL2) and induced to differentiate once they have arrived. Irrespective, it is evident that Ly6C expression on immigrating monocytes quickly changes at both sites, with downregulated Ly6C expression being the end point in both subsets. Thus, as shown in ours and other studies, Ly6C^{hi} monocytes arriving in response to infection quickly downregulate expression of this molecule (Sunderkotter et al., 2004; Leon et al., 2007; Getts et al., 2008; Davison & King, 2011). In contrast, at both sites, within 24h, immigrating Ly6C^{lo} monocytes become Ly6C^{hi} at the site, only to downregulate expression of this molecule again within a further 24h, while also upregulating CD11c to become DC. Furthermore, in the dermis, it is exclusively these cells originally entering the dermis as Ly6C^{lo} monocytes, that then migrate from the dermis to the DLN, presumably carrying viral antigen with them (Davison & King, 2011). Since so many Ly6C^{lo} cells also migrate from the BM to the DLN to become DC, it is tempting to speculate that these cells may differentiate into the final migratory couriers of antigen between the subcapsular sinus of the DLN, where DC arrive from the dermis via the afferent lymphatics, to the CD8α^{+} DC in the deep paracortex.

Early antiviral activity by Ly6C^{hi} monocyte-derived TipDC in the dermis may influence the outcome of infection by reducing virus titres locally; indeed, antiviral activity may account for the high survival rates observed in a mucosal model of flavivirus infection after intravaginal inoculation of a viral dose that is lethal by all other routes. In this model, large numbers of DC accumulate just beneath the epidermal site of infection, essentially separating infected epithelium from uninfected stroma below (Burke et al., 2004). Interestingly, CCL2 is also strongly expressed at this site (King, Unpublished observations).

4. Entry into the CNS

Virus undoubtedly spreads via the bloodstream at some point to further infect peripheral organs, including the CNS, where neurons are the main target (Xiao et al., 2001; Shrestha et al., 2003; Cheeran et al., 2005; Samuel & Diamond, 2009). However, the factors controlling these phases of virus spread are virtually unknown. The blood of acutely viraemic human donors shows substantial increases in IFN-γ and α as well as IFN-stimulated CXCL10 and CCL2. This upregulation of cytokines and chemokines occurs before IgM seroconversion and is therefore argued to be involved in the initial response to acute viraemia. On the other hand, this could be the result of chemokine gradients from the WNV-infected brain, since both chemokines are increased in the WNV-infected brain (Klein et al., 2005; Getts et al., 2008). Upregulated IL-4 was also detected in the same time frame, implicating IL-4 in early modulation of immune responses (Tobler et al., 2008).
How virus gains entry into the CNS is still unclear. In some models it is argued that breakdown of the blood-brain barrier (BBB) enables virus entry into the CNS. Toll-like receptors, TLR3, 7 and 8, are responsible for detecting RNA products of viral replication and although TLR3 and 7 are protective against WNV (Daffis et al., 2008; Town et al., 2009; (Daffis et al., 2008), TLR3 has also been implicated in aiding entry of WNV into the brain. TLR3 knockout mice have less BBB leakiness and significantly lower viral levels in the brain than wild type mice, with higher viral loads in the periphery, thought to be due to reduced production of TNF, a cytokine strongly implicated in BBB breakdown (T. Wang et al., 2004). Interestingly, macrophages isolated from young humans show a marked reduction in TLR3 levels during WNV infection, while those from elderly donors do not. TLR3 levels are controlled by a signal transducer and activator of transcription 1 (STAT1)-mediated pathway, which is downregulated by WNV E-protein in cells from young, but not elderly donors. Cells from elderly donors produced increased levels of inflammatory cytokines, including TNF (Kong et al., 2008), supporting the notion that TLR3 may play a role in immunopathology in the elderly, ironically via an overly aggressive immune response to WNV. Endothelial tight junction proteins (TJP), such as ZO-1 and claudin-1, are crucial components of BBB integrity and this seal is maintained, *inter alia*, by astrocytes, non-neuronal support cells of the CNS that are susceptible to WNV infection *in vitro* (Y. Liu et al., 1989; Cheeran et al., 2005; Verma et al., 2010). WNV-infected astrocytes increase matrix metalloproteinase (MMP) production to degrade TJP (Verma et al., 2010). However, astrocyte infection *in vivo* has not been reported and furthermore, BBB breakdown is quite variable in flavivirus infection (T.H. Liu et al., 2008; Verma et al., 2010). Alternative ways in which virus could cross the BBB include endothelial transcytosis and/or endothelial infection (German et al., 2006). However, there are few if any reports of endothelial infection itself *in vivo* by flaviviruses. Moreover, in 167 mice examined at various timepoints after intraperitoneal infection, where significant viraemia occurs within 6 h of inoculation, we saw unequivocal endothelial infection only once (King, Unpublished).

Trojan horse transmission into the brain by infected monocytes remains a possibility. Macrophages are susceptible to WNV infection (Cardosa et al., 1986; Shen et al., 1995a; Rios et al., 2006) and could be a crucial cell type contributing to transmission of virus into the brain. However, this has not been shown, and in our hands, while both human and mouse monocytes are readily infectable *in vitro*, they also very effectively control flavivirus infection, a point further supported *in vivo* by the lack of infected microglia (or for that matter, infiltrating macrophages) in flavivirus encephalitis (Getts et al., 2007; Getts et al., 2008). A recent study has shown that neutrophils, recruited to the intraperitoneal infection site in large numbers by CXCL-1 and -2 produced by WNV-infected macrophages, exhibited much higher viral loads than macrophages. The removal of these chemokines or depletion of neutrophils prior to WNV infection resulted in delayed death of animals and reduced viral levels, suggesting a possible role for neutrophils as reservoirs for viral replication and dissemination during the early stages of WNV infection (Bai et al., 2010). However, of the leukocytes attracted to the brain after intranasal infection, less than 3% are neutrophils (King, Unpublished). The intranasal route of infection enables the separation of systemic anti-viral responses from those mediated by the CNS. Thus, insignificant numbers are in and of themselves attracted to the brain during infection, making it unlikely that they are a primary source of virus in neuroinvasion, although they may be a source of spread to other organs. Notwithstanding the susceptibility of most cells to *in vitro* infection with flaviviruses, it has yet to be convincingly demonstrated that cells in the brain parenchyma other than neurons become infected in *in vivo* infection. This begs the question of how infected macrophages and neutrophils specifically contribute to neuronal infection. Furthermore, infection via a Trojan horse scenario would presumably occur only if infected leukocytes or monocytes were attracted by chemotactic signals originating in the parenchyma of the brain, whether or not the BBB was intact. This assumes a response to infection, either directly, *e.g.*, via infected neurons producing CCL2 (Getts et al., 2008), or indirectly via other leukocytes already attracted by infection producing chemokines that in turn attract infected neutrophils and monocytes, *i.e.*, once the immune response is well and truly under way. Increases in virus in the brain temporally consistent with this scenario have not to our knowledge been reported.

In vitro cellular adhesion molecules like E-selectin, VCAM-1 and ICAM-1 are upregulated in WNV infection and could support the extravasation of leukocytes into the brain (Shen et al., 1997). Expression of ICAM-1 and VCAM-1 is clearly increased on cerebrovascular endothelium in WNV-infected mice *in vivo* and this is also associated with infiltration of large numbers of macrophages and microglia into the brain (Figure 1). In primary human brain microvascular endothelial cells, an increase in VCAM-1 and E-selectin is induced when viral replication is at its highest (Verma et al., 2009). Together with TLR3-mediated BBB breakdown, upregulated adhesion molecules could facilitate the infiltration of infected leukocytes into the CNS. However, it is worth noting that WNV-infected IFN-γ knockout mice upregulate cerebrovascular endothelial ICAM-1 and VCAM-1 expression significantly, but have substantially fewer immigrant leukocytes than wild type mice (King, Unpublished). Moreover, although WNV induces BBB permeability in some models, it may not be the primary route of entry into the CNS. Mice and hamsters infected with WNV exhibited signs of BBB leakiness at the same timepoint they succumbed to virus, indicating that infection of the brain began prior to the BBB becoming compromised (Morrey et al., 2006; Morrey et al., 2008) (King, Unpublished). Similarly, in TBEV infection in mice, BBB breakdown occurs 2-3 days after virus is detectable in the brain (Růžek et al., 2011).

There is however, good evidence of centripetal nerve spread from the periphery (Engle & Diamond, 2003; Hunsperger & Roehrig, 2006; Getts et al., 2007). In the footpad model, viral infection occurs in the dermal layer of the epithelium in the footpad, which is enervated by sensory fibres of the dorsal root ganglion (DRG) of the peripheral nervous system (PNS). *In vitro*, PNS neurons support WNV infection and in mice the DRG is highly susceptible to WNV infection, suggesting that it may be involved in retrograde axonal transport of virus from the PNS to CNS (Hunsperger & Roehrig, 2005, 2006). This is consistent with our own studies using intraperitoneal inoculation of WNV in mice, where WNV is seen in the cervical spinal cord 1-2 days before it is seen in the brain parenchyma, spreading in a caudal to rostral manner. In contrast, intranasal infection results in rostral to caudal spread through the brain, with spread to various anatomical regions via known neural connections (King, Unpublished). If the sciatic nerve of golden hamsters is transected above the infection site, a systemic infection with less severe clinical symptoms of CNS invasion occurs (Samuel et al., 2007), denoting a contribution to spread by intact axons. Treatment of mice with nocodazole, a microtubule inhibitor that prevents retrograde axonal transport, prior to inoculation, delays virus spread to the CNS by 6 days (Hunsperger & Roehrig, 2009). However, taken together, it is likely that more than one pathway is involved in WNV spread to the CNS, with inoculation site, dose, age and genetics all influencing this.

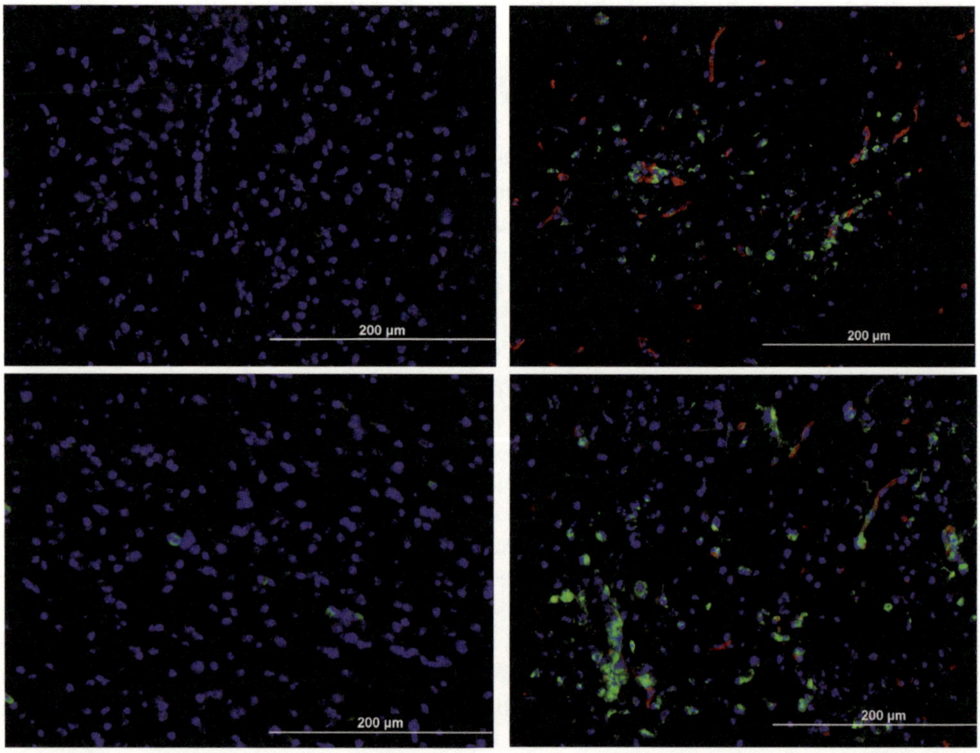

Fig. 1. WNV infection results in the upregulation of ICAM-1 and VCAM-1 on brain vasculature in WNV encephalitis. Green = macrophages and microglia (lectin staining), Red = ICAM-1 (top right), VCAM-1 (bottom right) Blue = DAPI.
Left panels = mock-infected, Right panels = d7 WNV-infected

5. CNS infection

In vitro, virions attaching to the plasma membrane enter cells via clathrin-mediated endocytosis to form endosomes. A lysosomal, pH-dependent fusion mechanism expels the nucleocapsid into the cytoplasm in close proximity to the ER where the virus is thought to replicate (Chu & Ng, 2004). All cells of the CNS are readily susceptible to WNV infection *in vitro* within 16-24 h, including neurons, Schwann cells and astrocytes, although microglia are more resistant (Y. Liu et al., 1989; Argall et al., 1991; Shrestha et al., 2003; Cheeran et al., 2005). In contrast, in animal models, detectable infection is seen in the brain between d3 and 6 post infection (p.i.), depending on the model, with virus in all cases evidently replicating exclusively within neurons, a behaviour distinguishing it from the encephalitic DNA viruses (Steele et al., 2000; Xiao et al., 2001; King et al., 2003; Shrestha et al., 2003; Getts et al., 2007; Brehin et al., 2008). Antibody labelling of monkey brain sections for neuron-specific endose, glial fibrillary acidic protein and WNV were argued to indicate WNV infection of both glia and neurons, but this interpretation is not well supported by the examples provided (He et al., 2009). In humans, viral antigen is found in neuronal cytoplasm and processes, usually at the centre of microglial nodules (Sampson et al., 2000; Guarner et al., 2004).

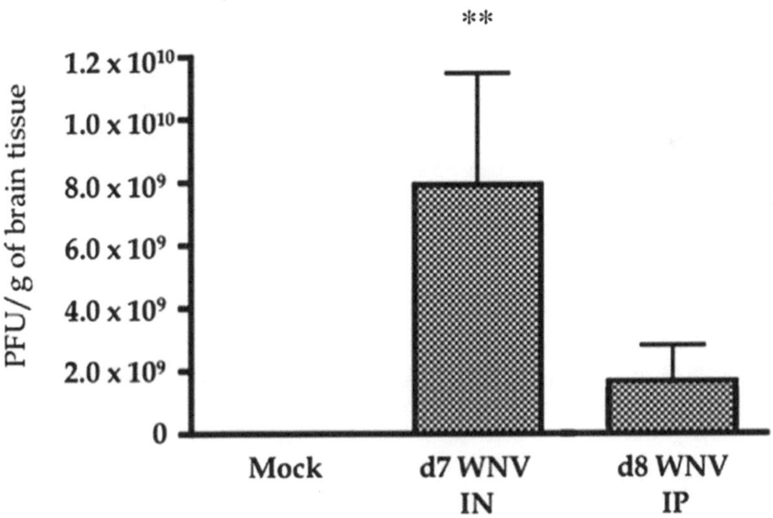

Fig. 2. Virus titres in the WNV-infected brain. IN = intranasal, IP = intraperitoneal infection

Following inoculation at the periphery, WNV replicates in lymphoid tissues, but once in the CNS, titres increase until the onset of encephalitis (Brehin et al., 2008). Plaque assays of brain tissue from mice intranasally infected with WNV show much higher viral titres at the time of death on d7 p.i. than peripherally inoculated animals (Figure 2). After footpad inoculation, virus RNA can be isolated from parts of the nervous system like the brainstem, as early as 24 h p.i., long before the peak of viraemia and symptoms are present. There are also indications that the virus may be cleared, only to be followed by re-emergence in that area (Hunsperger & Roehrig, 2006). In the murine model of WNV infection the brain structures most susceptible and showing the highest viral titres appear to be the cortex, hippocampus, brainstem and spinal cord (Xiao et al., 2001; Hunsperger & Roehrig, 2006). In humans, WNV seems to affect the brainstem and anterior horn of the spinal cord (Sejvar et al., 2003; Guarner et al., 2004). Neuroinvasion also occurs in animals that do not succumb to infection (Hunsperger & Roehrig, 2006; Appler et al., 2010). Damage to neurons can result from either excessive virus replication or an over-exuberant immune response, or both, with death ensuing in either eventuality. Increases in $CD45^+$ leukocyte numbers as well as viral antigen are associated with areas of neuronal injury, degeneration by apoptosis and onset of encephalitis, making it difficult to distinguish between viral and immune-mediated injury (Xiao et al., 2001; Shrestha et al., 2003; Brehin et al., 2008). In general, mice die soon after seizures become evident; if seizures can be suppressed, then survival may be extended several days and virus growth in the brain increases by a further 10-fold or more (Getts et al., 2007). This indicates that the neurons are capable of supporting much higher levels of virus replication than is usually evident at death. Microglial nodules, perivascular cuffing, principally comprised of infiltrating macrophages and T cells, and in advanced disease, neuronal loss, are prominent among the neurohistopathological and immunohistochemical findings (Steele et al., 2000; Guarner et al., 2004; Petzold et al., 2010). Significant leukocyte infiltration seems to occur around d5 p.i., irrespective of the model used, associated with full activation of the adaptive immune response.

Cells of the CNS each respond differently towards infiltrating virus. *In vitro* one of the responses to viral infection of astrocytes and microglia is the production of chemoattractants like CCL5 and CXCL10 (Cheeran et al., 2005), which recruit T cells and possibly monocytes; both astrocytes and microglia can produce CXCL9, which similarly attracts T cells (Muller et al., 2007) (Getts, Unpublished). Infected neurons produce copious amounts of CCL2, which recruit macrophages and microglia from the bone marrow (Getts et al., 2008). IFN-γ plays an important role in the formation of the seizure cascade during the development of the CNS, as IFN-γ knockout mice do not develop seizures during WNV infection. Seizures cannot be recapitulated by IFN-γ-producing T cells infiltrating into the brain in WNV-infected IFN-γ knockout chimeras previously reconstituted with wild type bone marrow. The role of the glutamate receptor, N-methyl-D-aspartate in the development of these seizures has also been shown (Getts et al., 2007). While it is clear that many soluble factors are produced in the brain, it is not so obvious which cells produce them *in vivo*. Much work will be required to fully characterise the sequence of inductive and inhibitory interactions between local cells, infected cells and immigrant leukocytes.

6. Microglial activation

Microglial activation is clearly associated with virus infection of neurons rather than immune leukocyte infiltration. After intraperitoneal inoculation, WNV can be seen in the brain by d6 p.i., when activated microglia are first observed, one day after leukocyte infiltration is first evident. However, in the intranasal model, microglial activation is seen at d3 p.i. when virus is first observed, while leukocyte infiltration is still seen first at d5 p.i., as in the intraperitoneal model (Getts et al., 2008) (King, Unpublished). Microglia form nodules around infected neurons soon after infection (King et al., 2003; Guarner et al., 2004; Petzold et al., 2010), presumably recruited by the soluble factor outputs from infected neurons, including CCL2. Consistent with this, microglia, at first dendritic, quickly lose these normal projections to assume a more motile amoeboid phenotype

(Getts et al., 2008). Interestingly, as the number of infected neurons increases, these nodules become less apparent, perhaps because the concentrations of these soluble factors reach a virtual equilibrium within the brain, thus abrogating the concentration gradients likely required for nodule formation (King, Unpublished). Whether the formation of nodules is protective or damaging to neurons is not known, but relatively few infected neurons at the centre of microglial nodules are TUNEL-positive in WNV encephalitis (Getts et al., 2007). There is a significant increase in microglial numbers in the brain during infection, with a decrease in resting microglial numbers. This increase is accounted for by bone marrow-derived monocyte immigration and is not due to *in situ* proliferation of microglia (Getts et al., 2008). Whether immigrant microglia subsequently return to a resting state in the brain if the host survives and/or whether these cells have a role in the causation of any subsequent neurological sequelae, remains to be elucidated.

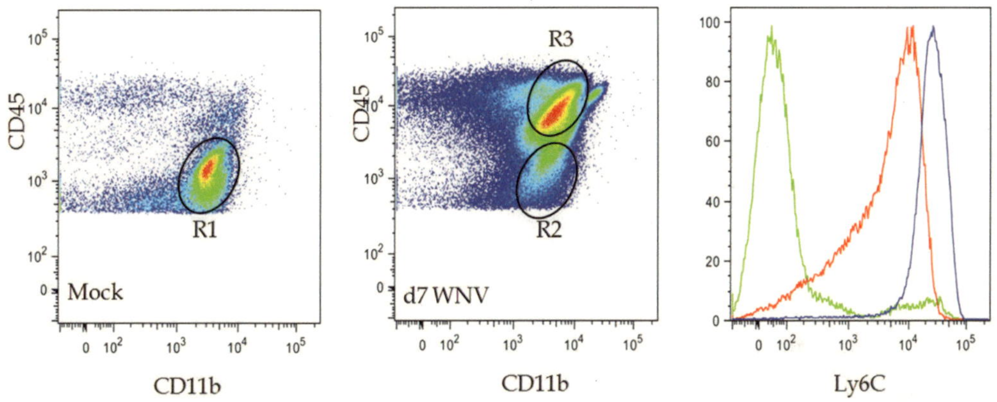

Fig. 3. Flow cytometry showing infiltration of macrophages and microglia in the WNV-infected and mock-infected mouse brain. R1 (green profile at right) = $CD45^{lo-int}$ microglia (mock-infected), R2 (red profile at right) = $CD45^{lo-int}$ microglia (WNV-infected), R3 (blue profile at right) = $CD45^{hi}$ macrophages (WNV-infected)

Usually by d6 p.i. the whole microglial population in the brain is activated and this can be detected as an increase in CD45 expression by flow cytometry (Figure 3) and by their amoeboid morphology using lectin immunohistochemistry (Brehin et al., 2008; Getts et al., 2008). Similar to infiltrating macrophages, activated microglia in the WNV-infected brain also express higher levels of Ly6C, compared to mock-infected mice. In Rhesus monkeys infected intracerebrally with three antigenically divergent flaviviruses, activated microglia are identified by their enlarged morphology, short thicker processes and CD68 expression. In this model, microglia are found next to dying neurons and neuronal debris where they perform a phagocytic function (Maximova et al., 2009). They also secrete various proinflammatory mediators and cytokines as part of the response to local and systemic infection. The increased microglial production of leukocyte-recruiting chemokines, CXCL10 and CCL2, is triggered by the activation of the p53-mitogen-activated protein kinase and extracellular signal-regulated kinase intracellular signaling pathways by WNV infection (Cheeran et al., 2005). Neutralisation of CCL2 by antibody on d6 p.i., results in prolonged survival, strongly implicating microglia as contributors to fatal neuropathology (Getts et al.,

2008). In Japanese encephalitis, bystander damage caused by activated microglia is a major contributor to the severity of the disease. Microglial activation is associated with elevation of proinflammatory mediators like TNF, IL-1β, IL-6, (inducible) nitric oxide synthase-2 (NOS2) and cyclooxygenase-2 (Cox-2), all of which have the potential to be neurotoxic (Ghoshal et al., 2007; Chen et al., 2010). Nitric oxide (NO), formed from the catalysis of arginine by sustained high levels of induced NOS2, can cause significant oxidative damage to neurons, while the production of Cox-2 results in reactive oxygen species as a byproduct that is also capable of inflicting irreversible damage on neurons (Ghoshal et al., 2007). TNF-induced endothelial expression of NOS2 and the formation of reactive nitrogen- and oxygen species is also implicated in the apoptosis of cells and development of hemorrhage in the murine model of dengue virus infection (Yen et al., 2008).

7. Macrophage infiltration

In mice infected with WNV by intranasal inoculation, virus is detectable only in the brain, making this model ideal to study brain responses to neuronal infection. In this model, the predominant leukocyte subtype immigrating into the brain in flavivirus encephalitis is the MDM (Figure 4, 5). By d7 p.i. large numbers of infiltrating macrophages can be seen surrounding infected neurons in the brains of WNV-infected mice. Neutralisation of CCL2 reduces macrophage immigration into the brain, indicating that CCL2, produced by infected neurons, is a major driver of MDM immigration into the CNS (Getts et al., 2008; Lim et al., 2011), however, this may later be supplemented with IL-23, which may intensify macrophage infiltration, or result in the recruitment of different functional macrophage subsets (Town et al., 2009). IL-23 is argued to originate from microglia, but this has not been shown. Some 35-50% of infiltrating leukocytes in the brain are $Ly6C^{hi}$ macrophages, with NK cells and $Ly6C^{+}$ immigrant microglia in each case making up approximately half these numbers (Figure 5).

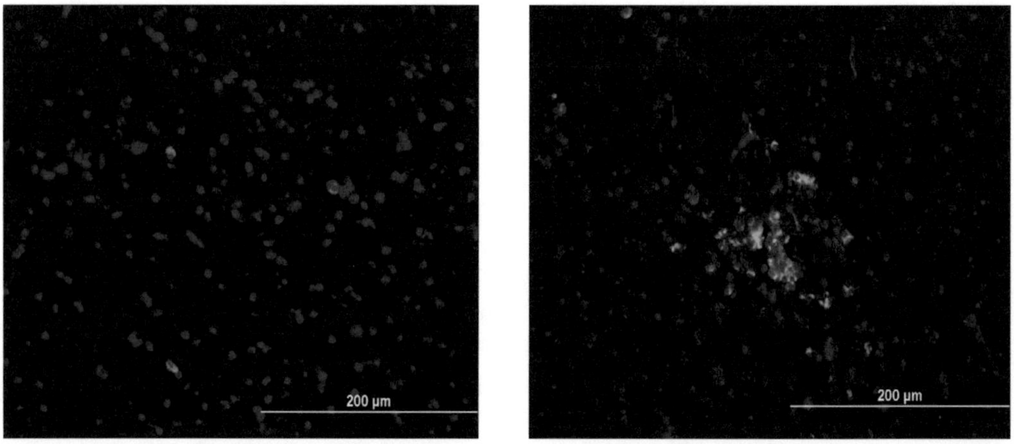

Fig. 4. Immunohistochemistry showing myeloid lineage cells infiltrating the WNV-infected brain. Green = macrophages and microglia (lectin staining); Red = anti-NS-1 (WNV-infected neurons); Blue = DAPI. Left = Mock-infected, Right = d7 p.i. WNV-infected

Once in the brain, both MDM and activated microglia can process antigen and reactivate WNV-specific memory T cells (Ford et al., 1996; Olson & Miller, 2004), but cannot initiate responses in naïve T cells (Getts, Unpublished). Both cell types produce significant amounts of NO, presumably via NOS2 induced by IFN-γ from infiltrating T cells (Schoneboom et al., 2000; Jana et al., 2001) (Figure 6). Pharmacological inhibition of NO at specific time points in an MVE model results in extended survival (Andrews et al., 1999). This is different from models in which NO is abrogated throughout infection, where survival is reduced (Fenyk-Melody et al., 1998; King et al., 2007). This highlights a crucial point about models used to determine susceptibility to lethal flavivirus infection. While the absence or presence of a particular gene may dictate susceptibility, the involvement of this gene in the disease process may vary significantly during the course of infection. It may be critical for virus control at one point, but be responsible for immunopathological damage at another. This is further emphasised by the fact that depletion of the macrophage population throughout the disease course results in accelerated death (Ben-Nathan et al., 1996), while temporally targeted inhibition of macrophage immigration into the brain in WNV encephalitis results in long term survival and immunity (Getts et al., 2008).

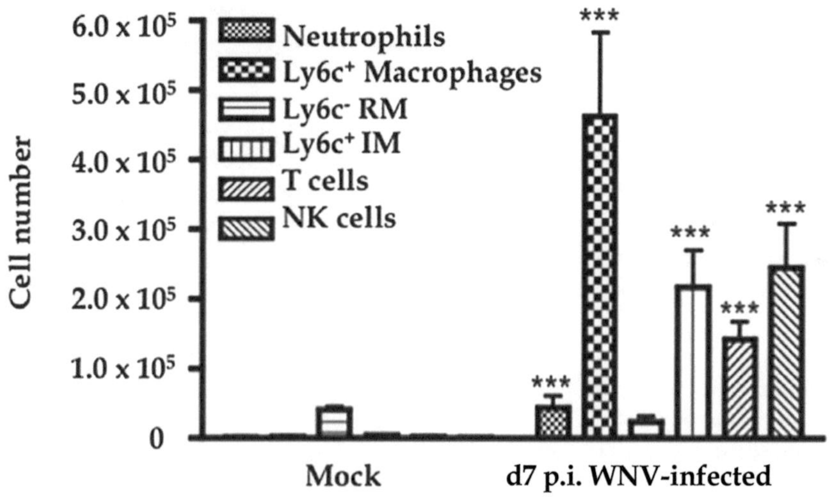

Fig. 5. Leukocyte subsets in the WNV-infected brain on d7 p.i. RM= resident microglia, IM= immigrant microglia

Peripheral production of NO is also involved in DC-programmed T cell responses. Bone marrow-derived DC from NOS2 knockout mice elicited a much stronger Th1 immune response with increased chemokine expression. Interestingly, lack of NO-mediated modulation resulted in expansion of a Ly6C^{hi} type inflammatory DC subset, implicating NO as a potential negative regulator of immune-mediated pathology (Giordano et al., 2010). On the other hand, in influenza infection, increased Th1 responses in the absence of NOS2 may result in higher antiviral antibody titres and more effective virus clearance with less immunopathology (Jayasekera et al., 2006). As with WNV encephalitis, neuroinflammation plays a significant role in the severity of experimental autoimmune encephalomyelitis (EAE). NOS2 knockout mice are much more susceptible to EAE than wild type mice (Fenyk-

Melody et al., 1998). This raises the question of the role of $Ly6C^{hi}$ inflammatory cells in the severity of neuropathology in WNV infection (Giordano et al., 2010).

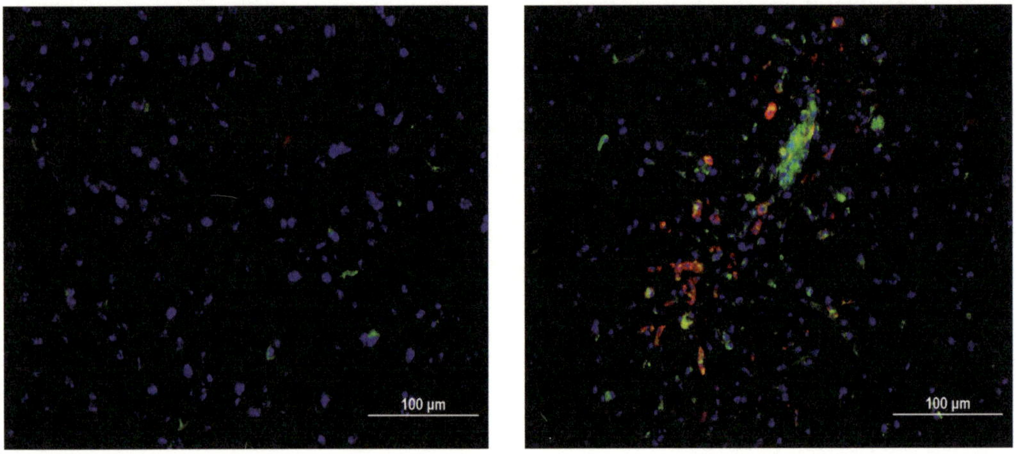

Fig. 6. Macrophages and microglia produce NO in response to WNV infection. Green = macrophages and microglia (lectin staining); Red = iNOS/NOS2; Blue = DAPI. Left = Mock infected, Right = d7 WNV

Mice and human peripheral blood monocytes are divided into circulating and inflammatory subsets. As mentioned above, inflammatory monocytes are recruited to inflamed tissue by chemokines like CCL2, while circulating monocytes may replace resident macrophages in the steady state. In the murine model, circulating monocytes have $Gr1^{-}(Ly6C^{lo})/CX3CR1^{+}$ phenotype; inflammatory monocytes have a $Gr1^{hi}(Ly6C^{hi})/CCR2^{+}$ phenotype (Geissmann et al., 2003; Tacke & Randolph, 2006). As mentioned, $Ly6C^{hi}$ monocytes can differentiate into DC in the spleen and lung as well as into LC and macrophages under inflammatory conditions, where they are capable of stimulating naïve T-cells (Geissmann et al., 2003; Leon et al., 2004; Ginhoux et al., 2006; Landsman et al., 2007). During WNV infection there is a substantial increase in $CD45^{int}/CD11b^{+}/CD11c^{-}$ activated microglia in the brain. Depletion of blood monocytes reduces numbers of activated microglia in the CNS and adoptive transfer of $Ly6C^{hi}$ inflammatory monocytes from the bone marrow confirms that activated microglia in the CNS are derived from inflammatory monocytes in WNV infection (Getts et al., 2008).

CCR2 and its ligand, CCL2, are important in the emigration of inflammatory monocytes from the bone marrow and migration to inflamed sites, including the CNS (Serbina & Pamer, 2006; Tsou et al., 2007; Getts et al., 2008; Lim et al., 2011). Immunohistochemical staining shows CCL2 expression by WNV-infected neurons, often with macrophages and microglia in close attendance (Figure 7). Recent findings however, indicate that CCR2 does not control the accumulation of $Ly6C^{hi}$ monocytes from blood to CNS directly, but rather by regulating the levels of monocytes in the blood (Lim et al., 2011). Interestingly the neutralisation of CCL2 leads to increased survival rates in WNV-infected mice, indicating the possible role that inflammatory cells play in the immunopathology of WNV encephalitis (Getts et al., 2008). CCR2 and CCR4 also seem to be involved in the pathogenesis of dengue virus disease. Dengue-infected CCR2 and CCR4 knockout mice show increased survival rates and have decreased levels of systemic cytokines like IL-6 and IFN-γ, as well as lower numbers of activated NKT, $CD4^+$, $CD8^+$ T cells and macrophages in the spleen compared to wild type mice. Although the viral load in the CCR4 knockout and wild type mice was similar, it was suggested that the reduced mortality rates in these mice is due to reduced damage to organs and tissues associated with the abrogated inflammatory response (Guabiraba et al., 2010).

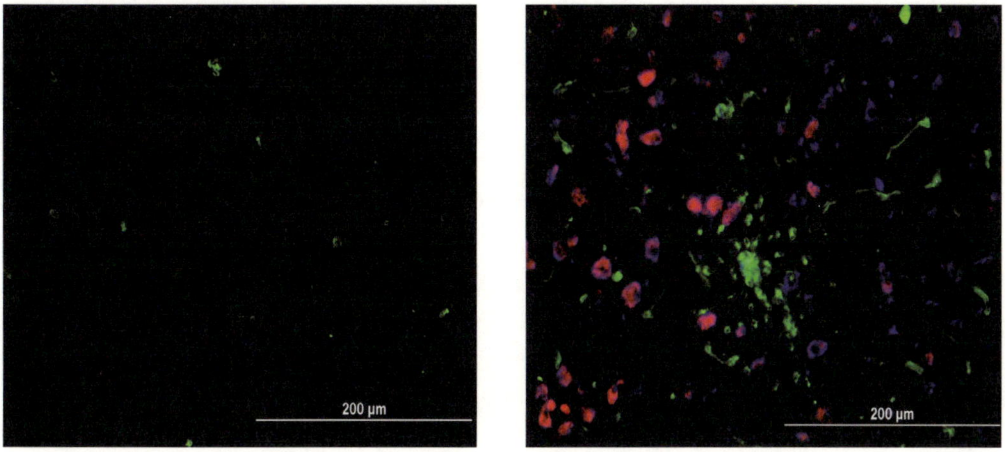

Fig. 7. Infected neurons produce CCL2 which recruits monocytes to the brain.
Green = macrophages and microglia (lectin staining); Red = NS-1 (actively infected neurons); Blue = CCL2. Left = Mock-infected, Right = d7 p.i. WNV-infected

8. Infiltration of other leukocyte subtypes

While up to 50% of leukocytes infiltrating into the CNS following infection are MDM, significant numbers of $CD4^+$, $CD8^+$ T cells (10-15%) and NK cells (10-20%) also immigrate into the brain, although there are relative few neutrophils (1-3%) (Figure 5, 8). T cells are recruited by increased astrocyte and microglial CXCL10 and CXCL9 expression, as well as CCL5 (Glass et al., 2005).

As for mice, T cell effector subsets migrate into the perivascular space and brain parenchyma during flavivirus infection of monkeys. T cells are seen spread evenly throughout the parenchyma and perivascular space, whereas labelling for $CD4^+$ and $CD8^+$ subsets shows a more compartmentalised distribution, with $CD4^+$ cells located mainly in the perivascular space. Either the $CD4^+$ or $CD8^+$ T cell subset may be the dominant lymphocyte present in CNS in infection (Kelley et al., 2003; Maximova et al., 2009). Whether they contribute to immunopathology or not, T cells are clearly crucial to virus clearance; mice deficient in this subpopulation exhibit higher mortality rates (Y. Wang et al., 2003; Y. Wang et al., 2006; Brien et al., 2008). Further highlighting these points, despite significantly lower myeloid cell infiltration in WNV infection in RAG knockout mice and prolonged survival, these animals die with high titres of virus in the CNS (King, Unpublished). In contrast to WNV, in TBEV infection in mice, immunopathology is evidently mediated by $CD8^+$ T-cells, although these cells are not responsible for BBB breakdown (Růžek et al., 2011). $CD4^+$ T cells evidently play a protective role in TBEV, possibly via secretion of IFN-γ and other pro-inflammatory cytokines and/or stimulation of 'macrophage-like' cells (Růžek et al., 2009).

The chemokine receptor CXCR3 is a key regulator of T-cell recruitment and thus plays a pivotal role in the pathogenesis of many diseases (Muller et al., 2007). During WNV encephalitis in mice the chemokine receptor CXCR3 enables recruitment of antiviral $CD8^+$ T cells to the CNS in a region-specific manner. Loss of this receptor leads to increased mortality rates in these animals (B. Zhang et al., 2008). TNF is also essential in the recruitment of antiviral $CD8^+$ T cells to the CNS in WNV infection (Shrestha et al., 2008).

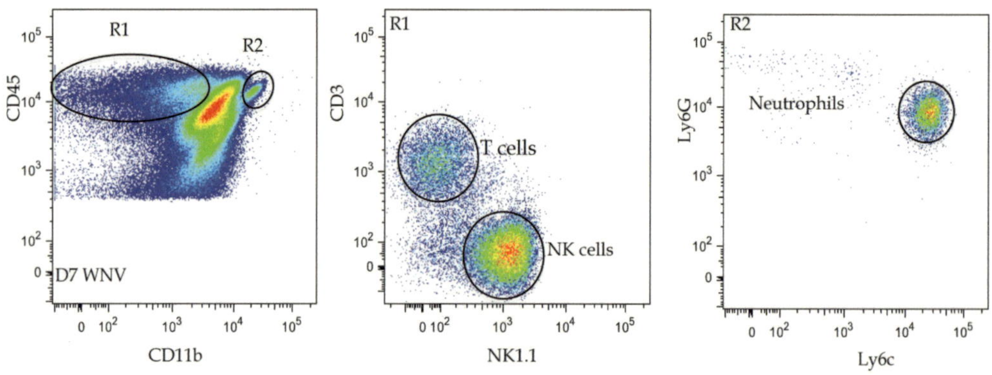

Fig. 8. Flow cytometry showing regional analysis of infiltrating leukocytes in murine brain. R1 denotes $CD45^{hi}$, $CD11b^{lo}$ lymphocytes, which can be further divided into T cells and NK cells; R2 denotes $CD45^{hi}$, $CD11b^{hi}$ neutrophils, which are $Ly6G^+$, $Ly6C^+$

Although B cells are also observed in the brain in some studies (Brehin et al., 2008), $CD20^+$ B cells are predominantly found in the perivascular space surrounding neurons. Proportions of B and T cells in the brain vary depending on the infecting flavivirus (Maximova et al., 2009). By flow cytometry, we find few B cells in the brain parenchyma and while the BBB is intact it seems unlikely that antibodies have a significant effect against WNV within the brain, although antibody is clearly important systemically in protection against WNV (Diamond et al., 2003). NK cells, while present in significant numbers in the brain parenchyma, have not been studied in any detail. Indeed, to date they have been regarded as redundant in flavivirus infection, since upregulated MHC expression on infected cells reduces NK cell recognition. However, *in vitro*, under artificially-stimulated conditions, NK cells are cytotoxic for WNV-infected cells (M. Zhang et al., 2010).

The lack of neutrophil infiltration is perhaps not surprising as there is little or no CXCL1 expression in the brain during infection. However, in MVE, infiltration of NO-producing neutrophils, attracted by TNF and N51/KC, are a significant part of the inflammatory leukocyte infiltration and contribute to the severity of disease. Neutrophil depletion and inhibition of NOS prolongs survival of infected animals and reduces the severity of pathology in the CNS (Andrews et al., 1999). Since the neutrophil-depleting antibody used also depletes monocytes, however, it is not clear to what extent immigrating macrophages may have contributed to lethal pathology. Nevertheless, this again highlights the point that temporally selective depletion may reduce pathology, while genetic deletion may exacerbate it.

9. Immunomodulating therapies

Despite the large amount of research in the field, there is currently no approved antiviral therapy against WNV in humans and treatment remains symptomatic. Currently, the only live flavivirus vaccines with a relatively good record of safety are against yellow fever (Monath, 2010) and JEV (X. Liu et al., 2011) and the only commercially available live vaccines against WNV are for horses. Two highly purified formalin-inactivated whole virus vaccines against TBEV have been used in Europe since 1976 (FSME Immun, Baxter) and 1999 (Encepur, Novartis) and an efficacy of 99% has been reported in Austria, with no difference between age groups, and no major safety issues reported (Barrett et al., 2003; Heinz et al., 2007). Another avenue that is currently being investigated is antivector vaccines that target mosquitoes or ticks directly (Kortekaas et al., 2010). Recently, stable infection with the bacterium, *Wolbachia*, has been achieved, with significant potential for limiting the transmission of dengue (McMeniman et al., 2009; Bian et al., 2010). Antivirals like Ribavirin can successfully act against WNV *in vitro* (Jordan et al., 2000; Anderson & Rahal, 2002), but have no notable antiviral effect when used to treat infected humans (Chowers et al., 2001). Although initial studies with antiviral medication appeared promising, increased mortality rates led to several candidates being disqualified. This and the fact that a significant amount of neuropathology is induced by the immune system itself has led to more research being conducted into modulation of the immune system. Indeed, general immunomodulators that inhibit inflammatory mediator synthesis and can cross the BBB are potential candidates. Patients infected with TBEV receiving the anti-inflammatory antibiotic, tetracycline, had reduced levels of IL-6, IL-1β, TNF, quicker improvement of symptoms and faster clinical recovery than untreated patients (Atrasheuskaya et al., 2003).

Because interferons play such a prominent role in mitigating viral infection and modulating the adaptive immune system, they have been prime candidates for immunomodulating therapies (Samuel & Diamond, 2005; Jiang et al., 2010). IFN-α2b has protective and therapeutic properties in Vero cells (Anderson & Rahal, 2002). IFN-γ and β play a role in inhibiting viral spread and replication in the periphery as well as the CNS and are also argued to reduce WNV-induced neuronal death (Samuel & Diamond, 2005). RNA for interferon-stimulated genes (ISG) and their protein expression are upregulated during viral infections (Wacher et al., 2007). Five of the IFN-α-induced ISG, namely Viperin, ISG20, protein kinase R (PKR) and IFN-induced transmembrane proteins 2 and 3 (IFITM2, IFITM3) have been shown to disrupt multiple steps in the dengue and WNV life cycle. IFITM2 and 3 in particular serve to inhibit viral entry into host cells (Jiang et al., 2010). The matrix metalloproteinase (MMP) inhibitor, GM6001 has been shown to reverse the damage to BBB integrity induced by MMPs with WNV infection (Verma et al., 2010). Cytotoxic T cells can eradicate WNV by lysing infected cells and this could potentially be used in developing treatment against WNV. The vaccination of individuals with a chimeric WNV/yellow fever vaccine, coding a WNV envelope antigen, results in the production of $CD8^+$ T cells that persist for up to a year with similar qualities to memory T cells (Smith et al., 2010). Cytotoxic T lymphocytes generated against WNV-specific epitopes are able to eradicate infected cells *in vitro* as well as increase survival rates when transferred into mice. This approach may thus result in a more targeted immune response and optimised eradication of virus (Purtha et al., 2007).

Neutralising antibodies have also been successful in treating and preventing early infection in animal models and humanised antibodies could provide the basis for treatment after known exposure to infection (Throsby et al., 2006; Vogt et al., 2009). The use of certain human single chain variable fragments fused with an IgG1 Fc region is able to confer some protection against lethal WNV in mice. The addition of Fc region to this protein is critical for the effectiveness of its neutralising function and suggests whole monoclonal antibodies (mAbs) may more effectively neutralise WNV (L.H. Gould et al., 2005). Further supporting this, the neutralising potential of mAb E16 is less effective in mice lacking the Fc receptor (Oliphant et al., 2005). It is tempting to speculate also, that NK cell-mediated antibody-dependent cell-mediated cytotoxicity may contribute to viral clearance in the periphery.

Of the myriad antibodies induced by WNV infection only a few neutralise WNV and have a possible therapeutic role. Neutralising antibodies are mainly directed against domain III of the WNV envelope-protein where they prevent the conformational change in the virus required to fuse to cellular membranes, consequently inhibiting it from entering the cell (Oliphant et al., 2005; Throsby et al., 2006; Morrey et al., 2007; S. Zhang et al., 2009). Polyclonal antibodies promote survival in B- and T cell-deficient mice, indicating their therapeutic potential (Engle & Diamond, 2003). The axonal spread of virus can also be blocked by neutralising antibodies *in vitro* and *in vivo* (Samuel et al., 2007). Two neutralising human monoclonal antibodies with therapeutic potential are CR4348 and CR4354, both capable of inhibiting WNV *in vitro* and *in vivo.* They bind to epitopes on the E-protein of the virus and neutralise the virus at the postattachment step, it is thought by preventing fusion of the virus to the endosomal membrane. Prophylactic treatment with these antibodies protects mice against lethal WNV infection (Vogt et al., 2009). On the other hand, humanised mAb E16 is able to increase survival of both mice and hamsters, even when administered after the CNS is infected (Oliphant et al., 2005; Morrey et al., 2007). The treatment of hamsters 5 days after WNV inoculation with this E16 antibody also results in decreased viral burden in the CNS and increased survival (Morrey et al., 2006). The affinity of neutralising antibodies has also been associated with neutralising efficacy. Affinity alone, however, does not ensure the efficacy of inhibiting WNV activity, as some non-neutralising antibodies bind with high affinity to their epitopes. Thus, not surprisingly, both the specific epitope and binding affinity play a role (Sanchez et al., 2005).

Other factors limiting antibody-mediated treatment include the poor movement of antibodies across an intact BBB to enable them to act on virus-infected neurons (Cheeran et al., 2005; Morrey et al., 2007) and the possibility that mutant virus strains might arise through antibody treatment. For example, mutations of the E16 epitope of the virus can abrogate the neutralising activity of monoclonal antibodies (Li et al., 2005; Sanchez et al., 2005). Thus, although resistant strains to specific mAbs are currently rare, they need to be considered in the design of antibody therapy (S. Zhang et al., 2009). Time of therapeutic administration and viable administration routes for human patients are also important considerations because of the possibility that antibodies could further exacerbate disease via antibody-dependent enhancement of infection. This classically occurs in a second dengue infection. Here, virus-specific antibodies from a first dengue infection with a low affinity for the second strain of dengue do not neutralise, but complex with virus. This enables virus to gain access to monocytes, macrophages and mature DC via Fcγ receptors typically borne by the myeloid lineage, resulting in increased viral loads in individual cells, as well as increasing numbers of productively-infected cells (Halstead & O'Rourke, 1977; Boonnak et al., 2011).

This currently leaves cell subset targeting as an immunomodulating therapy, but issues about which subset(s) to target, how to target them effectively and when to target them during disease remain to be resolved. However, the temporal targeting of immunopathological subsets and/or the enhancement of potentially anti-inflammatory subsets in viral encephalitis, with the idea of enabling successful virus clearance by the remaining elements of the adaptive immune response, remain a legitimate goal, since, unlike the long-term requirement for subset blockers in *e.g.*, multiple sclerosis, which may be associated with progressive multifocal leukoencephalopathy, short-term use is much less likely to have permanent sequelae.

10. Conclusion

Research on WNV and flaviviruses in general has increased dramatically in the last 10 years, since the advent of WNV in New York in August 1999. It has become clear that different flaviviruses have different interactions with the immune system and what may be pathogenic in one infection may prolong survival in another. This is undoubtedly further complicated by the variability of human (and mouse) genetics, as well as the variety of disease models. While it may eventually be possible to personalise treatments ranging from cancer to infectious disease, at this stage we do not know enough about the pathogenesis of these infections to inform the kind of generic approach required to intervene to prevent lethal disease in a meaningful number of patients successfully. While it seems likely that an effective vaccine will eventually be available, many issues have to be addressed before general immunisation is a viable proposition. Notwithstanding the success of this endeavour, there will always be individuals in which it will be necessary to intervene clinically, due to poor vaccine compliance, failure of vaccination, as well as other uncontrollable factors. Unlike species-specific viruses like smallpox, the pleotropic nature of flaviviruses, their carriage by migratory wild birds capable of amplifying them, the difficulty of eradicating their arthropod vectors, in addition to other factors, many of our own making, that continue to extend vector habitats, will make them virtually impossible to eradicate by vaccination.

11. References

Allan, R.S., Smith, C.M., Belz, G.T., Van Lint, A.L., Wakim, L.M., Heath, W.R. & Carbone, F.R. (2003) Epidermal viral immunity induced by CD8alpha+ dendritic cells but not by Langerhans cells. *Science*, 301, 5641, pp. 1925-1928, ISSN 0036-8075.

Anderson, J.F. & Rahal, J.J. (2002) Efficacy of interferon alpha-2b and ribavirin against West Nile virus in vitro. *Emerg Infect Dis*, 8, 1, pp. 107-108, ISSN 1080-6059.

Andrews, D.M., Matthews, V.B., Sammels, L.M., Carrello, A.C. & Mcminn, P.C. (1999) The severity of murray valley encephalitis in mice is linked to neutrophil infiltration and inducible nitric oxide synthase activity in the central nervous system. *J Virol*, 73, 10, pp. 8781-8790, ISSN 0022-538X.

Appler, K.K., Brown, A.N., Stewart, B.S., Behr, M.J., Demarest, V.L., Wong, S.J. & Bernard, K.A. (2010) Persistence of West Nile virus in the central nervous system and periphery of mice. *PLoS One*, 5, 5, pp. e10649, ISSN 1932-6203.

Argall, K.G., Armati, P.J., King, N.J.C. & Douglas, M.W. (1991) The effects of West Nile virus on major histocompatibility complex class I and II molecule expression by Lewis rat Schwann cells in vitro. *J Neuroimmunol*, 35, 1-3, pp. 273-284, ISSN 0165-5728.

Arnold, S.J., Osvath, S.R., Hall, R.A., King, N.J.C. & Sedger, L.M. (2004) Regulation of antigen processing and presentation molecules in West Nile virus-infected human skin fibroblasts. *Virology*, 324, 2, pp. 286-296, ISSN 0042-6822.

Atrasheuskaya, A.V., Fredeking, T.M. & Ignatyev, G.M. (2003) Changes in immune parameters and their correction in human cases of tick-borne encephalitis. *Clinical and experimental immunology*, 131, 1, pp. 148-154, ISSN 0009-9104.

Bai, F., Kong, K.F., Dai, J., Qian, F., Zhang, L., Brown, C.R., Fikrig, E. & Montgomery, R.R. (2010) A paradoxical role for neutrophils in the pathogenesis of West Nile virus. *J Infect Dis*, 202, 12, pp. 1804-1812, ISSN 1537-6613.

Bakonyi, T., Hubálek, Z., Rudolf, I. & Nowotny, N. (2005) Novel flavivirus or new lineage of West Nile virus, central Europe. *Emerg Infect Dis*, 11, 2, pp. 225-231, ISSN 1080-6059.

Barrett, P.N., Schober-Bendixen, S. & Ehrlich, H.J. (2003) History of TBE vaccines. *Vaccine*, 21 Suppl 1, pp. S41-49, ISSN 0264-410X.

Ben-Nathan, D., Huitinga, I., Lustig, S., Van Rooijen, N. & Kobiler, D. (1996) West Nile virus neuroinvasion and encephalitis induced by macrophage depletion in mice. *Arch Virol*, 141, 3-4, pp. 459-469, ISSN 0304-8608.

Bian, G., Xu, Y., Lu, P., Xie, Y. & Xi, Z. (2010) The endosymbiotic bacterium Wolbachia induces resistance to dengue virus in Aedes aegypti. *PLoS Pathog*, 6, 4, pp. e1000833.

Boonnak, K., Dambach, K.M., Donofrio, G.C., Tassaneetrithep, B. & Marovich, M.A. (2011) Cell type specificity and host genetic polymorphisms influence antibody-dependent enhancement of dengue virus infection. *J Virol*, 85, 4, pp. 1671-1683, ISSN 1098-5514.

Brehin, A.C., Mouries, J., Frenkiel, M.P., Dadaglio, G., Despres, P., Lafon, M. & Couderc, T. (2008) Dynamics of immune cell recruitment during West Nile encephalitis and identification of a new CD19+B220-BST-2+ leukocyte population. *J Immunol*, 180, 10, pp. 6760-6767, ISSN 0022-1767.

Brien, J.D., Uhrlaub, J.L. & Nikolich-Zugich, J. (2008) West Nile virus-specific CD4 T cells exhibit direct antiviral cytokine secretion and cytotoxicity and are sufficient for antiviral protection. *J Immunol*, 181, 12, pp. 8568-8575, ISSN 1550-6606.

Burke, S.A., Wen, L. & King, N.J.C. (2004) Routes of inoculation and the immune response to a resolving genital flavivirus infection in a novel murine model. *Immunol Cell Biol*, 82, 2, pp. 174-183, ISSN 0818-9641.

Byrne, S.N., Halliday, G.M., Johnston, L.J. & King, N.J.C. (2001) Interleukin-1beta but not tumor necrosis factor is involved in West Nile virus-induced Langerhans cell migration from the skin in C57BL/6 mice. *J Invest Derm*, 117, 3, pp. 702-709, ISSN 0022-202X.

Cardosa, M.J., Gordon, S., Hirsch, S., Springer, T.A. & Porterfield, J.S. (1986) Interaction of West Nile virus with primary murine macrophages: role of cell activation and receptors for antibody and complement. *J Virol*, 57, 3, pp. 952-959, ISSN 0022-538X.

Cdc (2010) West Nile Virus Activity – United States, 2009. *Morbidity and Mortality Weekly Report*, 59, 25, ISSN 0149-2195.

Cheeran, M.C., Hu, S., Sheng, W.S., Rashid, A., Peterson, P.K. & Lokensgard, J.R. (2005) Differential responses of human brain cells to West Nile virus infection. *J Neurovirol*, 11, 6, pp. 512-524, ISSN 1355-0284.

Chen, C.J., Ou, Y.C., Lin, S.Y., Raung, S.L., Liao, S.L., Lai, C.Y., Chen, S.Y. & Chen, J.H. (2010) Glial activation involvement in neuronal death by Japanese encephalitis virus infection. *J Gen Virol*, 91, Pt 4, pp. 1028-1037, ISSN 1465-2099.

Cheng, Y., King, N.J.C. & Kesson, A.M. (2004a) Major histocompatibility complex class I (MHC-I) induction by West Nile virus: involvement of 2 signaling pathways in MHC-I up-regulation. *J Infect Dis*, 189, 4, pp. 658-668, ISSN 0022-1899.

Cheng, Y., King, N.J.C. & Kesson, A.M. (2004b) The role of tumor necrosis factor in modulating responses of murine embryo fibroblasts by flavivirus, West Nile. *Virology*, 329, 2, pp. 361-370, ISSN 0042-6822.

Chowers, M.Y., Lang, R., Nassar, F., Ben-David, D., Giladi, M., Rubinshtein, E., Itzhaki, A., Mishal, J., Siegman-Igra, Y., Kitzes, R., Pick, N., Landau, Z., Wolf, D., Bin, H., Mendelson, E., Pitlik, S.D. & Weinberger, M. (2001) Clinical characteristics of the West Nile fever outbreak, Israel, 2000. *Emerg Infect Dis*, 7, 4, pp. 675-678, ISSN 1080-6059.

Chu, J.J. & Ng, M.L. (2004) Infectious entry of West Nile virus occurs through a clathrin-mediated endocytic pathway. *J Virol*, 78, 19, pp. 10543-10555, ISSN 0022-538X.

Daffis, S., Samuel, M.A., Suthar, M.S., Gale, M., Jr. & Diamond, M.S. (2008) Toll-like receptor 3 has a protective role against West Nile virus infection. *J Virol*, 82, 21, pp. 10349-10358, ISSN 1098-5514.

Davison, A.M. & King, N.J.C. (2011) Accelerated dendritic cell differentiation from migrating Ly6C(lo) bone marrow monocytes in early dermal West Nile virus infection. *J Immunol*, 186, 4, pp. 2382-2396, ISSN 1550-6606.

Diamond, M.S., Shrestha, B., Marri, A., Mahan, D. & Engle, M. (2003) B cells and antibody play critical roles in the immediate defense of disseminated infection by West Nile encephalitis virus. *J Virol*, 77, 4, pp. 2578-2586, ISSN 0022-538X.

Engle, M.J. & Diamond, M.S. (2003) Antibody prophylaxis and therapy against West Nile virus infection in wild-type and immunodeficient mice. *J Virol*, 77, 24, pp. 12941-12949, ISSN 0022-538X.

Fenyk-Melody, J.E., Garrison, A.E., Brunnert, S.R., Weidner, J.R., Shen, F., Shelton, B.A. & Mudgett, J.S. (1998) Experimental autoimmune encephalomyelitis is exacerbated in mice lacking the NOS2 gene. *J Immunol*, 160, 6, pp. 2940-2946, ISSN 0022-1767.

Ford, A.L., Foulcher, E., Lemckert, F.A. & Sedgwick, J.D. (1996) Microglia induce CD4 T lymphocyte final effector function and death. *J Exp Med*, 184, 5, pp. 1737-1745, ISSN 0022-1007.

Geissmann, F., Jung, S. & Littman, D.R. (2003) Blood monocytes consist of two principal subsets with distinct migratory properties. *Immunity*, 19, 1, pp. 71-82, ISSN 1074-7613.

German, A.C., Myint, K.S., Mai, N.T., Pomeroy, I., Phu, N.H., Tzartos, J., Winter, P., Collett, J., Farrar, J., Barrett, A., Kipar, A., Esiri, M.M. & Solomon, T. (2006) A preliminary neuropathological study of Japanese encephalitis in humans and a mouse model. *Trans R Soc Trop Med Hyg*, 100, 12, pp. 1135-1145, ISSN 0035-9203.

Getts, D.R., Matsumoto, I., Muller, M., Getts, M.T., Radford, J., Shrestha, B., Campbell, I.L. & King, N.J.C. (2007) Role of IFN-gamma in an experimental murine model of West Nile virus-induced seizures. *J Neurochem*, 103, 3, pp. 1019-1030, ISSN 0022-3042.

Getts, D.R., Terry, R.L., Getts, M.T., Muller, M., Rana, S., Shrestha, B., Radford, J., Van Rooijen, N., Campbell, I.L. & King, N.J.C. (2008) Ly6c+ "inflammatory monocytes" are microglial precursors recruited in a pathogenic manner in West Nile virus encephalitis. *J Exp Med*, 205, 10, pp. 2319-2337, ISSN 1540-9538.

Ghoshal, A., Das, S., Ghosh, S., Mishra, M.K., Sharma, V., Koli, P., Sen, E. & Basu, A. (2007) Proinflammatory mediators released by activated microglia induces neuronal death in Japanese encephalitis. *Glia*, 55, 5, pp. 483-496, ISSN 0894-1491.

Ginhoux, F., Tacke, F., Angeli, V., Bogunovic, M., Loubeau, M., Dai, X.M., Stanley, E.R., Randolph, G.J. & Merad, M. (2006) Langerhans cells arise from monocytes in vivo. *Nat Immunol*, 7, 3, pp. 265-273, ISSN 1529-2908.

Giordano, D., Li, C., Suthar, M.S., Draves, K.E., Ma, D.Y., Gale, M., Jr. & Clark, E.A. (2010) Nitric oxide controls an inflammatory-like Ly6ChiPDCA1+ DC subset that regulates Th1 immune responses. *J Leukoc Biol*, ISSN 1938-3673.

Glass, W.G., Lim, J.K., Cholera, R., Pletnev, A.G., Gao, J.L. & Murphy, P.M. (2005) Chemokine receptor CCR5 promotes leukocyte trafficking to the brain and survival in West Nile virus infection. *J Exp Med*, 202, 8, pp. 1087-1098, ISSN 0022-1007.

Gould, E.A. & Higgs, S. (2009) Impact of climate change and other factors on emerging arbovirus diseases. *Trans R Soc Trop Med Hyg*, 103, 2, pp. 109-121, ISSN 1878-3503.

Gould, L.H., Sui, J., Foellmer, H., Oliphant, T., Wang, T., Ledizet, M., Murakami, A., Noonan, K., Lambeth, C., Kar, K., Anderson, J.F., De Silva, A.M., Diamond, M.S., Koski, R.A., Marasco, W.A. & Fikrig, E. (2005) Protective and therapeutic capacity of human single-chain Fv-Fc fusion proteins against West Nile virus. *J Virol*, 79, 23, pp. 14606-14613, ISSN 0022-538X.

Guabiraba, R., Marques, R.E., Besnard, A.G., Fagundes, C.T., Souza, D.G., Ryffel, B. & Teixeira, M.M. (2010) Role of the chemokine receptors CCR1, CCR2 and CCR4 in the pathogenesis of experimental dengue infection in mice. *PLoS One*, 5, 12, pp. e15680, ISSN 1932-6203.

Guarner, J., Shieh, W.J., Hunter, S., Paddock, C.D., Morken, T., Campbell, G.L., Marfin, A.A. & Zaki, S.R. (2004) Clinicopathologic study and laboratory diagnosis of 23 cases with West Nile virus encephalomyelitis. *Hum Pathol*, 35, 8, pp. 983-990, ISSN 0046-8177.

Halstead, S.B. & O'Rourke, E.J. (1977) Dengue viruses and mononuclear phagocytes. I. Infection enhancement by non-neutralizing antibody. *J Exp Med*, 146, 1, pp. 201-217.

Hayes, C.G. (2001) West Nile virus: Uganda, 1937, to New York City, 1999. *Ann N Y Acad Sci*, 951, pp. 25-37, ISSN 0077-8923.

Hayes, E.B., Sejvar, J.J., Zaki, S.R., Lanciotti, R.S., Bode, A.V. & Campbell, G.L. (2005) Virology, pathology, and clinical manifestations of West Nile virus disease. *Emerg Infect Dis*, 11, 8, pp. 1174-1179, ISSN 1080-6059.

He, X., Ren, J., Xu, F., Ferguson, M.R. & Li, G. (2009) Localization of West Nile Virus in monkey brain: double staining antigens immunohistochemically of neurons, neuroglia cells and West Nile Virus. *Int J Clin Exp Pathol*, 3, 2, pp. 156-161, ISSN 1936-2625.

Heinz, F.X., Holzmann, H., Essl, A. & Kundi, M. (2007) Field effectiveness of vaccination against tick-borne encephalitis. *Vaccine*, 25, 43, pp. 7559-7567, ISSN 0264-410X.

Hildner, K., Edelson, B.T., Purtha, W.E., Diamond, M., Matsushita, H., Kohyama, M., Calderon, B., Schraml, B.U., Unanue, E.R., Diamond, M.S., Schreiber, R.D., Murphy, T.L. & Murphy, K.M. (2008) Batf3 deficiency reveals a critical role for CD8alpha+ dendritic cells in cytotoxic T cell immunity. *Science*, 322, 5904, pp. 1097-1100, ISSN 0036-8075.

Hunsperger, E.A. & Roehrig, J.T. (2005) Characterization of West Nile viral replication and maturation in peripheral neurons in culture. *J Neurovirol*, 11, 1, pp. 11-22, ISSN 1355-0284.

Hunsperger, E.A. & Roehrig, J.T. (2006) Temporal analyses of the neuropathogenesis of a West Nile virus infection in mice. *J Neurovirol*, 12, 2, pp. 129-139, ISSN 1355-0284.

Hunsperger, E.A. & Roehrig, J.T. (2009) Nocodazole delays viral entry into the brain following footpad inoculation with West Nile virus in mice. *J Neurovirol*, 15, 3, pp. 211-218, ISSN 1538-2443.

Iwamoto, M., Jernigan, D.B., Guasch, A., Trepka, M.J., Blackmore, C.G., Hellinger, W.C., Pham, S.M., Zaki, S., Lanciotti, R.S., Lance-Parker, S.E., Diazgranados, C.A., Winquist, A.G., Perlino, C.A., Wiersma, S., Hillyer, K.L., Goodman, J.L., Marfin, A.A., Chamberland, M.E. & Petersen, L.R. (2003) Transmission of West Nile virus from an organ donor to four transplant recipients. *N Engl J Med*, 348, 22, pp. 2196-2203, ISSN 1533-4406.

Jana, M., Liu, X., Koka, S., Ghosh, S., Petro, T.M. & Pahan, K. (2001) Ligation of CD40 stimulates the induction of nitric-oxide synthase in microglial cells. *J Biol Chem*, 276, 48, pp. 44527-44533, ISSN 0021-9258.

Jiang, D., Weidner, J.M., Qing, M., Pan, X.B., Guo, H., Xu, C., Zhang, X., Birk, A., Chang, J., Shi, P.Y., Block, T.M. & Guo, J.T. (2010) Identification of five interferon-induced cellular proteins that inhibit west nile virus and dengue virus infections. *J Virol*, 84, 16, pp. 8332-8341, ISSN 1098-5514.

Johnston, L.J., Halliday, G.M. & King, N.J.C. (1996) Phenotypic changes in Langerhans' cells after infection with arboviruses: a role in the immune response to epidermally acquired viral infection? *J Virol*, 70, 7, pp. 4761-4766, ISSN 0022-538X.

Johnston, L.J., Halliday, G.M. & King, N.J.C. (2000) Langerhans cells migrate to local lymph nodes following cutaneous infection with an arbovirus. *J Invest Dermatol*, 114, 3, pp. 560-568, ISSN 0022-202X.

Jordan, I., Briese, T., Fischer, N., Lau, J.Y. & Lipkin, W.I. (2000) Ribavirin inhibits West Nile virus replication and cytopathic effect in neural cells. *J Infect Dis*, 182, 4, pp. 1214-1217, ISSN 0022-1899.

Kelley, T.W., Prayson, R.A., Ruiz, A.I., Isada, C.M. & Gordon, S.M. (2003) The neuropathology of West Nile virus meningoencephalitis. A report of two cases and review of the literature. *Am J Clin Pathol*, 119, 5, pp. 749-753, ISSN 0002-9173.

Kesson, A.M. & King, N.J.C. (2001) Transcriptional regulation of major histocompatibility complex class I by flavivirus West Nile is dependent on NF-kappaB activation. *J Infect Dis*, 184, 8, pp. 947-954, ISSN 0022-1899.

King, N.J.C., Davison, A., Getts, D.R., Lu, D.P., Getts, M.T., Yeung, A., Peterson, J.K. & Kesson, A.M. (2009) Enhanced antigen processing or immune evasion? West Nile virus and the induction of immune recognition molecules. In: *West Nile Encephalitis Virus Infection: Viral Pathogenesis and the Host Immune Response* Diamond, M.S. (Ed.) pp. 309-339, Springer, sbn 978-0-387-79839-4, New York.

King, N.J.C., Getts, D.R., Getts, M.T., Rana, S., Shrestha, B. & Kesson, A.M. (2007) Immunopathology of flavivirus infections. *Immunol Cell Biol*, 85, 1, pp. 33-42, ISSN 0818-9641.

King, N.J.C. & Kesson, A.M. (1988) Interferon-independent increases in class I major histocompatibility complex antigen expression follow flavivirus infection. *J Gen Virol*, 69 (Pt 10), pp. 2535-2543, ISSN 0022-1317.

King, N.J.C. & Kesson, A.M. (2003) Interaction of flaviviruses with cells of the vertebrate host and decoy of the immune response. *Immunol Cell Biol*, 81, 3, pp. 207-216, ISSN 0818-9641.

King, N.J.C., Shrestha, B. & Kesson, A.M. (2003) Immune modulation by flaviviruses. In: *The Flaviviruses: Pathogenesis and Immunity.* Monath, T. & Chambers, T. (Eds.) pp. 121-155, Elsevier Academic Press, sbn 0-12-039860-5.

Kissenpfennig, A., Henri, S., Dubois, B., Laplace-Builhé, C., Perrin, P., Romani, N., Tripp, C.H., Douillard, P., Leserman, L., Kaiserlian, D., Saeland, S., Davoust, J. & Malissen, B. (2005) Dynamics and function of Langerhans cells in vivo: dermal dendritic cells colonize lymph node areas distinct from slower migrating Langerhans cells. *Immunity*, 22, 5, pp. 643-654, ISSN 1074-7613.

Klein, R.S., Lin, E., Zhang, B., Luster, A.D., Tollett, J., Samuel, M.A., Engle, M. & Diamond, M.S. (2005) Neuronal CXCL10 directs CD8+ T-cell recruitment and control of West Nile virus encephalitis. *J Virol*, 79, 17, pp. 11457-11466, ISSN 0022-538X.

Kong, K.F., Delroux, K., Wang, X., Qian, F., Arjona, A., Malawista, S.E., Fikrig, E. & Montgomery, R.R. (2008) Dysregulation of TLR3 impairs the innate immune response to West Nile virus in the elderly. *J Virol*, 82, 15, pp. 7613-7623, ISSN 1098-5514.

Kortekaas, J., Ergonul, O. & Moormann, R.J. (2010) Interventions against West Nile virus, Rift Valley fever virus, and Crimean-Congo hemorrhagic fever virus: where are we? *Vector Borne Zoonotic Dis*, 10, 7, pp. 709-718, ISSN 1557-7759.

Lanciotti, R.S., Roehrig, J.T., Deubel, V., Smith, J., Parker, M., Steele, K., Crise, B., Volpe, K.E., Crabtree, M.B., Scherret, J.H., Hall, R.A., Mackenzie, J.S., Cropp, C.B., Panigrahy, B., Ostlund, E., Schmitt, B., Malkinson, M., Banet, C., Weissman, J.,

Komar, N., Savage, H.M., Stone, W., Mcnamara, T. & Gubler, D.J. (1999) Origin of the West Nile virus responsible for an outbreak of encephalitis in the northeastern United States. *Science*, 286, 5448, pp. 2333-2337, ISSN 0036-8075.

Landsman, L., Varol, C. & Jung, S. (2007) Distinct differentiation potential of blood monocyte subsets in the lung. *J Immunol*, 178, 4, pp. 2000-2007, ISSN 0022-1767.

Leon, B., Lopez-Bravo, M. & Ardavin, C. (2007) Monocyte-derived dendritic cells formed at the infection site control the induction of protective T helper 1 responses against Leishmania. *Immunity*, 26, 4, pp. 519-531, ISSN 1074-7613.

Leon, B., Martinez Del Hoyo, G., Parrillas, V., Vargas, H.H., Sanchez-Mateos, P., Longo, N., Lopez-Bravo, M. & Ardavin, C. (2004) Dendritic cell differentiation potential of mouse monocytes: monocytes represent immediate precursors of CD8- and CD8+ splenic dendritic cells. *Blood*, 103, 7, pp. 2668-2676, ISSN 0006-4971.

Li, L., Barrett, A.D. & Beasley, D.W. (2005) Differential expression of domain III neutralizing epitopes on the envelope proteins of West Nile virus strains. *Virology*, 335, 1, pp. 99-105, ISSN 0042-6822.

Lim, J.K., Obara, C.J., Rivollier, A., Pletnev, A.G., Kelsall, B.L. & Murphy, P.M. (2011) Chemokine receptor Ccr2 is critical for monocyte accumulation and survival in West Nile virus encephalitis. *J Immunol*, 186, 1, pp. 471-478, ISSN 1550-6606.

Lindsey, N.P., Hayes, E.B., Staples, J.E. & Fischer, M. (2009) West Nile virus disease in children, United States, 1999-2007. *Pediatrics*, 123, 6, pp. e1084-1089, ISSN 1098-4275.

Liu, T.H., Liang, L.C., Wang, C.C., Liu, H.C. & Chen, W.J. (2008) The blood-brain barrier in the cerebrum is the initial site for the Japanese encephalitis virus entering the central nervous system. *J Neurovirol*, 14, 6, pp. 514-521, ISSN 1538-2443.

Liu, X., Yu, Y., Li, M., Liang, G., Wang, H., Jia, L. & Dong, G. (2011) Study on the protective efficacy of SA14-14-2 attenuated Japanese encephalitis against different JE virus isolates circulating in China. *Vaccine*, 29, 11, pp. 2127-2130, ISSN 0264-410X.

Liu, Y., King, N.J.C., Kesson, A.M., Blanden, R.V. & Mullbacher, A. (1989) Flavivirus infection up-regulates the expression of class I and class II major histocompatibility antigens on and enhances T cell recognition of astrocytes in vitro. *J Neuroimmunol*, 21, 2-3, pp. 157-168, ISSN 0165-5728.

Lobigs, M., Mullbacher, A. & Regner, M. (2003) MHC class I up-regulation by flaviviruses: Immune interaction with unknown advantage to host or pathogen. *Immunol Cell Biol*, 81, 3, pp. 217-223, ISSN 0818-9641.

Maximova, O.A., Faucette, L.J., Ward, J.M., Murphy, B.R. & Pletnev, A.G. (2009) Cellular inflammatory response to flaviviruses in the central nervous system of a primate host. *J Histochem Cytochem*, 57, 10, pp. 973-989, ISSN 0022-1554.

Mcmeniman, C.J., Lane, R.V., Cass, B.N., Fong, A.W.C., Sidhu, M., Wang, Y.-F. & O'neill, S.L. (2009) Stable introduction of a life-shortening Wolbachia infection into the mosquito Aedes aegypti. *Science*, 323, 5910, pp. 141-144, ISSN 0036-8075.

Merad, M., Manz, M.G., Karsunky, H., Wagers, A., Peters, W., Charo, I., Weissman, I.L., Cyster, J.G. & Engleman, E.G. (2002) Langerhans cells renew in the skin throughout life under steady-state conditions. *Nat Immunol*, 3, 12, pp. 1135-1141, ISSN 1529-2908.

Monath, T.P. (2010) Suspected yellow fever vaccine-associated viscerotropic adverse events (1973 and 1978), United States. *Am J Trop Med Hyg*, 82, 5, pp. 919-921, ISSN 0002-9637.

Morrey, J.D., Olsen, A.L., Siddharthan, V., Motter, N.E., Wang, H., Taro, B.S., Chen, D., Ruffner, D. & Hall, J.O. (2008) Increased blood-brain barrier permeability is not a primary determinant for lethality of West Nile virus infection in rodents. *J Gen Virol*, 89, Pt 2, pp. 467-473, ISSN 0022-1317.

Morrey, J.D., Siddharthan, V., Olsen, A.L., Roper, G.Y., Wang, H., Baldwin, T.J., Koenig, S., Johnson, S., Nordstrom, J.L. & Diamond, M.S. (2006) Humanized Monoclonal Antibody against West Nile Virus Envelope Protein Administered after Neuronal Infection Protects against Lethal Encephalitis in Hamsters *J Infect Dis*, 194, 9, pp. 1300-1308, ISSN 0022-1899.

Morrey, J.D., Siddharthan, V., Olsen, A.L., Wang, H., Julander, J.G., Hall, J.O., Li, H., Nordstrom, J.L., Koenig, S., Johnson, S. & Diamond, M.S. (2007) Defining limits of treatment with humanized neutralizing monoclonal antibody for West Nile virus neurological infection in a hamster model. *Antimicrob Agents Chemother*, 51, 7, pp. 2396-2402, ISSN 0066-4804.

Muller, M., Carter, S.L., Hofer, M.J., Manders, P., Getts, D.R., Getts, M.T., Dreykluft, A., Lu, B., Gerard, C., King, N.J.C. & Campbell, I.L. (2007) CXCR3 signaling reduces the severity of experimental autoimmune encephalomyelitis by controlling the parenchymal distribution of effector and regulatory T cells in the central nervous system. *J Immunol*, 179, 5, pp. 2774-2786, ISSN 0022-1767.

Oliphant, T., Engle, M., Nybakken, G.E., Doane, C., Johnson, S., Huang, L., Gorlatov, S., Mehlhop, E., Marri, A., Chung, K.M., Ebel, G.D., Kramer, L.D., Fremont, D.H. & Diamond, M.S. (2005) Development of a humanized monoclonal antibody with therapeutic potential against West Nile virus. *Nat Med*, 11, 5, pp. 522-530, ISSN 1078-8956.

Olson, J.K. & Miller, S.D. (2004) Microglia initiate central nervous system innate and adaptive immune responses through multiple TLRs. *J Immunol*, 173, 6, pp. 3916-3924, ISSN 0022-1767.

Petzold, A., Groves, M., Leis, A.A., Scaravilli, F. & Stokic, D.S. (2010) Neuronal and glial cerebrospinal fluid protein biomarkers are elevated after West Nile virus infection. *Muscle Nerve*, 41, 1, pp. 42-49, ISSN 1097-4598.

Poidinger, M., Hall, R.A. & Mackenzie, J.S. (1996) Molecular characterization of the Japanese encephalitis serocomplex of the flavivirus genus. *Virology*, 218, 2, pp. 417-421, ISSN 0042-6822.

Purtha, W.E., Myers, N., Mitaksov, V., Sitati, E., Connolly, J., Fremont, D.H., Hansen, T.H. & Diamond, M.S. (2007) Antigen-specific cytotoxic T lymphocytes protect against lethal West Nile virus encephalitis. *Eur J Immunol*, 37, 7, pp. 1845-1854, ISSN 0014-2980.

Rios, M., Zhang, M.J., Grinev, A., Srinivasan, K., Daniel, S., Wood, O., Hewlett, I.K. & Dayton, A.I. (2006) Monocytes-macrophages are a potential target in human infection with West Nile virus through blood transfusion. *Transfusion*, 46, 4, pp. 659-667, ISSN 0041-1132.

Růžek, D., Salát, J., Palus, M., Gritsun, T.S., Gould, E.A., Dykova, I., Skallova, A., Jelinek, J., Kopecký, J. & Grubhoffer, L. (2009) CD8+ T-cells mediate immunopathology in tick-borne encephalitis. *Virology*, 384, 1, pp. 1-6, ISSN 1096-0341.

Růžek, D., Salát, J., Singh, S.K. & Kopecký, J. (2011) Breakdown of the Blood-Brain Barrier during Tick-Borne Encephalitis in Mice Is Not Dependent on CD8 T-Cells. *PLoS ONE*, 6, 5, pp. e20472, ISSN: 1932-6203

Sampson, B.A., Ambrosi, C., Charlot, A., Reiber, K., Veress, J.F. & Armbrustmacher, V. (2000) The pathology of human West Nile Virus infection. *Hum Pathol*, 31, 5, pp. 527-531, ISSN 0046-8177.

Samuel, M.A. & Diamond, M.S. (2005) Alpha/beta interferon protects against lethal West Nile virus infection by restricting cellular tropism and enhancing neuronal survival. *J Virol*, 79, 21, pp. 13350-13361, ISSN 0022-538X.

Samuel, M.A. & Diamond, M.S. (2009) West Nile Virus Infection of the Central Nervous System. In: *West Nile Encephalitis Virus Infection: Viral Pathogenesis and the Host Immune Response.* Diamond, M.S. (Ed.) pp. 474, Springer, sbn 978-0-387-79839-4, New York.

Samuel, M.A., Wang, H., Siddharthan, V., Morrey, J.D. & Diamond, M.S. (2007) Axonal transport mediates West Nile virus entry into the central nervous system and induces acute flaccid paralysis. *Proc Natl Acad Sci U S A*, 104, 43, pp. 17140-17145, ISSN 0027-8424.

Sanchez, M.D., Pierson, T.C., Mcallister, D., Hanna, S.L., Puffer, B.A., Valentine, L.E., Murtadha, M.M., Hoxie, J.A. & Doms, R.W. (2005) Characterization of neutralizing antibodies to West Nile virus. *Virology*, 336, 1, pp. 70-82, ISSN 0042-6822.

Schneider, B.S., Mcgee, C.E., Jordan, J.M., Stevenson, H.L., Soong, L. & Higgs, S. (2007) Prior exposure to uninfected mosquitoes enhances mortality in naturally-transmitted West Nile virus infection. *PLoS One*, 2, 11, pp. e1171, ISSN 1932-6203.

Schneider, B.S., Soong, L., Coffey, L.L., Stevenson, H.L., Mcgee, C.E. & Higgs, S. (2010) Aedes aegypti saliva alters leukocyte recruitment and cytokine signaling by antigen-presenting cells during West Nile virus infection. *PLoS One*, 5, 7, pp. e11704, ISSN 1932-6203.

Schoneboom, B.A., Lee, J.S. & Grieder, F.B. (2000) Early expression of IFN-alpha/beta and iNOS in the brains of Venezuelan equine encephalitis virus-infected mice. *J Interferon Cytokine Res*, 20, 2, pp. 205-215, ISSN 1079-9907.

Sejvar, J.J., Haddad, M.B., Tierney, B.C., Campbell, G.L., Marfin, A.A., Van Gerpen, J.A., Fleischauer, A., Leis, A.A., Stokic, D.S. & Petersen, L.R. (2003) Neurologic manifestations and outcome of West Nile virus infection. *JAMA*, 290, 4, pp. 511-515, ISSN 1538-3598.

Serbina, N.V. & Pamer, E.G. (2006) Monocyte emigration from bone marrow during bacterial infection requires signals mediated by chemokine receptor CCR2. *Nat Immunol*, 7, 3, pp. 311-317, ISSN 1529-2908.

Shen, J., Devery, J.M. & King, N.J.C. (1995a) Adherence status regulates the primary cellular activation responses to the flavivirus West Nile. *Immunology*, 84, 2, pp. 254-264, ISSN 1365-2567.

Shen, J., Devery, J.M. & King, N.J.C. (1995b) Early induction of interferon-independent virus-specific ICAM-1 (CD54) expression by flavivirus in quiescent but not proliferating fibroblasts--implications for virus-host interactions. *Virology*, 208, 2, pp. 437-449, ISSN 0042-6822.

Shen, J., T-To, S.S., Schrieber, L. & King, N.J.C. (1997) Early E-selectin, VCAM-1, ICAM-1, and late major histocompatibility complex antigen induction on human endothelial cells by flavivirus and comodulation of adhesion molecule expression by immune cytokines. *J Virol*, 71, 12, pp. 9323-9332, ISSN 0022-538X.

Shrestha, B., Gottlieb, D. & Diamond, M.S. (2003) Infection and injury of neurons by West Nile encephalitis virus. *J Virol*, 77, 24, pp. 13203-13213, ISSN 0022-538X.

Shrestha, B., Zhang, B., Purtha, W.E., Klein, R.S. & Diamond, M.S. (2008) Tumor necrosis factor alpha protects against lethal West Nile virus infection by promoting trafficking of mononuclear leukocytes into the central nervous system. *J Virol*, 82, 18, pp. 8956-8964, ISSN 1098-5514.

Smith, H.L., Monath, T.P., Pazoles, P., Rothman, A.L., Casey, D.M., Terajima, M., Ennis, F.A., Guirakhoo, F. & Green, S. (2010) Development of antigen-specific memory CD8+ T cells following live-attenuated chimeric West Nile virus vaccination. *J Infect Dis*, 203, 4, pp. 513-522, ISSN 1537-6613.

Smithburn, K.C., Hughes, T.P., Burke, A.W. & Paul, J.H. (1940) A Neurotropic virus isolated from the blood of a native of Uganda. *Am J Trop Med Hyg*, 20, pp. 471-492, ISSN 0002-9637.

Steele, K.E., Linn, M.J., Schoepp, R.J., Komar, N., Geisbert, T.W., Manduca, R.M., Calle, P.P., Raphael, B.L., Clippinger, T.L., Larsen, T., Smith, J., Lanciotti, R.S., Panella, N.A. & Mcnamara, T.S. (2000) Pathology of fatal West Nile virus infections in native and exotic birds during the 1999 outbreak in New York City, New York. *Vet Pathol*, 37, 3, pp. 208-224, ISSN 0300-9858.

Steinman, R.M. (1991) The dendritic cell system and its role in immunogenicity. *Annu Rev Immunol*, 9, pp. 271-296, ISSN 0732-0582.

Sunderkotter, C., Nikolic, T., Dillon, M.J., Van Rooijen, N., Stehling, M., Drevets, D.A. & Leenen, P.J. (2004) Subpopulations of mouse blood monocytes differ in maturation stage and inflammatory response. *J Immunol*, 172, 7, pp. 4410-4417, ISSN 0022-1767.

Tacke, F. & Randolph, G.J. (2006) Migratory fate and differentiation of blood monocyte subsets. *Immunobiology*, 211, 6-8, pp. 609-618, ISSN 0171-2985.

Throsby, M., Geuijen, C., Goudsmit, J., Bakker, A.Q., Korimbocus, J., Kramer, R.A., Clijsters-Van Der Horst, M., De Jong, M., Jongeneelen, M., Thijsse, S., Smit, R., Visser, T.J., Bijl, N., Marissen, W.E., Loeb, M., Kelvin, D.J., Preiser, W., Ter Meulen, J. & De Kruif, J. (2006) Isolation and characterization of human monoclonal antibodies from individuals infected with West Nile Virus. *J Virol*, 80, 14, pp. 6982-6992, ISSN 0022-538X.

Tobler, L.H., Cameron, M.J., Lanteri, M.C., Prince, H.E., Danesh, A., Persad, D., Lanciotti, R.S., Norris, P.J., Kelvin, D.J. & Busch, M.P. (2008) Interferon and interferon-induced chemokine expression is associated with control of acute viremia in West Nile virus-infected blood donors. *J Infect Dis*, 198, 7, pp. 979-983, ISSN 0022-1899.

Town, T., Bai, F., Wang, T., Kaplan, A.T., Qian, F., Montgomery, R.R., Anderson, J.F., Flavell, R.A. & Fikrig, E. (2009) Toll-like receptor 7 mitigates lethal West Nile encephalitis via interleukin 23-dependent immune cell infiltration and homing. *Immunity*, 30, 2, pp. 242-253, ISSN 1074-7613.

Tsou, C.L., Peters, W., Si, Y., Slaymaker, S., Aslanian, A.M., Weisberg, S.P., Mack, M. & Charo, I.F. (2007) Critical roles for CCR2 and MCP-3 in monocyte mobilization from bone marrow and recruitment to inflammatory sites. *J Clin Invest*, 117, 4, pp. 902-909, ISSN 0021-9738.

Vazquez, A., Sanchez-Seco, M.P., Ruiz, S., Molero, F., Hernandez, L., Moreno, J., Magallanes, A., Tejedor, C.G. & Tenorio, A. (2010) Putative new lineage of West Nile virus, Spain. *Emerg Infect Dis*, 16, 3, pp. 549-552, ISSN 1080-6059.

Venter, M., Human, S., Zaayman, D., Gerdes, G.H., Williams, J., Steyl, J., Leman, P.A., Paweska, J.T., Setzkorn, H., Rous, G., Murray, S., Parker, R., Donnellan, C. & Swanepoel, R. (2009) Lineage 2 west nile virus as cause of fatal neurologic disease in horses, South Africa. *Emerg Infect Dis*, 15, 6, pp. 877-884, ISSN 1080-6059.

Verma, S., Kumar, M., Gurjav, U., Lum, S. & Nerurkar, V.R. (2010) Reversal of West Nile virus-induced blood-brain barrier disruption and tight junction proteins degradation by matrix metalloproteinases inhibitor. *Virology*, 397, 1, pp. 130-138, ISSN 1096-0341.

Verma, S., Lo, Y., Chapagain, M., Lum, S., Kumar, M., Gurjav, U., Luo, H., Nakatsuka, A. & Nerurkar, V.R. (2009) West Nile virus infection modulates human brain microvascular endothelial cells tight junction proteins and cell adhesion molecules: Transmigration across the in vitro blood-brain barrier. *Virology*, 385, 2, pp. 425-433, ISSN 1096-0341.

Vogt, M.R., Moesker, B., Goudsmit, J., Jongeneelen, M., Austin, S.K., Oliphant, T., Nelson, S., Pierson, T.C., Wilschut, J., Throsby, M. & Diamond, M.S. (2009) Human monoclonal antibodies against West Nile virus induced by natural infection neutralize at a postattachment step. *J Virol*, 83, 13, pp. 6494-6507, ISSN 1098-5514.

Wacher, C., Muller, M., Hofer, M.J., Getts, D.R., Zabaras, R., Ousman, S.S., Terenzi, F., Sen, G.C., King, N.J.C. & Campbell, I.L. (2007) Coordinated regulation and widespread cellular expression of interferon-stimulated genes (ISG) ISG-49, ISG-54, and ISG-56 in the central nervous system after infection with distinct viruses. *J Virol*, 81, 2, pp. 860-871, ISSN 0022-538X.

Wang, T., Town, T., Alexopoulou, L., Anderson, J.F., Fikrig, E. & Flavell, R.A. (2004) Toll-like receptor 3 mediates West Nile virus entry into the brain causing lethal encephalitis. *Nat Med*, 10, 12, pp. 1366-1373, ISSN 1078-8956.

Wang, Y., Lobigs, M., Lee, E., Koskinen, A. & Mullbacher, A. (2006) CD8(+) T cell-mediated immune responses in West Nile virus (Sarafend strain) encephalitis are independent of gamma interferon. *J Gen Virol*, 87, Pt 12, pp. 3599-3609, ISSN 0022-1317.

Wang, Y., Lobigs, M., Lee, E. & Mullbacher, A. (2003) CD8+ T cells mediate recovery and immunopathology in West Nile virus encephalitis. *J Virol*, 77, 24, pp. 13323-13334, ISSN 0022-538X.

Weiss, D., Carr, D., Kellachan, J., Tan, C., Phillips, M., Bresnitz, E. & Layton, M. (2001) Clinical findings of West Nile virus infection in hospitalized patients, New York and New Jersey, 2000. *Emerg Infect Dis*, 7, 4, pp. 654-658, ISSN 1080-6059.

Xiao, S.Y., Guzman, H., Zhang, H., Travassos Da Rosa, A.P. & Tesh, R.B. (2001) West Nile virus infection in the golden hamster (Mesocricetus auratus): a model for West Nile encephalitis. *Emerg Infect Dis*, 7, 4, pp. 714-721, ISSN 1080-6059.

Yen, Y.T., Chen, H.C., Lin, Y.D., Shieh, C.C. & Wu-Hsieh, B.A. (2008) Enhancement by tumor necrosis factor alpha of dengue virus-induced endothelial cell production of reactive nitrogen and oxygen species is key to hemorrhage development. *J Virol*, 82, 24, pp. 12312-12324, ISSN 1098-5514.

Zhang, B., Chan, Y.K., Lu, B., Diamond, M.S. & Klein, R.S. (2008) CXCR3 mediates region-specific antiviral T cell trafficking within the central nervous system during West Nile virus encephalitis. *J Immunol*, 180, 4, pp. 2641-2649, ISSN 0022-1767.

Zhang, M., Daniel, S., Huang, Y., Chancey, C., Huang, Q., Lei, Y.F., Grinev, A., Mostowski, H., Rios, M. & Dayton, A. (2010) Anti-West Nile virus activity of in vitro expanded human primary natural killer cells. *BMC Immunol*, 11, pp. 3, ISSN 1471-2172.

Zhang, S., Vogt, M.R., Oliphant, T., Engle, M., Bovshik, E.I., Diamond, M.S. & Beasley, D.W. (2009) Development of resistance to passive therapy with a potently neutralizing humanized monoclonal antibody against West Nile virus. *J Infect Dis*, 200, 2, pp. 202-205, ISSN 0022-1899.

3

Immunity Versus Immunopathology in West Nile Virus Induced Encephalitis

Tian Wang[1,2,3,4,5], Thomas Welte[1], Vandana Saxena[1] and Guorui Xie[1]
[1]*Department of Microbiology & Immunology,*
[2]*Department of Pathology,*
[3]*Center for Biodefense and Emerging Infectious Diseases,*
[4]*Institute for Human Infections and Immunity,*
[5]*Sealy Center for Vaccine Development, The University of Texas Medical Branch, Galveston, TX*
USA

1. Introduction

West Nile virus (WNV), a mosquito-borne neurotropic pathogen, belongs to the family of Flaviviridae, the genus Flavivirus, a group of plus-sense, single-stranded RNA viruses (Anderson *et al.*, 1999; Lanciotti *et al.*, 1999). WNV genome is a single-stranded, positive-sense RNA molecule, approximately 11,000 nucleotides in length that is translated into a single polypeptide, which is co- and post-translationally processed into ten proteins - three structural proteins (envelope (E), membrane and nucleocapsid) and seven nonstructural (NS) proteins (NS1, NS2A, NS2B, NS3, NS4A, NS4B and NS5) (Anderson *et al.*, 1999; Lanciotti *et al.*, 1999). The virus was originally isolated in Africa, and later caused epidemics with mainly a febrile illness in humans in Europe, the Middle East, and parts of Asia. In 1999, a more virulent WNV strain was detected in New York City. Since then, it has rapidly spread throughout the continental United States, southern Canada, Mexico, Guatemala, the Caribbean and to several countries in South America. It has become a public health concern in North America over the past decade (Campbell *et al.*, 2002). The virus is maintained in an enzootic cycle that involves mosquitoes and birds. Human infection results primarily from mosquito bites; blood transfusion, organ transplantation, breast feeding and *in utero* or occupational exposure have all been associated with viral infection (2002a; 2002b; Alpert *et al.*, 2003; Charatan, 2002). Although most WNV infections in humans are asymptomatic, severe neurological disease (including encephalitis) and death have been observed with a higher frequency in the elderly and immunocompromised (Campbell *et al.*, 2002; Pletnev *et al.*, 2006). Recent evidence also suggests that WNV can persist for years in humans and animals convalescing from infection (Appler *et al.*, 2010; Murray *et al.*, 2010; Tesh *et al.*, 2005). Currently, licensed vaccines are not yet ready to use in humans. Treatment is currently nonspecific and supportive (Campbell *et al.*, 2002).

WNV has been studied in various animal models, including mice, hamsters, monkeys and horses (Davis *et al.*, 2001; Kramer & Bernard, 2001; Ratterree *et al.*, 2004; Xiao *et al.*,

2001). Following the initial subcutaneous or intraperitoneal infection in mice, WNV induces a systemic infection, invades the central nervous system (CNS) and causes death rapidly when encephalitis develops, usually within 1–2 weeks (Beasley *et al.*, 2002; Kramer & Bernard, 2001; Wang *et al.*, 2001b). The severity and symptoms of lethal infection observed in mice mimic the symptoms caused by WNV infection in humans. The murine model has been an effective *in vivo* experimental model to investigate viral pathogenesis and the host immunity in humans. Based on information obtained from studies on animal models, cell culture and patient samples, this review will be focused on discussion of the role of several important immune factors, including pathogen recognition receptor (PRR) - mediated signaling pathways, cytokines, monocytes/microglia, $\gamma\delta$ T cells, $CD4^+$ and $CD8^+$ $\alpha\beta$ T cells in protection and pathogenesis of WNV-induced encephalitis.

2. Innate Immunity to WNV infection

2.1 PRR signaling pathways

The key players of the innate immune surveillance are the sensor molecules known as PRRs which recognize specific pathogen associated molecular patterns (PAMPs) and trigger the signaling cascade ultimately leading to the production of type 1 interferon (IFN)s and pro-inflammatory cytokines. Three classes of PRRs have been implicated for viral PAMPs: toll-like receptors (TLRs), retinoid acid-inducible gene-I (RIG-I) -like receptors (RLRs), and nucleotide oligomerization domain (NOD) -like receptors (NLRs) (Iwasaki & Medzhitov, 2010; Wilkins & Gale, 2010). Of these, several TLRs and RLRs are involved in WNV recognition.

2.1.1 TLRs

TLRs, a family of thirteen mammalian homologues of *Drosophila* Toll that recognize PAMPs, play an essential role in the initiation of innate immunity (Qureshi & Medzhitov, 2003). Most TLR signaling pathways (except TLR3) utilize myeloid differentiation factor 88 (MyD88) as the primary adaptor (Akira & Hemmi, 2003). TLR stimulation culminates in the synthesis of antiviral cytokines, such as type 1 IFN and proinflammatory cytokines, which may directly suppress viral replication. WNV is a positive ssRNA virus that produces dsRNA in its life cycle (Samuel, 2002). TLR3 recognizes dsRNA and is expressed in dendritic cells (DCs) and several CNS cell types, including neurons, astrocytes, and microglia (Daffis *et al.*, 2008; Town *et al.*, 2006; Wang *et al.*, 2004). TLRs 7 and 8 are implicated in MyD88-dependent recognition of ssRNA and ssRNA-producing viruses. Depending on the virus dose (lethal versus sub-lethal), passage history of the virus (Vero cell-derived versus insect cell- derived) or routes of inoculation, TLRs 3 and 7 are known to play important roles in host immunity to WNV infection, either pathogenic or protective. Following a sub-lethal dose of insect cell derived WNV infection either intraperitoneally or subcutaneously, TLR3 provides a protective effect against WNV infection, partially by restricting replication in neurons (Daffis *et al.*, 2008). WNV NS1 protein plays a role in viral pathogenesis by counteracting TLR3 signaling in *in vitro* cell culture (Wilson *et al.*, 2008). During an intraperitoneal infection of WNV, TLR7-mediated signaling promoted IL-12/IL-23-dependent immune cell homing to infected target cells, thereby contributing to a vital host defense mechanism (Town *et al.*, 2009). MyD88-mediated signaling was reported to restrict

WNV by inhibiting replication in neurons and modulating expression of chemokines that regulate immune cell migration into the CNS (Szretter *et al.*, 2010).

TLR3 and TLR7 -mediated signaling can also be pathogenic to host during WNV infection. For example, upon a lethal dose of a mammalian cell-passaged WNV challenge in mice via the intraperitoneal route, TLR3-dependent proinflammatory cytokines , including tumor-necrosis factor (TNF)-α were involved in blood brain barrier (BBB) compromise, and neuronal injury (Wang *et al.*, 2004). In young human donors, binding of the glycosylated WNV envelope protein to the C-type lectin DC-specific intercellular adhesion molecule 3 (ICAM3) grabbing nonintegrin (DC-SIGN) leads to a reduction in the expression of TLR3 in macrophages via the signal transducer and activator of transcription 1 (STAT1)-mediated pathway. This signaling was shown to be impaired in the elderly, which led to higher levels of TLR3 and proinflammatory cytokines. Thus, the alteration of the innate immune response with aging may lead to higher TLR3 levels and increased BBB permeability, which may suggest a possible mechanism for the increased severity of WNV infection in older individuals (Kong *et al.*, 2008). Another example, WNV permissive Langerhans cells (LCs) could migrate from the skin to the lymph nodes upon a cutaneous infection, a process that might contribute to WNV dissemination in early viral infection (Byrne *et al.*, 2001; Johnston *et al.*, 2000). TLR7 recognition of WNV in skin epidermal keratinocytes induced IFN-α, interleukin-1β (IL-1β), IL-6 and IL-12 responses were shown to promote LC migration from the skin and WNV dissemination from the skin to other peripheral organs to initiate systemic infection. This effect might compromise its protective effect during a systemic infection (Welte *et al.*, 2009).

2.1.2 RLRs

RLRs, which include RIG-I and melanoma differentiation antigen 5 (MDA-5) recognize dsRNA during viral infection. RIG-I is involved in the initial recognition of WNV infection and controls early virus replication. The wild-type WNV NY99 strain is known to evade the activation of interferon regulatory factor 3 (IRF3) through RIG-I-dependent and -independent pathways without antagonizing host defense signaling (Fredericksen & Gale, 2006). MDA-5 is needed to amplify and maintain the antiviral signals (Fredericksen *et al.*, 2008). Both MDA5 and RIG-I work in concert to maintain the induction of the antiviral genes, while IFN-α functions to amplify and/or expand the response in an attempt to control viral replication. They are responsible for triggering downstream gene expression in response to WNV infection by signaling through an adaptor, interferon promoter stimulator-1 (IPS-1), which leads to activation of transcription of IRFs and NF-κB (Fredericksen *et al.*, 2008). IPS-1 also plays a role to modulate adaptive immune response by providing effective antibody response and by restricting the expansion of regulatory T cells, though the mechanism needs to be deciphered. (Suthar *et al.*, 2010). RIG-I signaling is regulated by multiple host factors, including ubiquitination, autophagy or the RNA helicase LGP2 (Gack *et al.*, 2007; Jounai *et al.*, 2007; Saito *et al.*, 2007). Caspases are a family of aspartic acid–specific cysteine-dependent proteases mainly involved in apoptotic and inflammatory signaling pathways. During WNV infection, Caspase 12 has been found to be required for an effective antiviral innate response by regulating the ubiquitination of RIG-I through the tripartite motif (TRIM) 25 mediated pathway (Wang *et al.*, 2010).

2.2 Cytokines

2.2.1 IFNs

Type 1 IFNs, including IFN-α and IFN-β participate in the control of viral infections (Katze *et al.*, 2002) and *in vitro,* can partially protect fetal murine spinal cord tissues, neuroblastoma cells and primate cells from WNV infection (Anderson & Rahal, 2002; Lucas *et al.*, 2003; Samuel & Diamond, 2005; Shahar *et al.*, 1990). IFN-α/β $R^{-/-}$ mice were much more susceptible to WNV infection than controls (Samuel & Diamond, 2005). The production of type 1 IFNs after flavivirus infection is primarily triggered by viral RNA through several distinct PRRs including the cell surface and endosomal RNA sensors TLR3 and TLR7, and the cytoplasmic RNA sensors, RIG-I and MDA-5 (2002c; Daffis *et al.*, 2008; Fredericksen & Gale, 2006; Fredericksen *et al.*, 2008; Town *et al.*, 2009; Wang *et al.*, 2004). In older donors, the production of type 1 IFNs was significantly lower in DCs, compared with younger donors, which might contribute to their higher susceptibility to WNV encephalitis (Qian *et al.*, 2011). Type 2 IFN, such as IFN-γ was produced by γδ T cells, nature killer (NK) cells and CD8 T cells, which provide protective immunity against lethal WNV encephalitis (Shrestha *et al.*, 2006b; Wang *et al.*, 2003a). Several NS proteins have been reported to be associated with evasion of host innate immune defenses (Laurent-Rolle *et al.*, 2010; Puig-Basagoiti *et al.*, 2007; Rossi *et al.*, 2007), including inhibiting IFN signaling by the blockage of STAT1 and STAT2 activation (Evans & Seeger, 2007; Liu *et al.*, 2005; Munoz-Jordan *et al.*, 2005).

2.2.2 Proinflammatory and regulatory cytokines

Proinflammatory cytokines, such as TNF-α, IFN-γ or IL-1β can act synergistically with WNV to modulate the expression of immune recognition molecules, including class I and II major histocompatibility complex (MHC) and various adhesion molecules on endothelial cell surface, leading to increased recognition by the virus-specific cytotoxic T cells (King *et al.*, 2003). Neuronal TNF-α expression could diminish chemokine (C-X-C motif) ligand 10 (CXCL10) -induced death in the CNS (Zhang *et al.*, 2010a).

TNF-α and IL-1β were up-regulated with replication of the E protein-glycosylated virus indicating a relation to the neuroinvasive phenotype of E protein-glycosylated WNV (Shirato *et al.*, 2006). Microarray analysis of genes upregulated by neurovirulent strains of WNV also revealed the involvement of TNF-α and other inflammatory cytokines in both mouse (Venter *et al.*, 2005) and human cells (Cheeran *et al.*, 2005) following WNV infection. Consistent with these findings, WNV replication induced TNF-α and macrophage migration inhibitory factor (MIF) responses during systemic infection were shown to modulate the BBB permeability, which in turn may enable viral entry into the brain and induce lethal encephalitis (Arjona *et al.*, 2007; Wang *et al.*, 2004). Regulatory cytokines, such as IL-10 is known to be involved in WNV pathogenesis (Bai *et al.*, 2009; Schneider *et al.*, 2007). WNV infection was diminished in IL-10-deficient mice, and this ultimately increased the survival rate (Bai *et al.*, 2009; Schneider *et al.*, 2007). Another regulatory cytokine, transforming growth factor (TGF)-β was found to suppress the protective γδ T cell subsets expansion during WNV infection (Welte T. & Wang T, unpublished data).

2.2.3 Chemokines

Chemokines and chemokine receptors mediate leukocyte trafficking during WNV infection. Cxcr2 is important for early neutrophil migration to the initial site of virus entry (Bai *et al.*,

2010). Ccr2 is critical for monocyte recruitment to the CNS, acting mainly by regulating monocytosis in the blood (Lim *et al.*, 2011). Cxcr3 and Cxcl 10 appear to control $CD4^+$ and $CD8^+$ T lymphocyte accumulation in the brain (Klein *et al.*, 2005; Zhang *et al.*, 2008). CNS expression of the chemokine receptor CCR5 and its ligand CCL5 was prominently up-regulated by WNV, and this was associated with the infiltration of $CD4^+$ and $CD8^+$ T cells, $NK1.1^+$ cells and macrophages expressing the receptor (Glass *et al.*, 2005). In humans, CCR5 may function normally to limit disease due to WNV infection (Lim *et al.*, 2010). It is suggested that CCR5 deficiency is a strong and consistent risk factor for symptomatic WNV infection in the United States (Lim *et al.*, 2008).

2.3 Cellular players: Monocytes /macrophages, microglia, neutrophils, NK cells and γδ T cells

2.3.1 Monocytes /macrophages and microglia

Initial studies suggest that macrophages are important in the non-specific immediate defense system of WNV infection. *In vivo* depletion of macrophages had an exacerbating effect on the course of the infection by an attenuated WNV strain, exhibited by higher and extended viremia and accelerated development of encephalitis and death (Ben-Nathan *et al.*, 1996).

Nevertheless, the susceptibility of monocytes / macrophages to productive WNV infection *in vitro* (Cardosa *et al.*, 1983) is also compatible with a potential role in initial WNV replication and propagation in humans (Rios *et al.*, 2006). In support of this notion, silencing early viral replication in macrophages in mice seems to effectively suppress WNV induced encephalitis (Ye *et al.*, 2003). In the CNS, microglia and macrophage-associated inflammation are involved in neuropathology (Wang *et al.*, 2004). An attenuated microglia activation in *Tlr3*$^{-/-}$ brains was reported to contribute to the resistance of these mice to WNV encephalitis during systemic infection (Wang *et al.*, 2004). Although there were more microglia in the CNS during WNV infection, few of them were proliferating, which suggests that the increased numbers in the CNS might be derived from a migratory precursor cell. Indeed, a recent report shows that $Ly6c^+Gr1^{hi}Ly6C^{hi}CCR2^+$ "inflammatory monocytes" are microglial precursors recruited to the CNS during WNV infection (Getts *et al.*, 2008). Consistent with these findings, CCL2-dependent inflammatory monocyte migration was reported to be critical for increases in microglia during WNV infection and may play a pathogenic role during WNV encephalitis (Lim *et al.*, 2011).

2.3.2 Neutrophils

Neutrophils are the most abundant type of leukocytes in humans, a key component of the innate immune response, and the first immune cells to be recruited to inflammatory foci. Following a lethal dose of WNV challenge, neutrophils greatly expand as the virus invades the brain (Brehin *et al.*, 2008). Neutrophils play a paradoxical role during WNV infection. Depletion of these cells can be either beneficial or harmful during WNV infection, depending on the timing of depletion. Neutrophil depletion 1 or 2 days following infection resulted in increased susceptibility whereas unexpectedly, if neutrophils were depleted 1 day prior to infection, the opposite results were observed: increased resistance (Bai *et al.*, 2010).

2.3.3 NK cells

NK cells are a crucial component of the host innate immune system with anti-viral properties. The role of NK cells in WNV infection is controversial. They are reported to be important to control WNV infection by recognition and elimination of WNV infected cells. Infection of mice with WNV was accompanied by temporary activation of NK cells (Vargin & Semenov, 1986). Interaction of NKp44 with the WNV E protein is an important step in triggering NK cell activation during infection (Hershkovitz *et al.*, 2009). A more recent study shows that co-culture of peripheral blood mononuclear cells with K562D2 stimulatory cells is an efficient technique to prepare large quantities of pure and active human NK cells, and these expanded NK cells inhibited WNV infection of Vero cells through both cytolytic and noncytolytic activities, which may imply a potential role of NK cells in combating WNV infection (Zhang *et al.*, 2010b). Nevertheless, antibody depletion of NK cells in mice did not show enhanced susceptibility to WNV encephalitis (Chung *et al.*, 2007; Shrestha & Diamond, 2004).

2.3.4 γδ T cells

In mice and humans, γδ T cells comprise a minority of the $CD3^+$ T cells in lymphoid tissue and blood but are well represented at epithelial and mucosal sites (Hayday, 2000). They can rapidly produce Th1, Th2, or Th-17 type cytokines dependent upon the type of antigen or the subtype of γδ T cells stimulated (Carding & Egan, 2002; Hayday, 2000; Hayes & Love, 2002; Roark *et al.*, 2007) and have unique features, including a lack of MHC restriction and the potential capacity to respond to antigens without a requirement for conventional antigen processing, which together suggest a role in innate immunity against pathogen infection (Wang *et al.*, 2001a). γδ T cells are important for early control of WNV dissemination (Wang *et al.*, 2003a). $TCR\delta^{-/-}$ mice, which are deficient in γδ T cells had elevated viral loads and greater dissemination of the pathogen to the CNS, more severe encephalitis and thereby were much more susceptible to WNV infection than wild-type controls. This protection relied partially on their IFN-γ producing capacity. Adoptive transfer of wild-type or $TCR\beta^{-/-}$ mice splenocytes to naïve $TCR\delta^{-/-}$ mice enhanced survival, whereas $TCR\beta^{-/-}$ IFN-$\gamma^{-/-}$ splenocoytes did not. Further, irradiated mice reconstituted with IFN-γ-deficient γδ T cells had significantly higher levels of viral loads in blood, and brains throughout the time course compared to mice reconstituted with IFN-γ-sufficient γδ T cells (Shrestha *et al.*, 2006b). γδ T cells are further divisible into functionally distinct subsets in human and mouse, which have direct and indirect effects on host immunity to pathogen infection (Bank *et al.*, 1986). Following WNV challenge, $V\gamma1^+$ cells, the major subpopulation, expanded significantly and were the main resource for IFN-γ. Mice depleted of $V\gamma1^+$ cells had an enhanced viremia and higher mortality to WNV encephalitis. A major risk factor for fatality of WNV infection in humans is aging (Hayes & Gubler, 2006; Wang & Fikrig, 2004). Aged mice were more susceptible to WNV infection than young mice. $V\gamma1^+$ T cells in aged mice displayed a slower and reduced response following WNV infection, which might partially contribute to the enhanced host susceptibility to viral encephalitis (Welte *et al.*, 2008). Human γδ T cells are also known to display numerical and functional alteration in the elderly (Argentati *et al.*, 2002; Cardillo *et al.*, 1993; Weerkamp *et al.*, 2005). Nevertheless, whether the dysfunction of γδ T cells of older individuals leads to their higher susceptibility to WNV encephalitis remains undefined.

$V\gamma4^+$ cells, another peripheral $\gamma\delta$ T cell subset, had a higher potential for producing TNF-α, a cytokine known to be involved in BBB compromise and WNV entry into the brain. Depletion of $V\gamma4^+$ cells reduced TNF-α level in the periphery, accompanied by a decreased viral load in the brain and a lower mortality to WN encephalitis (Welte *et al.*, 2008).

3. DCs, the linkage between innate and adaptive immunity

DCs, macrophages, and B cells are the antigen presenting cells (APCs) involved during WNV infection (Kulkarni *et al.*, 1991). DCs represent the most important APCs exhibiting the unique capacity to initiate primary T cell responses. In particular, during cutaneous WNV infection, the bone-marrow-derived epidermal DCs - LCs are important APCs in the skin – where the pathogen is naturally deposited during mosquito transmission of the virus (Byrne *et al.*, 2001; Johnston *et al.*, 2000). These cells migrate from the epidermis by an IL-1β-dependent pathway and accumulate in the local draining lymph nodes, thereby playing an important role in T-cell activation and proliferation (Byrne *et al.*, 2001). Interestingly, a recent report shows that mosquito saliva contains factors that could alter the antiviral signaling of APCs, including macrophages and DCs, which may explain the enhancement of WNV diseases during a natural infection (Schneider *et al.*, 2010). Upon microbial infection, DC maturation is an innate response that leads to adaptive immunity to foreign antigens (Bennett *et al.*, 1998; De Smedt *et al.*, 1996). Maturation of DCs results in the expression of high levels of MHC and co-stimulatory molecules such as CD40, CD80 and CD86 and is often associated with the secretion of IL-12 (Fujii *et al.*, 2004; Inaba *et al.*, 2000). WNV-induced $\gamma\delta$ T-cell activation plays an important role in promoting DC maturation, which further initiates $CD4^+$ T-cell priming. Splenic DCs of WNV-infected $TCR\delta^{-/-}$ mice displayed lower levels of CD40, CD80, CD86 and MHC class II expression and IL-12 production than those of wild-type mice (Fang *et al.*, 2010).

WNV permissive LCs could migrate from the skin to the lymph nodes upon a cutaneous infection, which contributes to WNV dissemination in early viral infection (Byrne *et al.*, 2001; Johnston *et al.*, 2000). DC-SIGN is highly expressed in monocyte-derived DCs *in vitro* and at lower levels *in vivo* in subsets of macrophages and DCs (Geijtenbeek *et al.*, 2000; Krutzik *et al.*, 2005; Soilleux *et al.*, 2002). DC-SIGN plays an important role in the enhancement of infection by WNV glycosylated strains. Further, the location of the N-linked glycosylation sites on a virion determines the types of glycans incorporated, thus controlling viral tropism for DC-SIGN -expressing cells (Davis *et al.*, 2006).

4. Adaptive immunity

4.1 T cell responses

Both $CD4^+$ and $CD8^+$ $\alpha\beta$ T cells contribute to host survival during WNV infection. $CD4^+$ T cells respond vigorously in the periphery (Kulkarni *et al.*, 1991). They are known to provide help for antibody responses and to sustain WNV-specific $CD8^+$ T cell responses in the CNS enabling viral clearance (Sitati & Diamond, 2006). Among $CD4^+$ $\alpha\beta$ T cells, higher levels of peripheral Tregs after infection protect against severe WNV disease in immunocompetent animals and humans possibly by dampening the WNV-specific immune response and inflammation. In humans, WNV symptomatic donors exhibited lower Treg frequencies from 2 weeks through 1 year after index donation. Similarly, symptomatic WNV-infected mice also had lower Treg frequencies compared with asymptomatic mice at 2 weeks after infection (Lanteri *et al.*, 2009). In WNV-infected mice, $CD8^+$ T cell responses have been observed in both the spleen and brain (Liu *et al.*, 1989). $CD8^+$ T cells have important functions in clearing infection from peripheral tissues and CNS, and in preventing viral persistence (Brien *et al.*, 2007; Shrestha & Diamond, 2004). During WNV infection, chemokines secreted from CNS, including CXCL10 (Klein *et al.*, 2005) or CCL5 (Glass *et al.*, 2005) help to recruit the antigen specific $CD8^+$ effector T cells. CD40-CD40L interactions are also important for T cell trafficking into the CNS and for protection of the host from a low dose WNV challenge (Sitati *et al.*, 2007). Once inside CNS, these cells kill the virus infected target cells in perforin or FasL effector-dependent manners (Shrestha & Diamond, 2007; Shrestha *et al.*, 2006a). Both primary and memory $CD8^+$ T cells have been demonstrated to efficiently kill target cells that display WNV antigens restricted by a class I MHC (Shrestha & Diamond, 2004).

αβ T cells can also be pathogenic. For example, they can support a low but productive WNV replication. Following a systemic infection, WNV might cross the BBB and enter the CNS by being carried by infected infiltrating T cells (Wang *et al.*, 2008). Another study suggests that $CD8^+$ T cells contribute to immunopathology upon high-dose WNV challenge (Wang *et al.*, 2003b). Nevertheless, little is known about the role of T cell-mediated pathology in WNV-related brain damage. In the aged mouse model of WNV infection, defects in T cell responses against dominant WNV epitopes were shown to contribute to the enhanced susceptibility to WNV encephalitis (Brien *et al.*, 2009). Primary and memory T cell responses in old mice induced by RepliVAX WN, a single-cycle flavivirus vaccination were significantly lower than those seen in younger mice. However, this seems to be overcome by repeating *in vivo* stimulation of T cell responses in old mice (Uhrlaub *et al.*, 2011). In investigation of the correlation between T cell phenotype and disease severity, CD8 T cells of a terminally differentiated/cytolytic profile were found to be associated with neuroinvasion (Piazza *et al.*, 2010).

4.2 B cells, antibody and complement responses to WNV infection

B cells and specific antibodies are critical in the control of disseminated WNV infection, but are not sufficient to eliminate it from the host (Diamond *et al.*, 2003a; Diamond *et al.*, 2003b; Diamond *et al.*, 2003c; Roehrig *et al.*, 2001). In particular, induction of a specific, neutralizing IgM response early during infection limits viremia and dissemination into the CNS and protects the host against lethal infection (Diamond *et al.*, 2003c). Mice deficient in B cells and antibody (microMT mice) were vulnerable to lethal WNV infection (Engle & Diamond, 2003). Patients with defects in humoral immunity may not produce a serologic response and clear WNV infection permanently, which would result in persistent CNS infection (Penn *et al.*, 2006).

The complement system is made up of a complex pathway of more than 30 serum proteins and cell surface receptors that are involved in direct cell lysis and the enhancement of B and T cell responses (Avirutnan *et al.*, 2008; Carroll, 2004). Complement is activated by three different pathways: classical, lectin and alternative. All three share the common step of activating the central component C3, but they differ according to the nature of recognition. Although one early study suggests that complement could enhance IgM-dependent WNV replication in macrophages *in vitro* (Cardosa *et al.*, 1983), more evidence supports that it is required for control of WNV infection *in vivo*. Protection against WNV encephalitis requires an intact complement system as mice lacking C3 uniformly succumbed to infection (Mehlhop *et al.*, 2005). All complement activation pathways are required, as mice deficient in C1q (classical pathway) or fB (alternative pathway) (Mehlhop & Diamond, 2006), or mice deficient in lectin pathway recognition molecules (mannose binding lectin-A and mannose binding lectin-C or the effector enzyme mannan-binding lectin-associated serine protease-2) were more vulnerable to WNV infection (Fuchs *et al.*, 2011). The complement system is known to control WNV infection, in part through its ability to induce a protective antibody response and by priming adaptive immune responses through distinct mechanisms (Mehlhop & Diamond, 2006; Mehlhop *et al.*, 2005). Mice deficient of classical and lectin pathways had defects in WNV specific antibody production and T cell responses. In comparison, mice deficient of alternative pathway had normal B cell function but impaired $CD8^+$ T cell response (Mehlhop & Diamond, 2006).

5. Conclusions

Studies from animal models, cell culture and patient samples have suggested that both innate and adaptive immunity are involved in host protective immune responses. Among them, type 1 IFNs, $\gamma\delta$ T cells and humoral immunity are critical in controlling dissemination of WNV (Anderson & Rahal, 2002; Diamond *et al.*, 2003a; Fredericksen *et al.*, 2008; Klein *et al.*, 2005; Lucas *et al.*, 2003; Roehrig *et al.*, 2001; Wang *et al.*, 2003a). $CD4^+$ (Kulkarni *et al.*, 1991) and $CD8^+$ $\alpha\beta$ T-cells (Shrestha *et al.*, 2006a; Wang *et al.*, 2003b) contribute to host survival following WNV infection. Host immune responses may act as a double-edged sword during WNV infection. Depending on the virus dose (lethal versus sub-lethal), passage history of the virus (Vero cell-derived versus insect cell derived) or routes of inoculation, immune factors can be either pathogenic or protective in host immunity against WNV infection.

6. Acknowledgements

This work is supported by NIH grant AI072060 (T. Wang).

7. References

(2002a). Laboratory-acquired West Nile virus infections--United States, 2002. *MMWR Morb Mortal Wkly Rep* 51, 1133-1135.

(2002b). Possible West Nile virus transmission to an infant through breast-feeding--Michigan, 2002. *MMWR Morb Mortal Wkly Rep* 51, 877-878.

(2002c). West Nile virus activity--United States, August 21-28, 2002, and Illinois, January 1-August 27, 2002. *MMWR Morb Mortal Wkly Rep* 51, 764-766.

Akira, S. & Hemmi, H. (2003). Recognition of pathogen-associated molecular patterns by TLR family. *Immunol Lett* 85, 85-95.

Alpert, S. G., Fergerson, J. & Noel, L. P. (2003). Intrauterine West Nile virus: ocular and systemic findings. *Am J Ophthalmol* 136, 733-735.

Anderson, J. F., Andreadis, T. G., Vossbrinck, C. R., Tirrell, S., Wakem, E. M., French, R. A., Garmendia, A. E. & Van Kruiningen, H. J. (1999). Isolation of West Nile virus from mosquitoes, crows, and a Cooper's hawk in Connecticut. *Science* 286, 2331-2333.

Anderson, J. F. & Rahal, J. J. (2002). Efficacy of interferon alpha-2b and ribavirin against West Nile virus *in vitro*. *Emerg Infect Dis* 8, 107-108.

Appler, K. K., Brown, A. N., Stewart, B. S., Behr, M. J., Demarest, V. L., Wong, S. J. & Bernard, K. A. (2010). Persistence of West Nile virus in the central nervous system and periphery of mice. *PLoS One* 5, e10649.

Argentati, K., Re, F., Donnini, A., Tucci, M. G., Franceschi, C., Bartozzi, B., Bernardini, G. & Provinciali, M. (2002). Numerical and functional alterations of circulating gammadelta T lymphocytes in aged people and centenarians. *J Leukoc Biol* 72, 65-71.

Arjona, A., Foellmer, H. G., Town, T., Leng, L., McDonald, C., Wang, T., Wong, S. J., Montgomery, R. R., Fikrig, E. & Bucala, R. (2007). Abrogation of macrophage migration inhibitory factor decreases West Nile virus lethality by limiting viral neuroinvasion. *J Clin Invest* 117, 3059-3066.

Avirutnan, P., Mehlhop, E. & Diamond, M. S. (2008). Complement and its role in protection and pathogenesis of flavivirus infections. *Vaccine* 26 Suppl 8, I100-107.

Bai, F., Kong, K. F., Dai, J., Qian, F., Zhang, L., Brown, C. R., Fikrig, E. & Montgomery, R. R. (2010). A paradoxical role for neutrophils in the pathogenesis of West Nile virus. *J Infect Dis* 202, 1804-1812.

Bai, F., Town, T., Qian, F., Wang, P., Kamanaka, M., Connolly, T. M., Gate, D., Montgomery, R. R., Flavell, R. A. & Fikrig, E. (2009). IL-10 signaling blockade controls murine West Nile virus infection. *PLoS Pathog* 5, e1000610.

Bank, I., DePinho, R. A., Brenner, M. B., Cassimeris, J., Alt, F. W. & Chess, L. (1986). A functional T3 molecule associated with a novel heterodimer on the surface of immature human thymocytes. *Nature* 322, 179-181.

Beasley, D. W., Li, L., Suderman, M. T. & Barrett, A. D. (2002). Mouse neuroinvasive phenotype of West Nile virus strains varies depending upon virus genotype. *Virology* 296, 17-23.

Ben-Nathan, D., Huitinga, I., Lustig, S., van Rooijen, N. & Kobiler, D. (1996). West Nile virus neuroinvasion and encephalitis induced by macrophage depletion in mice. *Arch Virol* 141, 459-469.

Bennett, S. R., Carbone, F. R., Karamalis, F., Flavell, R. A., Miller, J. F. & Heath, W. R. (1998). Help for cytotoxic-T-cell responses is mediated by CD40 signalling. *Nature* 393, 478-480.

Brehin, A. C., Mouries, J., Frenkiel, M. P., Dadaglio, G., Despres, P., Lafon, M. & Couderc, T. (2008). Dynamics of immune cell recruitment during West Nile encephalitis and identification of a new CD19+B220-BST-2+ leukocyte population. *J Immunol* 180, 6760-6767.

Brien, J. D., Uhrlaub, J. L., Hirsch, A., Wiley, C. A. & Nikolich-Zugich, J. (2009). Key role of T cell defects in age-related vulnerability to West Nile virus. *J Exp Med* 206, 2735-2745.

Brien, J. D., Uhrlaub, J. L. & Nikolich-Zugich, J. (2007). Protective capacity and epitope specificity of CD8(+) T cells responding to lethal West Nile virus infection. *Eur J Immunol* 37, 1855-1863.

Byrne, S. N., Halliday, G. M., Johnston, L. J. & King, N. J. (2001). Interleukin-1beta but not tumor necrosis factor is involved in West Nile virus-induced Langerhans cell migration from the skin in C57BL/6 mice. *J Invest Dermatol* 117, 702-709.

Campbell, G. L., Marfin, A. A., Lanciotti, R. S. & Gubler, D. J. (2002). West Nile virus. *Lancet Infect Dis* 2, 519-529.

Cardillo, F., Falcao, R. P., Rossi, M. A. & Mengel, J. (1993). An age-related gamma delta T cell suppressor activity correlates with the outcome of autoimmunity in experimental Trypanosoma cruzi infection. *Eur J Immunol* 23, 2597-2605.

Carding, S. R. & Egan, P. J. (2002). Gammadelta T cells: functional plasticity and heterogeneity. *Nat Rev Immunol* 2, 336-345.

Cardosa, M. J., Porterfield, J. S. & Gordon, S. (1983). Complement receptor mediates enhanced flavivirus replication in macrophages. *J Exp Med* 158, 258-263.

Carroll, M. C. (2004). The complement system in regulation of adaptive immunity. *Nat Immunol* 5, 981-986.

Charatan, F. (2002). Organ transplants and blood transfusions may transmit West Nile virus. *Bmj* 325, 566.

Cheeran, M. C., Hu, S., Sheng, W. S., Rashid, A., Peterson, P. K. & Lokensgard, J. R. (2005). Differential responses of human brain cells to West Nile virus infection. *J Neurovirol* 11, 512-524.

Chung, K. M., Thompson, B. S., Fremont, D. H. & Diamond, M. S. (2007). Antibody recognition of cell surface-associated NS1 triggers Fc-gamma receptor-mediated phagocytosis and clearance of West Nile Virus-infected cells. *J Virol* 81, 9551-9555.

Daffis, S., Samuel, M. A., Suthar, M. S., Gale, M., Jr. & Diamond, M. S. (2008). Toll-like receptor 3 has a protective role against West Nile virus infection. *J Virol* 82, 10349-10358.

Davis, B. S., Chang, G. J., Cropp, B., Roehrig, J. T., Martin, D. A., Mitchell, C. J., Bowen, R. & Bunning, M. L. (2001). West Nile virus recombinant DNA vaccine protects mouse and horse from virus challenge and expresses in vitro a noninfectious recombinant antigen that can be used in enzyme-linked immunosorbent assays. *J Virol* 75, 4040-4047.

Davis, C. W., Mattei, L. M., Nguyen, H. Y., Ansarah-Sobrinho, C., Doms, R. W. & Pierson, T. C. (2006). The location of asparagine-linked glycans on West Nile virions controls their interactions with CD209 (dendritic cell-specific ICAM-3 grabbing nonintegrin). *J Biol Chem* 281, 37183-37194.

De Smedt, T., Pajak, B., Muraille, E., Lespagnard, L., Heinen, E., De Baetselier, P., Urbain, J., Leo, O. & Moser, M. (1996). Regulation of dendritic cell numbers and maturation by lipopolysaccharide in vivo. *J Exp Med* 184, 1413-1424.

Diamond, M. S., Shrestha, B., Marri, A., Mahan, D. & Engle, M. (2003a). B cells and antibody play critical roles in the immediate defense of disseminated infection by West Nile encephalitis virus. *J Virol* 77, 2578-2586.

Diamond, M. S., Shrestha, B., Mehlhop, E., Sitati, E. & Engle, M. (2003b). Innate and adaptive immune responses determine protection against disseminated infection by West Nile encephalitis virus. *Viral Immunol* 16, 259-278.

Diamond, M. S., Sitati, E. M., Friend, L. D., Higgs, S., Shrestha, B. & Engle, M. (2003c). A critical role for induced IgM in the protection against West Nile virus infection. *J Exp Med* 198, 1853-1862.

Engle, M. J. & Diamond, M. S. (2003). Antibody prophylaxis and therapy against West Nile virus infection in wild-type and immunodeficient mice. *J Virol* 77, 12941-12949.

Evans, J. D. & Seeger, C. (2007). Differential effects of mutations in NS4B on West Nile virus replication and inhibition of interferon signaling. *J Virol* 81, 11809-11816.

Fang, H., Welte, T., Zheng, X., Chang, G. J., Holbrook, M. R., Soong, L. & Wang, T. (2010). gammadelta T cells promote the maturation of dendritic cells during West Nile virus infection. *FEMS Immunol Med Microbiol.*

Fredericksen, B. L. & Gale, M., Jr. (2006). West Nile virus evades activation of interferon regulatory factor 3 through RIG-I-dependent and -independent pathways without antagonizing host defense signaling. *J Virol* 80, 2913-2923.

Fredericksen, B. L., Keller, B. C., Fornek, J., Katze, M. G. & Gale, M., Jr. (2008). Establishment and maintenance of the innate antiviral response to West Nile Virus involves both RIG-I and MDA5 signaling through IPS-1. *J Virol* 82, 609-616.

Fuchs, A., Pinto, A. K., Schwaeble, W. J. & Diamond, M. S. (2011). The lectin pathway of complement activation contributes to protection from West Nile virus infection. *Virology* 412, 101-109.

Fujii, S., Liu, K., Smith, C., Bonito, A. J. & Steinman, R. M. (2004). The linkage of innate to adaptive immunity via maturing dendritic cells *in vivo* requires CD40 ligation in addition to antigen presentation and CD80/86 costimulation. *J Exp Med* 199, 1607-1618.

Gack, M. U., Shin, Y. C., Joo, C. H., Urano, T., Liang, C., Sun, L., Takeuchi, O., Akira, S., Chen, Z., Inoue, S. & Jung, J. U. (2007). TRIM25 RING-finger E3 ubiquitin ligase is essential for RIG-I-mediated antiviral activity. *Nature* 446, 916-920.

Geijtenbeek, T. B., Torensma, R., van Vliet, S. J., van Duijnhoven, G. C., Adema, G. J., van Kooyk, Y. & Figdor, C. G. (2000). Identification of DC-SIGN, a novel dendritic cell-specific ICAM-3 receptor that supports primary immune responses. *Cell* 100, 575-585.

Getts, D. R., Terry, R. L., Getts, M. T., Muller, M., Rana, S., Shrestha, B., Radford, J., Van Rooijen, N., Campbell, I. L. & King, N. J. (2008). Ly6c+ "inflammatory monocytes" are microglial precursors recruited in a pathogenic manner in West Nile virus encephalitis. *J Exp Med* 205, 2319-2337.

Glass, W. G., Lim, J. K., Cholera, R., Pletnev, A. G., Gao, J. L. & Murphy, P. M. (2005). Chemokine receptor CCR5 promotes leukocyte trafficking to the brain and survival in West Nile virus infection. *J Exp Med* 202, 1087-1098.

Hayday, A. C. (2000). Gammadelta cells: a right time and a right place for a conserved third way of protection. *Annu Rev Immunol* 18, 975-1026.

Hayes, E. B. & Gubler, D. J. (2006). West Nile virus: epidemiology and clinical features of an emerging epidemic in the United States. *Annu Rev Med* 57, 181-194.

Hayes, S. M. & Love, P. E. (2002). Distinct structure and signaling potential of the gamma delta TCR complex. *Immunity* 16, 827-838.

Hershkovitz, O., Rosental, B., Rosenberg, L. A., Navarro-Sanchez, M. E., Jivov, S., Zilka, A., Gershoni-Yahalom, O., Brient-Litzler, E., Bedouelle, H., Ho, J. W., Campbell, K. S., Rager-Zisman, B., Despres, P. & Porgador, A. (2009). NKp44 receptor mediates interaction of the envelope glycoproteins from the West Nile and dengue viruses with NK cells. *J Immunol* 183, 2610-2621.

Inaba, K., Turley, S., Iyoda, T., Yamaide, F., Shimoyama, S., Reis e Sousa, C., Germain, R. N., Mellman, I. & Steinman, R. M. (2000). The formation of immunogenic major histocompatibility complex class II-peptide ligands in lysosomal compartments of dendritic cells is regulated by inflammatory stimuli. *J Exp Med* 191, 927-936.

Iwasaki, A. & Medzhitov, R. (2010). Regulation of adaptive immunity by the innate immune system. *Science* 327, 291-295.

Johnston, L. J., Halliday, G. M. & King, N. J. (2000). Langerhans cells migrate to local lymph nodes following cutaneous infection with an arbovirus. *J Invest Dermatol* 114, 560-568.

Jounai, N., Takeshita, F., Kobiyama, K., Sawano, A., Miyawaki, A., Xin, K. Q., Ishii, K. J., Kawai, T., Akira, S., Suzuki, K. & Okuda, K. (2007). The Atg5 Atg12 conjugate associates with innate antiviral immune responses. *Proc Natl Acad Sci U S A* 104, 14050-14055.

Katze, M. G., He, Y. & Gale, M., Jr. (2002). Viruses and interferon: a fight for supremacy. *Nat Rev Immunol* 2, 675-687.

King, N. J., Shrestha, B. & Kesson, A. M. (2003). Immune modulation by flaviviruses. *Adv Virus Res* 60, 121-155.

Klein, R. S., Lin, E., Zhang, B., Luster, A. D., Tollett, J., Samuel, M. A., Engle, M. & Diamond, M. S. (2005). Neuronal CXCL10 directs CD8+ T-cell recruitment and control of West Nile virus encephalitis. *J Virol* 79, 11457-11466.

Kong, K. F., Delroux, K., Wang, X., Qian, F., Arjona, A., Malawista, S. E., Fikrig, E. & Montgomery, R. R. (2008). Dysregulation of TLR3 Impairs the Innate Immune Response to West Nile Virus in the Elderly. *J Virol* 82, 7613-7623.

Kramer, L. D. & Bernard, K. A. (2001). West Nile virus infection in birds and mammals. *Ann N Y Acad Sci* 951, 84-93.

Krutzik, S. R., Tan, B., Li, H., Ochoa, M. T., Liu, P. T., Sharfstein, S. E., Graeber, T. G., Sieling, P. A., Liu, Y. J., Rea, T. H., Bloom, B. R. & Modlin, R. L. (2005). TLR activation triggers the rapid differentiation of monocytes into macrophages and dendritic cells. *Nat Med* 11, 653-660.

Kulkarni, A. B., Mullbacher, A. & Blanden, R. V. (1991). Functional analysis of macrophages, B cells and splenic dendritic cells as antigen-presenting cells in West Nile virus-specific murine T lymphocyte proliferation. *Immunol Cell Biol* 69 (Pt 2), 71-80.

Lanciotti, R. S., Roehrig, J. T., Deubel, V., Smith, J., Parker, M., Steele, K., Crise, B., Volpe, K. E., Crabtree, M. B., Scherret, J. H., Hall, R. A., MacKenzie, J. S., Cropp, C. B., Panigrahy, B., Ostlund, E., Schmitt, B., Malkinson, M., Banet, C., Weissman, J., Komar, N., Savage, H. M., Stone, W., McNamara, T. & Gubler, D. J. (1999). Origin of the West Nile virus responsible for an outbreak of encephalitis in the northeastern United States. *Science* 286, 2333-2337.

Lanteri, M. C., O'Brien, K. M., Purtha, W. E., Cameron, M. J., Lund, J. M., Owen, R. E., Heitman, J. W., Custer, B., Hirschkorn, D. F., Tobler, L. H., Kiely, N., Prince, H. E., Ndhlovu, L. C., Nixon, D. F., Kamel, H. T., Kelvin, D. J., Busch, M. P., Rudensky, A. Y., Diamond, M. S. & Norris, P. J. (2009). Tregs control the development of symptomatic West Nile virus infection in humans and mice. *J Clin Invest* 119, 3266-3277.

Laurent-Rolle, M., Boer, E. F., Lubick, K. J., Wolfinbarger, J. B., Carmody, A. B., Rockx, B., Liu, W., Ashour, J., Shupert, W. L., Holbrook, M. R., Barrett, A. D., Mason, P. W., Bloom, M. E., Garcia-Sastre, A., Khromykh, A. A. & Best, S. M. (2010). The NS5 protein of the virulent West Nile virus NY99 strain is a potent antagonist of type I interferon-mediated JAK-STAT signaling. *J Virol* 84, 3503-3515.

Lim, J. K., Louie, C. Y., Glaser, C., Jean, C., Johnson, B., Johnson, H., McDermott, D. H. & Murphy, P. M. (2008). Genetic deficiency of chemokine receptor CCR5 is a strong risk factor for symptomatic West Nile virus infection: a meta-analysis of 4 cohorts in the US epidemic. *J Infect Dis* 197, 262-265.

Lim, J. K., McDermott, D. H., Lisco, A., Foster, G. A., Krysztof, D., Follmann, D., Stramer, S. L. & Murphy, P. M. (2010). CCR5 deficiency is a risk factor for early clinical manifestations of West Nile virus infection but not for viral transmission. *J Infect Dis* 201, 178-185.

Lim, J. K., Obara, C. J., Rivollier, A., Pletnev, A. G., Kelsall, B. L. & Murphy, P. M. (2011). Chemokine receptor Ccr2 is critical for monocyte accumulation and survival in West Nile virus encephalitis. *J Immunol* 186, 471-478.

Liu, W. J., Wang, X. J., Mokhonov, V. V., Shi, P. Y., Randall, R. & Khromykh, A. A. (2005). Inhibition of interferon signaling by the New York 99 strain and Kunjin subtype of West Nile virus involves blockage of STAT1 and STAT2 activation by nonstructural proteins. *J Virol* 79, 1934-1942.

Liu, Y., Blanden, R. V. & Mullbacher, A. (1989). Identification of cytolytic lymphocytes in West Nile virus-infected murine central nervous system. *J Gen Virol* 70, 565-573.

Lucas, M., Mashimo, T., Frenkiel, M. P., Simon-Chazottes, D., Montagutelli, X., Ceccaldi, P. E., Guenet, J. L. & Despres, P. (2003). Infection of mouse neurones by West Nile virus is modulated by the interferon-inducible 2'-5' oligoadenylate synthetase 1b protein. *Immunol Cell Biol* 81, 230-236.

Mehlhop, E. & Diamond, M. S. (2006). Protective immune responses against West Nile virus are primed by distinct complement activation pathways. *J Exp Med* 203, 1371-1381.

Mehlhop, E., Whitby, K., Oliphant, T., Marri, A., Engle, M. & Diamond, M. S. (2005). Complement activation is required for induction of a protective antibody response against West Nile virus infection. *J Virol* 79, 7466-7477.

Munoz-Jordan, J. L., Laurent-Rolle, M., Ashour, J., Martinez-Sobrido, L., Ashok, M., Lipkin, W. I. & Garcia-Sastre, A. (2005). Inhibition of alpha/beta interferon signaling by the NS4B protein of flaviviruses. *J Virol* 79, 8004-8013.

Murray, K., Walker, C., Herrington, E., Lewis, J. A., McCormick, J., Beasley, D. W., Tesh, R. B. & Fisher-Hoch, S. (2010). Persistent infection with West Nile virus years after initial infection. *J Infect Dis* 201, 2-4.

Penn, R. G., Guarner, J., Sejvar, J. J., Hartman, H., McComb, R. D., Nevins, D. L., Bhatnagar, J. & Zaki, S. R. (2006). Persistent neuroinvasive West Nile virus infection in an immunocompromised patient. *Clin Infect Dis* 42, 680-683.

Piazza, P., McMurtrey, C. P., Lelic, A., Cook, R. L., Hess, R., Yablonsky, E., Borowski, L., Loeb, M. B., Bramson, J. L., Hildebrand, W. H. & Rinaldo, C. R. (2010). Surface phenotype and functionality of WNV specific T cells differ with age and disease severity. *PLoS One* 5, e15343.

Pletnev, A. G., Swayne, D. E., Speicher, J., Rumyantsev, A. A. & Murphy, B. R. (2006). Chimeric West Nile/dengue virus vaccine candidate: Preclinical evaluation in mice, geese and monkeys for safety and immunogenicity. *Vaccine* 24, 6392-6404.

Puig-Basagoiti, F., Tilgner, M., Bennett, C. J., Zhou, Y., Munoz-Jordan, J. L., Garcia-Sastre, A., Bernard, K. A. & Shi, P. Y. (2007). A mouse cell-adapted NS4B mutation attenuates West Nile virus RNA synthesis. *Virology* 361, 229-241.

Qian, F., Wang, X., Zhang, L., Lin, A., Zhao, H., Fikrig, E. & Montgomery, R. R. (2011). Impaired Interferon Signaling in Dendritic Cells From Older Donors Infected In Vitro With West Nile Virus. *J Infect Dis.*

Qureshi, S. T. & Medzhitov, R. (2003). Toll-like receptors and their role in experimental models of microbial infection. *Genes Immun* 4, 87-94.

Ratterree, M. S., Gutierrez, R. A., Travassos da Rosa, A. P., Dille, B. J., Beasley, D. W., Bohm, R. P., Desai, S. M., Didier, P. J., Bikenmeyer, L. G., Dawson, G. J., Leary, T. P., Schochetman, G., Phillippi-Falkenstein, K., Arroyo, J., Barrett, A. D. & Tesh, R. B. (2004). Experimental infection of rhesus macaques with West Nile virus: level and duration of viremia and kinetics of the antibody response after infection. *J Infect Dis* 189, 669-676.

Rios, M., Zhang, M. J., Grinev, A., Srinivasan, K., Daniel, S., Wood, O., Hewlett, I. K. & Dayton, A. I. (2006). Monocytes-macrophages are a potential target in human infection with West Nile virus through blood transfusion. *Transfusion* 46, 659-667.

Roark, C. L., French, J. D., Taylor, M. A., Bendele, A. M., Born, W. K. & O'Brien R, L. (2007). Exacerbation of Collagen-Induced Arthritis by Oligoclonal, IL-17-Producing {gamma}{delta} T Cells. *J Immunol* 179, 5576-5583.

Roehrig, J. T., Staudinger, L. A., Hunt, A. R., Mathews, J. H. & Blair, C. D. (2001). Antibody prophylaxis and therapy for flavivirus encephalitis infections. *Ann N Y Acad Sci* 951, 286-297.

Rossi, S. L., Fayzulin, R., Dewsbury, N., Bourne, N. & Mason, P. W. (2007). Mutations in West Nile virus nonstructural proteins that facilitate replicon persistence in vitro attenuate virus replication in vitro and in vivo. *Virology* 364, 184-195.

Saito, T., Hirai, R., Loo, Y. M., Owen, D., Johnson, C. L., Sinha, S. C., Akira, S., Fujita, T. & Gale, M., Jr. (2007). Regulation of innate antiviral defenses through a shared repressor domain in RIG-I and LGP2. *Proc Natl Acad Sci U S A* 104, 582-587.

Samuel, C. E. (2002). Host genetic variability and West Nile virus susceptibility. *Proc Natl Acad Sci U S A* 99, 11555-11557.

Samuel, M. A. & Diamond, M. S. (2005). Alpha/beta interferon protects against lethal West Nile virus infection by restricting cellular tropism and enhancing neuronal survival. *J Virol* 79, 13350-13361.

Schneider, B. S., McGee, C. E., Jordan, J. M., Stevenson, H. L., Soong, L. & Higgs, S. (2007). Prior exposure to uninfected mosquitoes enhances mortality in naturally-transmitted West Nile virus infection. *PLoS One* 2, e1171.

Schneider, B. S., Soong, L., Coffey, L. L., Stevenson, H. L., McGee, C. E. & Higgs, S. (2010). Aedes aegypti saliva alters leukocyte recruitment and cytokine signaling by antigen-presenting cells during West Nile virus infection. *PLoS One* 5, e11704.

Shahar, A., Lustig, S., Akov, Y., David, Y., Schneider, P. & Levin, R. (1990). Different pathogenicity of encephalitic togaviruses in organotypic cultures of spinal cord slices. *J Neurosci Res* 25, 345-352.

Shirato, K., Miyoshi, H., Kariwa, H. & Takashima, I. (2006). The kinetics of proinflammatory cytokines in murine peritoneal macrophages infected with envelope protein-glycosylated or non-glycosylated West Nile virus. *Virus Res.*

Shrestha, B. & Diamond, M. S. (2004). Role of CD8+ T cells in control of West Nile virus infection. *J Virol* 78, 8312-8321.

Shrestha, B. & Diamond, M. S. (2007). Fas ligand interactions contribute to CD8+ T-cell-mediated control of West Nile virus infection in the central nervous system. *J Virol* 81, 11749-11757.

Shrestha, B., Samuel, M. A. & Diamond, M. S. (2006a). CD8+ T Cells Require Perforin To Clear West Nile Virus from Infected Neurons. *J Virol* 80, 119-129.

Shrestha, B., Wang, T., Samuel, M. A., Whitby, K., Craft, J., Fikrig, E. & Diamond, M. S. (2006b). Gamma interferon plays a crucial early antiviral role in protection against West Nile virus infection. *J Virol* 80, 5338-5348.

Sitati, E., McCandless, E. E., Klein, R. S. & Diamond, M. S. (2007). CD40-CD40 ligand interactions promote trafficking of CD8+ T cells into the brain and protection against West Nile virus encephalitis. *J Virol* 81, 9801-9811.

Sitati, E. M. & Diamond, M. S. (2006). CD4+ T-cell responses are required for clearance of West Nile virus from the central nervous system. *J Virol* 80, 12060-12069.

Soilleux, E. J., Morris, L. S., Leslie, G., Chehimi, J., Luo, Q., Levroney, E., Trowsdale, J., Montaner, L. J., Doms, R. W., Weissman, D., Coleman, N. & Lee, B. (2002). Constitutive and induced expression of DC-SIGN on dendritic cell and macrophage subpopulations in situ and in vitro. *J Leukoc Biol* 71, 445-457.

Suthar, M. S., Ma, D. Y., Thomas, S., Lund, J. M., Zhang, N., Daffis, S., Rudensky, A. Y., Bevan, M. J., Clark, E. A., Kaja, M. K., Diamond, M. S. & Gale, M., Jr. (2010). IPS-1 is essential for the control of West Nile virus infection and immunity. *PLoS Pathog* 6, e1000757.

Szretter, K. J., Daffis, S., Patel, J., Suthar, M. S., Klein, R. S., Gale, M., Jr. & Diamond, M. S. (2010). The innate immune adaptor molecule MyD88 restricts West Nile replication and spread in neurons of the central nervous system. *J Virol.*

Tesh, R. B., Siirin, M., Guzman, H., Travassos da Rosa, A. P., Wu, X., Duan, T., Lei, H., Nunes, M. R. & Xiao, S. Y. (2005). Persistent West Nile virus infection in the golden hamster: studies on its mechanism and possible implications for other flavivirus infections. *J Infect Dis* 192, 287-295.

Town, T., Bai, F., Wang, T., Kaplan, A. T., Qian, F., Montgomery, R. R., Anderson, J. F., Flavell, R. A. & Fikrig, E. (2009). Toll-like receptor 7 mitigates lethal West Nile encephalitis via interleukin 23-dependent immune cell infiltration and homing. *Immunity* 30, 242-253.

Town, T., Jeng, D., Alexopoulou, L., Tan, J. & Flavell, R. A. (2006). Microglia recognize double-stranded RNA via TLR3. *J Immunol* 176, 3804-3812.

Uhrlaub, J. L., Brien, J. D., Widman, D. G., Mason, P. W. & Nikolich-Zugich, J. (2011). Repeated In Vivo Stimulation of T and B Cell Responses in Old Mice Generates Protective Immunity against Lethal West Nile Virus Encephalitis. *J Immunol* 186, 3882-3891.

Vargin, V. V. & Semenov, B. F. (1986). Changes of natural killer cell activity in different mouse lines by acute and asymptomatic flavivirus infections. *Acta Virol* 30, 303-308.

Venter, M., Myers, T. G., Wilson, M. A., Kindt, T. J., Paweska, J. T., Burt, F. J., Leman, P. A. & Swanepoel, R. (2005). Gene expression in mice infected with West Nile virus strains of different neurovirulence. *Virology* 342, 119-140.

Wang, L., Kamath, A., Das, H., Li, L. & Bukowski, J. F. (2001a). Antibacterial effect of human V gamma 2V delta 2 T cells in vivo. *J Clin Invest* 108, 1349-1357.

Wang, P., Arjona, A., Zhang, Y., Sultana, H., Dai, J., Yang, L., LeBlanc, P. M., Doiron, K., Saleh, M. & Fikrig, E. (2010). Caspase-12 controls West Nile virus infection via the viral RNA receptor RIG-I. *Nat Immunol* 11, 912-919.

Wang, S., Welte, T., McGargill, M., Town, T., Thompson, J., Anderson, J. F., Flavell, R. A., Fikrig, E., Hedrick, S. M. & Wang, T. (2008). Drak2 contributes to West Nile virus entry into the brain and lethal encephalitis. *J Immunol* 181, 2084-2091.

Wang, T., Anderson, J. F., Magnarelli, L. A., Wong, S. J., Koski, R. A. & Fikrig, E. (2001b). Immunization of mice against West Nile virus with recombinant envelope protein. *J Immunol* 167, 5273-5277.

Wang, T. & Fikrig, E. (2004). Immunity to West Nile virus. *Curr Opin Immunol* 16, 519-523.

Wang, T., Scully, E., Yin, Z., Kim, J. H., Wang, S., Yan, J., Mamula, M., Anderson, J. F., Craft, J. & Fikrig, E. (2003a). IFN-gamma-producing gammadelta T cells help control murine West Nile virus infection. *J Immunol* 171, 2524-2531.

Wang, T., Town, T., Alexopoulou, L., Anderson, J. F., Fikrig, E. & Flavell, R. A. (2004). Toll-like receptor 3 mediates West Nile virus entry into the brain causing lethal encephalitis. *Nat Med* 10, 1366-1373.

Wang, Y., Lobigs, M., Lee, E. & Mullbacher, A. (2003b). CD8+ T cells mediate recovery and immunopathology in West Nile virus encephalitis. *J Virol* 77, 13323-13334.

Weerkamp, F., de Haas, E. F., Naber, B. A., Comans-Bitter, W. M., Bogers, A. J., van Dongen, J. J. & Staal, F. J. (2005). Age-related changes in the cellular composition of the thymus in children. *J Allergy Clin Immunol* 115, 834-840.

Welte, T., Lamb, J., Anderson, J. F., Born, W. K., O'Brien, R. L. & Wang, T. (2008). Role of two distinct gammadelta T cell subsets during West Nile virus infection. *FEMS Immunol Med Microbiol* 53, 275-283.

Welte, T., Reagan, K., Fang, H., Machain-Williams, C., Zheng, X., Mendell, N., Chang, G. J., Wu, P., Blair, C. D. & Wang, T. (2009). Toll-like receptor 7-induced immune response to cutaneous West Nile virus infection. *J Gen Virol* 90, 2660-2668.

Wilkins, C. & Gale, M., Jr. (2010). Recognition of viruses by cytoplasmic sensors. *Curr Opin Immunol* 22, 41-47.

Wilson, J. R., de Sessions, P. F., Leon, M. A. & Scholle, F. (2008). West Nile virus nonstructural protein 1 inhibits TLR3 signal transduction. *J Virol* 82, 8262-8271.

Xiao, S. Y., Guzman, H., Zhang, H., Travassos da Rosa, A. P. & Tesh, R. B. (2001). West Nile virus infection in the golden hamster (Mesocricetus auratus): a model for West Nile encephalitis. *Emerg Infect Dis* 7, 714-721.

Ye, S. F., Ichimura, K., Wakame, K. & Ohe, M. (2003). Suppressive effects of Active Hexose Correlated Compound on the increased activity of hepatic and renal ornithine decarboxylase induced by oxidative stress. *Life Sci* 74, 593-602.

Zhang, B., Chan, Y. K., Lu, B., Diamond, M. S. & Klein, R. S. (2008). CXCR3 mediates region-specific antiviral T cell trafficking within the central nervous system during West Nile virus encephalitis. *J Immunol* 180, 2641-2649.

Zhang, B., Patel, J., Croyle, M., Diamond, M. S. & Klein, R. S. (2010a). TNF-alpha-dependent regulation of CXCR3 expression modulates neuronal survival during West Nile virus encephalitis. *J Neuroimmunol* 224, 28-38.

Zhang, M., Daniel, S., Huang, Y., Chancey, C., Huang, Q., Lei, Y. F., Grinev, A., Mostowski, H., Rios, M. & Dayton, A. (2010b). Anti-West Nile virus activity of in vitro expanded human primary natural killer cells. *BMC Immunol* 11, 3.

4

Dengue Encephalitis

Sandra Theresa Jackson, Justin Jang Hann Chu, Po-Ying Chia,
Owen St. Clair Morgan and Lee-Ching Ng
University of the West Indies
Jamaica

1. Introduction

Dengue encephalitis and other neurological manifestations of dengue infection have been documented with increased frequency since the early 1900's. Infections with the dengue virus present with a wide range of clinical manifestations which have been classified according to severity by the World Health Organization (WHO) as; non-specific febrile illness, classical dengue syndrome, dengue hemorrhagic fever (DHF) and dengue shock syndrome (DSS) (WHO 1997). In 2009, WHO adjustments in the classification of the disease resulted in the recognition of two main presentations of dengue. These are referred to as Dengue Fever and Severe Dengue. Neurological dengue is classified as a form of Severe Dengue (WHO 1997, 2009).

A member of the Flavivirus genus of the family Flaviviridae, there are 4 genetically and antigenically distinct serotypes of dengue (DENV 1–4). Co-circulation of multiple serotypes (hyperendemnicity) (Gubler D. 2006), serotype virulence and hyperimmune responses have been identified as risk factors for Severe Dengue, an emerging and major public health concern in the Americas and the Pacific (Bennett, 2010). The incidence and prevalence of dengue encephalitis and other forms of neurological dengue will vary according to the degree of endemnicity and epidemic activity of dengue within geographic regions. Increased documentation of evidence based dengue encephalitis has accompanied the resurgence of dengue infections with the prevalence of dengue encephalitis ranging from 4.2 % to 13% of central nervous system infections (Solomon et al., 2000 & Jackson, 2008). The morbidity and sometimes fatal outcome of dengue encephalitis necessitates a better understanding of the disease, early diagnosis and appropriate management. This chapter reviews the epidemiology, pathogenesis, clinical features, laboratory diagnosis and evidence supporting dengue encephalitis.

2.Epidemiology

2.1 Vector and geographic distribution

Outbreaks of dengue have been documented in the Eastern Mediterranean Region since 1799 in Egypt. William Smart documented descriptions of neurological manifestations of dengue as early as 1827. An example of such documentation is demonstrated in the excerpt which follows (Smart, 1877).

"In children, the attack may be ushered in with convulsions, and the resolution may be attended by sensorial depression, approaching more or less to "dementia", which last condition may attend the stage of resolution of the disease in elderly persons also" (Smart, 1877).

By then the disease had earned numerous names including that of "dandy fever" given to it by the West Indian negro slaves from the strange attitudes of the sufferers when it first appeared among them. It was translated as dengue in Spanish and altered into denguis for scientific classification (Smart, 1877, Thomas, 1880). J Thomas also described other names given to this disease of wide clinical presentations including: "break-bone fever," "el dengue," which means literally "affectation," denguis, aburunka-bah, which means "father of the knee," " scarlatinarheumatica," "eruptive articular fever," "eruptive rheumatic fever," "eruptive epidemic fever of India," " broken-wing fever," mudak-mariata, mudka meaning contraction or stiffness, and mariata, the name of an idol or Hindoo deity (Smart, 1877, Thomas, 1880).

Though sporadic prior to the World War II, the frequency of dengue outbreaks increased significantly after the war. It was accompanied by an increase in the incidence of complicated forms of dengue (DHF and DSS) in South East Asia (Halstead, 1966). Since then, there has been a worldwide surge in the number and severity of dengue cases. Currently, an estimated 50 million dengue infections occur annually and approximately 2.5 billion people live in dengue endemic countries (WHO, 2009a). It is the most rapidly spreading mosquito-borne viral disease in the world and in the last 50 years its incidence has increased 30-fold with increasing geographic expansion to new countries. Besides making a comeback in places such as the Americas and Singapore, where dengue was previously successfully controlled for decades (Koh et al., 2008, Guzman and Kouri, 2003), it breached the subtropical temperate barrier and expanded from urban to rural settings extending its reach into places as far north as Nepal (Pandey et al., 2008), Ningbo China (Xu et al., 2007) and France (Gould et al., 2010); and as far south as Bueno Aires in Argentina (Natiello et al., 2008). The Pacific islands, with much lower population densities, have also not been spared, with increasing dengue outbreaks since the 1970s (Singh et al., 2005).

Incidences in South East Asia and the Western Pacific account for greater than 75% of the global burden of dengue. Within the Americas the burden of dengue accounts for 64.6% in the Southern Cone countries, 19% in the Andean contries, 12.5% in Central America and Mexico and 3.9% in the Caribbean (WHO 2009). In North America dengue is frequently seen in Texas and Hawaii (WHO 2009). Other regions in which dengue is endemic include the Eastern Mediterranean and the East and West African Regions (WHO, 2009).

The increased intensity of dengue transmission is effected by the rise in number and size of densely populated urban cities, which are conducive for the spread of the disease and the adaptation and proliferation of dengue vectors; and by international travel which results in the continuous importation and exchange of dengue serotypes and genotypes that become established at various levels (Lee et al., 2010, Ng et al., 2009, Lambrechts et al., 2009). Although the efficiency of dengue virus transmission is affected by a complex interplay of multiple factors, the displacement of one genotype by another more "virulent" or "fit" type has been documented (Rico-Hesse, 2003). The epidemiology of dengue encephalitis and neurological dengue will therefore vary according to the interplay of virus virulence, transmissibility, host susceptibility, endemnicity and/or epidemic activity within geographic locations (Salazar et al., 2010).

2.2 Incidence of dengue encephalitis

Neurologic involvement occurs in 4%-5% of confirmed dengue cases (Puccioni-Sohler et al., 2009). The incidence of dengue infection in patients with suspected central nervous system

(CNS) infection is noted to range from 4.2% in southern Vietnam (Solomon et al., 2000) to 13.5% in Jamaica (Jackson et al., 2008). The higher frequency of neurological dengue (13.5%) reported by Jackson et al.,may be attributed to the inclusion of both adults and children in the study. In this study the frequency of dengue encephalitis among 401 patients with suspected viral central nervous system infections was found to be 6.9% (Jackson et.al., 2008). The incidence of dengue among patients with clinical manifestations of encephalitis-like illness ranges from 18% (Kankirawatana et al., 2000) to 22% (Jackson et al., 2008). Among confirmed neurological dengue cases studies have documented encephalitis to be the presenting clinical manifestation in 52% (Jackson et al., 2008) to 56% (Solomon et al., 2000).. Other neurological manifestations of dengue noted in the Jamaican study include; meningits (34%), seizures (11%), acute flaccid paralysis and Guillain-Barré syndrome (4%).

2.3 Transmission

The transmission of DENV includes a sylvatic, enzootic cycle between nonhuman primates and arboreal mosquitoes of the genus Aedes, and an urban, endemic/epidemic cycle between human reservoir hosts and peridomestic *Aedes spp.*, particularly mosquitoes with larval development in peridomestic water containers. Though the sylvatic dengue strains are associated with illness in Africa and Asia, they do not lead to sustained urban transmission. The *Aedes (Stegomyia) aegypti* (Egyptian tiger mosquito), a day-biting mosquito that is widespread along the tropical and subtropical belt, is the primary vector of the urban cycle. The *Aedes (Stegomyia) albopictus*, also known as the Asian tiger mosquito or forest day mosquito, is a secondary vector of dengue in Asia (Moncayo et al., 2004). In places such as China (including Hong Kong), Hawaii and France (Xu et al., 2007, Gould et al., 2010, Effler et al., 2005), where *Ae. aegypti* is absent, the Asian Tiger mosquito has been shown to be the vector of dengue transmission.

Humans are the main amplifying host of the virus in the urban cycle. DENV circulating in the blood of viraemic humans is ingested by female mosquitoes during feeding. The virus then infects the mosquito mid-gut and subsequently spreads systemically, including the salivary glands, over a period of 8-12 days. After this extrinsic incubation period, the virus can be transmitted to immunologically naive humans during subsequent probing or feeding. The extrinsic incubation period is influenced in part by environmental conditions, especially ambient temperature and the genetic make up of the virus. Thereafter the mosquito remains infective for the rest of its life. *Ae. aegypti* is one of the most efficient vectors for arboviruses because it is highly anthropophilic, frequently bites several times before completing oogenesis, and thrives in close proximity to humans. The eggs can remain viable for many months in the absence of water. Vertical transmission (transovarial transmission) of DENV has been documented with infected eggs remaining viable for many months in the absence of water. Factors influencing virus transmission include environmental and climate factors related to vector distribution and proliferation, host-pathogen interactions and population immunological factors.

Evolution and virus adaptation have resulted in endemic DENV-2 strains being more efficient than sylvatic strains at infecting the peridomestic DENV vectors *Ae. aegypti* and *Ae. albopictus*. Evolutionary DENV emergence events (DENV 1–4) suggest that adaptation of DENV to new vectors and hosts occurred repeatedly from 300 to 1,500 years ago in Asia or Oceania. Continued emergence of endemic DENV from sylvatic progenitor strains occurs in conjunction with the peridomestication of *Aedes* mosquitoes and virus adaptation to these anthropophilic vectors (Moncayo et al., 2004).

3. Dengue virus

Dengue virus (DENV) belongs to the Flavivirus genus of the family Flaviviridae. There are 4 genetically and antigenically distinct serotypes,(DENV 1-4). Infection with one genotype confers life long immunity to the serotype, but only temporary immunity to the other three. The virus is non-enveloped, spherical with a diameter of 50nm containing multiple copies of three structural proteins, a host-derived membrane bilayer and a single copy of a positive-sense, single-stranded RNA genome. The genome is cleaved by host and viral proteases in three structural proteins (capsid, prM, the precursor of membrane protein and envelope protein) and seven nonstructural proteins (NS).

4. Clinical manifestations of Dengue

4.1 Classification of Dengue disease spectrum

The significant contribution of dengue virus (DENV) as an etiological agent of central nervous system infections is evidenced by studies documenting the prevalence of dengue encephalitis of 4.2 % to 13% in dengue endemic regions and during dengue epidemics respectively (Solomon et al., 2000; Jackson, 2008). The 1997 World Health Organization (WHO) classification of symptomatic DENV infections defined dengue as:
i) undifferentiated fever, ii) dengue fever (DF), and iii) dengue haemorrhagic fever (DHF). In this classification system, DHF is further classified into four severity grades, with grades III and IV being defined as dengue shock syndrome (DSS). Plasma leakage with or without

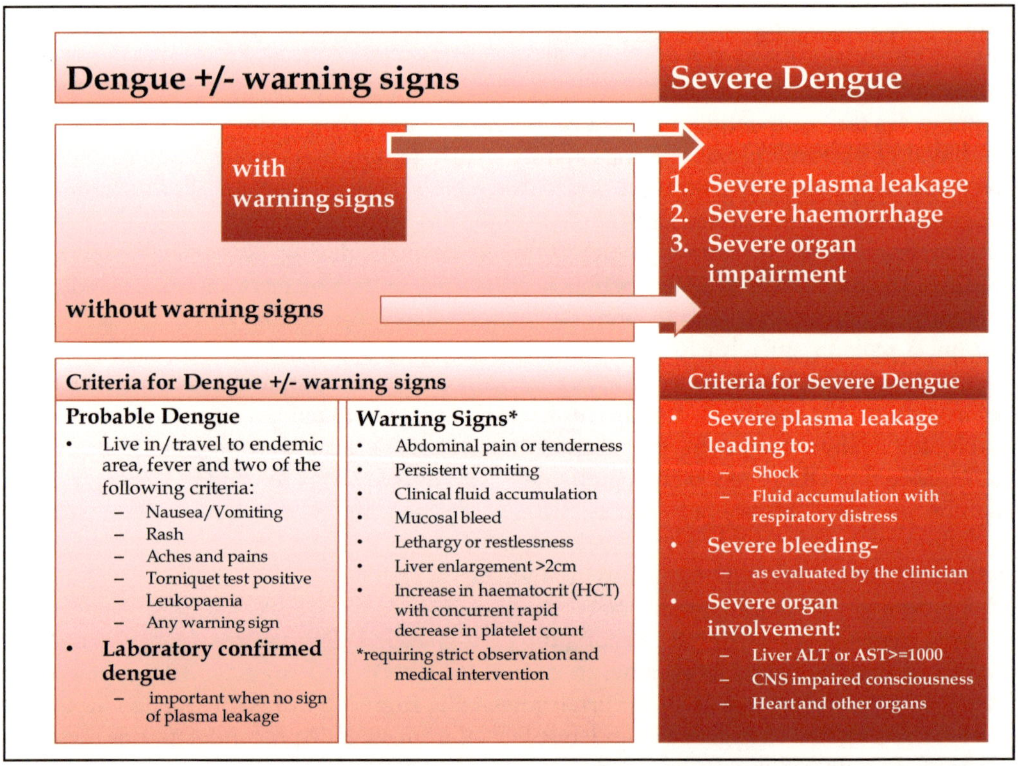

Fig. 1. WHO suggested dengue case classification and levels of severity, (WHO, 2009)

hemorrhage and thrombocytopenia (platelet count of less than 100,000mm^3) are important criteria of DHF/DSS (WHO, 1997) and assist in differentiating DHF/DSS from other arboviral encephalitides. Although this classification into DF/DHF/DSS continues to be widely used, changes in the epidemiology of dengue and difficulties in the use of the 1997 WHO classification (Deen et al., 2006), together with the increase in clinically severe dengue inclusive of neurological dengue resulted in the proposition of an adjusted case classification according to levels of severity by WHO in 2009 (WHO, 2009b).

The suggested classification system divides dengue infection into patients with severe dengue and those with non-severe dengue. Non-severe dengue is divided further into two subgroups -patients with warning signs and those without them (Figure 1). The challenge in classification and clinical diagnosis of dengue is indeed reflected by the statement made by the Expert Consensus Groups in Latin America (Havana, Cuba, 2007), South-East Asia (Kuala Lumpur, Malaysia, 2007), and at WHO headquarters in Geneva, Switzerland in 2008: "Dengue is one disease entity with different clinical presentations and often with unpredictable clinical evolution and outcome" (WHO, 2009b). Nevertheless, the proposed 2009 WHO classification acknowledges the evidence of research findings that dengue patients without warning signs may develop severe dengue and that central nervous system (CNS) impaired consciousness may be one of the presentations of severe dengue.

4.2 Clinical manifestations of Dengue encephalitis

Dengue encepahlitis is a severe form of dengue. Clinical manifestations of dengue encephalitis documented in early and present descriptions of the disease suggests that it is an infrequent but serious manifestation of dengue virus infection. It should be considered in the differential diagnosis of acute viral encephalitis in geographic regions in which dengue is known to occur. Patients with Dengue encephalitis may be at risk of developing complications of dengue haemorrhagic fever (Muzaffar et al., 2006) although some patients with encephalitis may not show any characteristic features of the disease (Solomon et al., 2000). It is possible that earlier descriptons of encephalitis may have been referred to as encephalomyelopathy because of failed attempts to demonstrate direct invasion of the central nervous system by the dengue virus (Muzaffar et al., 2006, Varatharaj, 2010).

Several forms of Dengue encephalitis have been described. These include focal-encephalitis, pan-encephalitis, acute disseminated encephalomyelitis and meningoencephalomyelitis. The onset of encephalitis is usually sudden with non-specific prodromal symptoms, which include myalgia, malaise, fever, vomiting and diarrhoea. Within a few days patients display headache, disorientation, depressed sensorium and seizures. Other features which have been identified include frontal release signs, abnormal posturing, facial nerve palsy and tetraparesis. Isolated case reports describe more esoteric features ranging from altered sensation to hippocampal encephalitis presenting as amnesia (Varatharaj, 2010, Newman Dorland, 2003).

5. Pathogenesis

5.1 Virus entry and replication

Though evidences for various mechanisms are emerging, there is no consensus on the pathogenesis of DENV. During the feeding of mosquitoes on humans, DENV is presumably injected into the bloodstream, with spillover in the epidermis and dermis, resulting in infection of keratinocytes and immature Langerhans cells (epidermal dendritic cells [DC]). Infected cells then migrate from site of infection to lymph nodes, where monocytes and macrophages are recruited, which become targets of infection (Martina et al., 2009).

The DENV envelope (E) glycoprotein is known to play a key role in the binding of the virions to cells, which is critical for infectivity (Anderson et al., 1992). The virus binds on the cell surface, via the E glycoprotein and viral receptors which may include heparan sulfate or the lectin Dendritic Cell-Specific Intercellular adhesion molecule-3- Grabbing Non-integrin (DC-SIGN) (Nielsen, 2009, Chen et al., 1997, Tassaneetrithep et al., 2003). The virus can also bind to cell surface immunoglobulin receptors in the presence of antibodies to the E glycoprotein or membrane precursor (pre-M) protein, (Morens, 1994). In mature dendritic cells, antibodies enhance dengue infection via Fc receptors.

Following fusion of viral and cell membranes in acidified endocytic vesicles, the viral RNA enters the cytoplasm. The viral proteins are then translated directly from the viral RNA as a single polyprotein, which is cleaved to yield three structural and seven nonstructural proteins (Henchal and Putnak, 1990). Cleavage of several of the viral proteins requires a functional viral protease encoded by the nonstructural protein NS3. The nonstructural protein NS5 is the viral RNA-dependent RNA polymerase, which assembles with several other viral proteins and several host proteins to form the replication complex. The complex transcribes the viral RNA to produce negative-strand viral RNA, which serves as the template for the production of the viral genomic RNA.

Viral protein and RNA synthesis occur predominantly in the cytoplasm of host cells. Replication begins within 15 hrs after infection. DENV replication does not significantly affect the metabolic function of the host cell as exemplified by normal levels of protein synthesis by the infected host cells (Noisakran and Perng, 2008). Replication of the virus results in amplification of infection and dissemination through the lymphatic system. As a result of this primary viremia, several cells of the mononuclear lineage, including blood-derived monocytes , myeloid DC and splenic and liver macrophages are infected (Martina et al., 2009). DENV's tropism for circulating mononuclear cells in blood and for cells residing in the spleen, lymph nodes, and bone marrow has been demonstrated in infected AG129 mice. Leukocytes also have been shown to be infected with DENV in experimentally infected nonhumans primates (Martina et al., 2009).

Downstream of dendritic cells, T-cells become activated and generate cytokines associated with vascular leakage and shock in addition to activating effector cells. Both the virus and the antibodies are involved in release of complement and anaphylatoxins which can cause or exacerbate DHF/DSS. These systems are inextricable and strongly associated with dengue pathogenesis (Nielsen, 2009). It should be noted that during secondary infections with heterologous DENV, high concentrations of DENV-specific immunoglobulin G (IgG) will complex newly produced virus that adheres to and is taken up by mononuclear cells. Following infection, mononuclear cells predominantly die by apoptosis , while abortively infected or bystander DC are stimulated to produce the bulk of mediators that are involved in inflammatory and hemostatic responses of the host. In this regard, factors that influence the amount of target cells infected, and consequently the levels of viremia, may determine the ratio of different proinflammatory and anti-inflammatory cytokines, chemokines, and other mediators, as well as the way in which the inflammatory response affects the hemostatic system (Martina et al., 2009).

5.2 Antibody response

At or a few days prior to the onset of illness, the virus can be detected in serum, plasma, circulating blood cells and other tissues for 4–5 days followed by the disappearance of DENV and antigens from the blood coincident with the appearance of specific antibodies.

The NS1 antigen may be detected in some patients for a few days after defervescence (WHO, 2009b, Pok et al., 2010). Antibody response to infection differs according to the past exposure of the host to dengue serotypes and/or other flaviviruses. Previously unexposed patients develop a primary response characterized by a slow increase of specific IgM antibodies between days 3 to 5 after the onset of illness. IgM levels peak about two weeks after the onset of symptoms and then decline generally to undetectable levels over 2-3 months. Anti-dengue serum IgG is generally detectable at low titres at the end of the first week of illness, increasing slowly and remains detectable after several months, and probably even for life. During a secondary dengue infection (a dengue infection in a host that has previously been infected by a dengue virus, or sometimes after non-dengue flavivirus vaccination or infection), IgG antibody titres rise rapidly to high levels, even in the acute phase and persists for periods lasting from 10 months to life. IgM levels at early convalescent stage are significantly lower in secondary infections than in primary ones and may be undetectable in some cases (WHO, 2009b).

5.3 Pathogenesis of severe Dengue

The pathogenesis of severe dengue is not completely understood but is likely to be multifactorial (Martina et al., 2009). Secondary infections are considered as one of the risk factors for severe dengue disease (DHF/DSS) (Thein et al., 1997, Guzman et al., 1991, Guzman et al., 1990) and form the basis of the antibody-mediated pathogenesis or antibody-dependent enhancement theory (Nielsen, 2009, Noisakran. & Perng, 2008, Martina et al., 2009). There have however been reports on the absence of association between secondary dengue or circulation of multiple serotypes and DHF/DSS (Harris et al., 2000, Morens et al., 1986). It is believed that antibody-mediated enhancement of infection either results in a high viral load or represents the link to type 2 cytokine responses (Martina et al., 2009).

Dengue cross-reactive T cells have been shown to lose their cytolytic activity (Martina et al.,2009) and once primed during primary infection with one of the dengue serotype or a member of the Flavivirus family respond vigorously (memory T-cell responses) upon exposure to a second infection releasing massive amounts of proinflammatory cytokines, which induce vascular endothelial cell activation and are the likely cause of the capillary leak syndrome and predispose to DHF and DSS (Noisakran and Perng, 2008). Involvements of the liver and endothelial cell lining of different organ systems are important factors in the pathogenesis of severe dengue. Vascular permeability is increased through mediators which promote the widening of adherens junctions. Disruption of vascular integrity and increase capillary fragility is also affected by; thrombocytopenia, platelet dysfunction and virus infection of the endothelial cells (Martine et al., 2009).

High levels of complement activation products C3a and C5a can be found in the plasma accompanied by accelerated consumption and a marked reduction of the complement components in DHF/DSS the time of defervescence and onset of plasma leakage. In severe dengue, complement can be directly activated by the NS1 dengue antigen or via the binding of heterotypic antibodies to NS1 expressed on infected cells. Production of the C5b-C9 complex subsequently triggers cellular reactions and stimulates the production of inflammatory cytokines that are associated with development of DHF/DSS. (Martina et al., 2009)

The virulence theory hypothesis states that certain dengue strains are responsible for more severe disease (Martina et al. 2009) with increased severity being associated with primary infection with DENV-1 followed by infection with DENV-2 or DENV-3. Intra-epidemic evolution of the virus has also been found to be responsible for increased severity of disease.

Hyperthermal factors, physical status of virus in viremic individuals, conditioning of neutralizing antibody assay in DENV infection, concept of vector transmission, serotype virulence, nutritional status and genetic attributes of the infected individual (Noisakran and Perng, 2008) are factors which have been associated with severe dengue (Martina et al. 2009).
The mechanism by which the dengue virus enters into the central nervous system in severe and non-severe dengue is not clearly understood. It is hypothesized that the increased capillary permeability and the effects of the "cytokine storm" play a role in the neuropathology of dengue. This is evidenced by the finding of cerebral edema even in cases of benign dengue, and which may explain the origin of severe headaches (Chaturvedi et al., 1991).

5.4 Pathogenesis of neurological Dengue

5.4.1 Primary and secondary infections

Several studies have refered to a pan-tropic nature of the dengue virus with increased documentation of its neurtopism in recent years. One pathogenesis theory of neurological dengue proposes secondary and systemic derangements as a cause. In such cases encephalopathy and not encephalitis is the primary manifestation. Although encephalopathy can exist in severe dengue as a result of multi-oragan involvement, there is a growing body of evidence in support of dengue neurotropism. This is evidenced by the documentation of neurological manifestations in both primary and secondary dengue infections (Cam et al., 2001, Hendarto and Hadinegoro, 1992, Solomon et al., 2000, Janssen et al., 1998, Thisyakorn et al., 1999). Several studies have also reported neurological manifestations as the presenting symptom of dengue infection (Pancharoen and Thisyakorn, 2001, Solomon et al., 2000, Soares et al., 2008, 2010).

5.4.2 Virus detection in the CNS

The early onset of neurological signs and symptoms in the viremic phase suggests direct CNS invasion by DENV (Lum et al., 1996, Soares st al. 2006). Studies with mice models have shown that with the intravenous inoculation of dengue Induced cytotoxic factor, there is transient compromise in the integrity of the blood brain barrier. This occurs in a dose-dependent manner, allowing leakage of protein and erythrocytes (Chaturvedi et al., 1991). Infiltration by DENV infected macrophages have also been proposed as one of the mechanisms of direct CNS invasion (Miagostovich et al., 1997).
There have been several reports of detection of dengue specific immunoglobulin IgM via enzyme linked immunoassay and dengue RNA via real-time polymerase chain reaction (RT-PCR) in the cerebrospinal fluid (Agarwal et al., 2009, Cam et al., 2001, Angibaud et al., 2001, Garcia-Rivera et al., 2009, Puccioni-Sohler et al., 2009, Thisyakorn et al., 1999). In addition studies have also supported the intrathecal synthesis of IgG (Puccioni-Sohler et al., 2009, Soares et al., 2006). Direct infection of the central nervous system (CNS) by dengue has been documented thorough virus antigen detection using immunoperoxidase stain in CNS biopsies in fatal encephalopathy cases with confirmed dengue infection (Miagostovich et al., 1997, Nogueira et al., 2002) and in CNS biopsies in fatal cases which presented with encephalitis (Pancharoen and Thisyakorn, 2001, Thisyakorn et al., 1999). Although the detection of viral antigens is not evidence of viral replication studies have identified dengue antigens in the neurons, astrocytes, microglia and Purkinje cells in autopsies and necropsies (Bhoopat et al., 1996, Ramos et al., 1998, Bordignon et al., 2008, Jessie et al., 2004). Encephalitis, apoptosis and CNS replication of dengue virus has also been observed in the neurons in the cortex and hippocampus following intracerebral inoculation of mice with

neuroadapted DENV1 viruses (Despres et al., 1998). Neuronal apoptosis has also been observed in fatal human DENV2 and DENV3 infections but the authors of the report attributed this to severe brain ischemia as dengue virus antigens were not detected via immunohistochemical staining in these cases (Limonta et al., 2007, Limonta et al., 2009).
Immunostaining for NS3 of all dengue serotypes has revealed the presence of dengue antigen in perivascular cells of the cerebrum in interferon-receptor deficient mouse models infected with dengue and in fatal cases of human dengue infection (Balsitis et al., 2009). However in the study by Balsitis et al., none of the fatal cases presented with signs of neurological involvement thus demonstrating that DENV-infected cells may be present in the central nervous system even in patients without neurological manifestations who present with classic DHF/DSS signs and symptoms (Balsitis et al., 2009).

5.4.3 Serotypes

Neurological manifestations have been documented to occur with all dengue serotypes (Kunishige et al., 2004, Ramos et al., 1998, Solomon et al., 2000), with more frequent identification of serotype 2 and 3 (Lum et al., 1996, Garcia-Rivera et al., 2009, Hendarto and Hadinegoro, 1992, Solomon et al., 2000) and less frequently with serotype 4 (Ramos et al., 1998). However in other serotype neurovirulence studies using parental and live attenuated DENV2 and DENVV3 in monkeys, specifically *Macacafascicularis* and *Macacamulatta,* lesions were less frequently observed in the central nervous system and clinical manifestations were not severe (Angsubhakorn et al., 1986, Angsubhakorn et al., 1987, Angsubhakorn et al., 1994).

5.4.4 Genetic diversity

It is important to note that most studies on clinical manifestations center on DENV serotypes as the main subdivision, with limited consideration to the genetic diversity among viruses within a serotype (Rico-Hesse, 1990, Lanciotti et al., 1994, Lanciotti et al., 1997). Animal studies using mice have shown that DENV3 genotype I , can cause neurological disease clinically and histologically if intracerebrally inoculated while genotype III (P1-64/2006) causes only asymptomatic disease with mild disease on histology (Ferreira et al., 2010). Infection with DENV3 genotype I is associated with decreased leukocytosis, the detection of viable virus concentrations in the brain and higher levels of interferon-gamma, interleukin-6 and monocyte chemoattractant protein 1 (Ferreira et al., 2010). The phenomenon that RNA viruses are known to be of low fidelity, forming numerous variants called quasispecies (Clyde et al., 2006), has been observed in acute dengue infections (Lauring and Andino, 2010).

5.4.5 Envelope protein

Substitution of aspartate-67 for asparagine-67 in DENV envelope sequences is associated with a greater electrostatically negative charge and this substitution has been identified in the sequences of viruses causing encephalitis (Barker et al., 2009). In contrast asparagine is found in the position corresponding to glycosylated asparagine-67 in DENV2, in all known flaviviruses causing hemorrhagic disease, and in 93% of sequences of viruses causing hemorrhagic fever . However, asparagine was only located in 33% (2/6) flaviviruses causing encephalitis and in 2.6% of the relevant encephalitic sequences (Barker et al., 2009).
Different amino acid substitutions have been described (Bordignon et al., 2007) and studies on the other DENV serotypes have shown an association of amino acid substitutions in E protein domain with neurovirulence (Bray et al., 1998, Kawano et al., 1993, Lee et al., 1997).

Amino acid substitution of glutamate to lysine at position 126 in E protein domain II, has been shown to contribute to DENV2 neurovirulence in mice (Hiramatsu et al., 1996, Gualano et al., 1998). Substitutions at position 62 and 203 of domain II of DENV2 E protein were also reported to alter neurovirulence (Zhao et al., 2003). Another amino acid substitution which occurs is in the alpha-helical region E400-412. This region participates in the conversion of E dimer to homotrimers and cellular attachment (Modis et al., 2004, Stiasny et al., 2005).
The position of isoleucine-209 on non-structural protein 3 (NS3) on domain 1 has been found in association with all viruses causing encephalitis (Xu et al., 2005). One such amino acid substitution observed in a study on mice neuroadapted DENV1, is valine-209 to isoleucine-209 (Bordignon et al., 2007). This coincides with the NTPase domain of DENV2 (Xu et al., 2005). A second significant neurovirulent amino acid substitution is observed in the NS3 domain II at position 435 (Bordignon et al., 2007, Despres et al., 1998) which corresponds to the beta-hairpin tip of the helicase domain (Duarte dos Santos et al., 2000).

5.4.6 Host factors

Reserch studies indicate that genetic factors are improtant and play a role in population susceptibility and disease severity (Martina et al., 2009). Host genetic predisposition has been proposed to be a risk factor in presentations such as monophasic neuromyelitis optica (NMO), a rare form of post-infectious acute disseminated encephalomyelitis (ADEM) (Miranda de Sousa et al., 2006). Non-HLA and HLA-associated genetic factors implied as predisposing factors for severe dengue include; Vitamin D receptor polymorphism, glucose-6-phosphate dehydrogenase (G6PD) deficiency, mannose-binding lectin (MBL)2, Fc_RIIa polymorphism, TNF-alpha (-308) A allele and IL-10 (-1082/-819/-592) ACC/ATA haplotype, CTLA- 4, transporters associated with antigen presentation and human platelet antigen, DC-SIGN polymorphism, HLA class I alleles A*01, A*0207, A*24, B*07, B*46, B*51 and HLA class II alleles DQ*1, DR*1, DR*4 (Martina et al., 2009). TNFalpha (-308) GG and TGFbeta1 (c25) GG genotypes have been shown to be associated with protection.

5.4.7 Ancillary studies

Ancillary investigations include lumbar puncture, neuroimaging and electroencephalogram (EEG). Lumbar puncture may be normal or may demonstrate pleocytosis with normal or mildly elevated protein and normal glucose (Muzaffar et al., 2006, Lum et al., 1996, Misra et al., 2006).
Cerebral edema has been the primary finding of neuroimaging studies using computed tomography and magnetic resonance imaging (MRI). In the prospective case control study by Cam and coworkers, MRI revealed cerebral edema (12/18) or no changes (4/18) in the majority of the patients with dengue encephalopathy, while only the minority (2/18) showed specifically scattered focal lesions (Cam et al., 2001,Muzaffar et al., 2006). EEG revealed slow background waves for the majority of the patients which resolves with clinical recovery (Angibaud et al., 2001, Arachchi et al., 2003, Lum et al., 1996, Misra et al., 2006, Wasay et al., 2008).

6. Laboratory diagnosis

Early laboratory confirmation of clinical diagnosis may be valuable as some patients progress from mild to severe disease and sometimes to death, within a short period of time. Early intervention may be life-saving. Several laboratory methodologies are available for confirming acute DENV infection and may be used singly or in combination. These include detection of the virus, viral nucleic acid, antigens and/or antibodies (Table 1). The hallmark for the laboratory diagnosis of encephalitis is the demonstration of the DENV or antigen in the tissues of the central nervous system and or the cerebrospinal fluid.

Diagnostic Method	Specimen	Time of collection after onset of symptoms	Diagnosis of acute infection
Virus isolation Serotype confirmation	Whole blood, serum, Tissue	1 to 5 days	Confirmed
Nucleic acid detection	Whole blood, serum, plasma, Tissue	1 to 5 days	Confirmed
NS1 antigen detection	Serum Tissue	1 to 6 days	Confirmed
IgM ELISA -paired seroconversion	Serum, plasma, whole blood	Acute sera (1-5 days) Convalescent sera (>15 days)	Confirmed
IgM ELISA-Single sera	Serum, plasma, whole blood	>5 days	Probable
IgM rapid test	Serum, plasma, whole blood	>5 days	Probable
IgG single serum , HI titre>1280	Serum, plasma, whole blood	>5 days	Probable
IgG (paired sera) by ELISA, HI or Neutralization test (seroconversion or 4 fold rise)	Serum, plasma, whole blood	Acute sera (1-5 days) Convalescent sera (>15 days)	Confirmed

Table 1. Summary of laboratory methods used in the diagnosis of dengue infection

Adapted from summary of operating characteristics and comparative costs of dengue diagnostic methods, and interpretation of dengue diagnostic tests from Dengue and Control (DENCO) and other studies (WHO, 2009b, Pok et al., 2010). To distinguish primary and secondary dengue infections, IgM/IgG antibody ratios are now more commonly used than the haemagglutination-inhibition test (HI) (WHO 2009).

7. Prognosis

The reported morbidity and mortality due to dengue encephalitis itself is low with most survivors recovering fully (Cam et al., 2001, Angibaud et al., 2001, Pancharoen and Thisyakorn, 2001). Documented sequelae from encephalitis included weakness and spasticity (Pancharoen and Thisyakorn, 2001) and, spasms (Soares et al., 2006). Encephalitis accompanied by post-infectious neurological manifestations however may have a prolonged recovery. Residual weakness can occur in patients with nerve palsies (Chappuis et al., 2004). Post-infectious myelitis may complicate encephalomyelitis. Myletis patients can remain symptomatic with urinary retention or spastic paraparesis (Puccioni-Sohler et al., 2009, Soares et al., 2006). Residual abnormalities in vision have been documented in cases of maculopathy, optic neuritis and neuropathy (Sanjay et al., 2008, Wen et al., 1989). The majority of deaths are associated with dengue hemorrhagic fever or dengue shock syndrome (DHF/DSS) and not with direct neurological involvement. Studies have documented an increase risk of developing DHF/DSS among patients with neurological dengue (Muzaffar et al., 2006 & Ramos et al., 1998). Infrequent causes of death have been attributed to tonsillar herniation secondary to cerebral edema (Wasay et al., 2008) and pontine hemorrhage with no underlying systemic derangement (Janssen et al., 1998).

8. Conclusion

The resurgence of dengue in the Americas and Pacific regions has been accompanied by a corresponding increase in frequency of documentation of dengue encephalitis. Dengue encephalopathy and dengue encephalitis are two distinct manifestations of neurological dengue. Although not a primary clinical manifestation, dengue encephalitis is a form of severe dengue which infrequently may occur without co-existing features of DHF and DSS. As the clinical presentation of dengue encephalitis is similar to that of other encephalitides, the diagnosis of this entity may be easily misdiagnosed. Identification of other criteria of severe and non-severe dengue will assist in greater accuracy of diagnosis of dengue encephalitis. Mortality associated with dengue encephalitis has been frequently associated with features of DHF and DSS. Although advances in unveiling the pathogenesis of dengue have been made, continued research is needed to fully elucidate the pathogenesis of the complex interplay of immunological responses, virus characteristics and host predisposing factors.

9. References

Agarwal, J. P., Bhattacharyya, P. C., Das, S. K., Sharma, M. & Gupta, M. (2009) Dengue encephalitis. *Southeast Asian Journal of Tropical Medicine and Public Health*, Vol.40, (January 2009), pp. 54-5.

Anderson, R., King, A. D. & Innes, B. L. (1992) Correlation of E protein binding with cell susceptibility to dengue 4 virus infection. *Journal General Virology*, Vol. 73 (August 1992), pp. 2155-9.

Angibaud, G., Luaute, J., Laille, M. & Gaultier, C. (2001) Brain involvement in Dengue fever. *Journal of Clinical Neuroscience*, Vol.8, (January 2001), pp.63-5.

Angsubhakorn, S., Moe, J. B., Latendresse, J. R., Ward, G. S., Ngamprochana, M., Sahaphong, S. & Bhamarapravati, N. (1986) The neurovirulence of flaviviruses in crab-eating monkeys (Macaca fascicularis). *Southeast Asian Journal of Tropical Medicine and Public Health*, Vol.17, (December 1986), pp.604-12.

Angsubhakorn, S., MOE, J. B., Marchette, N. J., Palumbo, N. E., Yoksan, S. & Bhamarapravati, N. (1987) Neurovirulence effects of dengue-2 viruses on the rhesus (Macaca mulatta) brain and spinal cord. *Southeast Asian Journal of Tropical Medicine and Public Health*, Vol. 18, (October 1987), pp.52-5.

Angsubhakorn, S., Yoksan, S., Pradermwong, A., Nitatpattana, N., Sahaphong, S. & Bhamarapravati, N. (1994) Dengue-3 (16562) PGMK 33 vaccine: neurovirulence, viremia and immune responses in Macaca fascicularis. *Southeast Asian Journal of Tropical Medicine Public Health*, Vol.25, (September 1994), pp.554-9.

Arachchi, J. K., Ajanthan, R., Lamabadusuriya, S. P. & Gunasena, S. (2003) Dengue encephalitis in a child. *Ceylon Medical Journal*, Vol.48, (December 2003), pp.144-5.

Balsitis, S. J., Coloma, J., Castro, G., Alava, A., Flores, D., Mckerrow, J. H., BEATTY, P. R. & HARRIS, E. (2009) Tropism of dengue virus in mice and humans defined by viral nonstructural protein 3-specific immunostaining. *American Journal of Tropical Medicine and Hygiene*, Vol.80, (March 2009), pp.416-24.

Barker, W. C., Mazumder, R., Vasudevan, S., Sagripanti, J. L. & WU, C. H. (2009) Sequence signatures in envelope protein may determine whether flaviviruses produce hemorrhagic or encephalitic syndromes. *Virus Genes,* Vol.39, (August 2009), pp.1-9.

Bennett, S.N., Drummond, A.J., Kapan, D.D., Suchard, M.A., Mun˜oz-Jorda´n, J.L., Pybus, O.G.,Holmes ,E.C., and Gubler, D.J.,(2010) Epidemic Dynamics Revealed in Dengue Evolution. *Molecular Biology and Evolution* Vol.27 (4), (April 2010), pp.811–818.

Bhoopat, L., Bhamarapravati, N., Attasiri, C., Yoksarn, S., Chaiwun, B., Khunamornpong, S. & Sirisanthana, V. (1996) Immunohistochemical characterization of a new monoclonal antibody reactive with dengue virus-infected cells in frozen tissue using immunoperoxidase technique. *Asian Pacific Journal of Allergy and Immunology,* Vol.14, (December 1996), pp.107-13.

Bordignon, J., Probst, C. M., Mosimann, A. L., Pavoni, D. P., Stella, V., Buck, G. A., Satproedprai, N., Fawcett, P., Zanata, S. M., DE Noronha, L., Krieger, M. A. & Duarte Dos Santos, C. N. (2008) Expression profile of interferon stimulated genes in central nervous system of mice infected with dengue virus Type-1. *Virology,* Vol.377, (August 2008), pp.319-29.

Bordignon, J., Strottmann, D. M., Mosimann, A. L., Probst, C. M., Stella, V., Noronha, L., Zanata, S. M. & DOS SANTOS, C. N. (2007) Dengue neurovirulence in mice: identification of molecular signatures in the E and NS3 helicase domains. *Journal of Medical Virology,* Vol.79, (October 2007), pp.1506-17.

Bray, M., Men, R., Tokimatsu, I. & Lai, C.-J. (1998) Genetic Determinants Responsible for Acquisition of Dengue Type 2 Virus Mouse Neurovirulence. *Journal of Virology.* Vol.72, (February 1998), pp.1647-1651.

Cam, B. V., Fonsmark, L., Hue, N. B., Phuong, N. T., Poulsen, A. & Heegaard, E. D. (2001) Prospective case-control study of encephalopathy in children with dengue hemorrhagic fever. *American Journal of Tropicalc Medicine and Hygiene,* Vol.65,(December 2001), pp.848-51.

Chappuis, F., Justafre, J. C., Duchunstang, L., Loutan, L. & Taylor, W. R. (2004) Dengue fever and long thoracic nerve palsy in a traveler returning from Thailand. *Journal of Travel Medicine,* Vol.11, (March 2004), pp.112-4.

Chaturvedi, U. C., Dhawan, R., Khanna, M. & Mathur, A. (1991) Breakdown of the blood-brain barrier during dengue virus infection of mice. *Journal of General Virology,* Vol.72, (April 1991), pp.859-866.

Chen, Y., Maguire, T., Hileman, R. E., Fromm, J. R., Esko, J. D., Linhardt, R. J. & Marks, R. M. (1997) Dengue virus infectivity depends on envelope protein binding to target cell heparan sulfate. *Nature Medicine,* Vol.3, (August 1997), pp.866-71.

Clyde, K., Kyle, J. L. & Harris, E. (2006) Recent Advances in Deciphering Viral and Host Determinants of Dengue Virus Replication and Pathogenesis. *Journal of Virology.* Vol.80,(August 2006), pp.11418-11431.

Deen, J. L., Harris, E., Wills, B., Balmaseda, A., Hammond, S. N., Rocha, C., Dung, N. M., Hung, N. T., Hien, T. T. & FARRAR, J. J. (2006) The WHO dengue classification and case definitions: time for a reassessment. *Lancet,* Vol.368, (July 2006), pp.170-3.

Despres, P., Frenkiel, M. P., Ceccaldi, P. E., Duarte Dos Santos, C. & Deubel, V. (1998) Apoptosis in the mouse central nervous system in response to infection with mouse-neurovirulent dengue viruses. *Journal of Virology*, Vol.72, (January 1998), pp.823-9.

Duarte dos Santos, C. N., Frenkiel, M. P., Courageot, M. P., Rocha, C. F., Vazeille-Falcoz, M. C., Wien, M. W., REY, F. A., DEUBEL, V. & DESPRES, P. (2000) Determinants in the envelope E protein and viral RNA helicase NS3 that influence the induction of apoptosis in response to infection with dengue type 1 virus. *Virology*, Vol.274, (September 2000), pp.292-308.

Effler, P. V., Pang, L., Kitsutani, P., Vorndam, V., Nakata, M., Ayers, T., Elm, J., Tom, T., Reiter, P., Rigau-Perez, J. G., Hayes, J. M., Mills, K., Napier, M., Clark, G. G. & Gubler, D. J. (2005) Dengue fever, Hawaii, 2001-2002. *Emerginging Infectious Disease*,Vol. 11, (May 2005), pp.742-9.

Ferreira, G. P., Figueiredo, L. B., Coelho, L. F., S, P. A., JR., Cecilio, A. B., Ferreira, P. C., Bonjardim, C. A., Arantes, R. M., Campos, M. A. & Kroon, E. G. (2010) Dengue virus 3 clinical isolates show different patterns of virulence in experimental mice infection. *Microbes and Infection*, Vol.12, (July 2010), PP.546-54.

Garcia-Rivera, E. J., Vorndam, V. & Rigau-Perez, J. G. (2009) Use of an enhanced surveillance system for encephalitis and aseptic meningitis for the detection of neurologic manifestations of dengue in Puerto Rico, 2003. *Porto Rico Health Sciences Journal*, Vol.28,(June 2009), pp.114-20.

Gould, E. A., Gallian, P., DE Lamballerie, X. & Charrel, R. N. (2010) First cases of autochthonous dengue fever and chikungunya fever in France: from bad dream to reality! *Clinical Microbiology and Infection*, Vol.16,(December 2010), pp.1702-4.

Gualano, R. C., Pryor, M. J., Cauchi, M. R., Wright, P. J. & Davidson, A. D. (1998) Identification of a major determinant of mouse neurovirulence of dengue virus type 2 using stably cloned genomic-length cDNA. *Journal of General Virology*, Vol.79 (Pt 3), (March 1998),pp.437-46.

Gubler D. 2006. Dengue/dengue haemorrhagic fever: history andcurrent status. *Novartis Found Symp*. Vol.277, pp.3–16.

Guzman, M. G. & Kouri, G. (2003) Dengue and dengue hemorrhagic fever in the Americas: lessons and challenges. *Journal Clinical Virology*,Vol. 27,(May 2003), pp.1-13.

Guzman, M. G., Kouri, G. P., Bravo, J., Soler, M., Vazquez, S. & Morier, L. (1990) Dengue hemorrhagic fever in Cuba, 1981: a retrospective seroepidemiologic study. *American Journal Tropical Medicine and Hygiene*,Vol. 42,(1990) pp.179-84.

Guzman, M. G., Kouri, G., Bravo, J., Soler, M. & Martinez, E. (1991) Sequential infection as risk factor for dengue hemorrhagic fever/dengue shock syndrome (DHF/DSS) during the 1981 dengue hemorrhagic Cuban epidemic. *Mem Inst Oswaldo Cruz*, Vol.86, (July 1991), pp.367.

Habot-Wilner, Z., Moisseiev, J., Bin, H. & Rubinovitch, B. (2005) A returned traveler with dengue fever and visual impairment. *Israel Medical Association Journal*, Vol.7, (March 2005), pp.200-1.

Halstead, S. B. (1966) Mosquito-borne haemorrhagic fevers of South and South-East Asia. *Buletin of World Health Orgaization*, Vol.35, pp. 3-15.

Harris, E., Videa, E., Perez, L., Sandoval, E., Tellez, Y., Perez, M. L., Cuadra, R., Rocha, J., Idiaquez, W., Alonso, R. E., Delgado, M. A., Campo, L. A., Acevedo, F., Gonzalez, A., Amador, J. J. & Balmaseda, A. (2000) Clinical, epidemiologic, and virologic features of dengue in the 1998 epidemic in Nicaragua. *American Journal of Tropical Medicine and Hygiene*,Vol. 63, (July 2000),pp. 5-11.

Henchal, E. A. & Putnak, J. R. (1990) The dengue viruses. *Clinical Microbiology Reviews*, Vol.3, (October 1990), pp.376-96.

Hendarto, S. K. & Hadinegoro, S. R. (1992) Dengue encephalopathy. *Acta Paediatrica Japonica*, Vol.34, (June 1992), pp.350-7.

Hiramatsu, K., Tadano, M., Men, R. & Lai, C. J. (1996) Mutational analysis of a neutralization epitope on the dengue type 2 virus (DEN2) envelope protein: monoclonal antibody resistant DEN2/DEN4 chimeras exhibit reduced mouse neurovirulence. *Virology*, Vol.224, (October 1996),pp. 437-45.

Jackson, S. T., Mullings, A., Bennett, F., Khan, C., Gordon-Strachan, G. & Rhoden, T. (2008) Dengue infection in patients presenting with neurological manifestations in a dengue endemic population. *West Indian Medical Journal*, Vol. 57, (September 2008), pp.373-6.

Janssen, H. L., Bienfait, H. P., Jansen, C. L., Van Duinen, S. G., Vriesendorp, R., Schimsheimer, R. J., Groen, J. & Osterhaus, A. D. (1998) Fatal cerebral oedema associated with primary dengue infection. *Journal of Infection*, Vol.36, (May 1998), pp.344-6.

Jessie, K., Fong, M. Y., Devi, S., Lam, S. K. & Wong, K. T. (2004) Localization of Dengue Virus in Naturally Infected Human Tissues, by Immunohistochemistry and in Situ Hybridization. *The Journal of Infectious Diseases*, Vol.189, (April 2004),pp. 1411-1418.

Kankirawatana P, Chokephaibulkit K, Puthavathana P, Yoksan S, Apintanapong S, Pongthapisit V. (2000) Dengue infection presenting with central nervous system manifestation. *Journal of Child Neurology*, Vol.15,(August 2000), pp.544-7

Kawano, H., Rostapshov, V., Rosen, L. & Lai, C. J. (1993) Genetic determinants of dengue type 4 virus neurovirulence for mice. *Journal of Virology.*, Vol.67,(November 1993), pp.6567-6575.

Koh, B. K., NG, L. C., Kita, Y., Tang, C. S., Ang, L. W., Wong, K. Y., James, L. & Goh, K. T. (2008) The 2005 dengue epidemic in Singapore: epidemiology, prevention and control. *Annals of the Academy of Medicine Singapore*, Vol.37, (July 2008), pp.538-45. Kumar, S. & Prabhakar, S. (2005) Guillain-Barre syndrome occurring in the course of dengue fever. *Neurology India*, Vol.53, (June 2005), pp.250-1.

Kunishige, M., Mitsui, T., Tan, B. H., Leong, H. N., Takasaki, T., Kurane, I., Mihara, A. & Matsumoto, T. (2004) Preferential gray matter involvement in dengue myelitis. *Neurology*, Vol.63, (November 2004),pp.1980-1.

Lambrechts, L., Chevillon, C., Albright, R. G., Thaisomboonsuk, B., Richardson, J. H., Jarman, R. G. & Scott, T. W. (2009) Genetic specificity and potential for local adaptation between dengue viruses and mosquito vectors. *BMC Evol utionary Biology*, Vol.9,(July 2009), pp.160.

Lanciotti, R. S., Lewis, J. G., Gubler, D. J. & Trent, D. W. (1994) Molecular evolution and epidemiology of dengue-3 viruses. *Journal of General Virology*, Vol.75, (January 1994), pp.65-75.

Lanciotti, R., Gubler, D. & Trent, D. (1997) Molecular evolution and phylogeny of dengue-4 viruses. Journal of General Virology, Vol.78,(September 1997), pp.2279-2284.

Lauring, A. S. & Andino, R. (2010) Quasispecies theory and the behavior of RNA viruses. *PLoS Pathogens*, Vol.6, (July 2010),e1001005.

Lee, E., Weir, R. C. & Dalgarno, L. (1997) Changes in the dengue virus major envelope protein on passaging and their localization on the three-dimensional structure of the protein. *Virology*, Vol.232, (June 1997), pp.281-90.

Lee, K. S., Lai, Y. L., Lo, S., Barkham, T., Aw, P., Ooi, P. L., Tai, J. C., Hibberd, M., Johansson, P., Khoo, S. P. & NG, L. C. (2010) Dengue virus surveillance for early warning, Singapore. *Emerging Infectious Diseases*, Vol.16,(May 2010), pp.847-9.

Limonta, D., CAPO, V., Torres, G., Perez, A. B. & Guzman, M. G. (2007) Apoptosis in tissues from fatal dengue shock syndrome. *Journal of Clinical Virology*, Vol.40, (September 2007), pp.50-4.

Limonta, D., Gonzalez, D., Capo, V., Torres, G., Perez, A. B., Rosario, D., Roche-Rodriguez, R., Alvarez, M. & Guzman, M. G. (2009) Fatal severe dengue and cell death in sickle cell disease during the 2001-2002 Havana dengue epidemic. *International Journal of Infectious Diseases*, Vol.13, (March 2009), e77-8.

Lum, L. C., Lam, S. K., Choy, Y. S., George, R. & Harun, F. (1996) Dengue encephalitis: a true entity? *American Journal of Tropical Medicine and Hygiene*, Vol.54,(March 1996), pp.256-9.

Martina, B. E., Koraka, P. & Osterhaus, A. D. (2009) Dengue virus pathogenesis: an integrated view. *Clinical Microbiol ogy Reviews*, Vol. 22, (October 2009),pp. 564-81.

Miagostovich, M. P., Ramos, R. G., Nicol, A. F., Nogueira, R. M., Cuzzi-Maya, T., Oliveira, A. V., Marchevsky, R. S., Mesquita, R. P. & Schatzmayr, H. G. (1997) Retrospective study on dengue fatal cases. *Clinical Neuropathology*, Vol.16, (July 1997), PP.204-8.

Miranda De Sousa, A., Puccioni-Sohler, M., Dias Borges, A., Fernandes Adorno, L., Papais Alvarenga, M. & Papais Alvarenga, R. M. (2006) Post-dengue neuromyelitis optica: case report of a Japanese-descendent Brazilian child. *Journal of Infection and Chemotherapy*, Vol.12, (December 2006), pp.396-8.

Misra, U. K., Kalita, J., Syam, U. K. & Dhole, T. N. (2006) Neurological manifestations of dengue virus infection. *Journal of Neurological Sciences*, Vol.244,(May 2006), pp.117-22.

Modis, Y., Ogata, S., Clements, D. & Harrison, S. C. (2004) Structure of the dengue virus envelope protein after membrane fusion. *Nature*, Vol.427, (January 2004),pp.313-319.

Moncayo, A. C., Fernandez, Z., Ortiz, D., Diallo, M., Sall, A., Hartman, S., Davis, C. T., Coffey, L., Mathiot, C. C., Tesh, R. B. & Weaver, S. C. (2004) Dengue emergence and adaptation to peridomestic mosquitoes. *Eme ging Infectious Diseases*, Vol.10, (October 2004), pp.1790-6.

Morens, D. M. (1994) Antibody-dependent enhancement of infection and the pathogenesis of viral disease. *Clinical Infectious Diseases*, Vol.19, (September 1994),pp. 500-12.

Morens, D. M., Rigau-Perez, J. G., Lopez-Correa, R. H., Moore, C. G., Ruiz-Tiben, E. E., Sather, G. E., Chiriboga, J., Eliason, D. A., Casta-Velez, A. & Woodall, J. P. (1986) Dengue in Puerto Rico, 1977: public health response to characterize and control an epidemic of multiple serotypes. *American Journal of Tropical Medicine and Hygiene*, Vol.35, (January 1986),pp.197-211.

Muzaffar, J., Venkata Krishnan, P., Gupta, N. & Kar, P. (2006) Dengue encephalitis: why we need to identify this entity in a dengue-prone region. *Singapore Medical Journal*, Vol.47, (November 2006), pp.975-7.

Natiello, M., Ritacco, V., Morales, M. A., Deodato, B., Picollo, M., Dinerstein, E. & Enria, D. (2008) Indigenous dengue fever, Buenos Aires, Argentina. *Emerging Infectious Diseases*, Vol.14, (September 2008), pp.1498-9.

Newman Dorland W.A., 2003. Dorland's Illustrated Medical Dictionary: 30th Edition. 608-9. Saunders W. B.,ISBN: 0-7216-0146-4, Philadelphia

Ng, L. C., Lam, S. & Teo, D. (2009) Epidemiology of dengue and chikungunya viruses and their potential impact on the blood supply. *ISBT Science Series* Vol. 4, (October 2009), pp.357-367.

Nielsen, D. G. (2009) The relationship of interacting immunological components in dengue pathogenesis. Virology Journal Vol. 6, (November 2009), pp.211.

Nogueira, R. M., Filippis, A. M., Coelho, J. M., Sequeira, P. C., Schatzmayr, H. G., Paiva, F. G., Ramos, A. M. & Miagostovich, M. P. (2002) Dengue virus infection of the central nervous system (CNS): a case report from Brazil. *Southeast Asian Journal of Tropical Medicine and Public Health*, Vol.33, (March 2002),pp.68-71.

Noisakran, S. & Perng, G. C. (2008) Alternate hypothesis on the pathogenesis of dengue hemorrhagic fever (DHF)/dengue shock syndrome (DSS) in dengue virus infection. *Experimental Biology and Medicine* (Maywood, N.J), Vol.233, (April 2008),pp. 401-8.

Pancharoen, C. & Thisyakorn, U. (2001) Neurological manifestations in dengue patients. Southeast *Asian Journal of Tropical Medicine and Public Health*, Vol.32, (June 2001), pp.341-5.

Pandey, B. D., Morita, K., Khanal, S. R., Takasaki, T., Miyazaki, I., Ogawa, T., Inoue, S. & Kurane, I. (2008) Dengue virus, Nepal. *Emerging Infectious Diseases*, Vol.14, (March 2008), pp.514-5.

Pok, K. Y., Lai, Y. L., Sng, J. & Ng, L. C. (2010) Evaluation of Nonstructural 1 Antigen Assays for the Diagnosis and Surveillance of Dengue in Singapore. *Vector Borne and Zoonotic Diseases*.Vol.10, (December 2010), pp.1009-16.

Puccioni-Sohler, M., Soares, C. N., Papaiz-Alvarenga, R., Castro, M. J., Faria, L. C. & Peralta, J. M. (2009) Neurologic dengue manifestations associated with intrathecal specific immune response. *Neurology* 2009 Vol 27,(October 2009) pp.1413-7

Ramos, C., Sanchez, G., Pando, R. H., Baquera, J., Hernandez, D., Mota, J., Ramos, J., Flores, A. & Llausas, E. (1998) Dengue virus in the brain of a fatal case of hemorrhagic dengue fever. *Journal of Neurovirology*, Vol.4, (August 1998), pp.465-8.

Rico-Hesse, R. (1990) Molecular evolution and distribution of dengue viruses type 1 and 2 in nature. *Virology*, Vol.174, (February 1990), pp.479-493.

Rico-Hesse, R. (2003) Microevolution and virulence of dengue viruses. *Advances Virus Research*, Vol.59,(2003), pp.315-41.

Salazar, M. I., Loroño-Pino, M. A., Farfán-ALE, J. A., Olson, K. E. & Beaty, B. J. (2010) American and American/Asian genotypes of dengue virus differ in mosquito infection efficiency: candidate molecular determinants ofproductive vector infection. *Revisita Biomed*, Vol.21, (September 2010), pp.121-1351.

Sanjay, S., Wagle, A. M. & Au Eong, K. G. (2008) Optic neuropathy associated with dengue fever. *Eye* (Lond), Vol.22, (May 2008),pp.722-4.

Singh, N., Kiedrzynski, T., Lepers, C. & Benyon, E. K. (September2005) Dengue in the Pacific--an update of the current situation. *Pacific Health Dialogue*, Vol.12, (2005), pp.111-9.

Smart, W. R. (1877) On Dengue or Dandy Fever. *British Medical Journal*, Vol. 1, (March 1877), pp.382-3.

Soares, C. N., Cabral-Castro, M. J., Peralta, J. M., Freitas, M. R. & Puccioni-Sohler, M. (2010) Meningitis determined by oligosymptomatic dengue virus type 3 infection: report of a case. *International Journal of Infectious Diseases*, Vol.14, (February 2010), e150-2.

Soares, C. N., Cabral-Castro, M., Oliveira, C., Faria, L. C., Peralta, J. M., Freitas, M. R. & Puccioni-Sohler, M. (2008) Oligosymptomatic dengue infection: a potential cause of Guillain Barre syndrome. *Arqivosde Neuro-psiquiatria*, Vol.66, (June 2008), pp.234-7.

Soares, C. N., Faria, L. C., Peralta, J. M., De Freitas, M. R. & Puccioni-Sohler, M. (2006) Dengue infection: neurological manifestations and cerebrospinal fluid (CSF) analysis. *Journal of Neurological Sciences*, Vol.249, (November 2006),pp.19-24.

Solomon, T., Dung, N. M., Vaughn, D. W., Kneen, R., Thao, L. T., Raengsakulrach, B., Loan, H. T., Day, N. P., Farrar, J., Myint, K. S., Warrell, M. J., James, W. S., Nisalak, A. & White, N. J. (2000) Neurological manifestations of dengue infection. *Lancet*, Vol.355,(March 2000), pp.1053-9.

Stiasny, K., kossl, C. & Heinz, F. X. (2005) Differences in the Postfusion Conformations of Full-Length and Truncated Class II Fusion Protein E of Tick-Borne Encephalitis Virus. *Journal of Virology*, Vol.79, (May 2005),pp.6511-6515.

Tassaneetrithep, B., Burgess, T. H., Granelli-Piperno, A., Trumpfheller, C., Finke, J., Sun, W., Eller, M. A., Pattanapanyasat, K., Sarasombath, S., Birx, D. L., Steinman, R. M., Schlesinger, S. & Marovich, M. A. (2003) DC-SIGN (CD209) mediates dengue virus infection of human dendritic cells. *The Journal of Experimental Medicine*, Vol.197, (April 2003), pp.823-9.

Thein, S., Aung, M. M., Shwe, T. N., Aye, M., Zaw, A., Aye, K., Aye, K. M. & Aaskov, J. (1997) Risk factors in dengue shock syndrome. *American Journal of Tropical Medicine and Hygiene*, Vol.56, (May 1997), pp.566-72.

Thisyakorn, U., Thisyakorn, C., limpitikul, W. & Nisalak, A. (1999) Dengue infection with central nervous system manifestations. *Southeast Asian Journal of Tropical Medicine and Public Health*, Vol.30, (September 1999), pp.504-6.

Thomas, J. G. (1880) Dengue. Public Health Papers and Reports, Vol.6, pp.136-53.

Varatharaj, A. (2010) Encephalitis in the clinical spectrum of dengue infection. *Neurology India*, Vol.58, (July 2010), pp.585-91.

Wasay, M., Channa, R., Jumani, M., Shabbir, G., Azeemuddin, M. & Zafar, A. (2008) Encephalitis and myelitis associated with dengue viral infection clinical and neuroimaging features. *Clinical Neurology Neurosurgery*, Vol.110,(June 2008), pp.635-40.

Wen, K. H., Sheu, M. M., Chung, C. B., Wang, H. Z. & Chen, C. W. (1989) [The ocular fundus findings in dengue fever].Kaohsiung *Journal of Medical Sciences*, Vol.5, (January 1989),pp.24-30.

WHO (1997) Dengue haemorrhagic fever: diagnosis, treatment, prevention and control. 2nd ed., Geneva: World Health Organization, 1997.

WHO (2009a) Dengue in the Western Pacific Region. Western Pacific Regional Office, World Health Organization.

WHO (2009b) Dengue: Guidelines for diagnosis, treatment, prevention and control. World Health Organisation and Special Programme for Research and Training in Tropical Diseases, 2009.

Xu, G., Dong, H., Shi, N., Liu, S., Zhou, A., Cheng, Z., Chen, G., Liu, J., Fang, T., Zhang, H., Gu, C., Tan, X., Ye, J., Xie, S. & Cao, G. (2007) An outbreak of dengue virus serotype 1 infection in Cixi, Ningbo, People's Republic of China, 2004, associated with a traveler from Thailand and high density of Aedes albopictus. *American Journal of Tropical Medicine and Hygiene*, Vol.76, (June 2007), pp.1182-8.

Xu, T., Sampath, A., Chao, A., Wen, D., Nanao, M., Chene, P., Vasudevan, S. G. & Lescar, J. (2005) Structure of the Dengue Virus Helicase/Nucleoside Triphosphatase Catalytic Domain at a Resolution of 2.4 *A. Journal of Virology*. Vol.79, (August 2005),pp.10278-10288.

Zhao, W., Fan, B., Hu, Z., Chen, S., Wang, P., Yuan, X., Li, X., Yu, M., Qin, E. & Yang, P. (2003) Study on the determinants of suckling mice neurovirulence of dengue 2 virus. *Sciences China Series C Life Sciences Chinese Academy of Science*.s Vol.46, (February 2003), pp.95-103.

5

Flaviviral Infections and Potential Targets for Antiviral Therapy

Andrea Baier
Department of Molecular Biology, Institute of Biotechnology, The John Paul II Catholic University of Lublin Poland

1. Introduction

The family *Flaviviridae* includes human and animal pathogenic viruses of global importance, e.g. the human flaviviruses West-Nile virus (WNV), dengue virus (DENV), Japanese encephalitis virus (JEV), tick-borne encephalitis virus (TBEV) and yellow fever virus (JEV) as well as hepacivirus hepatitis C virus (HCV). This virus family was named after the jaundice occurring in course of YFV infection, the first identified virus of the *Flaviviridae* (Monath, 1987; Halstead, 1992). In humans infections with *Flaviviridae* may lead to fulminant, hemorrhagic diseaes [YFV, DENV and omsk hemorrhagic fever virus (OHFV)], viral encephalitis [JEV, TBEV, WNV, St. Louis encephalitis virus (SLEV)] or chronic hepatitis C, formerly referred to as non-A, non-B hepatitis (HCV) (Monath & Heinz, 1996; Rice, 1996). Viruses belonging to the third genus, pestivirus, infect only animals, leading to severe disease of the host, usually followed by death [bovine viral diarrhea virus (BVDV), classical swine fever virus (CSFV) and border disease virus (BDV)] (Nettelton & Entrican, 1995).

The genus flavivirus consists of more than 70 species that are, on the basis of phylogenetic analyses, divided into 14 classes which in turn are grouped into three clusters: the mosquito-borne cluster, the tick-borne cluster and the non-vector cluster. All flaviviruses of human importance are mosquito- or tick-borne viruses. They enter through the skin by the bite of an infected arthropod, proliferating locally and spreading through the blood circulation and cross the blood-brain barrier and finally entering the central nervous system. This fact is important for further pathogenesis and unfavorable clinical outcome of the infection (King et al., 2007). Most pathogenic flaviviruses are associated with neurological diseases. The mosquito-borne encephalitic flaviviruses are grouped phylogenetically in the Japanese encephalitis serocomplex. Most tick-borne flaviviruses cause encephalitis and are mainly spread through Europe and Asia. Approximately up to 200 million new cases of infections caused by viruses of the *Flaviviridae* family are registered annually. Up to date, there is no effective antiviral therapy directed against *Flaviviridae* viruses.

Members of the family of *Flaviviridae* are small (40 to 50 nm), spheric, enveloped RNA viruses of similar structure. The genome of the viruses consists of one single-stranded, positive-sense RNA with a length of 9100 to 11000 bases [e.g. 10862 for YFV (strain 17D), 10477 for Russian spring-summer encephalitis virus (RSSEV) and approx. 9100 for HCV].

The RNA possesses a single open reading frame (ORF) flanked by 5′- and 3′- terminally located untranslated regions (5′UTR and 3′UTR respectively). In course of infection with flaviviruses the polyprotein is cleaved co- and post-translationally by proteases (Pryor et al., 1998). The amino terminus of the polyprotein is processed into 3 structural proteins. The spheric nucleocapsid is composed of one viral capsid protein (C-protein). Furthermore, it is surrounded by a lipid bilayer that is acquired for the budding of the virus particle into the lumen of intracellular vesicles. The lipid membrane contains two species of glycoproteins. Protein M, processed from a larger precursor protein (Pre-M), and the envelope protein (E-protein) form homodimers that determine the form of the virus particle. Beside the structural proteins the polyprotein is additionally processed into seven nonstructural proteins (NS1, NS2A, NS2B, NS3, NS4A, NS4B, NS5) (Westaway, 1987; Leyssen et al., 2000; Monath & Heinz, 1996; Rice, 1996). Figure 1 presents, schematically, the structure of the flavivirus polyprotein.

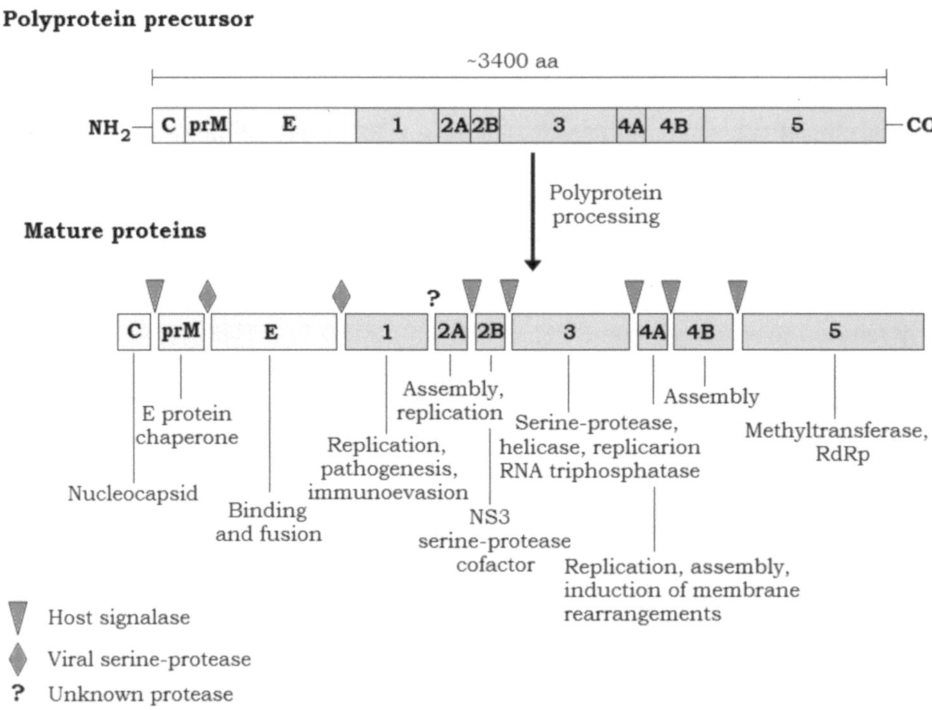

Fig. 1. Genome organization and functions of viral proteins. The polyprotein is co- and posttranslationally cleaved by host and viral proteases (as shown in the figure) into structural (light) and nonstructural (dark) protein. Putative functions of the viral proteins during viral replication are indicated

2. Viral life cycle

Genomic replication proceeds very similarly within the *Flaviviridae* family. After binding to the cell by specific receptors and entry of the virus *via* receptor-mediated endocytosis the viral RNA is uncoated by acid-catalyzed membrane fusion and translation is initiated by cap-mediated processes. The viral RNA is translated into one viral polyprotein which is co- and posttranslationally cleaved by viral and host proteases. RNA synthesis occurs in cytoplasmic replication complexes localized at the perinuclear membranes. All NS proteins appear to be involved in RNA replication. The blockade of their activities leads to inhibition of the virus propagation. The genomic RNA is encapsidated into the core shell consisting of capsid proteins, enveloped by viral surface protein embedded cellular derived lipid membranes.

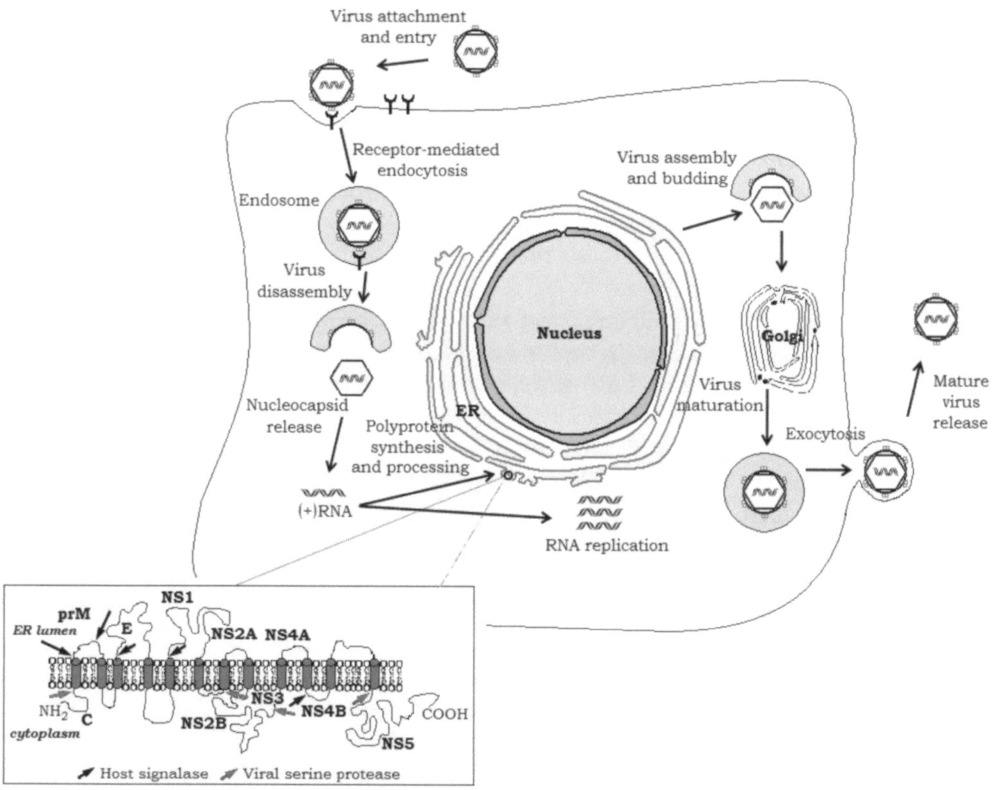

Fig. 2. Flaviviral replication cycle. After binding of the virion to the specific host receptor the virus enters the cell *via* receptor-mediated endocytosis. The low pH in the endosomes mediates fusion of viral membranes with endosomal membranes and lead to release of viral RNA. The viral RNA is translated into one polyprotein and proteolytically processed. Virus assembly consisting of coating and formation of immature virion occurs at the ER. Maturation of the immature virion particle to the mature virion occurs in the trans Golgi network. Mature virions are finally released by exocytosis

The virus particle is budded through intracellular membranes into cytoplasmic vesicles. By the cellular secretory pathway the virus particles are transported to the plasma membrane and undergo a maturation procedure. Virus release into the extracellular compartment is connected with fusion of the vesicles with the plasma membrane. Figure 2 presents the flaviviral life cycle.

3. Promising targets for antiviral therapy

The presumed replication cycle of flaviviruses consists of: I) Adsorption and receptor-mediated endocytosis; II) low pH-dependent fusion in lysosomes and uncoating; III) cap-mediated initiation of translation of the viral RNA into viral precursor polyprotein; IV) co- and post-translational proteolytic processing of the viral polyprotein by cellular and viral proteases; V) membrane-associated synthesis of template minus-strand RNA and progeny plus-strand RNA; VI) assembly of the nucleocapsid, budding of virions in the endoplasmic reticulum (ER), transport and maturation of virions in the ER and the Golgi complex, vesicle fusion and release of mature virions. Some of these steps could be potential targets for antiviral compounds.

3.1 Adsorption and receptor-mediated endocytosis

To date a broad range of receptors for members of the *Flaviviridae* have been identified. Predominantly there are oligo- and polysaccharides, particularly heparin, heparan sulfate and glycosoaminoglycans (GAGs) (Lee & Lobigs, 2000). Nevertheless, in some cases membrane proteins, especially receptor proteins, serve as binding site(s) for viruses of the *Flaviviridae* family.

The entry of flaviviruses into their target cells is mediated by the interaction of the E glycoprotein with cellular surface receptor molecules. Receptor usage is both cell type and virus-specific and contributes to host range, tissue tropism and viral pathogenicity. Highly sulfated, negatively charged glycosaminoglycans, such as heparan sulfate, can be utilized by several flaviviruses as low-affinity attachment factors that concentrate the virus on the cell surface (Agnello et al., 1999; Germi et al., 2002; Kroschewski et al., 2003; Lee & Lobings, 2008; Chen et al., 2010; Kozlovskaya et al., 2010). Similar to observations made for other *Flaviviridae,* low-density lipoprotein receptor may play a role as an attachment receptor of nonheparan sulfate adapted JEV strains in mammalian cells, and might be responsible for the neurovirulence of the virus (Chien et al., 2008). For WNV and JEV, $\alpha_v\beta_3$ integrin has been documented as a functional receptor in permissive mammalian cells. Recent studies have reported that WNV entry into embryonic mouse fibroblasts and hamster melanoma cells is independent from $\alpha_v\beta_3$ integrin, suggesting alternative receptor molecules for different cell types or strain differences (Medigeshi et al., 2008).

C-type lectin receptors (CLR) are host pathogen-recognition receptors (PRR) that are specialized in sensing invading pathogens. Several members of this family are highly expressed on myeloid cells, including monocytes macrophages and dendritic cells (DCs), and thus play a central role in activating host immune defenses (Robinson et al., 2006). Dendritic-cell specific ICAM-3-grabbing nonintegrin (DC-SIGN, CD209), one of the CLRs, possesses a critical function between viral replication in insect vectors and infection of the vertebrate host (Lozach et al., 2005; Navarro-Sanchez et al., 2003; Tassaneetrithep et al., 2003). DC-SIGN is a tetrameric C-type lectin specialized in pathogen capture and antigen presentation and is constitutively expressed on DCs, including those residing in the skin, the anatomical site of initial infection (van Kooyk & Geijtenbeek, 2003). DC-SIGN recognizes carbohydrate structures present on flavivirus glycoproteins. The remarkable capacity of DC-SIGN to distinguish between high-mannose glycans typical for insect-derived glycoproteins and the complex glycosylation of host-derived proteins (Lozach et al., 2005; van Kooyk & Geijtenbeek, 2003) implies that flaviviruses have evolved an elegant strategy to initiate infection of human cells by taking advantage of the ligand specificity of this PRR.

3.2 Low pH-dependent fusion in lysosomes and uncoating

After the attachment of an enveloped virus to the cell surface receptors, the fusion of the viral envelope with the host membrane follows. This process is mediated by virus-specific fusion proteins that merge the viral and cellular membranes. The fusion proteins contain a striking motif, so-called fusion peptide, that becomes exposed in course of conformational changes, and is inserted into the target membrane. To date two different classes of fusion proteins have been described. The proteins (class I and II) differ dramatically in their structure and molecular architecture (Weissenhorn et al., 1999; Colman & Lawrence, 2003). The fusion protein of class I is represented by hemagglutinin of influenza virus and of other related viruses (Wilson et al., 1981; Weissenhorn et al., 1999). Class II fusion protein is represented by the E protein of flaviviruses (Modis et al., 2003). The fusion of the viral and host membranes may occur at neutral or alternatively at lowered pH in endocytic vesicles. *Flaviviridae* require acidic pH for successful fusion with the cell membrane, followed by uncoating of the virus (Bressanelli et al., 2004). As demonstrated for DENV-2 and TBEV at neutral pH, the envelope glycoproteins (in the form of homodimers or homotrimers, respectively) are so closely packed that the viral membrane is practically inaccessible and fusion does not occur. The lowered pH leads to changes of the conformation of envelope glycoproteins. In course of these conformational alterations, fragments of the surface area of the viral membrane will be exposed, making penetration of the virus particle into the cell possible (Bressanelli et al., 2004). A major role in this process is given to several conserved histidine residues of protein E. Mutagenesis confirmed the function and importance of initial pH-sensing and fusion-protein refolding (Fritz et al., 2008; Harrison, 2008).

3.3 Cap-mediated initiation of translation of the viral RNA into viral precursor polyprotein

Signals required for replication of plus-strand RNA viruses are usually located in the 5'-terminal regions of the template strands. They act as promoter elements for initiation of minus- and plus-strand RNA synthesis. In flaviviruses, the translation is initiated by a process called capping. The cap is an unique structure found at the 5´-terminus of viral and cellular eukaryotic mRNA, which is important for mRNA stability and binding to the ribosome during translation. The viral mRNA capping is a cotranscriptional modification resulting from three reactions mediated by viral enzymes: (1) 5´-triphosphate of the mRNA is converted to diphosphate by an RNA triphosphatase (encoded in the NS3 protein). (2) Transfer of guanosine monophosphate (GMP) from GTP to the 5´-diphosphate RNA to form a 5′-5′ triphosphate linkage, typical for cap structures. This reaction is mediated by a guanylyltransferase. (3) The transferred guanosine moiety is methylated at the N7 position by guanine-N7 RNA MTase and forms the cap0 structure m^7GpppN (Egloff et al., 2002; Ray et al., 2006). A second methylation at the first nucleotide yields a cap1 m^7GpppN^m and additionally at the second to cap2 $m^7GpppN^mN^m$. Sequence analysis revealed the presence of RNA GTase, N7 MTase and 2′-O MTase within the NH_2-terminal domain of the NS5 protein of flaviviruses.

3.4 Co- and post-translational proteolytic processing of the viral polyprotein by cellular and viral proteases

The flaviviral polyprotein is processed by host and viral proteases. The viral trypsin-like serine protease is localized at the NH_2-terminal domain of NS3. The viral enzyme catalyzes the cleavages at C-prM, NS2A-NS2B, NS2B-NS3, NS3-NS4A, NS4A-NS4B and NS4B-NS5. It has a preference for basic amino acids, like Arg-Arg, Arg-Lys, Lys-Arg or Gln-Arg) at position P1 and P2 followed by Gly, Ala or Ser at P1′ (Chambers et al., 1990). The host signal peptidase is responsible for cleavage at prM-E and E-NS1 (Speight et al., 1988; Nowak et al., 1989; Falgout & Markoff, 1995). The NS3 protease activity is dependent from its cofactor, a 40-amino acid region of NS2B. This protein fulfils the function of a chaperone, like stabilization of the latter protein, and is responsible for membrane association of the NS2B/NS3 complex. It was shown that a non-cleavable, soluble form obtained by substitution of the linker between NS2B and NS3 revealed a very active protease (Leung et al., 2001). From this results that the cleavage of NS2B-NS3 is not necessary for protease activity. Comparison of NS2B/NS3 full-length protein and NS2B/NS3 protease domain demonstrated the marginal influence of the NS3 nucleoside triphosphatase (NTPase)/helicase domain towards the protease activity. On the opposite site, the unwinding activity of the NS3 protein is significantly decreased by fusion with NS2B using DNA substrate (Chernov et al., 2008). Since this protein is essentially involved in the formation of the replication complex, it is an attractive target for potential antivirals.

3.5 Metabolism of RNA - membrane-associated synthesis of templated minus-strand RNA and progeny plus-strand RNA

The negative-stranded RNA of viruses is synthesized with the use of the parental positive-strand RNA as template. The resulting negative-strand RNA is then used as template for the synthesis of the positive-strand progeny RNA, that is then assembled into viral particles. Since the negative and positive oriented RNA strands are complementary, the NS3-associated helicase activity appears to be necessary for strand separation. NTPase/helicases are in general nucleoside triphosphate-dependent ubiquitous proteins, capable of enzymatic unwinding of double-stranded DNA or RNA structures by disrupting the hydrogen bonds that keep the two strands together. Approximately 80% of all known plus-strand RNA viruses possess at least one NTPase/helicase. The protein consists of three equally-sized structural domains separated by deep clefts. Domains 1 and 3 share with each other a more extensive interface than either of them shares with domain 2. In consequence, the clefts between domains 1 and 2 and domains 2 and 3 are the largest. The domain 2 is flexibly linked to the other two and could undergo a rigid movement relative to domains 1 and 3.

Domains 1 and 2 host seven conserved amino acid sequences, characteristic for the majority of known NTPase/helicases within superfamily II (Kadare & Haenni, 1997).

Some of the motifs are attributed to defined function of the enzyme. The motifs I and II, so called Walker motifs A and B, have been described as a key part of the NTP binding pocket. Walker motif A binds to the terminal phosphate group of the NTP and the Walker motif B builds a chelate complex with the Mg^{2+} ion of the Mg^{2+} – NTP complex (Walker et al., 1982). In the absence of substrate, the residues of the Walker motifs bind one to the other, and to the residues of the conserved T-A-T sequence of motif III. This motif is part of a flexible "switch sequence" connecting domains 1 and 2, which transduces the energy resulting from NTP hydrolysis and participates in the conformational changes induced by NTP binding (Matson & Kaiser-Rogers, 1990).

Another main target for potential antivirals within the replication complex is the RNA-dependent RNA polymerase. The enzyme facilitates the synthesis of both the negative-strand RNA intermediate, complementary to the viral genome, and the the positive-strand RNA complementary to the negative-strand intermediate. The investigated fragment of NS5 is folded in the characteristic fingers, palm, and thumb subdomains. The finger subdomain contains a region, the "fingertips", that displays the same fold with reverse transcriptases (RTs). Comparison with the known structures of the RTs showed that residues from the palm and fingertips are structurally equivalent (Bressanelli et al., 1999). Conserved clusters between *Flaviviridae, Picornaviridae* families and retroviruses in defined regions of the molecular surface are: (1) the RNA and NTP binding groove, (2) the back of the thumb, (3) the NTP tunnel, and (4) acidic path at the top-front of the fingers. The back surface of the thumb could be conceivably a site of interaction with other components of the replication complex mentioned above or cellular proteins (Bressanelli et al., 1999). Due to the fact that human cells lack RNA-dependent RNA or DNA polymerases, this protein is the most promising and beside the protease activity best examined enzyme within the flaviviral nonstructural proteins.

3.6 Assembly of the nucleocapsid, budding of virions in ER, transport and maturation of virions in the ER and the Golgi complex, vesicle fusion and release of mature virions

Progeny virions are assembled by encapsidating the genomic RNA into the core shell of capsid proteins, enveloped by two viral surface proteins (prM and E) embedded into host-derived lipid membranes. Although the intracellular assembly of flaviviruses is not completely understood, the viral morphogenesis takes place by budding through intracellular membranes into cytoplasmic vesicles (Heinz & Allison, 2003). Virus assembly intermediates or nucleocapsid particles during the replication process of the flaviviruses have rarely been visualized by electron microscopy, and viral particles first become visible at the intracellular membrane compartment in infected cells. A study using cryo-immunoelectron microscopy has described the nucleocapsid particles of Kunjin virus. Intracellular viral particles appear to be present within the lumen of the rough endoplasmic reticulum, which are then transported to the plasma membrane *via* the cellular secretory pathway (Mackenzie & Westaway, 2001). During the transport to the plasma membrane, the intracellular viral particles undergo the maturation process. Glycans on prM and E proteins are modified by trimming and terminal addition of sugar residues (Mason, 1989; Heinz et al., 1994). The N-terminal fragment of prM is cleaved by furin or a related protease in the trans-Golgi apparatus, and this cleavage is prevented by elevation of the pH in acidic intracellular compartments (Heinz et al., 1994; Stadler et al., 1997). This prM cleavage is generally considered to distinguish extracellular viral particles from intracellular viral particles and is required for converting immature virions into mature virions characterized by the ability being highly infectious and to induce cell fusion (Allison et al., 1995; Elshuber et al., 2003). The uncleaved prM interacts with E protein, forms a fusion-inactive prM/E heterodimer, and keeps E protein from undergoing an acid-induced conformational change during the transport to the plasma membrane (Guirakhoo et al., 1991; 1992). Fusion of the vesicles with the plasma membrane releases the large amount of progeny virions into the extracellular compartment (Mason, 1989).

4. Potential inhibitors

4.1 Viral attachment and entry

The lowered pH leads to conformational changes of envelope glycoprotein. In course of these conformational alterations, fragments of the surface area of the viral membrane will be exposed, making penetration of the virus particle into the cell possible (Bressanelli et al., 2004). In this context, it is likely that compounds or short peptides competing with the regions of E protein which mediate the low pH-induced rearrangements of the structure of the virus surface would be potential antivirals. Another mechanism of action of potential flavivirus inhibitors of fusion and uncoating could be a reduction of the pH-gradient between acidified and pH-neutral cell compartments. The macrolide antibiotic bafilomycin A1 (Baf-A1, Fig. 3), a specific inhibitor of vacuolar-type H(+)-ATPase, is commonly used to demonstrate the requirement of low endosomal pH for viral uncoating (Bayer, et al., 1998; Nawa, 1998; Natale & McCullough, 1998). Treatment of the cell with the compound induced complete disappearance of acidified cell compartments. The effect of Baf-A1 is concentration-dependent. As demonstrated for JEV growth in Vero cells, the rate of infection decreases proportionally to the degree of depletion of the pH-lowered compartments (Andoh, 1998). Nevertheless, there are indications that Baf-A1 acts additionally on further intracellular processes, like blockade of transport from early to late endosomes. Since the early endosomes are suspected to lack components essential for uncoating, this activity of Baf-A1 could result in a further antiviral mechanism of action of the compound (Bayer et al., 1998).

Stem peptides and their interaction sites along the core trimer are potential targets for inhibition. The presence of a DENV derived peptide blocks infection by the flaviviruses DENV and WNV (Hrobowski et al., 2005). The hydrophobic pocket in the hinge region between domains I and II is thought to be a highly conserved structure amongst the flaviviruses. By virtual screening and followed biological tests Kampmann et al. identified two peptides (Fig. 3) which are able to block WNV and/or YFV infection with IC_{50} values in low micromolar range (Kampmann et al., 2009).

4.2 Enzyme activities associated with NS3 and NS5 proteins

The flavivirus proteases recognize cleavage sites containing dibasic amino acid residues (at positions P1 and P2) and a small amino acid side chain (position P1'). Therefore protease inhibitors like benzamidine and PMSF are inactive against flaviviral NS3 proteases. Several compounds capable of inhibiting the protease activity of NS3 have been identified. Some are short peptides that mimic the protease cleavage site, and thus competitively inhibit NS3 protease activity by binding to its catalytic site. Recently, experiments using palmatine (Fig. 3) as protease inhibitor showed inhibitory effects towards WNV (Jia et al., 2010).

Using a high-throuput system and molecular modelling a substrate competitive inhibitor (Fig. 3) of the WNV protease activity was detected by Mueller et al. (Mueller et al., 2008). An extensive study of pyrazole derivatives (Fig. 3) showed effectiveness in low micromolar range (Sidique et al., 2009). These tested analogues possess higher stability in aqueous buffer then former tested compounds (Johnston et al., 2007).

The NS3-associated NTPase is inhibited by a broad range of nucleotide analogues (Fig. 3) either with a modified nucleobase, e.g. ribavirin-5'-triphosphate, paclitaxel and some ring expanded nucleosides (RENs) triphosphates (Borowski et al., 2000; Borowski et al., 2002; Zhang et al., 2003a; Zhang et al., 2003b), or by nucleotide derivatives that possess a nonhydrolysable bound between the beta- and gamma-phosphates (unpublished data). Nevertheless, inhibition was mostly obtained under selective reaction conditions and the antiviral effect of the compounds as well as the exact *in vivo* mechanism of action is unclear.

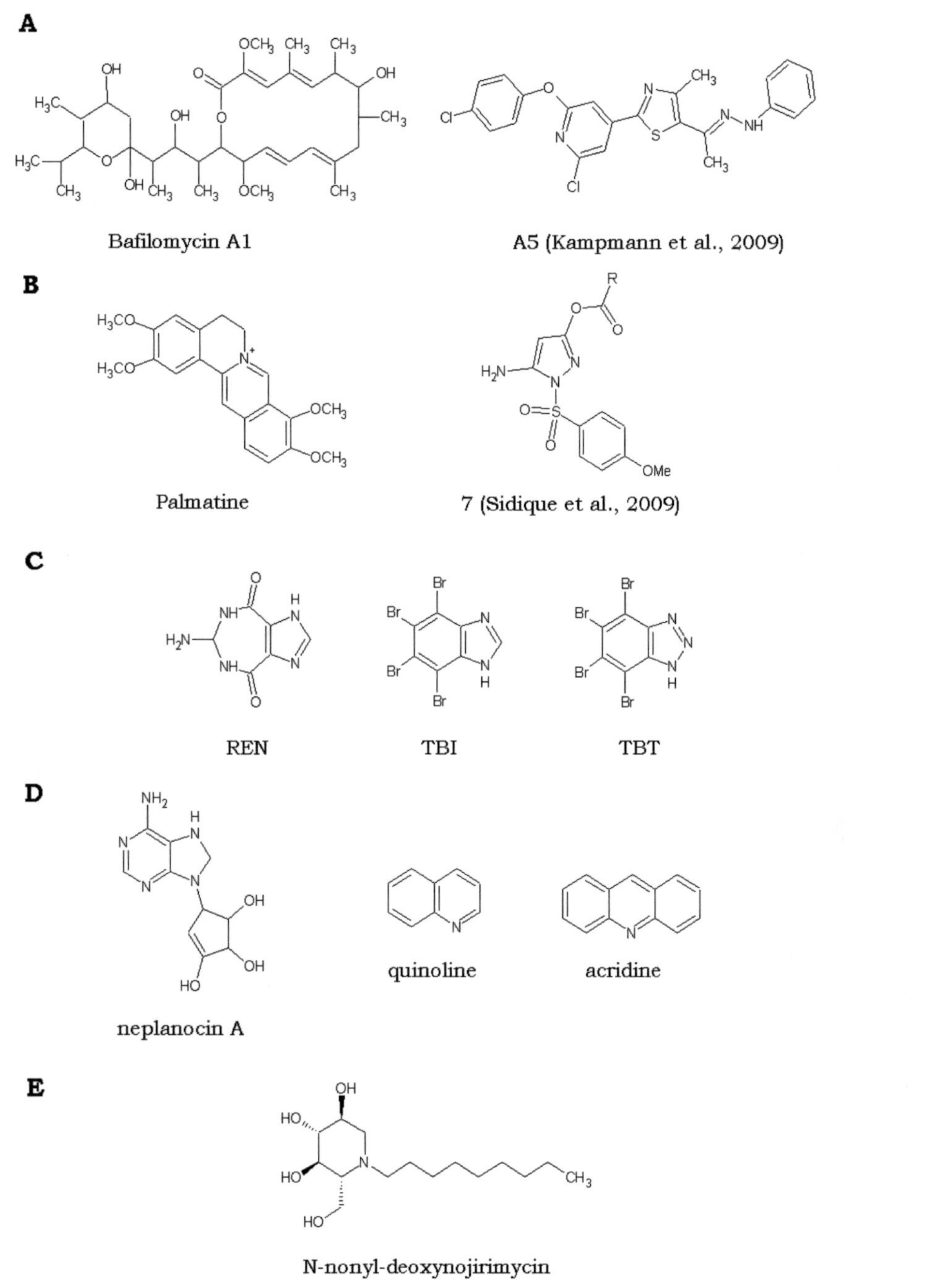

Fig. 3. Structures of antiflaviviral substances. Each panel shows inhibitors from different steps during viral replication: (A) entry, (B) polyprotein processing, (C) replication (NS3 NTPase/helicase activity), (D) replication (NS5 MTase/RdRp activities), and (E) viral maturation and release

The second promising target for potential antivirals is the viral NS5 protein-associated methyltransferase. The majority of the viral and cellular methyltransferases could be inhibited by derivatives of S-adenosylmethionine (SAM), the S-adenosylhomocysteine (SAH) (De Clercq, 1993). In this context, specific inhibitors of a cellular SAH hydrolase might inhibit the replication of *Flaviviridae* RNA, as demonstrated for rhabdoviruses or reoviruses (De Clercq, 1993). Such substances have already been found. For example, neplanocin A (Fig. 3), a naturally occurring carbocyclic nucleoside, and related abacavir and carbovir, in which the absence of a true glycosidic bond makes the compounds chemically more stable, as they are not susceptible to enzymatic cleavage by SAH hydrolase (Song et al., 2001). A further possibility to inhibit the interactions between cap-structure and its target protein, eucaryotic initiation factor 4E (eIF4E), is the reduction of the affinity of the last to the ligand. There are findings suggesting strongly that this affinity is regulated by intracellular protein phosphorylation taking place in the cap-structure-binding pocket of eIF4E (Scheper & Proud, 2002).

The majority of currently known HCV polymerase inhibitors fall into two main categories, according to their chemical structure and their mechanism of action. There are nucleoside analogue inhibitors and non-nucleoside inhibitors. Recently a third class of compounds, mimicking the pyrophosphate group and displaying an ability to inhibit RdRp, was separated.

All nucleoside analogues appear to inhibit the polymerase activity in a similar manner. After penetration into the cell, the compounds undergo intracellular phosphorylation to the corresponding triphosphate. Subsequently the nucleotide analogues are incorporated by the viral polymerase into the growing nucleic acid chain. This leads, in turn, to an increased error frequency of the polymerase and, in consequence, to early termination of the elongation reaction. The second category of RdRp inhibitors comprises structurally and chemically heterogenous compounds, not related to the non-nucleosides or nucleotides. The substances are not incorporated into growing DNA or RNA strand. The compounds inhibit the polymerase indirectly by binding to the enzyme in a reversible and non-competitive manner. A third category of polymerase inhibitors consists of the chemically and structurally homogenous pyrophosphate mimics possessing a diketo acid moiety. The mechanism by which the compounds exert their inhibitory effect is the blockade of the active site of the enzyme. Thus, the binding of the phosphoryl groups of the nucleotide substrate is blocked and formation of complexes Mg^{2+}-NTP or Mn^{2+}-NTP is abolished.

Recently, several small anti-WNV compounds were identified belonging to four different structural classes including pyrazolines, xanthanes, acridines, and quinolines (Goodell et al., 2006, Fig. 3).

4.3 Maturation and release

Endoplasmic reticulum alpha-glucosidase inhibitors block the trimming stem in the course of N-linked glycosylation, and eliminate the production of several ER-budding viruses. The iminosugar derivative N-nonyl-deoxynojirimycin (Fig. 3) was found to inhibit the replication of JEV and DENV significantly (Wu et al., 2002). This effect was probably mediated by inhibition of secretion of the viral glycoproteins E and NS1. The latter protein is known to be essential for flavivirus replication (Lindenbach & Rice, 1997).

5. Conclusion

Due to the fact that flaviviruses are arthropod-borne viruses their spreading around the world is difficult to control. Several strategies in case of YFV or DENV were successful for a short period but there is no way for complete eradication of all those arthropods. Especially the health infrastructure in most epidemic countries in South-East Asia, Africa or Latin America makes the fight against the arthropods and viruses difficult.

Our aims for the future should be to force all strength to develop vaccines against the most severe infection which are available for people living in endemic areas of the world, not only for industrial countries.

Until today no antiviral therapies are effective against flaviviruses. There is an urgent need for new molecules that block replication and/or modulate immune response. Much effort was done during last decades to resolve the virus structures and to examine their life cycles. Further step is the identification of potential antiviral targets. Screening of huge libraries of compounds for their inhibitory effect have been proven as the most promising strategy in the search of antiflaviviral therapy. Unfortunately, at the moment no candidates are detected possessing high activity on the one hand and being less toxic towards human cells. Furthermore, another problem which is already known from HIV therapy is the resistance development by viruses through mutation at the target site.

6. References

Agnello, V.; Abel, G.; Elfahal, M.; Knight, G.B. & Zhang, Q.X. (1999). Hepatitis C virus and other Flaviviridae viruses enter cells via low density lipoprotein receptor. *Proceedings of National Academy of the Sciences USA*, Vol.96, pp. 12766-12771

Allison, S.L.; Schalich, J.; Stiasny, K.; Mandl, C.W.; Kunz, C. & Heinz, F.X. (1995). Oligomeric rearrangement of tick-borne encephalitis virus envelope proteins induced by an acidic pH. *Journal of Virology*, Vol.69, pp. 695-700

Andoh, T.; Kawamata, H.; Umatake, M.; Terasawa, K.; Takegami, T. & Ochiai, H. (1998). Effect of bafilomycin A1 on the growth of Japanese encephalitis virus in Vero cells. *Journal of Neurovirology*, Vol.4, pp. 627-631

Bayer, N.; Schober, D.; Prchla, E.; Murphy, R.F.; Blaas, D. & Fuchs, R. (1998). Effect of bafilomycin A1 and nocodazole on endocytic transport in HeLa cells: implication for viral uncoating and infection. *Journal of Virol*ogy, Vol.72, pp. 9645-9655

Borowski, P.; Mueller, O.; Niebuhr, A.; Kalitzky, M.; Hwang, L.H.; Schmitz, H.; Siwecka, M. & Kulikowski, T. (2000). ATP-binding domain of NTPase/helicase as target for hepatitis C antiviral therapy. *Acta Biochimica Polonica*, Vol.47, pp. 173–180

Borowski, P.; Niebuhr, A.; Schmitz, P.; Hosmane, R.S.; Bretner, M.; Siwecka, M. & Kulikowski, T. (2002). NTPase/helicase of Flaviviridae: inhibitors and inhibition of the enzyme. *Acta Biochimica Polonica*, Vol.49, pp. 597–614

Bressanelli, S.; Tomei, L.; Roussel, A.; Incitti, I.; Vitale R.L.; Mathieu, M.; De Francesco, R. & Rey, F.A. (1999). Crystal structure of the RNA-dependent RNA polymerase of the hepatitis c virus. *Proceedings of the National Acadamy of Sciences USA*, Vol.96, pp. 13034-13039

Bressanelli, S.; Stiasny, K.; Allison, S.; Stura, E.; Duquerroy, S.; Lescar, J.; Heinz, F.X. & Rey, F. (2004). Structure of flavivirus envelope glycoprotein in its low-pH-induced membrane fusion conformation. *EMBO Journal*, Vol.23, pp. 728-738

Chambers, T.J.; Weir, R.C.; Grakoui, A.; McCourt, D.W.; Bazan, J.F.; Fletterick, R.J. & Rice, C.M. (1999). Evidence that the N-terminal domain of nonstructural protein NS3 from yellow fever virus is a serine protease responsible for site-specific cleavages in the viral polyprotein. *Proceedings of the National Academy of Sciences USA,* Vol.87, pp. 8898–8902

Chen, H.L.; Her, S.Y.; Huang, K.C.; Cheng, H.T.; Wu, C.W.; Wu, S.C. & Cheng, J.W. (2010). Identification of a heparin binding peptide from the Japanese encephalitis virus envelope protein. *Biopolymers,* Vol.94, pp. 331-338

Chernov, A.V.; Shiryaev, S.A.; Aleshin, A.E.; Ratnikov, B.I.; Smith, J.W.; Liddington, R.C. & Strongin, A.Y. (2008). The two-component NS2B-NS3 proteinase represses DNA unwinding activity of the West Nile virus NS3 helicase. *Journal of Biological Chemistry,* Vol.283, pp. 17270–17278

Chien, Y.J.; Chen, W.J.; Hsu, W.L. & Chiou, S.S. (2008). Bovine lactoferrin inhibits Japanese encephalitis virus by binding to heparan sulfate and receptor for low density lipoprotein. *Virology,* Vol.379, pp. 143-151

Chu, J.J. & Ng, M.L. (2003). Characterization of a 105-kDa plasma membrane associated glycoprotein that is involved in West Nile virus binding and infection. *Virology,* Vol.312, pp. 458–469

Chu, J.J. & Ng, M.L. (2004). Interaction of West Nile virus with alpha v beta 3 integrin mediates virus entry into cells. *Journal of Biological Chemistry,* Vol.279, pp. 54533-54541

Colman, P.M. & Lawrence, M.C. (2003). The structural biology of type I viral membrane fusion. *Nature Reviews in Molecular and Cellular Biology,* Vol.4, pp. 309-319

De Clercq E. (1993). Antiviral agents: characteristic activity spectrum depending on the molecular target with which they interact. *Advances in Virus Research,* Vol.42, pp. 1-55

Egloff, M.P.; Benarroch, D.; Selisko, B.; Romette, J.L. & Canard, B. (2002). An RNA cap (nucleoside-2′-O-)-methyltransferase in the flavivirus RNA polymerase NS5: crystal structure and functional characterization. *EMBO Journal,* Vol.21, pp. 2757–2768

Elshuber, S.; Allison, S.L.; Heinz, F.X. & Mandl, C.W. (2003). Cleavage of protein prM is necessary for infection of BHK-21 cells by tick-borne encephalitis virus. *Journal of General Virology,* Vol. 84, pp. 183-191

Falgout, B. & Markoff, L. (1995). Evidence that flavivirus NS1-NS2A cleavage is mediated by a membrane-bound host protease in the endoplasmic reticulum. *Journal of Virology,* Vol.69, pp. 7232–7243

Fritz, R.; Stiasny, K. & Heinz, F.X. (2008). Identification of specific histidines as pH sensors in flavivirus membrane fusion. *The Journal of Cell Biology,* Vol.183, pp. 353–361

Germi, R.; Crance, J.M.; Garin, D.; Guimet, J.; Lortat-Jacob, H.; Ruigrok, R.W; Zarski, J.P. & Drouet, E. (2002). Heparan sulfate-mediated binding of infectious dengue virus type 2 and yellow fever virus. *Virology,* Vol.292, pp. 162-168

Goodell, J.R.; Puig-Basagoiti, F.; Forshey, B.M.; Shi, P.Y. & Ferguson D.M. (2006). Identification of compounds with anti-West Nile Virus activity. *Journal of Medicinal Chemistry,* Vol.49, pp. 2127-2137

Guirakhoo, F.; Heinz, F.X.; Mandl, C.W.; Holzmann, H. & Kunz, C. (1991). Fusion activity of flaviviruses: comparison of mature and immature (prM-containing) tick-borne encephalitis virions. *Journal of General Virology,* Vol.72, pp. 1323-1329

Guirakhoo, F.; Bolin, R.A. & Roehrig, J.T. (1992). The Murray Valley encephalitis virus prM protein confers acid resistance to virus particles and alters the expression of epitopes within the R2 domain of E glycoprotein. *Virology*, Vol.191, pp. 921-931

Harrison, S.C. (2008). The pH sensor for flavivirus membrane fusion. *Journal of Cellular Biology*, Vol.183, pp. 177–179

Halstead, S.B. (1992). The XXth century dengue pandemic: need for survieillance and research. *World Health StatQ*, Vol.45, pp. 292-298

Heinz, F.X.; Stiasny, K.; Puschner-Auer, G.; Holzmann, H.; Allison, S.L.; Mandl, C. & Kunz, C. (1994). Structural changes and functional control of the tick-borne encephalitis virus glycoprotein E by the heterodimeric association with proteins prM. *Virology*, Vol.198, pp. 109-117

Heinz, F.X. & Allison, S.L. (2003). Flavivirus structure and membrane fusion. *Advances in Virus Research*, Vol.59, pp. 63-97

Hrobowski, Y.M.; Garry, R.F. & Michael, S.F. (2005). Peptide inhibitors of dengue virus and West Nile virus infectivity. *Virology Journal*, Vol.2,pp. 49

Jia, F.; Zou, G.; Fan, J. & Yuan, Z. (2010). Identification of palmatine as an inhibitor of West Nile virus. *Archives in Virology*, Vol.155, pp. 1325–1329

Johnston, P.A.; Phillips, J.; Shun, T.Y.; Shinde, S.; Lazo, J.S.; Huryn, D.M.; Myers, M.C.; Ratnikov, B.; Smith, J.W.; Su, Y.; Dahl, R.; Cosford, N.D.P.; Shiryaev, S.A. & Strongin, A.Y. (2007). *Assay and Drug Development Technologies*, Vol.5, pp. 737-750

Kadare, G. & Haenni, A. (1997). Virus-encoded RNA helicase. *Journal of Virology*, Vol.71, pp. 2583-2590

Kampmann, T.; Yennamallia, R.; Campbella, P.; Stoermerc, M.J.; airlie, D.P.; Kobea, B. & Young P.R. (2009). In silico screening of small molecule libraries using the dengue virus envelope E protein has identified compounds with antiviral activity against multiple flaviviruses. *Antiviral Research*, Vol.84, pp. 234–241

King, N.J.; Getts, D.R.; Getts, M.T.; Rana, S.; Shrestha, B. & Kesson, A.M. (2007). Immunopathology of flavivirus infections. *Immunology & Cell Biology*, Vol.85, pp. 33–42

Kozlovskaya, L.I.; Osolodkin, D.I.; Shevtsova, A.S.; Romanova, L.I.; Rogova, Y.V.; Dzhivanian, T.I.; Lyapustin, V.N.; Pivanova, G.P.; Gmyl, A.P.; Palyulin, V.A. & Karganova, G.G. (2010). GAG-binding variants of tick-borne encephalitis virus. *Virology*, Vol.398, pp. 262-272

Kroschewski, H.; Allison, S.L.; Heinz, F.X. & Mandl, C.W. (2003). Role of heparin sulfate for attachment and entry of tick-borne encephalitis virus. *Virology*, Vol.308, pp. 92-100

Lee, E. & Lobigs, M. (2008). E protein domain III determinants of yellow fever virus 17D vaccine strain enhance binding to glycosaminoglycans, impede virus spread, and attenuate virulence. *Journal of Virology*, Vol.82, pp. 6024-6033

Lee, E. & Lobigs, M. (2000). Substitutions at the Putative Receptor-Binding Site of an Encephalitic Flavivirus Alter Virulence and Host Cell Tropism and Reveal a Role for Glycosaminoglycans in Entry. *Journal of Virology*, Vol.74, pp. 8867-8875

Leung, D.; Schroder, K.; White, H.; Fang, N.X.; Stoermer, M.J.; Abbenante, G.; Martin, J.L.; Young, P.R. & Fairlie, D.P. (2001). Activity of recombinant dengue 2 virus NS3 protease in the presence of a truncated NS2B co-factor, small peptide substrates, and inhibitors. *Journal of Biology Chemistry*, Vol.276, pp. 45762–45771

Leyssen, P.; De Clercq, E. & Neyts, J. (2000). Perspectives for the treatment of infections with Flaviviridae. *Clinical Microbiology Reviews*, Vol.13, pp. 67-82

Lindenbach, B.D. & Rice, C.M. (1997). Trans-complementation of yellow fever virus NS1 reveal a role in early RNA replication. *Journal of Virology*, Vol.71, pp. 9608–9617

Lozach, P.Y.; Burleigh, L.; Staropoli, I.; Navarro-Sanchez, E.; Harriague, J.; Virelizier, J.L.; Rey, F.A.; Despres, P.; Arenzana-Seisdedos, F. & Amara, A. (2005). Dendritic cell-specific intercellular adhesion molecule 3-grabbing non-integrin (DC-SIGN)-mediated enhancement of dengue virus infection is independent of DC-SIGN internalization signals. *Journal of Biological Chemistry*, Vol.280, pp. 23698–23708

Mackenzie, J.M. & Westaway E.G. (2001). Assembly and Maturation of the Flavivirus Kunjin Virus Appear To Occur in the Rough Endoplasmic Reticulum and along the Secretory Pathway, Respectively. *Journal of Virology*, Vol.75, pp. 10787–10799

Mason, P.W. (1989). Maturation of Japanese encephalitis virus glycoproteins produced by infected mammalian and mosquito cells. *Virology*, Vol. 169, pp. 354-364

Matson, S.W. & Kaiser-Rogers, K.A. (1990). DNA helicases. *Annual Reviews in Biochemistry*, Vol.59, pp. 289–329

Medigeshi, G.R.; Hirsch, A.J.; Streblow, D.N.; Nikolich-Zugich, J. & Nelson, J.A. (2008). West Nile virus entry requires cholesterol-rich membrane microdomains and is independent of avb3 integrin. *Journal of Virology*, Vol.82, 5212-5219

Modis, Y.; Ogata, S.; Clements, D. & Harrison, S.C. (2003). A ligand-binding pocket in the dengue virus envelope glycoprotein. *Proceedings of the National Academy of Sciences USA*, Vol.100, pp. 6899-6901

Monath, T.P. & Heinz, F.X. (1996). Flaviviruses. In *Fields virology*, Fields, B.N.; Knipe, D.M. & Howley, P.M. (Eds.), pp. 961-1034, Lippincott-Raven Publishers, Philadelphia

Monath, T.P. (1987). Yellow fever: a medically neglected disease. Report on a seminar. *Reviews in Infectious Diseases*, Vol.9, pp. 165-175

Mueller, N.H.; Pattabiraman, N.; Ansarah-Sobrinho, C.; Viswanathan, P.; Pierson, T.C. & Padmanabhan, R. (2008). Identification and Biochemical Characterization of Small-Molecule Inhibitors of West Nile Virus Serine Protease by a High-Throughput Screen. *Antimicrobial Agents and Chemotherapy*, Vol.52, pp. 3385–3393

Natale, V.A.; McCullough, K.C. (1998). Macrophage cytoplasmic vesicle pH gradient and vacuolar H+-ATPase activities relative to virus infection. *Journal of Leukocyte Biology*, Vol.64, pp. 302-310

Navarro-Sanchez, E.; Altmeyer, R.; Amara, A.; Schwartz, O.; Fieschi, F.; Virelizier, J.L.; Arenzana-Seisdedos, F. & Despres, P. (2003). Dendritic-cell-specific ICAM3-grabbing non-integrin is essential for the productive infection of human dendritic cells by mosquito-cell-derived dengue viruses. *EMBO Reports*, Vol.4, pp. 723–728

Nawa, M. (1998). Effect of bafilomycin A1 on Japanese encephalitis virus in C6/36 mosquito cells. *Archives of Virology*, Vol.148, pp. 1555-1568

Nettelton, P.E. & Entrican, G. (1995). Ruminant pestiviruses. *British Veterinary Journal*, Vol.151, pp. 615-642

Nowak, T.; Farber, P.M. & Wengler, G. (1989). Analyses of the terminal sequences of West Nile virus structural proteins and of the in vitro translation of these proteins allow the proposal of a complete scheme of the proteolytic cleavages involved in their synthesis. *Virology*, Vol.169, pp. 365–376

Pryor, M.J.; Gualano, R.C.; Lin, A.D.; Davidson, A.D. & Wright, P.J. (1998). Growth restriction of dengue virus type 2 by site-specific mutagenesis of virus-encoded glycoproteins. *Journal of General Virology*, Vol.79, pp. 2631-2639

Ray, D.; Shah, A.; Tilgner, M.; Guo, Y.; Zhao, Y.W.; Dong, H.P.; Deas, T.S.; Zhou, Y.S.; Li, H.M. & Shi, P.Y. (2006). West Nile virus 5└-cap structure is formed by sequential guanine N-7 and ribose 2'-O methylations by nonstructural protein 5. *Journal of Virology*, Vol.80, pp. 8362–8370

Rice, M.C. (1996). Flaviviridae: the viruses and their replication. In: *Fields virology*, Fields, B.N.; Knipe, D.M. & Howley, P.M. (Eds), pp. 931-960, Lippincott-Raven Publishers, Philadelphia

Robinson, M.J.; Sancho, D.; Slack, E.C.; LeibundGut-Landmann, S. & Reis e Sousa, C. (2006). Myeloid C-type lectins in innate immunity. *Nature Immunology*,Vol.7, pp. 1258–1265

Scheper, G. & Proud, C. (2002). Does phosphorylation of the cap-binding protein eIF4E play a role in translation initiation? *European Journal of Biochemistry*, Vol.269, pp. 5350-5359

Sidique, S.; Shiryaev, S.A.; Ratnikov, B.I.; Herath, A.; Su, Y.; Strongin, A.Y. & Cosford, N.D.P. (2009). Structure–activity relationship and improved hydrolytic stability of pyrazole derivatives that are allosteric inhibitors of West Nile Virus NS2B-NS3 proteinase. *Bioorganic & Medicinal Chemistry Letters*, Vol.19, pp. 5773–5777

Song, G.Y.; Paul, V.; Choo, H.; Morrey, J.; Sidwell, R.W.; Schinazi, R.F. & Chu, C.K. (2001). Enantiomeric synthesis of D- and L- cyclopentyl nucleosides and their antiviral activity against HIV and West Nile virus. *Journal of Medicinal Chemistry*, Vol.44, pp. 3985–3993

Speight, G.; Coia, G.; Parker, M.D. & Westaway, E.G. (1988). Gene mapping and positive identification of the non-structural proteins NS2A, NS2B, NS3, NS4B and NS5 of the flavivirus Kunjin and their cleavage sites. *Journal of General Virology*, Vol.69, pp. 23–34

Stadler, K.; Allison, S.L.; Schalich, J. & Heinz, F.X. (1997). Proteolytic activation of tick-borne encephalitis virus by furin. *Journal of Virology*, Vol.71, pp. 8475–8481

Steffens, S.; Thiel, H.J. & Behrens, S.E. (1999). The RNA-dependent RNA polymerases of different members of the family *Flaviviridae* exhibit similar properties in vitro. *Journal of General Virology*, Vol.80, pp. 2583–2590

Tassaneetrithep, B.; Burgess, T.H.; Granelli-Piperno, A.; Trumpfheller, C.; Finke, J.; Sun, W.; Eller, M.A.; Pattanapanyasat, K.; Sarasombath, S., Birx, D.L., Steinman, R.M.; Sclesinger S. & Marovich M.A. (2003). DC-SIGN (CD209) mediates dengue virus infection of human dendritic cells. *The Journal of Experimental Medicne*, Vol.197, pp. 823–829

van Kooyk, Y. & Geijtenbeek, T.B. (2003). DC-SIGN: escape mechanism for pathogens. *Nature Reviews in Immunology*, Vol.3, pp. 697–709

Walker,J. E.; Saraste, M.; Runswick, M. J. & Gay, N.J. (1982). Distantly related sequences in the alpha- and beta-subunits of ATP synthase, myosin, kinases and other ATP-requiring enzymes and a common nucleotide binding fold. *EMBO Journal*, Vol.1, pp. 945-951

Weissenhorn, W.; Dessen, A.; Calder, I.J.; Harrison S.C.; Skehel, J.J. & Wiley, D.C. (1999). Structural basis for membrane fusion by enveloped viruses. *Molecular Membrane Biology*, Vol.16, pp. 3-9

Westaway, E.G. (1987). Flavivirus replication strategy. *Advances in Virus Research*, Vol.33, pp. 45-90

Wilson, I.A.; Skehel, J.J. & Wiley, D.C. (1981). Structure of the hemagglutinin membrane glycoprotein of influenza virus at 3Å resolution. *Nature*, Vol.289, pp. 366-378

Wu, S.F.; Lee, C.J.; Liao, C.L.; Dwek, R. & Zitzmann, N. (2002). Antiviral effects of an iminosugar derivative on flavivirus infections. *Journal of. Virology*, Vol.76, pp. 3596–3604.

Zhang, N.; Chen, H.M.; Koch, V.; Schmitz, H.; Liao, C.L.; Bretner, M.; Bhadti, V.S.; Fattom, A. I.; Naso, R.B.; Hosmane, R.H. & Borowski, P. (2003a). Ring-expanded (''fat'') nucleoside and nucleotide analogues exhibit potent in vitro activity against Flaviviridae NTPase/helicases, including those of West Nile virus, hepatitis C virus and Japanese encephalitis virus. *Journal of Medicinal Chemistry*, Vol.46, pp. 4149–4164

Zhang, N.; Chen, H.M.; Koch, V.; Schmitz, H.; Minczuk, M.; Stepien, P.; Fattom, A.I.; Naso, R.B.; Kalicharran, K.; Borowski, P. & Hosmane, R.S. (2003b). Potent inhibition of NTPase/helicase of the West Nile virus by ring-expanded (''fat'') nucleoside analogues. *Journal of Medicinal Chemistry*, Vol.46, pp. 4776–4789

6

Mosquito-Borne Arboviral Surveillance and the Prediction of Disease Outbreaks

Jonathan F. Day[1] and Jeffrey Shaman[2]
[1]*University of Florida, IFAS, Florida Medical Entomology Laboratory, Vero Beach, FL,*
[2]*Department of Environmental Health Sciences, Mailman School of Public Health, Columbia University, New York*
USA

1. Introduction

Mosquito-borne viruses (arboviruses) have the capacity to cause widespread epidemics in humans, as well as epizootics in domestic animals and wildlife. These epidemics and epizootics can be extremely costly and disruptive. Because most mosquito-borne arboviruses can cause encephalitis and encephalomyelitis in host vertebrates, healthcare issues associated with human infections can result in significant economic impact on local economies and health care providers (Villari et al., 1995). Likewise, the loss of domestic animals to encephalitis infection can produce significant adverse financial impacts on local agricultural industries (Wilson et al., 1986; Anon, 2003). Recent mosquito-borne epidemics caused by West Nile virus (family *Flaviviridae*, genus *Flavivirus*, WNV) in North America and Chikungunya virus (family *Togaviridae*, genus *Alphavirus*, CHIKV) in the islands of the Indian Ocean are examples of how mosquito-borne viruses can severely impact local, regional, and national economies.

All mosquito-borne virus disease transmission cycles are driven by four factors: 1) the annual cycle of the pathogen (the specific arbovirus), 2) the annual cycle of the mosquito vector, 3) the annual cycle of the amplification, reservoir, and secondary vertebrate hosts that are infected with a specific viral pathogen, and 4) the environmental factors that drive each biological cycle independently and at times cause these three cycles to synchronize in ways that produce epidemics and epizootics (Day, 2001). Because three biological cycles, pathogen, vector and host, inform the transmission dynamics of a specific arboviral disease, surveillance protocols have been developed to monitor each of these cycles in order to estimate the local risk of arboviral transmission for a specific region. For example, it is possible to use sentinel animals to detect and measure the spatial and temporal distributions of specific arboviruses. Sentinel chickens, pheasants, quail, pigeons, and hamsters have been successfully used to monitor the transmission of St. Louis encephalitis virus (family *Flaviviridae*, genus *Flavivirus*, SLEV), WNV, eastern equine encephalitis virus (family *Togaviridae*, genus *Alphavirus*, EEEV), and Venezuelan equine encephalitis virus (family *Togaviridae*, genus *Alphavirus*, VEEV). Likewise, competent mosquito vectors can be identified for each mosquito-borne arbovirus transmission cycle. Once regional mosquito vectors have been identified, their populations can be tracked and important factors such as abundance, population age structure, and infection status can be monitored and used to assess disease transmission risk. Similarly, the age structure and infectivity status of known amplification hosts can be monitored and used to measure arboviral transmission risk (Day and Stark, 1999). Finally, the environmental conditions that influence vector and amplification host population structures can be tracked and used to predict how and when vector, amplification host, and viral populations will synchronize and escalate to a point where epidemic disease transmission is inevitable (Shaman and Day, 2005; Day and Shaman, 2009).

A thorough knowledge of the three biological cycles (virus, vector, and amplification host) and the environmental factors that drive these cycles can allow the skillful prediction of when and where mosquito-borne arboviral disease outbreaks will occur (i.e. spatio-temporal disease transmission patterns). In this chapter we present a detailed analysis of the disease transmission cycles of SLEV, WNV, and EEEV in Florida, USA and WNV in Colorado, USA. We use these examples to illustrate how an intimate knowledge of the biotic cycles and the abiotic drivers of these biological cycles facilitate the accurate prediction of regional and local disease outbreaks. For example, SLEV was first isolated during an epidemic of human encephalitis in St. Louis, MO in the summer of 1933. Since 1933 at least 20 SLE epidemics have been reported in North America. In south Florida an SLE epidemic developed in 1990, lasted from August 1990 through January 1991, and resulted in 226 clinical cases and 11 deaths. A complete understanding of the SLEV transmission cycle in south Florida, including the mosquito and avian hosts responsible for SLEV amplification early in the summer of 1990, enabled prediction of epidemic transmission (an unusually elevated level of virus transmission to humans) eight weeks before the first human case was reported (Day and Lewis, 1992). In theory, all mosquito-borne encephalitis epidemics should have distinct biological and physical signatures that enable prediction of the spatio-temporal distribution of arboviral transmission risk prior to the appearance of human cases. To facilitate such real-time monitoring and risk prediction it is critical that these signatures are identified.

Epidemic prediction of vector-borne encephalitis diseases should be a priority for local vector control and public health programs. The development of systems for the skillful forecast of epidemic arboviral transmission is a desirable and attainable goal. Such forecasts help to minimize the impact of these dangerous disease agents on humans, domestic animals, and wildlife. Furthermore, the accurate early warning of impending arboviral epidemics allows increased vector control efforts and increased public awareness in the areas of highest risk for virus transmission. These predictive factors may allow vector control and public health officials the luxury of mitigating a potential arboviral epidemic before large numbers of humans and domestic animals are infected.

2. Biotic and abiotic factors associated with arboviral transmission cycles

Mosquito-borne viral cycles depend on the interaction of four distinct agents; three are biological (biotic) and one is a group of environmental factors (abiotic) that directly influence the biotic cycles. Under certain environmental conditions the three biotic cycles interact in ways that enhance viral abundance resulting in increased viral transmission. Depending on the exact local environmental conditions, viral transmission can be focal, sporadic, or epidemic. Focal transmission is constrained spatially and temporally and produces a localized outbreak of virus transmission. Sporadic transmission occurs intermittently over a broader geographic area than focal transmission but is often less locally intense. Epidemic transmission occurs when virus is transmitted intensely over a wide geographic area for an extended timeframe. These distinctions are somewhat qualitative but provide a loose framework for assessing the distribution and duration of an outbreak of arbovirus transmission to humans and domestic animals.

There are a number of well-known mosquito-borne arboviruses. These include yellow fever virus (family *Flaviviridae,* genus *Flavivirus,* YFV), dengue viruses (four serotypes in the family *Flaviviridae,* genus *Flavivirus,* DENV), and the mosquito-borne encephalitis viruses including WNV, SLEV, and EEEV. Mosquito-borne arboviruses are usually restricted to specific habitats and are seasonally abundant with transmission corresponding to the abundance of competent vector species.

Mosquito vector species are generally matched to specific arboviruses in different regions of the world. For example, DENV (serotypes 1, 2, 3, and 4) are most commonly transmitted by *Aedes aegypti* (Linnaeus) in the tropics and subtropics around the world. However, a second DENV vector, *Aedes albopictus* (Skuse), has been responsible for recent epidemics in Hawaii (Kolivras 2006) and Singapore (Ooi et al. 2006). Likewise, WNV was introduced into North America in 1999 and rapidly spread across the continent (Marfin and Gubler 2001). In different parts of North America, WNV encountered and exploited different mosquito species that became the dominant vector for the virus in that particular part of the continent. *Culex pipiens pipiens* Linnaeus became the primary WNV vector in the north-eastern quarter of the continent, while *Cx. pipiens quinquefasciatus* Say became one of the primary vectors in the southern half of the continent. In Florida, the primary WNV vector is *Cx. nigripalpus* Theobald, and in the western half of the continent the primary WNV vectors are *Cx. pipiens quinquefasciatus* and *Cx. tarsalis* Coquillett.

The ability of a mosquito vector to acquire and then transmit a virus is referred to as vector competence (Hardy et al. 1983, Tabachnick 1994). To function as a competent mosquito vector, ingested virus must be able to escape the mosquito midgut, infect other organs, replicate, and eventually infect the mosquito's salivary glands from where it is then transmitted with each subsequent probe or blood meal. Intrinsic factors in all mosquitoes regulate viral escape from infected organs, the penetration of virus into new organs, and viral replication within those organs (Black et al. 2002). Extrinsic factors including the amount of virus ingested by the mosquito with its first infective blood meal and ambient temperature, which determines how quickly the virus replicates in the mosquito and infects the salivary glands (a process known as the extrinsic incubation period (EIP)), also influence mosquito vector competence (Anderson et al. 2010, Richards et al. 2009, 2010). Most mosquito species are poor arboviral vectors, primarily because of intrinsic and extrinsic factors that disfavor viral replication and mosquito infection processes. For example, there are currently 80 mosquito species known to occur in Florida. However, only two of these (*Cx. nigripalpus* and *Cx. quinquefasciatus*) serve as epidemic vectors of WNV in the state.

There are three types of vertebrate hosts involved in arboviral transmission cycles: amplification hosts, reservoir hosts, and dead-end hosts. Once infected, amplification hosts produce a viremia (virus in the circulating blood) at levels (titers) sufficient to infect competent vector mosquitoes. In the case of SLEV, wild birds serve as amplification hosts. Efficient amplification hosts need to be susceptible to viral infection, capable of producing a high level viremia, spatially and temporally abundant, and easily accessible to vector mosquitoes. Many species of wild birds are susceptible to infection with SLEV; however, few wild avian species serve as efficient amplification hosts for the virus, primarily because most avian species produce a viremia insufficient to infect vector mosquitoes. Viral titers above 4.0 logs (10,000 viral particles (virions) per millilitre of blood) are usually necessary to infect mosquitoes. In addition, efficient amplification hosts need to be abundant and have a wide spatial distribution that insures frequent contact with infected and susceptible mosquito vectors. For instance, rare avian species may be infected, develop high viremias, and infect mosquitoes, but due to low prevalence in the environment, their mosquito contact rate is low and they are unlikely to infect mosquitoes at the levels necessary to sustain epidemic arboviral transmission. The major avian hosts involved in the amplification of SLEV in south Florida are Northern Cardinals, Common Grackles, Blue Jays, and Mourning Doves (Day and Stark 1999). These four avian species share three important characteristics that typify superior arboviral amplification hosts: 1) they are susceptible to SLEV infection, 2) they circulate virus at high enough titers to infect mosquito vectors, and 3) they are seasonally abundant and widely dispersed. This broad distribution and seasonal abundance ensures that these avian species have recurrent contact with mosquito vectors, which increases the probability that SLEV will be acquired by uninfected mosquitos from infected birds and that infected mosquitoes will contact susceptible birds and transmit SLEV. This cascade of viral transmission between infected mosquitoes and susceptible birds and, conversely, between infected birds and susceptible mosquitoes results in the amplification of virus in nature (Figure 1). As will be explained later in this chapter, the efficient amplification of an arbovirus, i.e. intense zoonotic transmission that increases arbovirus prevalence among vector mosquitoes and avian hosts, is a prerequisite for arboviral epidemics.

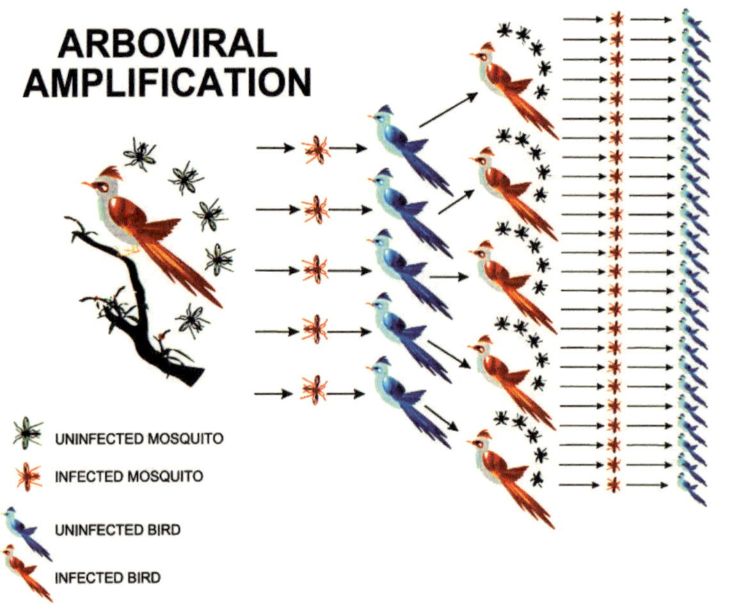

Fig. 1. An illustration depicting the sequence of events necessary for efficient arboviral amplification in nature. Epidemic amplification breaks down when there are too few competent mosquito vectors and when there are too few susceptible avian amplification hosts

A virus remains in an amplification host's circulating blood for a relatively short time, usually on the order of days. This is because the vertebrate host immune system usually clears the virus, rendering the infected host immune for life. In some cases there are vertebrate species that maintain long-term viremias at levels sufficient to infect vector mosquitoes. Such hosts are sometimes referred to as reservoir hosts because they serve as a long-term local source for the virus. Garter snakes are known to maintain long-term viremias when infected with western equine encephalitis virus (family *Togaviridae,* genus *Alphavirus,* WEEV). It has been proposed that WEEV infected snakes may be the reservoir that allows WEEV to survive winters in temperate habitats (Burton et al., 1966).

Secondary or dead-end hosts are vertebrate hosts that do not have a high enough virus titer in the circulating blood to infect mosquitoes. Dead-end host infections are wasted in terms of viral survival and propagation. Humans are dead-end hosts for SLEV. Though a human infected with SLEV may show clinical signs of infection resulting from replication of virus in the nervous system, the amount of virus in the circulating blood is not sufficient to infect mosquito vectors. The normal SLEV amplification cycle in nature occurs between wild birds and mosquitoes. The fact that humans are involved at all in the SLEV transmission cycle is an accident resulting from the nonspecific blood feeding behavior of some vector species that feed readily on humans as well as wild birds. Blood meals by infective mosquitoes on susceptible wild birds may result in the transmission of virus to the bird and a new avian infection. Infected birds can infect additional susceptible mosquitoes. On the other hand, SLEV transmission to susceptible humans results in a dead-end infection for the virus; it is transmitted to a host where virus titers in the host's circulating blood remain too low to infect mosquito vectors.

The three biotic cycles discussed above are all influenced by environmental factors. The environmental factors that most directly impact arbovirus transmission cycles include rainfall, surface water accumulation, relative humidity, temperature, and land use practices. These environmental factors directly impact the reproductive biology and survivorship of mosquito vectors and vertebrate amplification hosts. By influencing the reproduction and longevity of vectors and amplification hosts, select environmental factors also influence arboviral abundance and transmission rates. For this reason, arboviral transmission cycles go through long periods when the viruses are rare and difficult to detect and quantify in nature. Likewise, due to environmental conditions that favor viral amplification and transmission, there are periods when arboviruses become extremely abundant and are transmitted at epidemic levels.

2.1 Biology of the virus

Most arboviruses are endemic to a particular environment in a specific region of the world. This means that arboviruses have integrated themselves into ecological habitats where they have coevolved with local mosquito vectors and vertebrate amplification hosts. For example, Ross River virus (family *Togaviridae,* genus *Alphavirus,* RRV) is found throughout Australia, Papua New Guinea, and other South Pacific Islands where it has coevolved with local mosquito vectors, especially *Aedes camptorhynchus* (Thomson), and large marsupial mammals that serve as amplification hosts (Russell 2002). The ecological conditions that occur throughout the distribution range of RRV, including the presence of suitable mosquito vectors and vertebrate amplification hosts, identify the environment most conducive for the seasonal amplification and transmission of this virus. Within this range, the RRV remains endemic and can survive throughout the year.

Survival from year to year is a prerequisite for viral endemicity. In the tropics and sub-tropics viruses survive from wet seasons, when mosquitos and amplification hosts are abundant, through dry seasons, when mosquitoes and amplification hosts are less abundant and arboviral transmission is less intense. For example, SLEV transmission to sentinel chickens, used to monitor and document arboviral transmission in specific habitats throughout Florida, has been reported during every month of the year, indicating a year-round viral transmission pattern. In temperate habitats, arboviral survival through the winter is more problematic. In some cases, as for WNV in New York City, the virus survives in overwintering infected female mosquitoes (Nasci et al. 2001). For other viral cycles, like La Crosse virus (family *Bunyaviridae*, genus *Orthobunyavirus*, LACV) in the upper Midwest of the USA, the virus survives through a process known as transovarial transmission in which the LACV survives through winter in cold- and drought-resistant eggs deposited by infected female mosquitoes during the previous autumn (Watts et al. 1973). In other situations, viruses may be re-seeded into habitats by infected migrating birds. This may be the case for EEEV in Florida where infected birds that overwinter in tropical habitats where EEEV is endemic carry the virus north during spring migration and infect local mosquitoes in areas where the migrating birds stop to rest.

In some cases, viruses may be reintroduced into habitats where they have been absent for years or even decades. This happened in Key West, Florida sometime during 2009 when locally acquired human dengue (serotype 1) cases were reported for the first time in more than 50 years. The DENV may have been reintroduced through an infected human visiting the area. Whatever the source, the reintroduced DENV encountered an environment favorable for amplification (in susceptible humans) and transmission. The virus has since survived in a local transmission cycle in Key West for two years (MMWR 2010). It remains to be seen whether DENV will remain endemic in Key West for an extended period of time.

In other situations a virus may be introduced into a completely new habitat where the ecology favors viral amplification and transmission. This happened with WNV in New York City in 1999 (Marfin and Gubler, 2001). The virus may have been introduced by an infected mosquito, an infected bird, or an infected human. Regardless of the mode of introduction, WNV found a habitat conducive for amplification and transmission in NYC. Not only did the WNV find the biotic and abiotic conditions in NYC favorable for long-term establishment, the virus spread and became established throughout the USA in less than four years.

2.2 Biology of the vector

To be an optimal epidemic arboviral vector, a mosquito species needs to be susceptible to infection, spatially and temporally abundant, long lived, and willing to blood feed on amplification as well as dead-end hosts. As discussed above, mosquito vectors need to be susceptible to viral infection such that, once ingested, virus must escape the blood meal in the midgut, penetrate the midgut wall, enter the mosquito hemolymph, infect and reproduce in other mosquito organs and tissues including the salivary glands, and exit the salivary glands with saliva during subsequent mosquito probing and blood feeding. This cycle of virus ingestion to salivary gland infection constitutes the mosquito extrinsic incubation period (EIP) discussed above (Figure 2). The EIP is temperature dependent. In general, warmer ambient temperatures result in shorter EIPs. Typical EIPs range from as low as 5 days for *Culiseta melanura* (Coquillett) infected with EEEV (Scott and Weaver 1989) to more than three weeks in SLEV-infected *Cx. nigripalpus*.

Competent mosquito vectors need to be spatially and temporally abundant in areas where they are sympatric with the arboviruses they transmit. For example, *Culex salinarius* Coquillett and *Cx. restuans* Theobald are both competent vectors of WNV in eastern North America. However, in south Florida these mosquito species are most abundant during the spring and adult numbers decline steadily throughout the summer months. It is possible that both species are involved in the early season amplification of WNV in south Florida. But neither species is abundant during the mid-summer months when WNV is amplified and transmitted by the *Cx. nigripalpus* populations that are highly synchronized with avian amplification hosts.

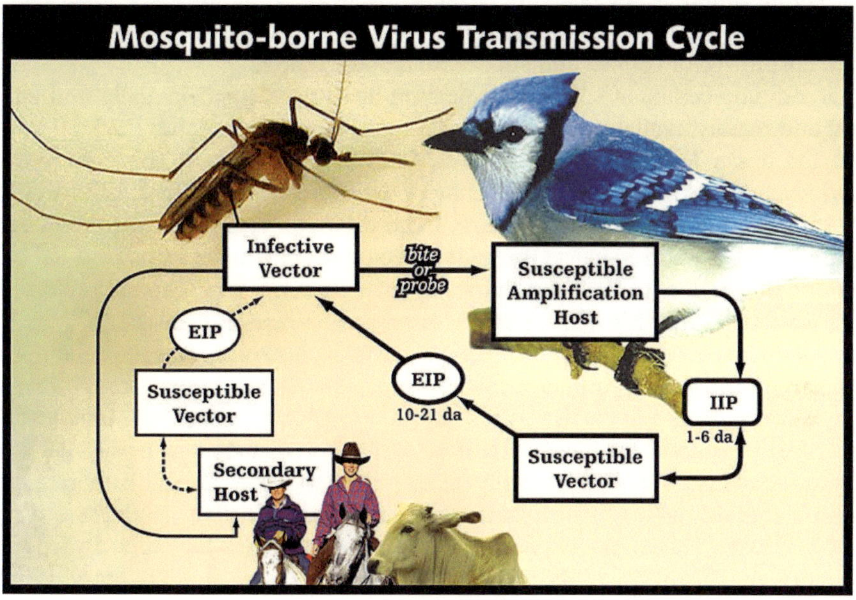

Fig. 2. An illustration depicting a typical mosquito-borne virus transmission cycle (e.g. SLEV). Abbreviations: IIP = intrinsic incubation period, EIP = extrinsic incubation period, secondary hosts are also often referred to as dead-end hosts

Short-lived mosquito species seldom serve as efficient arboviral vectors. This is because short-lived species do not have sufficient time to complete the temperature-dependent EIP. One of the most abundant mosquito species along the east coast of North America is *Aedes taeniorhynchus* (Wiedemann). Occasionally this species is found infected with SLEV or WNV; however, this mosquito species has never been implicated as a major arboviral vector along the east coast of North America. A major reason for this is that *Ae. taeniorhynchus* is a short-lived mosquito species, usually surviving as an adult for only two to three weeks. This short adult lifespan typically does not provide sufficient time for females to acquire an infective blood meal, complete the EIP, and blood feed a second time.

A final characteristic of an optimal arboviral vector is the willingness to blood feed on a variety of vertebrate hosts. Some mosquito species are efficient zoonotic vectors, that is, they feed selectively on certain vertebrate species, establishing an arboviral transmission cycle with those select species. For example, *Cs. melanura* feeds almost exclusively on birds. In areas of eastern North America where this mosquito species is abundant in hardwood swamps, efficient enzootic EEEV transmission cycles are readily established between resident wild birds and *Cs. melanura*. However, the transmission of EEEV to mammals involves secondary vectors, often referred to as "bridge vectors." Highly effective epidemic vectors blood feed willingly on amplification hosts as well as dead-end vertebrate hosts. *Culex nigripalpus* is an efficient epidemic vector of SLEV in south Florida where it readily blood feeds on avian amplification hosts as well as dead-end hosts including humans. In this instance a single mosquito species serves as both the amplification and the epidemic vector.

2.3 Biology of the amplification host

Many of the characteristics that make certain mosquito species optimal epidemic vectors are also characteristics that make some vertebrate hosts optimal arboviral amplification hosts. Efficient amplification hosts have to be susceptible to viral infection, maintain a high viremia in the peripheral blood, and maintain high viremias for a period of time that is long enough to ensure vector contact and successful blood feeding.

As with mosquito vectors, efficient amplification hosts need to be spatially and temporally abundant and readily available to host seeking mosquitoes. The primary mosquito vector of LACV in the upper Midwest of the USA is *Aedes triseriatus* (Say). This mosquito is day-active, which matches the day-active behavior pattern of the major LACV amplification host, the eastern chipmunk (*Tamias striatus*). In addition, the mosquito vector and vertebrate amplification host overlap in space through exploitation of similar woodland habitats. This spatio-temporal overlap of the mosquito and amplification host habitat preferences and behaviors maximizes the efficiency of LACV amplification and transmission.

The reproductive behavior of amplification hosts is also an important component of arboviral amplification and transmission. Young animals are highly susceptible to viral infection. Altricial birds are particularly susceptible to infection because they are virtually defenceless against blood feeding mosquitoes while on the nest and newly hatched birds have immune systems that are highly susceptible to viral infection. Many arboviral transmission cycles are synchronized with the reproductive patterns of primary amplification hosts. This is particularly true of arboviral cycles that rely on wild birds as their primary amplification hosts. As a consequence, years of high amplification host reproductive output may result in high levels of arboviral transmission. Avian and small mammal populations can cycle between years of extraordinary reproductive output and years of average or below average reproduction (Day and Stark 1999). When years of high amplification host reproductive output are synchronized with high vector output and high viral abundance, epidemic arboviral transmission can result. The vertebrate host and mosquito vector reproductive cycles are driven by environmental factors. Fortunately, it is uncommon for all three of the biological cycles associated with arboviral transmission patterns to be perfectly synchronized. This makes widespread arboviral epidemics rare events.

2.4 Environmental drivers of arboviral amplification and transmission

Arboviral cycles vary dramatically in their spatial and temporal distributions. There are times when it is difficult to find virus in habitats where specific viruses are known to be endemic. During tropical and subtropical dry seasons and during temperate winters it is almost impossible to make arboviral isolations from any source. During the hot summer months the appearance of virus may be focal, sporadic, or, at times, epidemic. The amount of virus present in an area during high volume transmission months is both directly and indirectly affected by the environmental factors that drive the biological cycles of the virus, the vector, and the amplification host. Perhaps the most important environmental factor affecting arboviral transmission cycles is rainfall. This is because rainfall directly impacts the reproduction, flight, and longevity of vector species. Mosquito larvae and pupae are fully aquatic, so eggs are laid in, on, or near water. Immature mosquitoes are aquatic, so eggs are laid on or near water, and larvae and pupae are fully aquatic. The lifecycle of all mosquitoes thus depends on the availability of standing water and it is precipitation that ultimately provides the land surface wetness that supports such standing waters. Similarly, rainfall cycles support the insect populations on which many birds rely for the nourishment of nestlings. As will be discussed below, the cycling of rainfall and drought can directly impact the viral EIP in infected vectors.

Rainfall and drought also influence mosquito longevity and flight behavior, and have two direct effects on mosquito lifecycles and behavior. First, most small insects, and mosquitoes in particular, are subject to desiccation. The surface humidity associated with rainfall increases the potential flight range of host searching mosquitoes and their ability to blood feed once a host is located by reducing the desiccation rate in these small, fragile insects. Second, rainfall directly influences the abundance and quality of mosquito oviposition sites. Mosquito species that rely on temporary pools of water for oviposition are at the mercy of local rainfall events. During long periods of drought, these temporary oviposition sites are totally absent. This forces gravid female mosquitoes that deposit eggs directly in water or on the water surface to wait for a rainfall event sufficient to produce acceptable oviposition sites. Such drought-enforced oviposition delay may greatly enhance the transmission of certain arboviruses. For example, SLEV is transmitted by *Cx. nigripalpus* in Florida. This mosquito species depends on temporary pools of water for oviposition. In the absence of such pools, gravid female mosquitos will sit for weeks waiting for the proper oviposition cues. If a female mosquito is infected with SLEV during her first blood meal, she may complete the 15-21 day EIP before the occurrence of a rainfall event suitable to produce the temporary oviposition sites necessary for egg laying. Under these conditions, infected female mosquitoes can become infective in a single gonotrophic cycle. This makes it possible for an infected mosquito to transmit virus during her second blood meal.

This drought-delayed oviposition behavior serves two important epidemiological functions. First, extended periods of drought force infected gravid female mosquitoes to retain their eggs while they await the rains necessary to produce suitable oviposition sites. Once egg retention extends beyond the EIP, these infected female mosquitoes are ready to biologically transmit virus. Second, the drought-induced egg retention by infected mosquitoes serves to synchronize blood feeding once oviposition occurs. This means that virus transmission is focused into discrete time periods by patterns of rainfall and drought.

When oviposition sites are readily available to gravid *Cx. nigripalpus* females, eggs can be deposited five days after an infective blood meal and female mosquitoes are ready to immediately resume host searching behavior. In this situation, an infected female mosquito could potentially go through three or four gonotrophic cycles before she becomes infective. Host searching is one of the most dangerous activities undertaken by a female mosquito. Predation, vertebrate host defensive behavior (including the eating of attracted mosquitoes), and desiccation are all factors that terminate mosquito host searching flights. The ability to become infective after a single gonotrophic cycle greatly enhances the efficiency of arboviral amplification and transmission by vector mosquitoes.

Temperature is another environmental factor that can greatly influence arboviral transmission cycles. Because the EIP is temperature-dependent, even a small increase in daily ambient temperature can reduce the overall EIP in an infected female mosquito. Reduction of the EIP from 17 to 14 days may increase the probability that the mosquito will survive to become infective and transmit virus with subsequent host contacts (Watts et al. 1987). Environmental temperatures may also impact avian nesting behavior and reproductive success (Day and Stark 1999). Severe winter freezes in south Florida have been shown to enhance avian nesting, foraging, and reproductive success during the following spring (Day and Shaman, 2009). The exact ways in which winter freezes in south Florida impact avian nesting success the following spring will be discussed in detail in the SLEV in Florida section below.

A final environmental driver of arboviral transmission involves changes in landscape management practices. Human land management has long been known to influence mosquito species diversity, abundance, and age structure. Agricultural practices in particular are known to produce huge mosquito populations. Japanese encephalitis virus (family *Flaviviridae*, genus *Flavivirus*, JEV) is endemic to Southeast Asia and the Far East where the primary vector is *Culex tritaeniorhynchus* Giles and domestic pigs and wild birds serve as amplification hosts (Erlanger et al. 2009). The JEV is the leading cause of mosquito-borne encephalitis in Asia where 30,000 to 50,000 cases are reported annually, primarily in rural settings. Rice paddies serve as the preferred oviposition site for *Cx. tritaeniorhynchus* and rice cultivation and associated agricultural practices, especially the production of domestic swine in areas adjacent to the rice paddies, greatly enhances the abundance, age structure, and JEV infection status of this important mosquito vector.

3. Specific examples of arboviral transmission cycles

To substantiate further the points discussed in Section 2, we will present examples of four mosquito-borne arboviral cycles from North America. These include: eastern equine encephalitis virus in the eastern USA; St. Louis encephalitis virus in Florida, USA; West Nile virus in eastern Colorado, USA; and West Nile virus in Florida, USA.

3.1 Eastern Equine Encephalitis virus in the Eastern USA

Eastern equine encephalitis virus is a complex of four viral lineages. Group I is endemic throughout the eastern half of the USA and the Caribbean Basin and is responsible for most human disease. Groups IIA, IIB, and III are endemic in Central and South America where they are primarily responsible for equine infections. In the USA, EEEV transmission occurs primarily east of the Mississippi River. As the name implies, EEE is primarily a disease of equines. Major epizootics that were consistent with the clinical definition of EEE infection in horses were reported in 1845 (Long Island and New York), 1902 (North Carolina), 1905 (New Jersey), 1908 (Florida), and 1912 (Maryland, New Jersey, and Virginia). In 1933 the EEEV was first isolated from the brain of an infected horse and recognized as the etiologic agent of EEE infection. Additional equine epizootics caused by EEEV were reported in 1933 (New Jersey), 1934 (Virginia), and 1935 (North Carolina). The largest equine epizootic in the USA occurred in 1947 in southern Louisiana and Texas where there were an estimated 14,334 equine cases with 11,727 deaths (Scott and Weaver 1989).

An average of six human EEE cases is reported annually in the USA. Most human cases are reported by health workers in coastal states from Texas east to Florida and north to New Hampshire. The first major human EEE epidemic was reported in eastern Massachusetts in 1938. During that year 34 human infections were reported with a case-fatality rate of 74%. A second human epidemic with 32 cases was reported in New Jersey during 1959 (Scott and Weaver 1989). Eastern equine encephalitis epidemics of this magnitude are exceedingly rare. In general, human EEE cases appear sporadically. For example, the highest number of human EEE cases reported during a single transmission season in Florida is five (this occurred on four separate occasions in 1978, 1980, 1991, and 2005). These annual groupings of five human cases were never clustered and during most years they were spread over three or four Florida counties.

The low number of human cases is a direct reflection of the complexity of the EEEV transmission cycle and the obstacles that this complexity places in the way of large-scale

EEEV amplification in vector mosquitoes. In the eastern USA, EEEV is endemic in hardwood freshwater swamps where the virus is cycled between resident and migratory wild birds by *Cs. melanura*. Because this mosquito species feeds almost exclusively on birds, mammals are rarely involved in the enzootic cycling of virus in these swamp habitats. If this were the extent of the EEEV amplification and transmission cycle, humans and horses would never be involved. However, the virus has two ways it can escape enzootic hardwood swamp habitats. First, it can move out of the swamp in infected birds as they disperse after fledging (Crans et al. 1994). Second, under the proper environmental conditions, where heavy rains saturate the open habitats surrounding the swamps, infected *Cs. melanura* and infected secondary mosquito vectors (bridge vectors) can disperse out of the swamps carrying the EEEV with them. Infected bridge vectors can blood feed on susceptible horses or humans in habitats adjacent to the swamps. In addition, infected bridge vectors and infected *Cs. melanura* females can blood feed on avian hosts at sites some distance from the original infection site and establish a secondary amplification focus. Once secondary mosquito vectors and amplification hosts become infected, new amplification foci are established. In Florida, secondary mosquito vectors include *Cx. nigripalpus, Coquillettidia perturbans* (Walker), *Mansonia* spp., and spring floodwater *Aedes* spp. All of these mosquito species are opportunistic blood feeders that will readily feed on a variety of wild bird species as well as mammals.

It is this two-tiered EEEV transmission cycle that makes it difficult to realize the large number of infected mosquito vectors required for epidemic transmission on the scale observed for WNV and DENV. Virus never escapes the hardwood swamps during many arboviral transmission seasons. During years when the virus does escape, secondary transmission foci need to become established or large numbers of infective bridge vectors need to escape the swamp habitats before human and horse cases appear. By their very nature, these transmission events involve fewer infected mosquitoes than what has been observed during epidemics caused by WNV. As a consequence, EEEV transmission foci remain small and isolated resulting in focal or sporadic transmission of virus to humans and horses.

3.2 St. Louis Encephalitis virus in Florida

St. Louis encephalitis virus is related to JEV, but its distribution is restricted to the New World. Transmission of SLEV has been reported throughout the USA and in Canada, Mexico, Central America, the Caribbean Islands, and South America. Transmission in North America is most commonly reported along the Mississippi and Ohio River basins. In Florida, SLEV is most commonly reported in the southern half of the state where epidemics were reported in 1959, 1961, 1962, 1977, and 1990 (Day 2001).

Prior to 1977 most SLEV transmission to humans in Florida occurred in urban transmission foci. The epidemics in 1959, 1961, and 1962 occurred in cities along the central west coast of Florida including St. Petersburg, Tampa, Clearwater, and Sarasota. Human infections during the 1977 and 1990 epidemics occurred mainly in suburban and rural settings. The shift of SLEV transmission from urban to rural foci may be a reflection of changes in urban public health practices, changes in the distribution and bionomics of the primary epidemic vector, *Cx. nigripalpus*, or changes in south Florida land use patterns.

The zoonotic transmission of SLEV occurs year round in south Florida where vector mosquitoes transmit virus to susceptible wild birds. The primary zoonotic vector is *Cx. nigripalpus*, a mosquito species that is present in a wide variety of Florida habitats throughout the year. Secondary zoonotic vectors may also be involved in the low level transmission and maintenance of SLEV during the south Florida dry season (November-May) and during years where environmental factors do not favor the amplification and transmission of SLEV during the south Florida wet season (June-October). Secondary zoonotic vectors may include: *Cx. salinarius, Cx. restuans, Cx. erraticus* (Dyar and Knab), and *Anopheles crucians* Wiedemann. Low level viral transmission occurs between primary and secondary zoonotic vectors and wild birds. Transmission levels increase during the south Florida avian nesting season (April-June amplification) when nestling birds provide a steady source of blood for mosquitoes infected with SLEV.

Sentinel chickens serve as the best means of documenting viral transmission in the field (Day and Lewis, 1992). Flocks of 8 to 12 chickens are placed into different habitats throughout Florida where they are exposed continually to blood feeding mosquitoes. Weekly blood samples are drawn from each chicken and analysed for antibody to SLEV, WNV, EEEV, and Highlands J virus (family *Togaviridae,* genus *Alphavirus,* HJV). A positive antibody test is indicative of recent arboviral transmission to the chicken. Depending on environmental conditions, SLEV transmission, as measured by sentinel chickens, may be absent, focal, sporadic, or epidemic. The Florida sentinel chicken surveillance program provides a weekly spatial analysis of the distribution of virus transmission throughout Florida. More than 30 years of sentinel chicken arboviral surveillance in Florida has shown that the major SLEV transmission period occurs between August and October.

Occasionally, environmental conditions favor the enhanced early season amplification of SLEV. In particular, the Florida SLEV cycle appears to be sensitive to patterns of drought and rainfall. Spring droughts seem to be particularly important because drought and landscape fragmentation conspire to constrict vector activity to the more humid hammock environments exploited by nesting birds. Some surface waters remain within and at the fringes of these habitats, often in channels and canals that *Cx. nigripalpus* can exploit without having to travel far (and risking desiccation). The drought-forced cohabitation of vector mosquitoes and avian hosts, including nestlings, facilitates a rapid increase in the infection rate among both vector and host (Shaman et al., 2002). Late spring rainfall then facilitates the dispersal of these infectious mosquitoes and birds, enabling the establishment of secondary amplification foci.

When late spring and summer rainfalls occur at an optimal rate of once every 10-14 days, *Cx. nigripalpus* populations will increase efficiently. Furthermore, should temperatures be high, such that viral EIP is reduced, and major rainfall events are appropriately spaced, EIP will be completed in a single gonotrophic cycle and SLEV transmission will proceed optimally. *Culex nigripalpus* is a flood water species that prefers freshly flooded oviposition habitats. Rainfall cycles that temporarily flood oviposition sites, allowing mosquito egg-laying and the completion of immature mosquito development before the oviposition sites dry down, produce the maximum number of mosquitoes in age structure cohorts that favor viral transmission (Day and Curtis 1999). When rainfall, mosquito reproduction, and avian reproduction coincide early in the summer, the viral amplification and transmission begun during spring drought is further maximized. When such environmental conditions favorable for amplification persist through the summer, large numbers of infected vectors are produced resulting in epidemic SLEV transmission in the late summer and early fall.

There are additional environmental factors that may favor enhanced mosquito and avian reproduction. For example, flood irrigation in Florida citrus groves often occurs during the dry months of April and May. During this process, thousands of acres of citrus trees are flooded producing suitable *Cx. nigripalpus* oviposition sites that allow the mosquitoes to begin reproducing early in the year, during the spring dry season, a period when there would normally be no available oviposition sites. In addition, it has also been shown (Day and Shaman 2009) that there is a significant relationship between severe south Florida winter freezes and avian reproduction during the three breeding seasons following the freeze. It is proposed that severe winter freezes clear cold-sensitive vegetation from the understories of woodland habitats. By clearing the understory vegetation, these habitats are opened to foraging by ground feeding birds, many of which are important SLEV amplification hosts that dramatically increase in abundance due to this increase in foraging and nesting habitat. It takes about three years for the understory vegetation to regrow after which avian reproductive rates return to normal (Day and Stark 1999).

The realization of epidemic SLEV transmission in south Florida depends on the precise synchronization of three biological cycles. The presence and abundance of virus depends on the abundance, distribution, and age structure of vector and amplification host populations. These population fluctuations are driven by winter freezes, spring drought, and the cycling of rainfall in a manner that produces periodic *Cx. nigripalpus* oviposition sites throughout summer.

3.3 West Nile virus in Eastern Colorado

West Nile virus is part of the Japanese encephalitis antigenic complex. Until 1999 the virus was enzootic throughout Africa and much of Asia, the Middle East, and the Mediterranean. A subtype of WNV is found in Australia where it is referred to as Kunjin virus (family *Flaviviridae*, genus *Flavivirus*, KUNV). In dramatic fashion, WNV was reported in New York City during the summer of 1999 (CDC, 1999). By 2001 the virus had spread west to the Mississippi River, north into Canada, and south to Florida. By 2002 it had spread to the front range of the Rocky Mountains, south into Mexico, and throughout the Caribbean Basin. By 2004 it was reported in all of the Continental United States (Hayes et al. 2005). Extremely large urban and rural epidemics were reported as WNV moved west across the USA. For example, in 2003 more than 6000 human clinical cases were reported in the Great Plains of the U.S. (i.e. Colorado, Nebraska, South Dakota, Wyoming, and Montana). West Nile virus and SLEV share similar viral transmission cycles, and states like Illinois, Louisiana, Texas, and California that had reported large SLE epidemics during the second half of the 20th century also reported large WN epidemics associated with establishment of the virus in those states.

Human cases of WN first manifested in Colorado during 2002. The following year, a major outbreak of WNV took place in Colorado with 2,947 human cases reported, and since then annual human cases in Colorado have numbered in the hundreds. The majority of cases have been in the eastern high plains of the state east of the Rocky Mountains (Shaman et al., 2010). This region is dominated by grasslands interspersed with river riparian zones that appear to be the nexus of WNV activity. These riparian zones provide habitat for avian host species and *Cx. tarsalis* and *Cx. pipiens,* the dominant vectors of WNV in the region (Bolling et al. 2007). In these riparian environments, WNV can be amplified and zoonotically transmitted between these vector mosquitoes and co-habitating avian hosts.

Both *Cx. tarsalis* and *Cx. pipiens* have been found to be more abundant in the riparian regions of the eastern Colorado plains than in the riparian regions of the foothills and higher elevations of the Rocky Mountains (Eisen et al., 2008; Barker et al., 2009). Thus, the geographic distribution of *Culex* vector abundance is consistent with higher WNV transmission risk in eastern Colorado (Winters et al., 2008). The distribution of *Culex* vectors and the environments that support them provides an indication of where in space WNV transmission is more likely to occur; however, to understand *where and when* WNV activity will occur, temporal variations in environmental conditions must also be considered.

When environmental conditions are more favorable for mosquito breeding, increased vector abundance within riparian zones increases the ratio of vectors to hosts. This change facilitates the proliferation and amplification of WNV in both the vector and host populations (Shaman, 2007). In eastern Colorado, changes to local soil moisture conditions appear to be the catalyst for vector mosquito population increases. Specifically, wetter than usual spring conditions, including waters derived from the melting of late winter snow storms, and drier than usual summer conditions presage increased human WN cases (Shaman et al., 2010).

The wetter spring conditions provide a greater abundance of the cleaner, less eutrophic waters preferred by *Cx. tarsalis.* These vector mosquitoes then proliferate and in the presence of normal or above-normal numbers of avian hosts, as well as the virus, *Cx. tarsalis* can initiate early springtime epizootic amplification of WNV. Dry summer conditions then reduce stream flow and facilitate puddling and ponding of stagnant waters within the riparian zones. These eutrophic waters are favored by the other dominant vector, *Cx. pipiens* (Savage and Miller 1995), which can increase in abundance and continue the amplification and zoonotic transmission of WNV.

The eastern Colorado WNV transmission cycle appears to be further complicated by irrigation practices, which divert riparian flow into agricultural fields, in effect spreading water resources out and providing more eutrophic habitats during the summer. Areas with agricultural irrigation in eastern Colorado have been associated with increased incidence of human WN cases (Eisen et al., 2010). In addition, the watering of lawns and golf courses, as well as the presence of golf course water hazards, in the towns and cities along the Front Range in eastern Colorado (e.g. Fort Collins, Denver) provide additional habitats favorable for vector mosquitoes and avian amplification hosts. These land irrigation and management practices put humans in greater contact with infectious vector mosquitoes and support the heightened transmission of WNV to humans evident in this region. Thus, a combination of hydrological and land management practices appear to facilitate WNV transmission to humans in eastern Colorado.

3.4 West Nile virus in Florida

Florida is the only state with a history of SLE epidemics that has yet to see a major WN epidemic (Gubler 2007). West Nile virus entered Florida in late 2000 or early 2001 and was first detected in July, 2001 in Jefferson County, located in the Florida Panhandle. Horses and dead wild birds were the first animals from which WNV was isolated in Florida. There was no WN horse vaccine available in 2001 and the entire Florida horse population was naïve and susceptible to infection as WNV moved through the state. The vulnerable condition of the Florida horse population is evidenced by the WNV transmission data reported for 2001 through 2010. In 2001 there were 491 WNV-positive horses reported in the state. An experimental horse vaccine was introduced into Florida late in 2001, but the availability of the vaccine did not slow WNV transmission in 2002 when 499 positive horses were reported in the state. The number of WNV-positive horses started to decline in 2003 when 117 positive horses were reported (USDA—APHIS 2011). The number of WNV-positive horses remained low from 2004-2010 with an annual average of 6 positive horses per year. A combination of the availability of an efficacious vaccine along with environmental conditions that did not favor the amplification of WNV in Florida appears to have been responsible for the reduced transmission observed between 2004 and 2010.

As was the case with WNV invasion in other states, human cases were associated with the first reports of virus in Florida. There were 12 clinical WN cases reported in Florida during 2001. These cases were reported from the western Florida Panhandle south to the Florida Keys, indicating that the virus was well-established in the state prior to the appearance of human cases. In 2002 there were 28 clinical human cases reported from throughout the state. The highpoint of WNV transmission to humans in Florida occurred in 2003 when a total of 94 clinical cases were reported from throughout the state. Since 2003 human cases have rarely been reported in Florida (CDC 2011).

The zoonotic transmission of WNV, as measured by sentinel chickens, is similar to that of SLEV and occurs year round in Florida. A major difference between the transmission cycles of the two viruses is the number of zoonotic mosquito vectors that transmit WNV. The WNV has been isolated from a wide variety of mosquito species in Florida and it is likely that many of these species can support the transmission of WNV to wild birds in nature. For example, *Deinocerites cancer* Theobald is a prolific mosquito species found in saltmarshes along the east coast of Florida where it blood feeds on marsh birds. Isolates of WNV have been made from pools of *De. cancer* collected in the Florida Keys (Hribar et al. 2004). It is very likely that this mosquito species supports WNV transmission in saltmarshes all along the east coast of Florida.

Even though a major WN epidemic has not yet been reported in Florida, the biological components of the WNV transmission cycle are already in place throughout the state. *Culex nigripalpus* is a proven vector of both SLEV and WNV in Florida (Shroyer 1991; Rutledge et al. 2003). The interaction of this mosquito species with WNV and avian amplification hosts, as well as the environmental drivers that affect WNV transmission, are very similar to those already reported for SLEV transmission in south Florida (Shaman et al. 2005).

As is the case with SLEV, the environmental conditions that favor a WN epidemic are rare occurrences. The exact sequence of events necessary to produce large numbers of nestlings along with abundant *Cx. nigripalpus* populations of just the right age structure are seldom realized. However, a knowledge of the biological and environmental conditions necessary to create a WN epidemic—winter freeze, ample bird abundance, spring drought and summer rainfall cycling—allow researchers to track seasonal biological events and predict when and where outbreaks may occur. Exactly how this is done is discussed in detail below.

4. Spatial-temporal arboviral surveillance and prediction

A thorough understanding of the biological and environmental components associated with any arboviral transmission cycle allows the tracking of those components and the formulation of a prediction about where and when arboviral amplification and transmission might occur. The biological components of an arboviral transmission cycle that can be tracked include: the abundance and spatio-temporal distribution of the virus; the abundance, spatio-temporal distribution, and age structure of all mosquito vectors involved with viral amplification and transmission; and the abundance, spatio-temporal distribution, and age structure of all amplification hosts associated with viral amplification and transmission. The physically-based components of an arboviral transmission cycle that can be easily tracked include: meteorological conditions (daily rainfall, temperature, and relative humidity; rainfall deviations from long term averages; and temperature deviations from long term averages), hydrological conditions (soil moisture levels, land surface ponding and puddling, as well as the relationship between physical factors including topography, soil type, incident radiation, vegetation, rainfall, and temperature with surface groundwater levels), and land use (forest clearing and regrowth, housing and business development, agricultural practices including irrigation and ground surface manipulation, and other land management practices). Sampling techniques that assist the tracking of these biological and environmental components are discussed below.

4.1 Viral sampling

The abundance and spatio-temporal distribution of arboviruses can be measured in three ways: sentinel animal surveillance, isolation of virus from vectors, and virus and viral antibody isolation from wild and domestic animals.

Sentinel animal surveillance provides one of the easiest, cheapest, and most effective ways to detect and monitor arboviruses in the field. For most sentinel programs, naïve animals are placed in the field prior to the beginning of the arboviral transmission season and maintained at a fixed site for the duration of the transmission season. Weekly blood samples are collected from each sentinel animal and analysed for arboviral-specific antibody. Confirmation of antibody indicates recent arboviral transmission to that sentinel at that site. One of the most frequently used sentinel animals is the domestic chicken. Sentinel chickens have proven highly versatile for monitoring SLEV, WNV, EEEV, and HJV in Florida, where the state-wide program was initiated following the 1977 Florida SLE epidemic (Day and Lewis 1992). A great advantage of sentinel chicken surveillance for mosquito-borne encephalitis viruses is that the chickens serve as dead-end hosts without further amplifying the viruses in the environment.

The value of arboviral surveillance through well-run sentinel animal programs is that the sentinels are caged at predetermined sites in the field. When these sites remain constant from year to year, long term baseline seroconversion data sets can be established. Once baseline data sets are known for individual surveillance sites, monthly, or even weekly, deviations from normal can be calculated and monitored for each site. An arboviral surveillance program based on sentinel chickens was established in Indian River County (IRC), Florida in 1978. There are sentinel chicken flock sites in IRC that have been in the same location for nearly 35 years. These long term data sets prove invaluable during years when unusual levels of viral transmission are detected. They accurately measure weekly differences in viral transmission levels and also provide a spatial measurement that identifies viral transmission hotspots throughout the county.

Occasionally, completely naïve animal populations detect arboviral introductions into new areas. This happened in Florida in 2001 when WNV first entered the state. At that time, the sentinel chicken program was already in place for SLEV and provided a ready network for tracking the appearance and spread of WNV. In addition, in 2001 local horse populations were unvaccinated and previously unexposed to WNV. In many Florida counties, WNV-positive local horses (both antibody positive horses and WNV isolations from horses that died of WN infection) were the first to detect the presence of WNV. Once WNV became endemic in Florida and an efficacious WNV vaccine was introduced, the value of horses for monitoring the presence and movement of WNV was greatly reduced.

Horses are highly susceptible to infection with EEEV. Even though there is a highly efficacious EEEV vaccine, many horses remain unvaccinated and the monitoring of dead horses in EEEV endemic areas sometimes provides the first indication of seasonal EEEV transmission in regions along the east coast of North America. Humans also sometimes serve as arboviral sentinels. The re-introduction of DENV into Key West, Florida in 2009 was first detected through an infected human because there are no avian or non-human reservoir or amplification hosts in the DENV transmission cycle in Key West, Florida.

In general, the isolation of virus from infected vectors provides a less sensitive measure of the spatiotemporal distribution of an arbovirus. Mosquitoes are able to fly and may move considerable distances from the point of infection. Still, viral isolation from an infected vector is a good way to detect the regional presence of a virus. Generally, mosquito species are assayed in groups or 'pools' of 50-100 mosquitoes. An increased number of infected mosquito pools collected at a site over a short period of time may be indicative of on-going arboviral amplification. However, positive mosquito pools do not provide evidence that the mosquito, or mosquitoes, responsible for the positive pool were able to transmit virus (Rutledge et al., 2003). During much of the year, mosquito infection rates are so low that viral detection in mosquito pools is difficult. Because mosquito pooling is labor intensive and expensive, it is more cost-effective to let sentinel animals screen large numbers of mosquitoes and to monitor viral presence and distribution through seropositive sentinels.

Because some viruses are highly pathogenic to certain vertebrate hosts, the mortality of these hosts sometimes provides a measure of viral transmission. For example, WNV can be highly pathogenic to many avian species, especially those in the Family Corvidae (crows, ravens, jays, and magpies). Thus, it is possible to analyse the tissues of dead birds for WNV to detect the presence of virus in an area (Nemeth et al. 2007) or to provide early warning of WNV amplification (Eidson et al. 2001). As with mosquito pooling, dead bird surveillance is labor intensive and expensive. Because birds can disperse from the original infection site, data interpretation is also sometimes difficult. However, dead bird surveillance was one of the major ways that the movement of WNV across the USA was monitored between 1999 and 2004 (Nemeth et al. 2007).

4.2 Vector sampling

Many mosquito control programs rely on adult and larval sampling to assess the spatial and temporal abundance of mosquito populations. Surveillance protocols are designed to monitor vector as well as nuisance species. A large number of adult and larval monitoring techniques, trapping devices, and sampling protocols have been developed (Service 1993). Each technique has its strengths and weaknesses, and individual surveillance programs rely on the technique that works best for the mosquito vectors and pests in their jurisdictions.

Light traps are among the most popular methods for sampling adult mosquitoes. The New Jersey light trap and the CDC light trap have both been used for decades by mosquito control programs to monitor adult mosquito populations. CDC light traps are commonly baited with CO_2 (in the form of dry ice or as bottled gas metered into the trap) as a secondary attractant. A disadvantage of light traps is that they capture a wide variety of non-target species including moths, beetles, and wasps. Non-target species in the collection greatly slows the sorting process. Carbon dioxide-baited suction traps usually make a pure collection of biting arthropods including mosquitoes and biting midges. Modified suction traps designed to capture gravid mosquitoes attracted to a tray containing oviposition media collect female mosquitoes that are more likely to be infected with an arbovirus because they have taken at least one blood meal and matured an egg batch. Mosquito control programs sometimes rely on landing rate count to quickly assess biting fly populations in selected areas of concern. Finally, mosquito control programs also rely on sampling techniques designed to capture immature mosquitoes (larvae and pupae). Mosquito dippers are used to survey aquatic habitats for the presence of immature mosquitoes, usually in targeted larval habitats. Skilled technicians can easily identify the mosquito species, its abundance, the age (in days) of the immature mosquitoes, and the projected emergence date of the adult mosquitoes (Service 1993). When field identifications are in question, immature mosquitoes can be returned to the laboratory where they are allowed to mature and emerge as adults that are generally easier to identify.

One of the most versatile adult mosquito sampling techniques for monitoring vector populations is the ground aspiration of resting mosquitoes (Day and Curtis 1993, 1999). This technique relies on a battery powered aspirator that is used to make sweep collections of resting mosquitoes. These collections include newly emerged and older males as well as females in a number of different life stages including: newly emerged, unfed, freshly blood fed, half blood/half gravid, and gravid. By tracking the proportions of females in different life stages it is possible to calculate the age structure of a vector population and in so doing assess the risk of viral transmission (Day and Curtis 1994). Ground aspiration adult mosquito surveillance is most effective for monitoring nocturnally active mosquitoes that congregate in daytime resting sites. For example, many species of *Anopheles* mosquitoes rest in and around human habitations where they can be easily collected by aspiration during the daytime (Service 1993). Likewise, many *Culex* species congregate in humid, heavily-vegetated habitats where they are easily collected in large numbers by ground aspiration (Day and Curtis 1993).

4.3 Vertebrate host sampling

In cases where the species of an arboviral amplification host is known, it is possible to monitor individual populations to assess amplification risk. In Florida several wild bird species are known amplification hosts for WNV and SLEV. With the proper State and Federal permits, wild birds can be trapped, handled, banded, and bled. Blood samples can be analysed for virus and virus-specific antibody. The appearance of virus or antibody in recently fledged birds is an indication of recent local viral transmission and is sometimes helpful in assessing transmission risk. Avian sampling is also helpful in determining species abundance, population age structure, and the viral immune status of adult and immature birds (Day and Stark 1999). As is the case with infected mosquitoes, seropositive wild birds are usually rare and the collection and handling of wild birds is labor intensive, with a low yield of positive results, especially during inter-epidemic periods.

4.4 Meteorological, hydrological, and other environmental data

A wealth of meteorological and hydrological data is available from university, governmental, and international resources. These data are typically compiled by national meteorological services and, in some instances (e.g. the United States), are available free of charge (NCDC 2011). Typical records may include hourly or daily measurements of 2-meter above-ground temperature, precipitation rates, and 2-meter above-ground humidity, all of which may influence the abundance and distribution of arboviral pathogens, vectors, and hosts in a particular region. In addition, estimates of soil moisture content and land surface wetness and water pooling are routinely derived from both satellite observations and physically-based hydrology models that numerically simulate hydrological conditions. Maps of the distribution of soil and vegetation type, as well as land use classifications are also available from a variety of sources. These maps are increasingly available in digital format through resources such as Google Earth.

Temperature is typically measured at meteorological stations on a sub-hourly, hourly, or daily basis at a height of 1-2 meters above ground. These stations are distributed across the landscape at a density that usually reflects the level of funding provided to a nation's meteorological service. Dense networks replete with hourly temperature records are available in many developed countries. These temperature data can be used to derive an estimate of the local EIP for a given arbovirus vector and to document the magnitude and duration of local freezes and the level of vegetation die-off. As temperatures can vary considerably from the surface to several meters above ground and from the understory to open areas, such estimates of EIP would need to be qualified. Indeed, the arboviral pathogen, vector, and host are only subject to the conditions in their immediate surroundings, i.e. their microclimate, which can vary considerably over short distances. Both vectors and hosts can in part control this microclimate (e.g. temperature conditions) by simply moving.

Records of hourly or daily total precipitation are also often maintained by national meteorological station networks. Daily precipitation is the more commonly available measure, though this 24-hour measure does not always correspond with the end of the day; rather, not infrequently it represents the 24-hour rainfall accumulated prior to some unspecified hour (e.g. 7 am local time).

Humidity is much less commonly recorded than either temperature or precipitation, as not all meteorological stations are routinely equipped with hygrometers. Standard humidity measurements, where available, are taken 1-2 meters above the ground. There are numerous measures of humidity, which fall into two distinct categories: 1) relative humidity, which measures the amount of water vapor in the air relative to saturation, which is the point at which rates of evaporation and condensation are equivalent and a cloud or fog begins to form; 2) absolute humidity, which provides a mass-based measure of the amount of water vapor in the air. Relative humidity is typically given as a percent of saturation; absolute humidity comes in multiple forms such as vapor pressure and specific humidity.

There also exist many estimates of drought (NIDIS 2011). Some of these are very simple algorithms or indices that derive a measure of drought from recent meteorological conditions, including precipitation and temperature. Other measures are derived from networks of soil moisture monitoring stations. Satellite sensors can be used to estimate soil moisture content directly from bare soil or to infer water availability by measuring the greenness of land surface vegetation (Anyamba et al. 2009). In addition, hydrology models can provide more sophisticated and comprehensive physically-based estimates of the movement and pooling of water beneath the surface and at the land-atmosphere interface (e.g. Koster and Suarez 1996). All these estimates suffer shortcomings that must be recognized and accounted for when using these data.

Measurements are very often automated, which can lead to gaps in a record due to equipment failure; however, automated stations, when functional, provide more frequent measures of conditions and are not subject to certain human-related measurement errors. Biases within automated stations still may exist, for example due to instrumental bias or placement of the station in the shade or near building ventilation systems. It is best when using environmental data derived from national network sources, to investigate the specific collection protocols and placement for the station data to be used.

In addition, thermometers, hygrometers, rain gauge stations and soil moisture sensors are readily available for purchase from a variety of scientific supply companies. These systems are easy to install and use, provide regular measures in the field at the site of interest, and typically come with software systems for automatically recording measured meteorological conditions. All systems should be calibrated prior to use.

4.5 The use of surveillance protocols to predict and mitigate arboviral transmission

A thorough knowledge of the biological and environmental components of an arbovirus transmission cycle allows the spatial and temporal tracking of the virus and a skillful prediction of where and when virus transmission will occur. The virus itself is tracked in a number of different ways. Sentinel surveillance uses virus-specific antibody in sentinel animals to narrow the spatio-temporal timeframe of viral amplification and transmission. An advantage of this technique is that it allows a better understanding of exactly where and when virus is being transmitted. A disadvantage is that there is often a significant time lag between the infective mosquito bite on the sentinel animal and the confirmation of positive virus-specific antibody in the sentinel's blood. Depending on the blood collection protocol, the delay may range from 10 days to a month (Day and Lewis 1992). Amplification host surveillance is a second way that specific viruses can be tracked in the field. Virus or antibody isolation from the blood of a known amplification host may help to determine recent viral transmission in the field. Disadvantages of this technique include the mobility of wild amplification hosts (they may be captured considerable distances from the original infection site), positive antibody tests in an adult animal that may represent an old infection, and the extensive permitting required for the handling and manipulation of most vertebrate amplification hosts.

The pooling of known mosquito vector species and subsequent viral isolation attempts is a third way that virus can be detected and monitored in the field. During inter-epidemic periods vector infection rates are usually very low. However, during epidemics or epizootics vector infection rates increase dramatically, especially during the early amplification phase of an epidemic, and it is possible to collect vectors in the field, pool them, and analyse the pools for the presence of virus (Day and Stark 1996). A positive mosquito pool indicates that virus was present in at least one of the mosquitoes contained in the pool. Large numbers of virus-specific positive mosquito pools from a localized area indicates that viral amplification may be on-going in that area (Shroyer 1991). Disadvantages of this technique are that vectors, like vertebrate amplification hosts, may disperse from the original infection site making it difficult to identify the exact geographical confines of the outbreak. In addition, a positive mosquito pool is not necessarily indicative of viral transmission by that mosquito species in the field (Rutledge et al. 2003) and positive mosquito pools may not accurately measure the viral transmission risk.

Dead animal surveillance is a fourth way that virus transmission can be monitored in the field. Focal die-offs of susceptible vertebrate species may indicate recent local viral transmission. Disadvantages of this technique include the fact that most amplification hosts do not die as a result of arboviral infection and there is a danger to the general public associated with the handling of animals that have died as the result of an arboviral infection.

The environmental forces that influence the movement and infection of vectors and vertebrate hosts can be monitored to better understand the risks associated with viral amplification and transmission. Hydrological and surface wetness models have proven to be valuable in the monitoring and prediction of WNV transmission in Florida (Shaman and Day 2005; Day and Shaman 2008) and eastern Colorado (Shaman et al. 2010). It is important to understand and monitor the exact environmental drivers for individual arboviral transmission cycles. For example, the environmental conditions responsible for high levels of WNV transmission in Texas are different than those responsible for WNV transmission in California. A careful study of the habitat-specific dynamics of viruses, vectors, and amplification hosts along with an understanding of the environmental conditions responsible for driving each of these cycles is necessary before transmission patterns are understood and outbreaks can be predicted.

Once the biological components of a transmission cycle and the environmental factors responsible for driving those biological components are understood, it is possible to attempt mitigation of an impending arboviral epidemic. Perhaps one of the best examples of how a thorough understanding of an arboviral transmission cycle can translate into epidemic mitigation comes from Pinellas County, Florida where a focal outbreak of WNV transmission resulted in 18 human cases in 2005 (Day and Shaman 2008). Pinellas County is located on the west coast of central Florida and consists of a peninsula that extends into the Gulf of Mexico to the west and Tampa Bay to the east. The main metropolitan districts in Pinellas County include St. Petersburg, Largo, and Clearwater. Pinellas County Mosquito Control (PCMC) is responsible for the arboviral surveillance program and mosquito control throughout the county. The Pinellas County Health Department (PCHD) and the PCMC are responsible for assessing arboviral transmission risk to humans and issuing mosquito-borne disease advisories and warnings. The first indication of a possible WNV transmission problem in Pinellas County during the summer of 2005 came on July 11, when seven sentinel chickens from three flocks located in the south western quarter of the county tested positive for WNV antibody. On July 25 an additional 12 sentinel chickens from the same flocks tested positive for WNV antibody, and on August 1 eight more sentinels from the same flocks tested positive. This intense, early season transmission of WNV to sentinel chickens indicated that WNV 1) was more abundant than normal in Pinellas County, 2) had undergone an efficient early season amplification cycle in the south western quadrant of the county, and 3) had infected mosquitoes that had completed the EIP and were transmitting the virus to sentinel chickens. In addition, a GIS modification of a hydrologic groundwater model developed for south Florida (Figure 3) (Shaman et al., 2005) indicated that the ground water conditions in the southern half of Pinellas County were favorable for WNV amplification during springtime, i.e. drought-induced restriction of *Cx. nigripalpus* activity to habitats exploited by nesting avian hosts (Day and Shaman, 2008).

The collection and analysis of arboviral surveillance data by PCMC initiated a series of events that most likely greatly reduced the impact of WNV transmission on the humans living in and visiting Pinellas County during the summer of 2005. As a result of the first group of WN-positive sentinel chickens reported on July 11, a West Nile Virus Advisory was issued by the PCHD in consultation with PCMC. On July 20, PCMC began extra mosquito control efforts focused around the area identified by the three positive sentinel chicken flocks. On August 1, 2005 the first human WN case was reported, and on that same day the PCHD upgraded the West Nile Virus Advisory to a Mosquito-borne Disease Alert. Elevated focused mosquito control efforts continued throughout August. The onset dates for the 18 human WN infections ranged from July 9 through August 12, 2005. It is suggested that the rapid responses to the WN surveillance data by PCMC and the PCHD mitigated a potential WN epidemic in Pinellas County during 2005. The peak WNV transmission months in Florida are July, August, and September. The fact that the final onset date for a human case in Pinellas County during the 2005 outbreak was August 12 indicates that the WNV transmission cycle was broken by a failure of sufficient rainfall cycling through the summer and aggressive mosquito control efforts coupled with a public health campaign designed to alert and educate the residents of Pinellas County about the risk of an impending WN epidemic. The outbreak and control of WNV in Pinellas County, Florida during the summer of 2005 is one of the best examples of how a well-designed arboviral surveillance program can be used to monitor and mitigate a potentially severe mosquito-borne arbovirus transmission event.

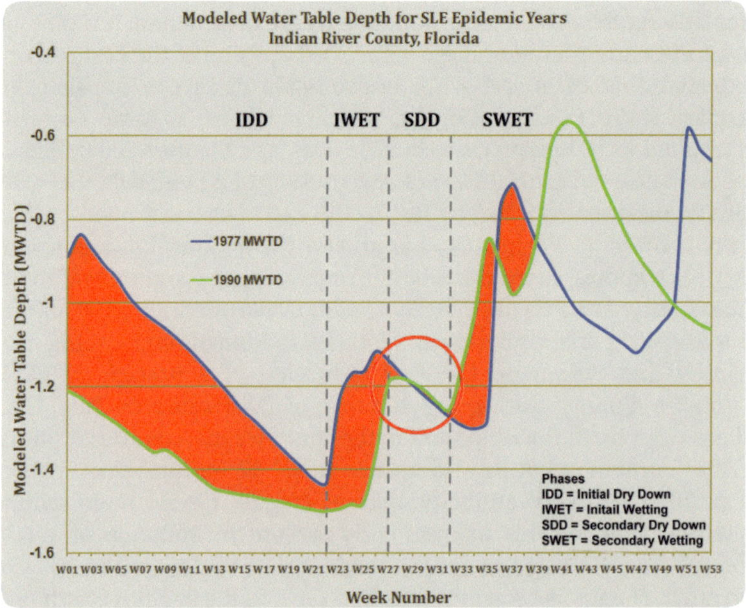

Fig. 3. Weekly Modeled Water Table Depth (MWTD) values in Indian River County, Florida for the SLE epidemic years 1977 (blue line) and 1990 (green line). The Florida Medical Entomology Laboratory Arboviral Epidemic Risk Model values (highlighted in orange) are compared to real-time WTD values collected throughout peninsular Florida. Modeled WTD values that fall continuously within the shaded area through the Initial Dry Down (IDD) and Initial Wetting (IWET) phases are favorable for the successful amplification of SLE and WN viruses. Areas where MWTD data closely follow the trends of the first two phases are considered at high risk for *focal* arboviral transmission. The Secondary Dry Down (SDD) phase, circled in red, along with a Secondary Wetting (SWET) phase, are considered critical for *epidemic* arboviral transmission. The last two phases provide conditions conducive for a second round of amplification followed by dispersal of virus out of the secondary amplification foci

5. Conclusions

Arboviral transmission cycles can be tracked in real time and the risk of an arboviral epidemic, based on surveillance data, can be predicted. The ability to accurately predict an arboviral outbreak is linked to the quality of the surveillance data, which depends greatly on an understanding of the biology and environmental conditions unique to each local disease transmission cycle. Our ability to mitigate arboviral transmission events is tied to the quality of the local long-term baseline data sets associated with annual measurements of virus abundance and transmission; vector abundance, age structure, and infectivity status; and amplification host abundance and susceptibility to viral infection. Superimposed on these three biological cycles are the environmental factors that regulate the population biology of the virus, vector, and amplification hosts. There is a continued need to fine-tune our understanding of local arboviral transmission cycles. In a constantly changing environment, the importance of the primary vectors and amplification hosts to the dynamics of viral transmission are ever-changing. Vectors that were previously important to disease transmission become rare and disappear, while new vectors invade habitats where they were previously unknown. Amplification host populations that were previously important to transmission cycles may become less significant while new amplification hosts emerge and become important to the continuation of arboviral transmission cycles. Finally, viruses that were once abundant in particular habitats disappear and re-emerge to become major players in new habitats, sometimes on new continents. It is important that surveillance programs remain strong and vital in order to track these continually changing biological and environmental cycles that are responsible for disease outbreaks in humans, domestic animals, and wildlife around the World.

6. Acknowledgments

We thank Roxanne Connelly, Joan Giustino, Timothy Hope, and Gregg Ross for their thoughtful suggestions regarding this manuscript. Figure credits: Figures 1 and 2, design: Jonathan Day, production: James Newman; Figure 3, design: Jonathan Day, production: Gregg Ross. This work was funded in part through grants from the Florida Department of Agriculture and Consumer Services.

7. References

Anderson, S.; Richards, S.; Tabachnick, W. & Smartt, C. (2010). Effects of West Nile virus dose and extrinsic incubation temperature on temporal progression of vector competence in *Culex pipiens quinquefasciatus*. *Journal of the American Mosquito Control Association*, Vol. 26, pp. 103-107

Anon (2003). Study: West Nile virus cost equine industries in Colorado, Nebraska millions in 2002. *Journal of the American Veterinary Medical Association*, Vol. 222, pp. 1669

Anyamba, A.; Chretien, J.; Small, J.; Tucker, C. J.; Formenty, P. B. & et al. (2009). Prediction of a Rift Valley fever outbreak. *Proceedings of the National Academy of Science*, Vol. 106, pp. 955-959

Barker, C.M.; Bolling, B.G.; Black, W.C.; Moore, C.G.; Eisen, L. (2009). Mosquitoes and West Nile virus along a river corridor from prairie to montane habitats in eastern Colorado. *Journal of Vector Ecology*, Vol. 34, pp. 276-293

Black, W.; Bennett, K.; Gorrochótegui-Escalante, N.; Barrillas-Mury, C. & et al. (2002). Flavivirus susceptibility in *Aedes aegypti*. *Archives of Medical Research*, Vol. 33, pp. 379-388

Bolling, B.G.; Moore, C.G.; Anderson, S.L.; Blair, C.D. & Beaty, B.J. (2007) Entomological studies along the Colorado Front Range during a period of intense West Nile virus activity. *Journal of the American Mosquito Control Association*, Vol. 23, pp. 37-46

Burton, A.; McLintock, J. & Rempel, J. (1966). Western equine encephalitis in Saskatchewan garter snakes and leopard frogs. *Science*, Vol. 154, pp. 1029-1031

CDC -- Centers for Disease Control (1999). Outbreak of West Nile-like viral encephalitis – New York, 1999. *MMWR-Morbidity and Mortality Weekly Report*, Vol. 48, pp. 845-849

CDC -- Centers for Disease Control (2011). West Nile virus-statistics, surveillance, and control archive: http://www.cdc.gov/ncidod/dvbid/westnile/surv&control_archive.htm

Crans, W.; Caccamise, D. & McNelly, J. (1994). Eastern equine encephalomyelitis virus in relation to the avian community of a coastal cedar swamp. *Journal of Medical Entomology*, Vol. 31, pp. 711-728

Day, J. F. (2001). Predicting St. Louis encephalitis virus epidemics : Lessons from recent, and not so recent, outbreaks. *Annual Review of Entomology*, Vol. 46, pp. 111-138

Day, J. F. & Curtis, G. A. (1993). Annual emergence patterns of *Culex nigripalpus* females before, during and after a widespread St. Louis encephalitis epidemic in south Florida. *Journal of the American Mosquito Control Association*, Vol. 9, pp. 249-255

Day, J. F. & Curtis, G. A. (1994). When it rains, they soar—and that makes *Culex nigripalpus* a dangerous mosquito. *American Entomologist*, Vol. 40, pp. 162-167

Day, J. F. & Curtis, G. A. (1999). *Culex nigripalpus* (Diptera: Culicidae) blood feeding and oviposition before, during and after a widespread St. Louis encephalitis epidemic in Florida, USA. *Journal of Medical Entomology*, Vol. 36, pp. 176-181

Day, J. F. & Lewis, A. L. (1992). An integrated approach to St. Louis encephalitis surveillance in Indian River County, Florida. *Florida Journal of Public Health*, Vol. 4, pp. 12-16

Day, J. F. & Shaman, J. (2008). Using hydrologic conditions to track the risk of focal and epidemic arboviral transmission in peninsular Florida. *Journal of Medical Entomology*, Vol. 45, pp. 458-493

Day, J. F. & Shaman, J. (2009). Severe winter freezes enhance St. Louis encephalitis virus amplification and epidemic transmission in peninsular Florida. *Journal of Medical Entomology*, Vol. 45, No. 6, pp. 1498-1506

Day, J. F. & Stark, L. M. (1996). Eastern equine encephalitis transmission to emus (*Dromaius novaehollandiae*) in Volusia County, Florida: 1992 through 1994. *Journal of the American Mosquito Control Association*, Vol. 12, pp. 429-436

Day, J. F. & Stark, L. M. (1999). Avian serology in a St. Louis encephalitis epicenter before, during, and after a widespread epidemic in South Florida, USA. *Journal of Medical Entomology*, Vol. 36, pp. 614-624

Eidson, M.; Kramer, L.; Stone, W. & Hagiwara, Y. (2001). Avian mortality surveillance as an early warning system for West Nile virus. *Emerging Infectious Diseases*, Vol. 7, pp. 631-635

Eisen, L.; Bolling, C.D.; Blair, B.J. & Moore, C.G. (2008). Mosquito species richness, composition and abundance along habitat-climate-elevation gradients in the northern Colorado Front Range. *Journal of Medical Entomology*, Vol. 45, pp. 800-811

Eisen, L.; Barker, C. M., Moore, C. G.; Pape, W. J.; Winters, A. M. & Cheronis, N. (2010). Agriculture is an important risk factor for West Nile virus disease in the hyperendemic Larimer-Boulder-Weld area of north central Colorado. *Journal of Medical Entomology*, Vol. 47, pp. 939-951

Erlanger, T. E.; Weiss, S.; Keiser, J.; Utzinger, J. & Wiedenmayer, K. (2009). Past, present, and future of Japanese encephalitis. *Emerging Infectious Diseases*, Vol. 15, pp. 1-7

Gubler, D. (2007). The continuing spread of West Nile virus in the Western Hemisphere. *Emerging Infections*, Vol. 45, pp. 1039-1046

Hardy, J.; Houk, E.; Kramer, L. & Reeves, W. (1983). Intrinsic factors affecting vector competence of mosquitoes for arboviruses. *Annual Review of Entomology*, Vol. 28, pp. 229-262

Hayes, E. B.; Komar, N.; Nasci, R. S.; Montgomery, S. P.; O'Leary, D. R. & Campbell, G. L. (2005). Epidemiology and transmission dynamics of West Nile virus disease. *Emerging Infectious Diseases*, Vol. 11, pp. 1167-1173

Hribar, L. J.; Stark, L. M.; Stoner, R. L.; DeMay, D. J.; Nordholt, A. L. & et al. (2004). Isolation of West Nile virus from mosquitoes (Diptera: Culicidae) in the Florida Keys, Monroe County, Florida. *Caribbean Journal of Science*, Vol. 40, pp. 362-367

Kolivras, K. N. (2006). Mosquito habitat and dengue risk potential in Hawaii: A conceptual framework and GIS application. *The Professional Geographer*, Vol. 58, pp. 139-154

Koster, R.D. & Suarez, M.J. (1996). Energy and water balance calculations in the Mosaic LSM. *NASA Technical Memo. 104606*, Vol. 9, pp. 1-58

Marfin, A.A. & Gubler, D.J. (2001). West Nile encephalitis: an emerging disease in the United States. *Clinical Infectious Disease*, Vol. 33, pp. 1713-1719

Morbidity and Mortality Weekly Report. (2010). Locally acquired dengue—Key West, Florida, 2009-2010. *MMWR*, Vol. 59, pp. 577-581

Nasci, R. S.; Savage, H. M.; White, D. J.; Miller, J. R.; Cropp, B. C. & et al. (2001). West Nile virus in overwintering *Culex* mosquitoes, New York City, 2000. *Emerging Infectious Diseases*, Vol. 4, pp. 1-3

NCDC--National Climate Data Center (2011). NOAA Satellite and Information Service: http://www.ncdc.noaa.gov/oa/ncdc.html

Nemeth, N.; Beckett, S.; Edwards, E.; Klenk, K. & Komar, N. (2007). Avian mortality surveillance for West Nile virus in Colorado. *American Journal of Tropical Medicine and Hygiene*, Vol. 76, pp. 431-437

NIDIS-National Integrated Drought Information System. (2011). *U.S. Drought Portal.* Online data repository: http://www.drought.gov/portal/server.pt/community/drought_gov/202;jsessionid=0E3F955A70124FBF5AE9F39D949AEBD2

Ooi, E-E.; Goh, K-T & Gubler, D. J. (2006). Dengue prevention and 35 years of vector control in Singapore. *Emerging Infectious Diseases*, Vol. 12, pp. 888-893

Richards S.; Lord, C.; Pesko, K. & Tabachnick, W. (2009). Mosquito age, incubation temperature, viremia and *Culex pipiens quinquefasciatus* Say (Diptera: Culicidae) vector competence for West Nile and St. Louis encephalitis viruses. *American Journal of Tropical Medicine and Hygiene*, Vol. 81, pp. 264-272

Richards S.; Lord, C.; Pesko, K. & Tabachnick, W. (2010). Environmental and biological factors influencing *Culex pipiens quinquefasciatus* (Diptera: Culicidae) vector competence for West Nile virus. *American Journal of Tropical Medicine and Hygiene*, Vol. 83, pp. 126-134

Russell, R. C. (2002). Ross River virus: Ecology and distribution. *Annual Review of Entomology*, Vol. 47, pp. 1-31

Rutledge, C.; Day, J.; Lord, C.; Stark, L. & Tabachnick, W. (2003). *Culex nigripalpus* Theobald (Diptera: Culicidae) transmission of West Nile virus in Florida: Infection rates in Florida *Culex* mosquitoes do not accurately reflect transmission rates in nature. *Journal of Medical Entomology*, Vol. 40, pp. 253-258

Savage, H. & Miller, B. (1995). House Mosquitoes of the U.S.A., *Culex pipiens* complex. *Wing Beats*, Vol. 6, pp. 8-9

Scott, T. & Weaver, S. (1989). Eastern equine encephalomyelitis virus: epidemiology and evolution of mosquito transmission. *Advances in Virus Research*, Vol. 37, pp. 277-328

Service, M. (1993). *Mosquito Ecology Field Sampling Methods*, Elsevier Applied Science, 1-85166-798-9, New York, New York

Shaman J. (2007). Amplification due to spatial clustering in an individual-based model of mosquito-avian arbovirus transmission. *Transactions of the Royal Society of Tropical Medicine and Hygiene*, Vol. 101, pp. 469-483

Shaman, J. & Day, J. (2005). Achieving operational hydrologic monitoring of mosquito-borne diseases. *Emerging Infectious Diseases*, Vol. 11, pp. 1343-1350

Shaman, J.; Day, J. & Stieglitz, M. (2002). Drought-Induced amplification of St. Louis encephalitis virus, Florida. *Emerging Infectious Diseases*, Vol. 8, pp. 575-580

Shaman, J.; Day, J. & Stieglitz, M. (2005). Drought-Induced amplification and epidemic transmission of West Nile Virus in south Florida. *Journal of Medical Entomology*, Vol. 42, pp. 134-141

Shaman J.; Day, J. F. & Komar, N. (2010). Hydrologic conditions describe West Nile virus risk in Colorado. *International Journal of Environmental Research and Public Health*, Vol. 7, pp. 494-508, doi:10.3390/ijerph7020494

Shroyer, D. A. (1991). The 1990 Florida epidemic of St. Louis encephalitis: virus infection rates in *Culex nigripalpus*. *Journal of the Florida Mosquito Control Association*, Vol. 62, pp. 69-71

Tabachnick W. (1994). Genetics of insect vector competence for arboviruses, In: *Advances in Disease Vector Research Vol. 10*, K. Harris K, pp. 93-108, Springer-Verlag, New York, New York

USDA - United States Department of Agriculture (2011). Animal health monitoring and surveillance—West Nile virus surveillance: http://www.aphis.usda.gov/vs/nahss/equine/wnv/

Villari, P. ; Spielman, A. ; Komar, N. ; McDowell, M. & Timperi, R. (1995). The economic burden imposed by a residual case of eastern encephalitis. *American Journal of Tropical Medicine and Hygiene*, Vol. 52, pp. 8-13

Watts, D. M.; Burke, D. S.; Harrison, B. A.; Whitmire, R. E. & Nisalak, A. (1987). Effect of temperature on the vector efficiency of *Aedes aegypti* for dengue 2 virus. *American Journal of Tropical Medicine and Hygiene*, Vol. 36, pp. 143-152

Watts, D. M.; Pantuwatana, S.; DeFoliart, G. R.; Yuill, T. M. & Thompson, W. H. (1973). Transovarial transmission of LaCrosse virus (California Encephalitis Group) in the mosquito, *Aedes triseriatus*. *Science*, Vol. 182, pp. 1140-1141

Wilson, J.; Rubin, H.; Lane, T. & Gibbs, P. (1986). A survey of eastern equine encephalomyelitis in Florida horses: Prevalence, economic impact, and management practices, 1982-1983. *Preventive Veterinary Medicine*, Vol. 4, pp. 261-271

Winters, A.M.; Boiling, B.G.; Beaty, B.J.; Blair, C.D.; Eisen, R.J.; Meyer, A.M; Paper, W.J.; Moore, C.G. & Eisen, L. (2008) Combining mosquito vector and human disease data for improved assessment of spatial West Nile virus disease risk. *American Journal of Tropical Medicine and Hygiene*, Vol. 78, pp. 654-665

Part 2

Tick-Borne Encephalitis

7

Tick-Borne Encephalitis Virus: A General Overview

Oliver Donoso-Mantke[1], Luidmila S. Karan[2] and Daniel Růžek[3]
[1]*German Consultant Laboratory for Tick-borne Encephalitis, Robert Koch Institute, Berlin,*
[2]*Laboratory of Epidemiology of Zoonoses, Central Research Institute of Epidemiology, Moscow,*
[3]*Institute of Parasitology, Biology Centre of the Czech Academy of Sciences, České Budějovice,*
[1]*Germany*
[2]*Russia*
[3]*Czech Republic*

1. Introduction

Tick-borne encephalitis (TBE) virus is classified as one species with three subtypes, namely the European subtype, the Siberian subtype and the Far Eastern subtype. TBE is distributed in an endemic pattern of so-called natural foci over a wide geographical area from Western Europe to the northern part of Japan. It is the most important flavivirus infection of the central nervous system in Europe and Russia, with about 13,000 estimated human cases per year. The epidemiology of TBE is closely related to the ecology and biology of ixodid ticks. In nature, TBE virus is propagated in a cycle involving permanently infected ticks and wild vertebrate hosts. Currently, the diagnosis of TBE is mainly based on the detection of specific antibodies in serum and cerebrospinal fluid. No specific treatment for the disease is available to date, but it can be prevented by active immunization.

2. Ecology of TBE virus

According to the concept of Pavlovskij, TBE virus is maintained in a cycle involving ticks and wild vertebrate animals in forested natural foci under certain botanical, zoological, climatical and geo-ecological conditions (Pavlovskij, 1939). The development of a TBE natural focus depends on the coincidence of all these factors.

The principal carrier (vector) as well as the reservoir of the European TBE virus subtype is the tick *Ixodes ricinus* (Rampas and Gallia, 1949), a dominant hard tick across Europe. However, the virus has been isolated also from several other tick species (Grešíková and Nosek, 1966; Křivanec et al., 1988; Grešíková and Kaluzová, 1997). *I. ricinus* ticks live preferentially in the dense undergrowth of the forests where the relative humidity is high. Oak, hornbeam as well as beech and fir woods with rich undergrowth of weeds, ferns, elder, hazel, and bramble bushes provide an ideal habitat for these ticks (Süss, 2003).

TBE virus strains from Far Eastern and Siberian subtypes are transmitted predominantly by *I. persulcatus*. This tick, which aggressively attaches to humans, comprises 80–97% of all tick species in the Ural, Siberia and the Far East region of Russia (Gritsun et al., 2003a). The habitat of *I. persulcatus* is mainly distributed in different taiga forest types. Key factors affecting *I. persulcatus* ticks are relatively warm and humid climate conditions. In the event of high humidity the ticks are frequent in warm and drained spruce and small-leaved forests. Under low humidity and warm conditions, the ticks are frequent in broad-leaved coniferous forests and in shaded places. The natural (boreal) habitat of *I. persulcatus* ticks spreads from the Baltic States to the Pacific. On the border of habitats (Baltic States, Finland, Karelia, and several regions of the European part of Russia) sympatric habitations of *I. persulcatus* and *I. ricinus* were observed (Votiakov et al., 2002).

The TBE natural foci do not expand beyond the natural habitats. However, TBE virus has been isolated also from 18 other tick species in Russia (e.g. frequently from *Dermacentor marginatus* in some steppe regions), but sporadically also from other parasitic invertebrates, e.g. fly, flea and lice (Gritsun et al., 2003b).

The life cycle of ticks (Fig. 1) consists of three stages: the larva, nymph and adult. Each stage feeds on a different individual vertebrate host, usually for a period of a few days. E.g., the infection rate of fed adult ticks and their immediate progenies depends on the bigger mammalian hosts: cattle and wild hares, foxes, boars and deer. Therefore, these hosts are of primary importance for the existence and transmission of TBE virus.

Each stage of *I. ricinus* takes approximately one year to develop to the next stage. Thus, the shortest life cycle takes 3 years on average to complete. However, it may vary from 2 to 6 years throughout the geographical range, depending on the availability of hosts and climatic conditions (Süss, 2003). Following copulation, the female spends six to eleven days feeding on blood and, during subsequent months, deposits 500 to 5,000 eggs. Several weeks later, larvae measuring 0.6–1.0 mm hatch from the eggs. The molting occurs only twice. Six-legged larva develops into an eightlegged nymph, which in turn molts to produce a similar but larger adult (Süss, 2003). TBE virus can be transmitted to man or other hosts by all the tick stages, i.e. larvae, nymphs, as well as adult ticks.

The virus infects ticks chronically for the duration of their life. Nevertheless, ticks themselves do not develop the disease. The virus is transmitted from one developmental stage of the tick to the next (transstadial transmission). In the period that precedes molting, the virus multiplies in the tick and invades almost all the tick's organs (Benda, 1958). TBE virus can be also transmitted transovarially (from infected fertilized female to egg) (Benda, 1958) and during co-feeding of ticks on the same host (Labuda et al., 1993; 1997). Despite the fact that the percentage of transovarial transmission of members of the European TBE virus subtype in *I. ricinus* is much lower than of Siberian and Far Eastern strains in *I. persulcatus*, it is sufficient under certain conditions to ensure the continuity of virus population. Co-feeding of both infected and naïve ticks on the same host allows TBE virus transmission even in the absence of systemic viremia. Results from laboratory experiments suggested that in this case viremia could be a product, rather than a prerequisite, of TBE virus transmission (Labuda et al., 1997). Frequently, it is observed that different stages of ticks belonging to various generations feed on the same host. Therefore, the virus is transmitted efficiently between generations of carriers for at least 5 consecutive years (Korenberg et al., 1991).

The prevalence of TBE virus infected *I. ricinus* ticks varies from 0.5% to 5%, whereas in *I. persulcatus* in certain regions of Russia prevalence up to 40% was recorded (Charrel et al., 2004).

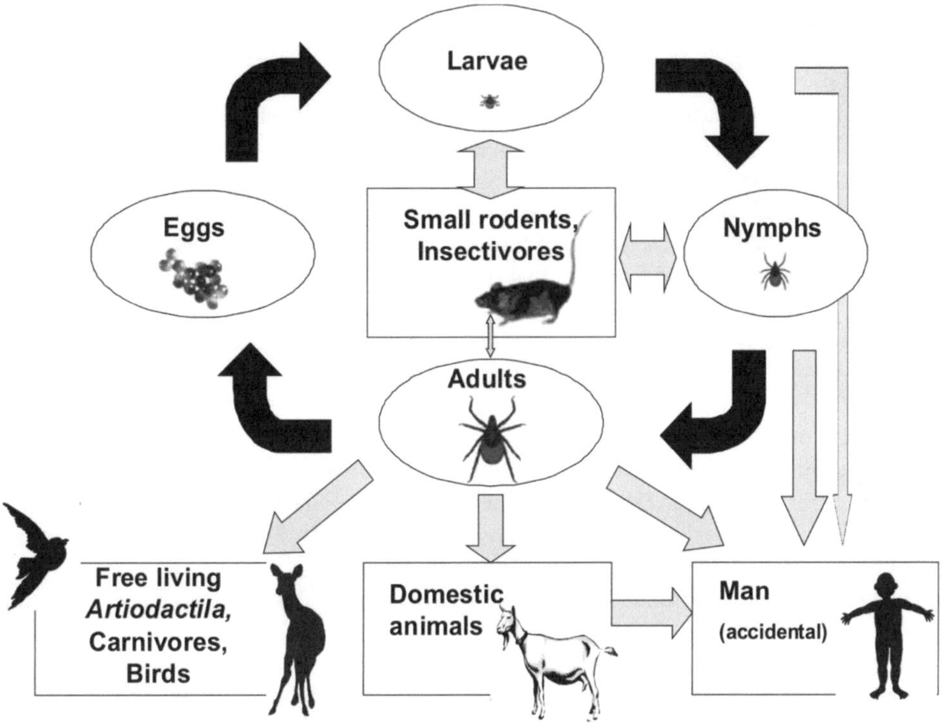

Fig. 1. Life cycle of ixodid tick and transmission cycle of TBE virus. Black lines show the cycle of ticks with different developmental stages. At each stage, a blood meal is needed to develop into the next stage. Therefore, each tick stage feeds on suitable hosts. Further, adult female ticks need a blood meal for egg production. Grey lines show the possible transmission of TBE virus. Thickness of grey arrows shows the most probable routes

Horizontal TBE virus transmission between ticks and their vertebrate reservoir hosts is necessary for virus endemism (Fig. 1) (Nuttall and Labuda, 2003). The duration of viremia in hosts is crucial for TBE virus transmission to ticks, because the virus is mostly ingested by ticks just while engorging on a viremic host. Generally, the hosts are divided into three groups: reservoir, indicator, and accidental hosts. Natural reservoir hosts of TBE virus, i.e. animals that are sensitive to the virus, exhibiting viremia for long period of time without becoming clinically ill and thus important for the transmission of the virus to ticks, include rodents (*Clethrionomys, Apodemus, Mus, Microtus, Micromys, Pitymys, Arvicola, Glis, Sciurus* and *Citellus*) (Kožuch et al., 1967), insectivores (*Sorex, Talpa, Erinaceus*) (Kožuch et al., 1967) and carnivores (*Vulpes, Mustela*) (Süss, 2003; Karabatsos, 1985). Insectivores and rodents harbor the virus also during the winter. The long-lasting viremia can be restored after the awakening of the animals after the winter sleep (posthibernation viremia). Indicator hosts have only brief viremia with low virus production and are not able to transmit the virus to vectors.

Humans are accidental hosts of TBE virus, i.e. they can develop a disease with viremia, but they do not participate in virus circulation in nature and are, therefore, a dead end of the natural TBE virus cycle.

People can be infected (i) by a bite of an infected tick, (ii) by drinking infected unboiled milk, or (iii) by inhaling infected aerosol or by needle-stick injury. In general, most frequently TBE virus infection of humans occurs following the bite of an infected tick, which is unnoticed in about a third of cases (Kaiser, 1999). The tick usually attaches itself to man while walking in dense vegetation in forests. The virus is transmitted by saliva during first minutes of feeding. On humans, ticks prefer to attach themselves to the hair-covered portion of the head, to the arm and knee bends, hand, feet and ears as well as the gluteal and genital regions. In children, 75% of ticks are situated on the head as children are closer to vegetation than adults (Süss, 2003). The incidence of human TBE cases correlates with the activity of the ticks. The seasonal activity of *I. ricinus* has two peaks: April–May and September–October. Comparison of the tick population curves and the morbidity rate in humans shows that there is approximately 14 days' difference between the peaks of the two curves. The gap between the peak of tick activity and the highest morbidity rate in humans corresponds to the incubation period of the disease that is between 4 and 14 days. The activity of *I. persulcatus* has only one peak and lasts from the end of April to the beginning of June. During July only some sporadic cases can be seen. When the summer is very hot, sporadic cases can be observed even in September, but not later (Grešíková and Kaluzová, 1997). The duration of epidemic season in the Southern Far East is 6 to 7 months, since imago molt from nymphs become active at once (Leonova et al., 1996).

Another natural route of human TBE virus infection is associated with the consumption of nonpasteurized milk from viremic livestock (goats, sheep and cows). The virus can pass from the blood of the livestock into the mammary gland. Experiments and epidemiological studies have revealed that antibodies to TBE virus are readily eliminated, and one and the same goat may be repeatedly infected and may excrete TBE virus with its milk (Korenberg, 1976). If a human drinks unboiled milk from infected animals, it can lead to the development of a form of biphasic meningoencephalitis, called 'biphasic milk fever'. The virus remains stable for a relative long period also in various milk products such as yoghurt, cheese and butter (Grešíková, 1959). Persistent infectivity in gastric juice is observed after ingestion of such products for up to 2 h (Charrel et al., 2004). With the aim to decrease the risk of TBE infection in humans by alimentary route, a candidate life attenuated TBE virus vaccine for goats was developed (Mayer, 1966). However, recent molecular analysis of the vaccine strain revealed that this vaccination strain is not an attenuated variant of TBE virus, but a strain of virus Langat, possibly a result of laboratory contamination of cell cultures (Růžek et al., 2006).

Single cases of laboratory TBE virus infections from needle-stick injuries or associated with aerosol infection of laboratory personnel were also described (Gallia et al., 1949; Molnár and Fornosi, 1952; Hoffmann, 1973; Bodemann et al., 1977; Avšič-Županc et al., 1995).

3. Geographical distribution

TBE occurs in many parts of Central Europe and Scandinavia, particularly, in Austria, Czech Republic, Estonia, Finland, Germany, Hungary, Latvia, Lithuania, Poland, Russia, Slovak Republic, Slovenia, Sweden, Switzerland, and also Northern Asia (Fig. 2) (Donoso Mantke et al., 2008; Süss, 2008; Lu et al., 2008). Recently, probable TBE cases were described in Turkey (Ergünay et al., 2011). Further, new TBE foci are emerging and latent ones re-emerging in a number of other European countries (Bröker and Gniel, 2003; Petri et al. 2010). In Russia, the highest TBE incidence is reported in Western Siberia and Ural (Grešíková and Kaluzová, 1997). No TBE cases have been reported e.g. in Great Britain, Ireland, Iceland, Belgium, the

Netherlands, Luxemburg, Spain and Portugal. Whereas Bulgaria, Croatia, Denmark, France, Greece, Italy, Norway, Romania, Serbia, China and Japan are countries with only sporadic TBE occurrence. Because of the increased mobility of people travelling to the risk areas, TBE has become an international public health problem with relation to travel medicine. The risk of an infection is especially high for people living in endemic areas or visiting them for leisure activities in nature (Bröker and Gniel, 2003).

Although TBE virus is a growing concern in Europe, surveillance and notification schemes are not uniform within the European countries. There is a lack of Europe-wide standard case definition and the quality of national surveillance programs differs considerably. Therefore, surveillance data from different countries are difficult to compare (Donoso Mantke et al., 2008).

Generally, the distribution of TBE virus correlates with ixodid tick vectors. *I. ricinus* occurs in most parts of Europe, and the distribution extends to the southeast (Turkey, Northern Iran, and Caucasus). *I. persulcatus* is seen in the wide area extending from Eastern Europe to China and Japan. Parallel occurrence of both tick species was reported in North-Eastern Europe and the east of Estonia and Latvia as well as in several European regions of Russia (Bormane et al., 2004; Golovljova et al., 2004).

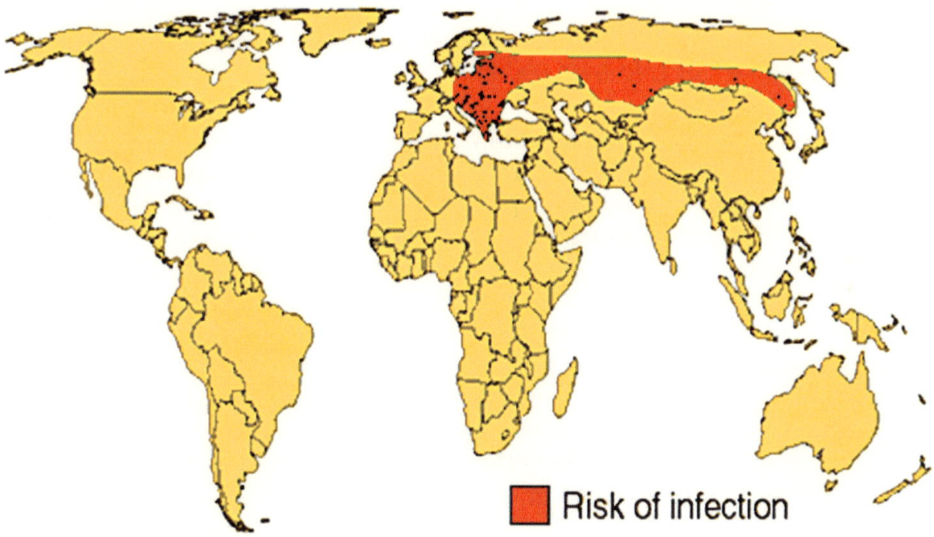

Fig. 2. Geographical distribution of TBE.
(http://www.traveldoctor.info/files/disease/10_ImageFile_KrxuNAAeGEcvwVLPnxks U.gif; date of access April 11, 2011)

The increase of TBE virus incidence in most European countries during the last decades is due to a complex interrelation of several factors that include ecological (effect of climate change on the vectors), agricultural, social (changes in human leisure activities), as well as technological factors (advanced diagnostics and increased medical awareness) (Donoso Mantke et al., 2008). It has been reported that there is an increase (i) in the number of cases in areas well known for TBE in humans; (ii) a reemergence of TBE in areas where it had previously occurred but had not or only sporadically been observed since the 1970s, or (iii) the emergence of TBE in areas where it had not been known to occur previously. Shift of the upper limit of the geographical habitats of ticks to higher altitudes was observed in Central Europe and Sweden (Daniel et al., 2003). Previously, the limit of ticks' occurrence was at 700–750 m above sea level and ticks were not able to finish their developmental cycle at higher altitudes. However, recent studies have shown that ticks (including TBE virus infected ones) shifted to the altitudes up to 1,000 m above sea level. This shift is in a clear correlation with an increased average temperature since the numbers of game animals, socio-economical factors or land-usage did not change in these areas (Danielová et al., 2008). Since these mountain zones are often used for recreation and outdoor activities, the risk of TBE virus infections in these areas increased considerably (Daniel et al., 2003).

4. Clinical picture

Serological surveys suggest that 70–95% of human TBE virus infections are either sub-clinical or asymptomatic (Shapoval, 1976, 1977; Pogodina et al., 1979).

While courses and symptoms are quite similar in the early stage of disease, TBE caused by viruses of the different subtypes may vary not only in the frequency of development of certain disease forms (febrile, meningeal, meningoencephalitic, polyencephalitic, poliomyelitic, polioradiculoneuritic, and chronic forms), but also in the severity of each form.

Siberian and Far Eastern TBE virus subtypes can be the cause of chronic disease (Pogodina et al., 2004; Voronkova and Zakharycheva, 2007). For the Far Eastern TBE virus subtype, the frequency of focal encephalitic symptoms is 31–64%, meningeal forms amount to nearly 26%, febrile forms 14–16% and biphasic forms 3–8%. Complete recovery occurs in 25% of all cases (Votiakov et al., 2002). The current increase in the proportion of patients with a febrile form is likely to be associated with the improved diagnostics. Case fatality rate is up to 35% (Dumpis et al., 1999). Chronic disease develops in less than 0.5% of cases.

The Siberian subtype is associated with focal encephalitic forms in 5% incidents, meningeal forms nearly 47%, febrile forms 40% and biphasic forms about 21%. Complete recovery occurs in 80% of all cases. Case fatality rate is nearly 2% (Votiakov et al., 2002). Nevertheless, infections with the Siberian subtype have a tendency for patients to develop chronic or extremely prolonged infections accompanied by diverse neurological and/or neuropsychiatric symptoms (Poponnikova, 2006).

However, due to differences in seroprevalence rates in Europe and in Russia, the higher morbidity of Eastern TBE forms could, at least partly, be the result of selective notification of mainly severe cases (Süss, 2003).

In contrast to the forms mentioned above, infections caused by European strains typically take a biphasic course in 72–87% of patients (Kaiser, 1999; Günther et al., 1997; Holzmann, 2003): After a short incubation period (usually 7–14 days, with extremes of 4–28 days), the first (viremic) phase presents as an uncharacteristic influenza-like illness lasting 2–4 days (range 1–8 days) with fever, malaise, headache, myalgia, gastrointestinal symptoms, leukocytopenia, thrombocytopenia and elevated liver enzymes as frequent symptoms. This is often followed by a symptom-free interval of about one week (range 1–33 days) before the second phase. Seroconversion without prominent morbidity is common.

The second phase of TBE occurs in 20–30% of infected patients (Gustaffson et al., 1992) and is marked by four clinical features of different severity (meningitis, meningoencephalitis, meningoencephalomyelitis or meningoencephaloradiculitis) and the appearance of specific antibodies in the serum and cerebrospinal fluid (CSF). This is usually the time when patients

with high fever and severe headache seek medical advice. Neurological symptoms at this stage principally do not differ from other forms of acute viral meningoencephalitis (Lindquist and Vapalathi, 2008).
The fatality rate in adult patients is less than 2%. However, severe courses of TBE infection with higher mortality and long-lasting sequelae often affecting the patient's quality of life have been correlated with increased age (Lindquist and Vapalathi, 2008; Mickiene et al., 2002). Further factors associated with severe forms are severity of illness in the viremic phase and low neutralizing antibody titers at onset of disease (Kaiser and Holzmann, 2000).

5. Outbreaks history

Although the first hints of the existence of TBE date back to Scandinavian church records from the 18th century (Åland islands, Finland), the first medical description of the disease was given by the Austrian physician H. Schneider in 1931 (Schneider, 1931).
In 1937–39, the Russian Ministry of Health organized three successive expeditions to the Far East with the purpose to elucidate the origin of severe infections of the central nervous system (CNS), called 'taiga encephalitis' or 'biphasic meningoencephalitis', a disease that had been observed there since 1914, but more frequently occurred since 1933. Initially, the disease was misdiagnosed as a toxic form of influenza. The expeditions revealed viral origin of the disease and the tick *I. persulcatus* as the main vector of the virus (Zilber, 1939). The newly described disease was called 'Russian spring-summer encephalitis' (or Far East or taiga encephalitis). The virus became known as Russian spring-summer encephalitis virus and lately tick-borne encephalitis virus. After TBE virus strains were isolated, the clinical picture and human pathology aspects were described, and in 1940 the first vaccine was tested.
In the Ural, cases of Kozhevnikov's epilepsy (*epilepsia corticalis sive partialis continua*; for details see Vein and van Emde Boas, 2011), a supposed complication of TBE that develops after acute meningoencephalitis, were described by V.P. Pervushin in 1901 and by M.G. Polykovsky in 1917- 1920 (Votiakov et al., 2002). There, TBE virus was isolated for the first time from the brain of a deceased patient in 1939 by M.P. Chumakov and N.A. Zeitlenok (1940). The history of the discovery of TBE virus in the European part of Russia started with the investigation of a TBE outbreak in the Volkhov Front's armies in 1942–1943. In the same period, the role of *I. ricinus* for virus transmission was demonstrated (Petrishcheva and Levkovich, 1945), and TBE virus of the Siberian subtype was isolated from this tick (Pogodina et al., 2004). In 1946, an expedition headed by L. Zilber isolated TBE virus from *I. ricinus* ticks and from patients in Belarus. This virus was proved to be in close relationship with the then known Louping ill virus rather than with the Far Eastern TBE virus strains. Lately, the virus was named the 'Western tick-borne encephalitis virus'.
In Central Europe, TBE virus was first isolated from human patients in Czechoslovakia after the Second World War in 1948 (Gallia et al., 1949; Krejčí, 1949a) when the incidence of clinical manifestations caused by the virus was so high that it was noticed by infectiologists in affected regions (Krejčí, 1949b). Simultaneously, the virus was also isolated from *I. ricinus* suggesting the role of the tick as a vector of the disease (Rampas and Gallia, 1949).
Retrospective analysis, however, revealed the presence of a clinically similar disease not only in Czechoslovakia, but also in a number of other European countries for several decades before the first isolation, because many clinical neurologists and physicians have

observed and described the disease without knowing the etiology (reviewed by Izbický, 1954). In Czechoslovakia, this disease was previously known as '*Encephalitis epidemica*'. Since 1945, there was nearly a tenfold increase in the incidence of this disease (Izbický, 1954).

Shortly, after the description of TBE in Czechoslovakia, the virus was isolated in Hungary (Fornosi and Molnár, 1952), Poland (Szajna, 1954), Bulgaria (Vaptsarov et al., 1954), Yugoslavia (Bedjanič et al., 1955), Austria (Pattyn and Wyler, 1955), Romania (Draganescu, 1959), Germany (Sinnecker, 1960), but also in Finland (Oker-Blom, 1956) and Sweden (Kaäriainen et al., 1961). Simultaneously, the virus was also revealed in Northern China and Japan (Ando et al., 1952). Recently, a successful detection of TBE virus in South Korea was reported (Kim et al., 2009; Ko et al., 2010).

The clinical course of the disease, its pathology and epidemiology, as well as the properties of the virus, its ecology, and ecology of the vectors have been studied in detail. Most of the studies were carried out in Russia, Czechoslovakia and Austria (Kunz and Heinz, 2003).

The incidence of TBE varies from year to year in different geographic regions. Across Eurasia, more than 13,000 human cases are reported annually. Over the last two decades, the most dramatic changes of all were the sudden increases (2- to 30-fold) in 1992–3 in Latvia, Lithuania, Poland and Belarus, and with marked but lesser increases in Estonia, Germany, Slovakia, and the Czech Republic. TBE cases have increased steadily since the mid-1970s in Russia, and since the mid-1980s in Switzerland, Sweden, and Finland. In Austria, the only country with extensive systematic vaccination coverage, TBE incidence has decreased progressively since the early 1980s (Randolph, 2002).

Russia is the country with the largest geographical range of TBE virus and the highest TBE incidence. In the early period of descriptive TBE studies in the 1930s-1940s, 200 cases were reported annually in average (with some divergences in 1941 and 1942). The analysis of data collected since 1948 demonstrates a registered shift in 1948 followed by a peak in 1956 (5,163 cases), and by a relative plateau thereafter (3,500 cases per year in average), with the next peak in 1964 (5,204 cases). From 1964 to 1974, the incidence dropped to 1,119 cases per year. The year 1975 brought a new shift that lasted till 1999 with peaks in 1993 (7,250 cases), 1996 (10,298 cases), and 1999 (9,955 cases). In some regions, the incidence rate reached 70 per 100,000 inhabitants. A negative trend in the incidence has been observed since 2000, with 2,796 cases reported in 2008. Since 2000, the average incidence showed a two-time decrease. It should be noted that at the same time the registered trends are of opposite direction. In the extreme north-west region of Russian TBE habitats, from 1997 to 2007 a continuous positive trend was observed. In Karelia and Vologda regions, the incidence increased twice, and in the neighboring Arkhangelsk region increased five times. But since most of the cases in Russia are reported for Ural, Siberia and some Volga regions, the data for the north-west region has not material impact on the incidence rate in the country as a whole. The data on TBE incidences for Russia are based on the reports of the Federal Center of Hygiene and Epidemiology in Moscow.

In Europe, the Czech Republic ranks among the countries with the highest incidence rate of TBE. In this country, the incidence of the illness noticeably varied during the monitored period, i.e. since 1950s. The high occurrence of the infection in 1960s gradually decreased and in 1970s and 1980s reached values of 139–400 cases annually. Sporadically, there were more than 400 cases per year in 1970, 1973, and 1979. A steep increase took place in 1990s (according to data from EPIDAT, National Institute of Public Health in Prague – www.szu.cz), when the annual incidence was more than two-fold higher in comparison with the preceding period, 400–600 cases per year with a maximum of 745 cases in 1995 and

706 in 2000 (Daniel et al., 2004). In the year 2006, the incidence (1,026 cases) of TBE in the Czech Republic was almost twice as high than in the preceding years, the highest ever recorded, indicating significantly increased epidemic activity of this important human pathogen (Daniel et al., 2008). A similar increase in number of cases was observed also in other regions of Europe (www.isw-tbe.info). This phenomenon is not definitely explained. One hypothesis dealing with the increased incidence of the last years is based on impact of climatic changes on the biology of the vector *I. ricinus* (Gray et al., 2009). Gradual raise of the temperature in the last decades caused prolongation of the period of the tick development within a year and, subsequently, acceleration of its development and increase of the density of its population (Daniel et al., 2004). This allowed the intensification of the circulation of TBE virus, more frequent contact of man with infected ticks, and caused dissemination of the ticks and TBE to regions with no or rare previous records of their incidence (Daniel et al., 2003, 2006).

A particularly unusual outbreak was caused by infected goat milk in the Rožňava district of Slovakia in 1951–52, when at least 660 people became infected (Blaškovič, 1954; Růžek et al., 2010). Other milk-borne TBE virus outbreaks occurred in Petersburg and Moscow regions (Drozdov, 1959) in Russia and in the Styrian region of Austria (Grešíková and Kaluzová, 1994). More recently, a relatively small outbreak of TBE by alimentary route was reported in 1999 in the Czech Republic. In this case, 22 people were infected by consumption of sheep cheese. Some of the cases were severe (Daneš, 2000). In 2007, outbreak of alimentary TBE after consumption of unpasteurized raw goat milk involving 25 patients of 154 exposed persons occurred in Hungary in August 2007 (Balogh et al., 2010). Lastly, an outbreak of TBE due to consumption of goat cheese from an alpine pasture of high altitude (1564 m above sea level) was reported in 2008 from an area in Vorarlberg, Austria, in which 6 persons were infected. Four of them were hospitalized with typical TBE symptoms, 2 were clinically asymptomatic (Holzmann et al., 2009).

6. Virology

TBE virus is the medically most important member of the tick-borne group of the genus *Flavivirus*, family *Flaviviridae* (Thiel et al., 2005). Besides TBE virus, three other tick-borne flaviviruses, i.e. Louping ill virus, Langat virus and Powassan virus, also cause encephalitis in humans and/or animals, but these infections are infrequent and the viruses do not produce significant outbreaks (Gritsun et al., 2003b).

TBE virus is subdivided into three subtypes: European (previously Central European encephalitis), Far Eastern (previously Russian spring and summer encephalitis) and Siberian (previously Western Siberian encephalitis) (Ecker et al., 1999).

Based on the antigenic similarity, the European TBE virus subtype is closely related rather to Louping ill virus than to the Far Eastern and Siberian subtypes (Hubálek et al., 1995). Moreover, on the basis of the comparison of genetic similarity of complete genomes, inclusion of Louping ill virus, Turkish sheep tick-borne encephalitis virus, and Spanish sheep encephalitis virus as different genotypes of TBE virus was proposed (Grard et al., 2007), but this classification has not been generally accepted so far, mostly because of important biological differences between these viruses.

Although TBE virus strains isolated from field collected ticks exhibit high heterogeneity with respect to their biological properties (Růžek et al., 2008), sequence analyses of various virus isolates have shown that the TBE virus is fairly homogeneous in endemic areas of Europe and is not subject to significant antigenic variations. On the other hand, the diversity of TBE virus from Siberian and Far Eastern subtypes is much higher. Currently, at least two groups in the Siberian genotype were identified (European and Asian groups, separated by Ural mountains) (Pogodina et al., 2007). Nevertheless, the antigenic similarity is still high enough to be sufficient for the cross-protection in the event of infection by TBE virus of the different subtypes.

The virions of TBE virus are spherical particles, approximately 50–60 nm in diameter (Slávik et al., 1967) with a nucleocapsid composed of a (+)ssRNA genome enclosed in a capsid (C) protein and surrounded by a host cell-derived lipid bilayer. The genome is approximately 11 kb in length and contains one large open reading frame which is flanked by 5′ and 3′ untranslated regions, with 5′-cap but no 3′-poly(A) tail. The untranslated regions form conserved secondary stem-loop structures that probably serve as *cis*-acting elements for genome amplification, translation and packaging (Gritsun et al., 2003b). Translation yields a 3414 amino acids long polyprotein that is co- and post-translationally cleaved by cellular and viral proteases into three structural proteins (C, prM, E) and seven non-structural proteins (NS1, NS2A, NS2B, NS3, NS4A, NS4B and NS5). The lipid envelope carries two surface proteins, the large envelope protein (E) and a small membrane protein (M). M protein is derived from its larger precursor, prM.

C protein binds viral DNA to form the virion nucleocapsid. The immature C protein contains a CTHD (C-terminal hydrophobic domain), i.e. a 20 amino acid length polypeptide, which is split off by serine protease to form a short CTHD polypeptide during polyprotein processing (Yamshchikov and Compans, 1993). The proteolysis site modification in this region is likely to predetermine the maturity rate of virions in the infected cells (Loktev et al., 2007).

The E protein is the major antigenic and virulence determinant of TBE virus and acts both as the ligand to the cell receptor and as the fusion protein (Lindenbach and Rice, 2003).

The viral non-structural proteins have several functions, i.e. the NS1 protein soluble homodimer is known as a complement-binding antigen; NS2A, NS4A and NS4B proteins are involved in the function as a replicative complex (Loktev et al., 2007); the complex of NS2B-NS3 proteins serves as viral serine protease; and NS5 is a RNA-dependent RNA polymerase (Lindenbach and Rice, 2003).

The infection of the host cell begins with the binding of the virus to a cell receptor, which has not been sufficiently identified till now (Kopecký et al., 1999). Apparently, just the ability to use multiple receptors can be responsible for the very wide host range of flaviviruses, which replicate in arthropods and in a broad range of vertebrates. After binding to the receptor, the virus is internalized by endocytosis. Acidification of the interior of the endosomal vesicle changes the conformation of the E protein and rearranges its dimers to trimeric forms. These changes result in fusion of the viral envelope and the membrane of the endosomal vesicle (Holzmann et al., 1995) and the release of the viral nucleocapsid into the cytoplasm. After uncoating, translation of the positive-stranded genome occurs, in parallel to synthesis of minus-strand RNA that serves as a template for RNA replication. Processing of the polyprotein yields the individual viral proteins (Mandl, 2005).

In vertebrate cells, virus assembly takes place in endoplasmatic reticulum and leads to formation of immature virions that contain the proteins C, prM and E. These immature particles are transported through the cellular secretory pathway and, shortly before release, prM is cleaved by furin or a similar enzyme in the acidic compartment of the trans-Golgi network to yield mature and fully infectious virions (Mandl, 2005).

However, the TBE virus maturation process in tick cells is completely different than in the cells from vertebrate hosts. In cell lines derived from the tick *Rhipicephalus appendiculatus* infected with TBE virus, nucleocapsids occur in cytoplasm and the envelope is acquired by budding on cytoplasmic membrane or into cell vacuoles (Šenigl et al., 2006). The studies focused on the adaptation of TBE virus to *Hyalomma marginatum* ticks and mammals described the presence of respective adaptive mutations within the second domain of E protein (Romanova et al., 2007).

Most of the studies on TBE pathogenesis have been done on laboratory mice that are susceptible to TBE virus and develop lethal infection of CNS (Simon et al., 1966), analogous to severe cases of TBE in humans (Mandl, 2005).

After the tick bite, the virus replicates in subcutaneous tissues (Fig. 3). Dendritic cells in the skin are likely to serve as a vehicle for the transport of the virus to draining lymph nodes (Labuda et al., 1996). The lymph nodes play an important part in the pathogenesis of TBE. However, virus replication is not accompanied by any virus-specific histological changes including any destruction of cells in the nodes (Málková and Filip, 1968). On the model of Syrian hamsters inoculated intracerebrally with TBE virus strains differing in virulence, specific involvement of the organs of the immune system (spleen, lymph nodes, and thymus) was established and morphological features of the process described. The most severe destructive changes of these organs (mass disintegration of lymphocytes, inhibition of their migration, almost complete inhibition of regeneration processes up to the complete elimination of germinal centers) were found in the hamsters inoculated with highly virulent strains (Karmysheva and Pogodina, 1990). TBE virus can be isolated from blood leucocytes during the first days after the tick bite indicating virus replication in immunocompetent blood cells (Leonova and Maistrovskaya, 1996).

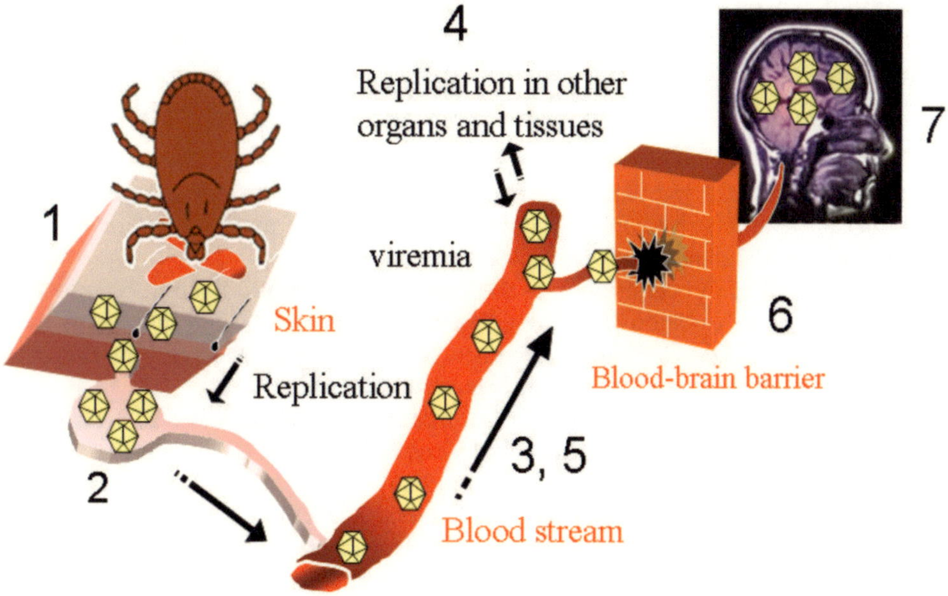

Fig. 3. Schematic drawing of the steps during TBE virus infection. (1) TBE virus transmission from an infected tick, (2) TBE virus replication in regional lymph node, (3) primary viremia, (4) replication of the virus in other organs and tissues, (5) secondary viremia, (6) TBE virus crossing of the blood-brain barrier, and (7) virus infection of the brain

Massive viral multiplication in the nodes leads to the spreading of virus into the blood stream and induction of viremia (Málková et al., 1969). Temporary leukopenia in the white blood picture is observed. A significant decrease is recorded in all cellular elements. In regional lymph nodes, a significant decrease in lymphocytes appears (Málková et al., 1961). Many extraneural tissues are infected during the viremic phase and, subsequently during the secondary viremia, the virus invades the CNS by still unknown mechanism. Mice dying due TBE exhibite severe systemic stress response, and increased levels of TNF-alpha compared with recovering mice (Hayasaka et al., 2009). Characteristic, but not disease-specific, are neuropathologic changes in CNS that include meningitis and polioencephalomyelitis accentuated in spinal cord, brainstem and cerebellum associated with inflammatory cell infiltration of infected animals (Gelpi et al., 2005). In mice, as well as in human post-mortem cases, prominent inflammatory infiltrates and cytotoxic T-cells were observed in close contact with morphologically intact neurons suggesting a key role for cytotoxic T-cells in the development of encephalitis (Gelpi et al., 2006; Růžek et al., 2009). Recent studies confirmed, that the host $CD8^+$ T-lymphocytes infiltrating brain parenchyma mediate immunopathology in TBE (Růžek et al., 2009). Thus, the host immune system contributes significantly to the development and higher severity of the disease.

TBE virus infection, in addition to causing fatal encephalitis in mice, induces considerable breakdown of the blood-brain barrier (BBB). The permeability of the BBB increases at later stages of TBE infection when high virus load is present in the brain (i.e., BBB breakdown was not necessary for TBE virus entry into the brain), and at the onset of the first severe clinical symptoms of the disease. The increased BBB permeability is in association with dramatic upregulation of proinflammatory cytokine/chemokine mRNA expression in the brain. Breakdown of the BBB can be also observed in mice deficient in $CD8^+$ T-cells, indicating, that these cells are not necessary for the increase in BBB permeability that occurs during TBE (Růžek et al., 2011).

7. Laboratory diagnosis

Since TBE shows clinical and laboratory findings similar to other CNS diseases which may require special treatment, microbiological laboratories have to perform specific diagnostics mainly for differential diagnosis (Donoso Mantke et al., 2007a).

This can be done (i) as direct detection of the virus or viral RNA in the first (viremic) phase of infection, by virus isolation in mammalian cell culture or RT-PCR, or (ii) as indirect detection of specific IgM and IgG antibodies with serological methods as enzyme immunoassay, immunofluorescence assay or neutralization test.

As the majority of patients come for medical attention when neurological symptoms are manifest, it is the current experts' opinion that virus isolation and RT-PCR at this time are of minor importance for the diagnosis of TBE, because at the beginning of the second phase of illness the virus itself is only rarely detectable in blood and CSF. Therefore, the diagnosis of TBE is mainly done by serological methods, usually enzyme-linked immunosorbent assay (ELISA) based on purified virions or recombinant virus-like particles, which have been developed towards higher specificity and sensitivity in the last decade (Holzmann, 2003; Sonnenberg et al., 2004; Günther and Haglund, 2005; Ludolfs et al., 2009).

However, detection by PCR methods could be valuable for an early differential diagnosis of TBE (Saksida et al., 2005; Schultze et al., 2007). This is particularly true for patients living in or coming from areas where more than one tick-transmitted disease is endemic. Detection of specific nucleic acid from blood and CSF depends on the sampling at the right time. The highest yield of TBE virus specific RNA is obtained during the transient viremia in the first week of the disease, much less in the second week after the appearance of antibodies and only occasionally later on (Holzmann, 2003; Puchhammer-Stöckl et al., 1995).

The benefit of molecular detection methods depends on the attention that affected people and clinicians pay to tick bites and symptoms. The earlier a correct diagnosis is obtained (e.g. TBE or other etiology), the earlier an appropriate therapy can be introduced. This could have dramatic influence upon survival and outcome of a suspected CNS disease.

RT-PCR can also be of great diagnostic help when the patient has not developed antibodies at the beginning of the second phase, has a severe case of TBE or has died after a relatively short course of infection (Gelpi et al., 2005; Schwaiger and Cassinotti, 2003).

Both serological and molecular detection methods for TBE are useful as single applications or in combination for clinical diagnosis, immunity testing, epidemiological surveillance and survey of virus prevalence in ticks and vertebrate hosts.

Although ELISA is currently the method of choice, due to its simple performance and ease of automation, and new commercial serological assays have been developed with higher sensitivity and specificity, certain restrictions have to be taken into consideration for the application of serological methods (Table 1).

Method	Serology	RT-PCR
Advantages	-Allows reliable detection of IgM and IgG antibodies in serum and CSF up from the 2nd week of disease - High throughput of clinical specimens is possible - Commercial kits are available	- Allows early diagnosis by detection of TBE virus specific RNA in the first phase of infection, if patient is hospitalized at this time point - Provides opportunity to discriminate between TBE virus subtypes - Provides opportunity to quantify viral load
Disadvantages	- Cross-reactions with antibodies elicited by other flaviviruses - Neutralization test has a high specificity, but requires higher containment laboratory	- Requires trained laboratory personnel for proper handling

Table 1. Advantages and disadvantages of serology and RT-PCR for the diagnosis of TBE (modified from Donoso Mantke et al., 2007a)

An early diagnosis by detecting only IgM is questionable, since IgM antibodies can persist for up to 10 months in vaccinees or individuals who acquired the infection naturally. Therefore, confirmation by detection of specific IgG is recommended, but may turn out negative in the first phase of infection. The necessary monitoring of an increase of IgG titers

1–2 weeks later is rarely done. Moreover, a major problem when using ELISA and immunofluorescence assays lays in the high cross-reactivity of the flaviviral antigenic structure. Possible diagnostic difficulties may arise due to cross-reactions of antibodies elicited by other flavivirus infections or vaccinations. This could happen in areas where other flaviviruses co-circulate (e.g. West Nile virus in the southern parts of the TBE endemic area), in patients recently returned from areas endemic for other flaviviruses (e.g. dengue virus endemic areas) or in individuals being vaccinated against TBE virus, Japanese encephalitis or yellow fever virus (Holzmann, 2003; Niedrig et al., 2001).

Thus, verification of positive results by neutralization test is advised which, due to the use of infectious virus particles, requires the handling in higher containment laboratories which makes this test time-consuming and expensive.

As mentioned, the molecular diagnostics for TBE are restricted to the first (viremic) phase of infection. But, in combination with a higher awareness of the disease, this fact could be more an advantage than an obstacle, leading to an early diagnosis of TBE (Table 1).

Also, the RT-PCR provides the opportunity to discriminate between all subtypes of TBE. This could be an important aspect while facing co-circulation of the different subtypes in some European regions (Růžek et al., 2007; Achazi et al., 2011). Unfortunately, a negative PCR result in serum or CSF of a patient is not predictive for the absence of a TBE infection. This may be caused either by the short viremia of the infection, by sampling at inappropriate times and/or by improper handling of diagnostic specimens. The lack of commercial assays of standardized quality provides another reason why RT-PCR has not been established so far in microbiological laboratories for TBE diagnosis (Donoso Mantke et al., 2007a). The presence of many in-house assays especially for the molecular detection of TBE requires quality control studies in order to avoid false positive and/or negative results and to achieve the same diagnostic quality among the different assays (Donoso Mantke et al., 2007b).

8. Prevention and treatment

Besides general preventive measures, like wearing appropriate clothing or checking the skin for attached ticks, TBE can be successfully prevented by active immunization (Kunz, 2003; Heinz et al., 2007).

In Russia, several vaccines are produced by using Far Eastern TBE subtype viruses: e.g. the vaccine of the Institute of Poliomyelitis and Viral Encephalitis (IPVE), in Moscow with strain Sofjin, and EnceVir by Virion, in Tomsk with strain 205.

In Europe two vaccines are available which are based on European TBE virus strains: FSME-IMMUN by Baxter Bioscience, Orth an der Donau, Austria with strain Neudoerfl, and Encepur by Novartis Vaccines and Diagnostics, Marburg, Germany with strain K23.

The large envelope protein E induces the production of neutralizing antibodies important for the protective immunity. Due to the highly conserved structure of this antigen broad cross-protection by the vaccines could be shown against TBE viruses of all three subtypes (Ecker et al., 1999; Leonova and Maistrovskaya, 1996; Klockmann et al., 1991; Holzmann et al., 1992; Hayasaka et al., 2001).

Since their introduction both European vaccines have undergone several modifications and are manufactured by the same steps during the production process (Rendi-Wagner, 2008). Viral antigens are propagated in chick embryo cells, filtered and inactivated by formaldehyde, and purified by ultracentrifugation. During the formulation the antigens are adsorbed to aluminium hydroxide and stabilized with human albumin (FSME-IMMUN) or sucrose (Encepur). Thiomersal was removed from both vaccine formulations in the 1990s to fulfill high safety and tolerability standards (Barrett et al., 2003).

The conventional immunization schedules for primary immunization are similar for both vaccines, with three intramuscular doses given on 0, 21 days–3 months and 9–12 months. Thus, both vaccines induce antibody concentrations that are believed to be protective in over 90% of children and adults (Lindquist and Vapalathi, 2008). Due to the high homology of the antigens and demonstrated cross-boostering in clinical studies, the two TBE vaccines seem interchangeable after a complete primary immunization (Rendi-Wagner et al., 2004; Bröker and Schöndorf, 2006). So far, the protective amount of antibodies is not clearly defined and standardized for both vaccines. Also, occasional vaccine breakthroughs have been reported (Bender et al., 2004; Kleiter et al., 2007; Andersson et al., 2010).

Besides vaccines for adults, both European vaccine manufacturers offer pediatric vaccine formulations containing half the dose of viral antigen of the adult ones to improve tolerability in children (Zent et al., 2003; Pavlova et al., 2003; Pöllabauer et al., 2010).

An age-dependent immune response after vaccination could be shown, with children having an enhanced response in comparison to adults (Girgsdies et al., 1996), whereas especially vaccinees aged over 60 years frequently have a poor antibody response (Hainz et al., 2005).

Data regarding the persistence of post-immunization antibodies led the manufacturers to change their recommendations (Rendi-Wagner, 2008). Regular boosters are recommended every 5 years for age-groups ≤ 49 years of age (except for the first booster after 3 years). In age-groups > 49 years of age a 3-year-booster interval is recommended due to the significantly gradual decline of post-immunization antibodies.

Rapid immunization schedules have been introduced by both vaccine producers for people who require immunity at short notice, such as travelers travelling to TBE-endemic areas or when the tick season has already started. However, since the experience with TBE vaccines is mainly based on the conventional immunization schedules, these should be always applied wherever possible.

In Russia, IPVE vaccine is applied for adults and children of three years and over, the vaccine is given in two doses over 5–7 months with the revaccination after 1 year, and then every 3 years. EnceVir vaccine is administered to adults aged 18 years and more, the vaccine is also given in two doses over 5–7 months, with the revaccination after 1 year and every 3 years thereafter. This vaccine is also available for the rapid immunization schedule: two doses over 1–2 months.

Clinical therapy is only symptomatic with strict bed rest, usually in an intensive care unit, until the fever and neurological symptoms have subsided. Maintenance of water and electrolyte balances, sufficient caloric intake, and administration of analgesics, vitamins, and antipyretics are the central pillars of clinical treatment of TBE patients.

Since there is no specific treatment for TBE available to date, and the administration of hyperimmunoglobulin for a passive post-exposure prophylaxis is highly questionable concerning the virtue and not recommended anymore due to concerns about antibody-dependent enhancement of infection (Kaiser, 1999; Waldvogel et al., 1996; Jones et al., 2007), active immunization should always be recommended for people living in or travelling to TBE endemic areas.

9. Future trends

Since the first descriptions of TBE and its viral etiology in the 1930s/1940s the scientific development in this research area has been tremendous. Today, we have knowledge about the structure and molecular biology of TBE virus and the biotic and non-biotic factors underlying its natural cycle. Also, there are effective and safe purified inactivated vaccines available on the market, which made vaccination an extremely successful measure for preventing the disease.

However, there are several issues in the context of TBE which need to be deepened in the future, like:

1. Further development of rapid differential diagnosis of TBE virus in combination with other tick-borne pathogens by detecting both the nucleic acids and viral antigens.
2. Further efforts in identifying the genetic basis of TBE virulence.
3. Study of interaction of virus and immune cells for further prognosis of clinical course and outcome of TBE and, if possible, for better treatment.
4. Establishment of international databases for TBE virus: epidemic risks, individual risks, mapping and characterization of natural foci, circulating genotypes, circulation of other tick-borne pathogens in TBE foci.
5. The taxonomic position of Louping ill virus (and subtypes Turkish sheep-, Spanish sheep encephalitis virus) and Greek goat encephalitis virus is under consideration.

10. Acknowledgements

We acknowledge financial support by the Czech Science Foundation project No. P302/10/P438 and No. P502/11/2116, and grants Z60220518 and LC06009 from the Ministry of Education, Youth, and Sports of the Czech Republic.

11. References

Achazi, K., Nitsche, A., Patel, P., Radonić, A., Donoso Mantke, O., and Niedrig, M. 2011. Detection and differentiation of tick-borne encephalitis virus subtypes by a reverse transcription quantitative real-time PCR and pyrosequencing. *J. Virol. Methods* 171(1):34-9.

Andersson CR, Vene S, Insulander M, Lindquist L, Lundkvist A, Günther G. Vaccine failures after active immunisation against tick-borne encephalitis. *Vaccine*. 2010 Apr 1;28(16):2827-31.

Ando, K., Kuratsuka, K., Arima, S., Hironaka, N., Honda, Y., and Ishii, K. 1952. Studies on the viruses isolated during epidemic of Japanese B encephalitis in 1948 in Tokyo area. *Kitasato. Arch. Exp. Med.* 24: 49–61.

Avsic-Zupanc, T., Poljak, M., Maticic, M., Radsel-Medvescek, A., LeDuc, J.W., Stiasny, K., Kunz, C., and Heinz, F.X. 1995. Laboratory acquired tick-borne meningoencephalitis: characterisation of virus strains. *Clin. Diagn. Virol.* 4: 51-9.

Balogh, Z., Ferenczi, E., Szeles, K., Stefanoff, P., Gut, W., Szomor, K.N., Takacs, M., and Berencsi, G. 2010. Tick-borne encephalitis outbreak in Hungary due to consumption of raw goat milk. *J. Virol. Methods* 163(2):481-5.

Barrett, P.N., Schober-Bendixen, S., and Ehrlich, H.J. 2003. History of TBE vaccines. *Vaccine* 21 (Suppl 1): S41-9.

Bedjanič, M., Rus, S., Kmet, J., Vesenjak-Zmijanac, J. 1955 Virus meningo-encephalitis in Slovenia. *Bull. World Health Organ.* 12: 503-12.

Benda, R. 1958. [The common tick "*Ixodes ricinus*" as a reservoir and vector of tick-borne encephalitis. I. Survival of the virus (strain B3) during the development of ticks under laboratory condition]. *J. Hyg. Epidemiol.* (Prague) 2: 314-30.

Bender, A., Jäger, G., Scheuerer, W., Feddersen, B., Kaiser, R., and Pfister, H.W. 2004. Two severe cases of tickborne encephalitis despite complete active vaccination - the significance of neutralizing antibodies. *J. Neurol.* 251: 353-4.

Blaškovič, D. 1954 [Outbreak of tick-borne encephalitis in Rožňava natural focus]. Bratislava: Vydavatelstvo SAV. [Book in Slovak]

Bodemann, H., Pausch, J., Schmitz, H., and Hoppe-Seyler, G. 1977. [Die Zeckenenzephalitis (FSME) als Laborinfektion]. *Med. Welt* 28: 1779-81. [Article in German]

Bormane, A., Lucenko, I., Duks, A., Mavtchoutko, V., Ranka, R., Salmina, K., and Baumanis, V. 2004. Vectors of tick-borne diseases and epidemiological situation in Latvia in 1993-2002. *Int. J. Med. Microbiol.* 293(Suppl 37): 36-47.

Bröker, M., and Gniel, D. 2003. New foci of tick-borne encephalitis virus in Europe: consequences for travellers from abroad. *Travel Med. Infect. Dis.* 1: 181-4.

Bröker, M., and Schöndorf, I. 2006. Are tick-borne encephalitis vaccines interchangeable? *Expert Rev. Vaccines* 5: 461-6.

Charrel, R.N., Attoui, H., Butenko, A.M., Clegg, J.C., Deubel, V., Frolova, T.V., Gould, E.A., Gritsun, T.S., Heinz, F.X., Labuda, M., Lashkevich, V.A., Loktev, V., Lundkvist, A., Lvov, D.V., Mandl, C.W., Niedrig, M., Papa, A., Petrov, V.S., Plyusnin, A., Randolph, S., Süss, J., Zlobin, V.I., and de Lamballerie X. 2004. Tick-borne virus diseases of human interest in Europe. *Clin. Microbiol. Infect.* 10: 1040-55.

Chumakov, M.P., and Zeitlenok, N.A. 1940 [Tick-borne Spring-Summer encephalitis in the Ural region. In: Neuroinfections in the Ural]. Sverdlovsk; pp. 23-30. [Chapter in Russian]

Daneš, L. 2000. [Human infections with tick-borne encephalitis virus]. *Medicína* 3: 16. [Article in Czech]

Daniel, M., Danielová, V., Kříž, B., and Beneš, Č. 2006. In: Menne B, Ebi KL, Eds. Climate change and adaptation strategies for human health. Steinkopff, Darmstadt, Springer, pp. 189-205.

Daniel, M., Danielová, V., Kříž, B., and Kott, I. 2004. An attempt to elucidate the increased incidence of tick-borne encephalitis and spread to higher altitudes in the Czech Republic. *Int. J. Med. Microbiol.* 293(Suppl 37): 55–62.

Daniel, M., Danielová, V., Kříž, B., Jirsa, A., and Nožička, J. 2003. Shift of the tick *Ixodes ricinus* and tick-borne encephalitis to higher altitudes in Central Europe. *Eur. J. Clin. Microbiol. Infect. Dis.* 22: 327–8.

Daniel, M., Kříž, B., Danielová, V., and Beneš, C. 2008 Sudden increase in tick-borne encephalitis cases in the Czech Republic, 2006. *Int. J. Med. Microbiol.* 298(Suppl. 1): 81-7.

Danielová, V., Kliegrová, S., Daniel, M., and Beneš, Č. 2008. Influence of climate warming on tick-borne encephalitis expansion to higher altitudes over the last decade (1997-2006) in the Highland Region (Czech Republic). *Cent. Eur. J. Public Health* 16: 4-11.

Donoso Mantke, O., Aberle, S.W., Avsic-Zupanc, T., Labuda, M., and Niedrig, M. 2007b. Quality control assessment for the PCR diagnosis of tick-borne encephalitis virus infections. *J. Clin. Virol.* 38: 73-7.

Donoso Mantke, O., Schädler, R., and Niedrig, M. 2008. A survey on cases of tick-borne encephalitis in European countries. *Euro Surveill.* 13(17). pii: 18848.

Donoso-Mantke, O., Achazi, K., and Niedrig, M. 2007a. Serological versus PCR methods for the detection of tick-borne encephalitis virus infections in humans. *Future Virology* 2: 565-72.

Draganescu, N. 1959. [Inframicrobial meningoencephalitis belonging to the group transmitted by arthropods. Identification of the pathogenic agent and study of the nerve lesions induced in white mice] *Stud. Cercet. Inframicrobiol.* 10: 363-9. [Article in Romanian]

Drozdov, S.G. 1959. [Role of domestic animals in epidemiology of diphasic milk fever]. *Zh. Microbiol. Epidemiol. Immunobiol.* 30: 102-8. [Article in Russian]

Dumpis, U., Crook, D., and Oksi, J. 1999. Tick-borne encephalitis. *Clin. Infect. Dis.* 28: 882-90.

Ecker, M., Allison, S.L., Meixner, T., and Heinz, F.X. 1999. Sequence analysis and genetic classification of tick-borne encephalitis viruses from Europe and Asia. *J. Gen. Virol.* 80: 179-85.

Ergünay, K., Saygan, M.B., Aydoğan, S., Litzba, N., Sener, B., Lederer, S., Niedrig, M., Hasçelik, G., and Us, D. 2011. Confirmed exposure to tick-borne encephalitis virus and probable human cases of tick-borne encephalitis in central/northern anatolia, Turkey. *Zoonoses Public Health* 58(3):220-7.

Fornosi, F., and Molnár, E. 1952. [Meningoencephalitis in Hungary] *Orv. Hetil.* 93: 993-6. [Article in Hungarian]

Gallia, F., Rampas, J., and Hollender, L. 1949. [Laboratory infection caused by tick-borne encephaltis virus]. *Čas. Lék. čes.* 88: 224-9. [Article in Czech]

Gelpi, E., Preusser, M., Garzuly, F., Holzmann, H., Heinz, F.X., and Budka, H. 2005. Visualization of Central European tick-borne encephalitis infection in fatal human cases. *J. Neuropathol. Exp. Neurol.* 64: 506-12.

Gelpi, E., Preusser, M., Laggner, U., Garzuly, F., Holzmann, H., Heinz, F.X., and Budka, H. 2006. Inflammatory response in human tick-borne encephalitis: analysis of postmortem brain tissue. *J. NeuroVirol.* 12: 322-7.

Girgsdies, O.E., and Rosenkranz, G. 1996. Tick-borne encephalitis: development of a paediatric vaccine. A controlled, randomized, double-blind and multicentre study. *Vaccine* 14: 1421-8.

Golovljova, I., Vene, S., Sjölander, K.B., Vasilenko, V., Plyusnin, A., and Lundkvist, A. 2004. Characterization of tickborne encephalitis virus from Estonia. *J. Med. Virol.* 74: 580-8.

Grard, G., Moureau, G., Charrel, R.N., Lemasson, J.J., Gonzalez, J.P., Gallian, P., Gritsun, T.S., Holmes, E.C., Gould, E.A., and de Lamballerie, X. 2007. Genetic characterization of tick-borne flaviviruses: new insights into evolution, pathogenetic determinants and taxonomy. *Virology* 361: 80-92.

Gray, J.S., Dautel, H., Estrada-Peña, A., Kahl, O., and Lindgren, E. 2009. Effects of climate change on ticks and tick-borne diseases in Europe. *Interdiscip. Perspect. Infect. Dis.* 2009: 593232.

Grešíková, M. 1959. [Persistence of tick-borne encephalitis virus infection in milk and milk products]. *Čs. Epidem. Mikrobiol. Immunol.* 8: 26-32. [Article in Czech]

Grešíková, M., and Kaluzová, M. 1997. Biology of tick-borne encephalitis virus. *Acta Virol.* 41: 115-24.

Grešíková, M., and Nosek, J. 1966. Isolation of tick-borne encephalitis virus from *Haemaphysalis inermis* ticks. *Acta Virol.* 10: 359-61.

Gritsun, T.S., Frolova, T.V., Zhankov, A.I., Armesto, M., Turner, S.L., Frolova, M.P., Pogodina, V.V., Lashkevich, V.A., and Gould, E.A.2003a. Characterization of a Siberian virus isolated from a patient with progressive chronic tick-borne encephalitis. *J. Virol.* 77: 25-36.

Gritsun, T.S., Lashkevich, V.A., and Gould, E.A. 2003b. Tick-borne encephalitis. *Antiviral Res.* 57: 129-46.

Günther, G., and Haglund, M. 2005. Tick-borne encephalopathies: epidemiology, diagnosis, treatment and prevention. *CNS Drugs* 19: 1009-32.

Günther, G., Haglund, M., Lindquist, L., Forsgren, M., and Sköldenberg, B. 1997. Tick-borne encephalitis in Sweden in relation to aseptic meningoencephalitis of other etiology: a prospective study of clinical course and outcome. *J. Neurol.* 244: 230-8.

Gustafson, R., Svenungsson, B., Forsgren, M., Gardulf, A., and Granstrom, M. 1992. Two-year survey of the incidence of *Lyme borreliosis* and tick-borne encephalitis in a high-risk population in Sweden. *Eur. J. Clin. Microbiol. Infect. Dis.* 11: 894-900.

Hainz, U., Jenewein, B., Asch, E., Pfeiffer, K.P., Berger, P., and Grubeck-Loebenstein, B. 2005. Insufficient protection for healthy elderly adults by tetanus and TBE vaccines. *Vaccine* 23: 3232-5.

Hayasaka, D., Goto, A., Yoshii, K., Mizutani, T., Kariwa, H., and Takashima, I. 2001. Evaluation of European tick-borne encephalitis virus vaccine against recent Siberian and far-eastern subtype strains. *Vaccine* 19: 4774-9.

Hayasaka, D., Nagata, N., Fujii, Y., Hasegawa, H., Sata, T., Suzuki, R., Gould, E.A., Takashima, I., and Koike, S. 2009. Mortality following peripheral infection with tick-borne encephalitis virus results from a combination of central nervous system pathology, systemic inflammatory and stress responses. *Virology* 390(1):139-50.

Heinz, F.X., Holzmann, H., Essl, A., Kundi, M. 2007. Field effectiveness of vaccination against tick-borne encephalitis. *Vaccine* 25: 7559-67.

Hoffmann, H. 1973. [Die unspezifische Abwehr bei neurotropen Arbovirusinfektionen]. *Zbl. Bakt. Hyg. I. Abt.* [Orig. A] 223: 143-63. [Article in German]

Holzmann, H. 2003. Diagnosis of tick-borne encephalitis. *Vaccine* 21(Suppl 1): S36-40.

Holzmann, H., Aberle, S.W., Stiasny, K., Werner, P., Mischak, A., Zainer, B., Netzer, M., Koppi, S., Bechter, E., and0 Heinz, F.X. 2009. Tick-borne encephalitis from eating goat cheese in a mountain region of Austria. Emerg *Infect. Dis.* 15(10):1671-3.

Holzmann, H., Stiastny, K., York, H., Dorner, F., Kunz, C., and Heiz, F.X. 1995. Tick-borne encephalitis virus envelope protein E-specific monoclonal antiobodies for the study of low pH-induced conformational changes and immature virions. *Arch. Virol.* 140: 213-21.

Holzmann, H., Vorobyova, M.S., Ladyzhenskaya, I.P., Ferenczi, E., Kundi, M., Kunz, C., and Heinz, F.X. 1992. Molecular epidemiology of tick-borne encephalitis virus: cross-protection between European and Far Eastern subtypes. *Vaccine* 10: 345-9.

Hubálek, Z., Pow, I., Reidl, H.W., and Hussain, M.H. 1995. Antigenic similarity of Central European encephalitis and louping-ill viruses. *Acta Virol.* 39: 251-6.

Izbický, A. [Current situation in the research of epidemiology of Czechoslovak tick-borne encephalitis]. Dissertation Thesis in Czech. Prague: Prof. Raška Institute of Epidemiology and Microbiology 1954.

Jones, N., Sperl, W., Koch, J., Holzmann, H., and Radauer, W. 2007. Tick-borne encephalitis in a 17-dayold newborn resulting in severe neurologic impairment. *Pediatr. Infect. Dis. J.* 26: 185-6.

Kaäriainen, L.E., Hirvonen, E., and Oker-Blom, N. 1961. Geographical distribution of biphasis tick-borne encephalitis in Finland. *Ann. Med. Exp. Fenn.* 39: 316-28.

Kaiser, R. 1999. The clinical and epidemiological profile of tick-borne encephalitis in southern Germany 1994-98: a prospective study of 656 patients. *Brain* 122(Pt 11): 2067-78.

Kaiser, R., and Holzmann, H. 2000. Laboratory findings in tick-borne encephalitis – correlation with clinical outcome. *Infection* 28: 78-84.

Karabatsos, N. (Ed.) International Catalogue of Arboviruses. Including certain other viruses of vertebrates. 3rd ed. San Antonio: American Society of Tropical Medicine and Hygiene, 1985.

Karmysheva, V.Ia., and Pogodina, V.V. 1990. [Thymus involvement in the pathogenesis of experimental tick-borne encephalitis]. *Vopr. Virusol.* 35: 144-6. [Article in Russian]

Kim, S.Y., Jeong, Y.E., Yun, S.M., Lee, I.Y., Han, M.G., and Ju, Y.R. 2009. Molecular evidence for tick-borne encephalitis virus in ticks in South Korea. *Med. Vet. Entomol.* 23: 15-20.

Kleiter, I., Jilg, W., Bogdahn, U., and Steinbrecher, A. 2007. Delayed humoral immunity in a patient with severe tick-borne encephalitis after complete active vaccination. *Infection* 35: 26-9.

Klockmann, U., Křivanec, K., Stephenson, J.R., and Hilfenhaus, J. 1991. Protection against European isolates of tick-borne encephalitis virus after vaccination with a new tick-borne encephalitis vaccine. *Vaccine* 9: 210-2.

Ko, S., Kang, J.G., Kim, S.Y., Kim, H.C., Klein, T.A., Chong, S.T., Sames, W.J., Yun, S.M., Ju, Y.R., and Chae, J.S. 2010. Prevalence of tick-borne encephalitis virus in ticks from southern Korea. *J. Vet. Sci.* 11(3):197-203.

Kopecký, J., Grubhoffer, L., Kovář, V., Jindrák, L., and Vokurková, D. 1999. A putative host cell receptor for tick-borne encephalitis virus identified by antiidiotypic antibodies and virus affinoblotting. *Intervirology* 42: 9-16.

Korenberg, E.I. 1976. Some contemporary aspects of natural focality and epidemiology of tick-borne encephalitis. *Folia Parasitol.* 23: 357-366.

Korenberg, E.I., Kuznetsova, R.I., Kovalevskiĭ, Iu.V., Vasilenko, Z.E., and Mebel', B.D. 1991. [The basic epidemiological traits of Lyme disease in the northwestern USSR]. *Med. Parazitol.* (Mosk) 3: 14-7. [Article in Russian]

Kožuch, O., Grešíková, M., Nosek, J., Lichard, M., and Sekeyová, M. 1967. The role of small rodents and hedgehogs in a natural focus of tick-borne encephalitis. *Bull. World Health Organ.* 36(Suppl 1): 61-6.

Krejčí, J. 1949a. Isolement d'un virus noveau en course d'un epidémie de meningoencephalite dans la region de Vyškov (Moraviae). *Presse Méd.* (Paris) 74: 1084. [Article in French]

Krejčí, J. 1949b. Epidemie virusových encefalitid na Vyškovsku [Outbreak of encephalitis virus in the region of Vyškov]. *Lék. Listy* (Brno) 4: 73-5, 112-6, 132-4. [Articles in Czech]

Křivanec, K., Kopecký, J., Tomková, E., and Grubhoffer, L. 1988. Isolation of TBE virus from the tick *Ixodes hexagonus*. *Folia Parasit.* 35: 273-6.

Kunz, C. 2003. TBE vaccination and the Austrian experience. *Vaccine* 21 (Suppl 1): S50-5.

Kunz, C., and Heinz, F.X. 2003. Tick-borne encephalitis. *Vaccine* 21(Suppl 1): S1–2.

Labuda, M., Austyn, J.M., Žuffová, E., Kožuch, O., Fuchsberger, N., Lysý, J., and Nuttall, P.A. 1996. Importance of localized skin infection in tick-borne encephalitis virus transmission. *Virology* 219: 357-66.

Labuda, M., Jones, L.D., Williams, T., Danielová, V., and Nuttall, P.A. 1993. Efficient transmission of tick-borne encephalitis virus between cofeeding ticks. *J. Med. Entomol.* 30: 295-9.

Labuda, M., Kožuch, O., Žuffová, E., Elečková, E., Hails, R.S., and Nuttall, P.A. 1997. Tick-borne encephalitis virus transmission between ticks cofeeding on specific immune natural rodent hosts. *Virology* 235: 138-43.

Leonova, G.N., and Maistrovskaya, O.S. 1996b. [Viremia in patients with tick-borne encephalitis and in patients with sucking ixodidae ticks]. *Vopr. Virusol.* 5: 224-8. [Article in Russian]

Leonova, G.N., and Maistrovskaya, O.S., and Borisevich, V.B. 1996a. [Antigenemia in subjects infected with tickborne encephalitis virus]. *Vopr. Virusol.* 6: 260-3. [Article in Russian]

Lindenbach, B.D., and Rice, C.M. 2003. Molecular biology of flaviviruses. *Adv. Virus. Res.* 59: 23-61.

Lindquist, L., and Vapalahti, O. 2008. Tick-borne encephalitis. *Lancet* 371: 1861-71.

Loktev, V.B., Ternovoĭ, V.A., and Netesov, S.V. 2007. [Molecular genetic characteristics of tick-borne encephalitis virus]. *Vopr. Virusol.* 52: 10-6. [Article in Russian]

Lu, Z., Bröker, M., and Liang, G. 2008. Tick-borne encephalitis in mainland China. *Vector Borne Zoonotic Dis.* 8: 713-20.

Ludolfs D, Reinholz M, Schmitz H. Highly specific detection of antibodies to tick-borne encephalitis (TBE) virus in humans using a domain III antigen and a sensitive immune complex (IC) ELISA. *J Clin Virol.* 2009 Jun; 45(2):125-8.

Málková, D., and Filip, O. 1968. Histological picture in the place of inoculation and in lymph nodes of mice after subcutaneous infection with tick-borne encephalitis virus. *Acta Virol.* 12: 355-60.

Málková, D., Mayer, V., and Vrubel, J. 1969. The significance of the regional lymphatic system in penetration of an attenuated strain of tick-borne encephalitis virus into blood of experimentally infected animals. *Acta Virol.* 13: 309-14.

Málková, D., Pala, F., and Šidák, Z. 1961. Cellular changes in the white cell count, regional lymph node and spleen during infection with tick-borne encephalitis virus in mice. *Acta Virol.* 5: 101-11.

Mandl, C.W. 2005. Steps of tick-borne encephalitis virus replication cycle that affect neuropathogenesis. *Virus Res.* 111: 161-74.

Mayer, V. 1966. A mutant of tick-borne encephalitis (TE) virus with lost neurovirulence for monkeys. *Acta Virol.* 10: 561.

Mickiene, A., Laiskonis, A., Günther, G., Vene, S., Lundkvist, A., and Lindquist, L. 2002. Tickborne encephalitis in an area of high endemicity in Lithuania: disease severity and long-term prognosis. *Clin. Infect. Dis.* 35: 650-8.

Molnár, E., and Fornosi, F. 1952. [Accidental laboratory infection with the Czechoslovakian strain of tick encephalitis]. *Orv. Hetil.* 93: 1032-3. [Article in Hungarian]

Niedrig, M., Vaisviliene, D., Teichmann, A., Klockmann, U., and Biel, S.S. 2001. Comparison of six different commercial IgG-ELISA kits for the detection of TBEV-antibodies. *J. Clin. Virol.* 20: 179-82.

Nuttall, P.A., and Labuda, M. 2003. Dynamics of infection in tick vectors and at the tick-host interface. *Adv. Virus Res.* 60: 233-72.

Oker-Blom, N. 1956. Kumlinge disease; a meningoencephalitis occuring in the Aaland Islands. *Ann. Med. Exp. Biol. Fenn.* 34: 309-18.

Pattyn, S.R., and Wyler, R. 1955. Viral meningoencephalitis in Austria. IV. Virus in blood in experimental infection; attempted transmission by mosquitoes. *Bull. World Health Organ.* 12: 581-9.

Pavlova, B.G., Loew-Baselli, A., Fritsch, S., Poellabauer, E.M., Vartian, N., Rinke, I., and Ehrlich, H.J. 2003. Tolerability of modified tick-borne encephalitis vaccine FSME-IMMUN "NEW" in children: results of post-marketing surveillance. *Vaccine* 21: 742-5.

Pavlovskij, E.N. 1939. [On natural focality of infectious and parasitic diseases]. *Vestn. Akad. Nauk SSSR* 10: 98-108. [Article in Russian]

Petri E, Gniel D, Zent O. Tick-borne encephalitis (TBE) trends in epidemiology and current and future management. *Travel Med Infect Dis.* 2010 Jul;8(4):233-45.

Petrishcheva, P.A., and Levkovich, E.N. 1945. [Spring-Summer encephalitis in Leningrad region. Papers of Medical Officers of Volkhov Front]. Leningrad, Russia. [Book in Russian]

Pogodina, V.V., Bochkova, N.G., and Karan', L.S., Frolova, M.P., Trukhina, A.G., Malenko, G.V., Levina, L.S., and Platonov, A.E. 2004. [Comparative analysis of virulence of the Siberian and Far-East subtypes of the tick-born encephalitis virus]. *Vopr. Virusol.* 49: 24-30. [Article in Russian]

Pogodina, V.V., Frolova, M.P., and Erman, B.A. 1979. [Chronic Tick-Borne Encephalitis]. Nauka, Moscow, Russia. [Book in Russian]

Pogodina, V.V., Karan', L.S., Koliasnikova, N.M., Levina, L.S., Malenko, G.V., Gamova, E.G., Lesnikova, M.V., Kiliachina, A.S., Esiunina, M.S., Bochkova, N.G., Shopenskaia, T.A., Frolova, T.V., Andaev, E.I., and Trukhina, A.G. 2007. [Evolution of tick-borne encephalitis and a problem of evolution of its causative agent]. *Vopr. Virusol.* 52: 16-21. [Article in Russian]

Pöllabauer EM, Pavlova BG, Löw-Baselli A, Fritsch S, Prymula R, Angermayr R, Draxler W, Firth C, Bosman J, Valenta B, Harmacek P, Maritsch F, Barrett PN, Ehrlich HJ. Comparison of immunogenicity and safety between two paediatric TBE vaccines. *Vaccine.* 2010 Jun 23;28(29):4680-5.

Poponnikova, T.V. 2006. Specific clinical and epidemiological features of tick-borne encephalitis in Western Siberia. *Int. J. Med. Microbiol.* 296(Suppl 40): 59-62.

Puchhammer-Stöckl, E., Kunz, C., Mandl, C.W., and Heinz, F.X. 1995. Identification of tick-borne encephalitis virus ribonucleic acid in tick suspensions and in clinical specimens by a reverse transcriptionnested polymerase chain reaction assay. *Clin. Diagn. Virol.* 4: 321-6.

Rampas, J., and Gallia, F. 1949. [Isolation of tick-borne encephalitis virus from ticks *Ixodes ricinus*]. *Čas. Lék. čes.* 88: 1179-80. [Article in Czech]

Randolph, S. 2002. The changing incidence of tick-borne encephalitis in Europe. *Euro Surveill* 6: pii=1953. Available online: http://www.eurosurveillance.org/ViewArticle.aspx?Articleld=1953.

Rendi-Wagner, P. 2008. Advances in vaccination against tick-borne encephalitis. Expert Rev Vaccines 7: 589-96.

Rendi-Wagner, P., Kundi, M., Zent, O., Banzhoff, A., Jaehnig, P., Stemberger, R., Dvorak, G., Grumbeck, E., Laaber, B., and Kollaritsch, H. 2004. Immunogenicity and safety of a booster vaccination against tick-borne encephalitis more than 3 years following the last immunisation. *Vaccine* 23: 427-34.

Romanova, L.Iu., Gmyl, A.P., Dzhivanian, T.I., Bakhmutov, D.V., Lukashev, A.N., Gmyl, L.V., Rumyantsev, A.A., Burenkova, L.A., Lashkevich, V.A., and Karganova, G.G. 2007. Microevolution of tick-borne encephalitis virus in course of host alternation. *Virology* 362: 75-84.

Růžek, D., Dobler, G., and Donoso Mantke, O. 2010. Tick-borne encephalitis: pathogenesis and clinical implications. *Travel Med. Infect. Dis.* 8(4):223-32.

Růžek, D., Gritsun, T.S., Forrester, N.L., Gould, E.A., Kopecký, J., Golovchenko, M., Rudenko, N., and Grubhoffer, L. 2008. Mutations in the NS2B and NS3 genes affect mouse neuroinvasiveness of a Western European field strain of tick-borne encephalitis virus. *Virology* 374: 249-55.

Růžek, D., Salát, J., Palus, M., Gritsun, T.S., Gould, E.A., Dyková, I., Skallová, A., Jelínek, J., Kopecký, J., and Grubhoffer, L. 2009. $CD8^+$ T-cells mediate immunopathology in tick-borne encephalitis. *Virology* 384: 1-6.

Růžek, D., Salát, J., Singh, S.K., Kopecký, J. 2011. Breakdown of the Blood-Brain Barrier During Tick-Borne Encephalitis in Mice Is Not Dependent on $CD8^+$ T-cells. *PLoS One*, 6(5):e20472.

Růžek, D., Šťastná, H., Kopecký, J., Golovljova, I., and Grubhoffer, L. 2007. Rapid subtyping of tick-borne encephalitis virus isolates using multiplex RTPCR. *J. Virol. Methods* 144: 133-7.

Růžek, D., Štěrba, J., Kopecký, J., and Grubhoffer, L. 2006. The supposedly attenuated Hy-HK variant of highly virulent Hypr strain of tick-borne encephalitis virus is obviously a strain of Langat virus. *Acta Virol.* 50: 277-8.

Saksida, A., Duh, D., Lotric-Furlan, S., Strle, F., Petrovec, M., and Avsic-Zupanc, T. 2005. The importance of tick-borne encephalitis virus RNA detection for early differential diagnosis of tick-borne encephalitis. *J. Clin. Virol.* 33: 331-5.

Schneider, H. 1931. [Über epidemische akute „Meningitis serosa"]. *Wien. Klin. Woch.* 44: 350-2. [Article in German]

Schultze D, Dollenmaier G, Rohner A, Guidi T, Cassinotti P. Benefit of detecting tick-borne encephalitis viremia in the first phase of illness. *J. Clin. Virol.* 2007; 38: 172-5.

Schwaiger M, Cassinotti P. Development of a quantitative real-time RT-PCR assay with internal control for the laboratory detection of tick borne encephalitis virus (TBEV) RNA. *J. Clin. Virol.* 2003; 27: 136-45.

Šenigl, F., Grubhoffer, L., and Kopecký, J. 2006. Differences in maturation of tick-borne encephalitis virus in mammalian and tick cell line. *Intervirology* 49: 236-48.

Shapoval, A.N. 1976. [Chronic Forms of Tick-Borne Encephalitis]. Medicina, Leningrad, Russia. [Book in Russian]

Shapoval, A.N. 1977. [Inapparent forms of tick-borne encephalitis]. *Zh. Mikrobiol. Epidemiol. Immunobiol.* 5:11-7. [Article in Russian]

Simon, J., Slonim, D., and Zavadova, H. 1966. [Experimentelle Untersuchungen von klinischen und subklinischen Formen der Zeckenencephalitis an unterschiedlich empfänglichen Wirten: Mäusen, Hamstern und Affen. II. Hamster]. *Acta Neuropathol.* 7: 89-100. [Article in German]

Sinnecker, H. 1960. [Zeckenencephalitis in Deutschland]. *Zbl. Bakt. Orig.* 180: 12-8. [Article in German]

Slávik, I., Mayer, V., and Mrena, E. 1967. Morphology of purified tick-borne encephalitis virus. *Acta Virol.* 11: 66.

Sonnenberg, K., Niedrig, M., Steinhagen, K., Rohwäder, E., Meyer, W., Schlumberger, W., Müller-Kunert, E., and Stöcker, W. 2004. State-of-the-art serological techniques for detection of antibodies against tick-borne encephalitis virus. *Int. J. Med. Microbiol.* 293(Suppl 37): 148-51.

Süss, J. 2003. Epidemiology and ecology of TBE relevant to the production of effective vaccines. *Vaccine* 21(Suppl 1): S19–35.

Süss, J. 2008. Tick-borne encephalitis in Europe and beyond - the epidemiological situation as of 2007. *Euro Surveill* 13(26). pii: 18916.

Szajna, M. 1954. [Tick-borne encephalitis in Poland]. *Pol. Tyg. Lek.* (Wars.) 9: 1625-7. [Article in Polish]

Thiel, H.J., Collett, M.S., Gould, E.A., Heinz, F.X., Houghton, M., Meyers, G. et al. 2005. In: Fauquet CM, Mayo MA, Maniloff J, Desselberger U, Ball LA, Eds. Virus Taxonomy: Classification and Nomenclature, Eighth Report of the International Committee on the Taxonomy of Viruses. Amsterdam, Boston, Heidelberg, London, New York, Oxford, Elsevier Academic Press; pp. 981-98.

Vaptsarov, I., Turpomanov, A., Spasov, Z., Nikov, D., and Dragiev, M. 1954. [Recurrent viral meningoencephalitis in southern Bulgaria]. *Surv. Med.* (Sofiia) 5: 86-103. [Article in Bulgarian]

Vein, A.A., and van Emde Boas, W. 2011. Kozhevnikov epilepsy: the disease and its eponym. *Epilepsia* 52(2):212-8.

Voronkova, G.M., and Zakharycheva, T.A. 2007. [The condition of tick-borne infections problem in Khabarovsk region]. *Bulletin SORAMN* 4: 82-88. [Article in Russian]

Votiakov, V.I., Zlobin, V.I., and Mishayeva, N.P. 2002. [Tickborne encephalitis of Eurasia. Ecology, molecular epidemiology, nosology, evolution]. *Nauka,* Novosibirsk, Russia. [Book in Russian]

Waldvogel, K., Bossart, W., Huisman, T., Boltshauser, E., and Nadal, D. 1996. Severe tick-borne encephalitis following passive immunization. *Eur. J. Pediatr.* 155: 775-9.

Yamshchikov, V.F., and Compans, R.W. 1993. Regulation of the late events in flavivirus protein processing and maturation. *Virology* 192: 38-51.

Zent, O., Banzhoff, A., Hilbert, A.K., Meriste, S., Słuzewski, W., and Wittermann Ch. 2003. Safety, immunogenicity and tolerability of a new pediatric tickborne encephalitis (TBE) vaccine, free of proteinderived stabilizer. *Vaccine* 21: 3584-92.

Zilber, L.A. 1939. [Spring (spring–summer) epidemical tick-borne encephalitis]. *Arch. biol. Nauk* 56: 9-37. [Article in Russian]

8

The Development of Encephalitis Following Tick-Borne Encephalitis Virus Infection in a Mouse Model

Daisuke Hayasaka
Department of Virology, Institute of Tropical Medicine, Nagasaki University
Japan

1. Introduction

Tick-borne encephalitis virus (TBEV) belongs to the genus *Flavivirus* in the family *Flaviviridae*. TBEV is transmitted through the bite of an infected tick and causes acute central nervous system (CNS) disease in humans (Dumpis, Crook, and Oksi, 1999; Lindquist and Vapalahti, 2008). TBEV is prevalent over a wide area of Europe and Asia, and is geographically and genetically divided into three subtypes, the European, Siberian and far eastern subtypes (Ecker et al., 1999; Hayasaka et al., 2001b). The endemic areas of Europe and Asia correspond to the geographical distribution of *Ixodes* tick species (Burke and Monath, 2001; Dumpis, Crook, and Oksi, 1999).

Tick-borne encephalitis (TBE) cases exhibit neurological symptoms including fever, headache, meningitis, meningoencephalitis and meningoencephalomyelitis, the latter being evident in the most severe cases (Dumpis, Crook, and Oksi, 1999). These non-specific clinical features of TBE may be due to widespread occurrence of neuronal dysfunction at different sites in the CNS. Hence, laboratory diagnosis is required to distinguish TBE from other neurological disorders (Charrel et al., 2004; Holzmann, 2003).

The laboratory mouse model is commonly employed to elucidate the mechanism of disease development following TBEV infection *in vivo*. The pathogenetic process following experimental infection with TBEV is fundamentally similar to that of other encephalitic flaviviruses including Japanese encephalitis virus (JEV), West Nile virus (WNV) and Murray Valley encephalitis virus (MVEV) (Albrecht, 1968; Burke and Monath, 2001; Garcia-Tapia et al., 2007). In the mouse model, the CNS pathology of TBEV and other encephalitic flaviviruses consists of two distinct features: neuroinvasiveness and neurovirulence. It is generally considered that death following peripheral infection represents neuroinvasiveness, whereas mortality following direct intracerebral infection represents neurovirulence (Mandl, 2005; Monath, 1986).

Recent works have proposed that CNS pathology following TBEV infection is a consequence of viral infection of the corresponding cells and the resulting inflammatory response. Direct viral infection of neurons is considered to be the major cause of neurological disease because viral infections cause apoptosis or degeneration of neurons *in vivo* and *in vitro* (Couderc et al., 2002; Liao et al., 1997; Prikhod'ko et al., 2001; Shrestha, Gottlieb, and Diamond, 2003). In addition, recent studies have demonstrated that immunopathological effects also contribute to the severity of CNS pathology (Hayasaka et al., 2009; Ruzek et al., 2009; Wang et al., 2003).

In this chapter, we discuss the multiple mechanisms of disease development observed in a mouse model following peripheral and intracerebral infection with TBEV.

2. Experimental infection in mice

2.1 Peripheral infection

Peripheral infection such as subcutaneous, foot-pad or intradermal route is considered to be a replica of natural infection resulting from the bite of an infected tick. From studies of encephalitic flavivirus infections, it is believed that initial virus replication occurs in dendritic cells (DCs) such as Langerhans cells at the site of infection, and infected DCs migrate to draining lymph nodes. After viremia and replication in peripheral organs, the virus invades the CNS and the host develops CNS disease, although the mechanism by which the blood-brain-barrier is crossed is not completely understood (Byrne et al., 2001; Dumpis, Crook, and Oksi, 1999; Robertson et al., 2009; Samuel and Diamond, 2006). Thus, peripheral infection is generally regarded as a model for neuroinvasiveness.

Following subcutaneous infection with low challenge dose (10^3 PFU) of TBEV, infectious virus is first detected in peripheral organs such as blood, spleen, thymus, lung (Hayasaka et al., 2009), liver and kidney (Hayasaka et al., unpublished data) at 1 to 3 days post-infection (p.i.), and subsequently appears in the CNS at 5 to 7 days p.i.. However, virus replication in peripheral organs does not appear to correlate with the progression of disease, because mice did not have apparent clinical signs during the peak stages of infectious virus in peripheral organs (Hayasaka et al., 2009).

2.2 Intracerebral infection

Intracerebral infection is commonly performed to examine direct neuronal virulence and pathogenicity in the CNS. Intracerebral infection usually results in high mortality rates, and 50% lethal doses (LD_{50}) are often below 1PFU (Chiba et al., 1999a; Monath et al., 1980). Thus, it is believed that the ensuing intracerebral infection and lethal encephalitis after viral entry into the CNS directly represent neurovirulence.

We previously showed that following intracerebral infection with TBEV, virus replication occurred almost simultaneously in peripheral and CNS organs, and acute viral replication was observed throughout the CNS (Hayasaka et al., 2010). Thus, mortality following intracerebral infection is directly related to the severity of viral infection in the CNS (Hayasaka et al., 2010).

2.3 Virus tropism within CNS

Interestingly, virus tropism has been observed in the CNS following TBEV infection. After subcutaneous infection with low virus challenge doses of TBEV Oshima strain, the brain cortex or cerebellum was infected at early or late stage of infection, respectively (Hayasaka et al., 2009). In particular, disappearance of Purkinje cells was observed at late periods post-infection. On the other hand, subcutaneous infection with high virus challenge doses resulted in acute and widespread neuronal infection without significant differences between the brain cortex, thalamus, cerebellum, brainstem and spinal cord (Hayasaka et al., 2009).

This virus tropism of TBEV within the CNS is clearly distinguished from the tropism of other encephalitic flaviviruses, e.g. JEV infection, in which infectious virus is mainly detected in the brain cortex regardless of inoculation route and challenge dose (Hayasaka, unpublished data).

2.4 Mortality as an index of virulence and pathogenesis

It has been generally accepted that CNS infection causes lethal encephalitis. Thus, death has been used as an index of pathogenesis, and mortality is considered as a measure of neuroinvasiveness or neurovirulence following peripheral or intracerebral infection, respectively. 50% lethal dose (LD_{50}) is often determined to compare the virulence of different virus strains or the pathogenesis in different conditions of infection.

However, the role of neuroinvasiveness in mortality is controversial because some mice recovered from illness with neuropathological sequelae following peripheral infection (Chiba et al., 1999a; Hayasaka et al., 2001b; Hayasaka et al., 1999). Thus, viral neuroinvasion following peripheral infection does not simply determine whether or not the mice will die; rather, mortality is determined after the development of CNS disease. In other words, the mechanism of mortality following peripheral infection differs from that of intracerebral infection.

2.4.1 Dose-independent mortality

LD_{50} is determined based on the correlation of increased challenge doses and increased mortality rates (Reed and Muench, 1938). However, with some strains of encephalitic flavivirus including TBEV, mice do not exhibit a normal dose response curve of mortality following peripheral infection. This phenomenon was first reported in the 1940's (Lennette, 1944), but the reason for these apparent discrepancies is not fully understood.

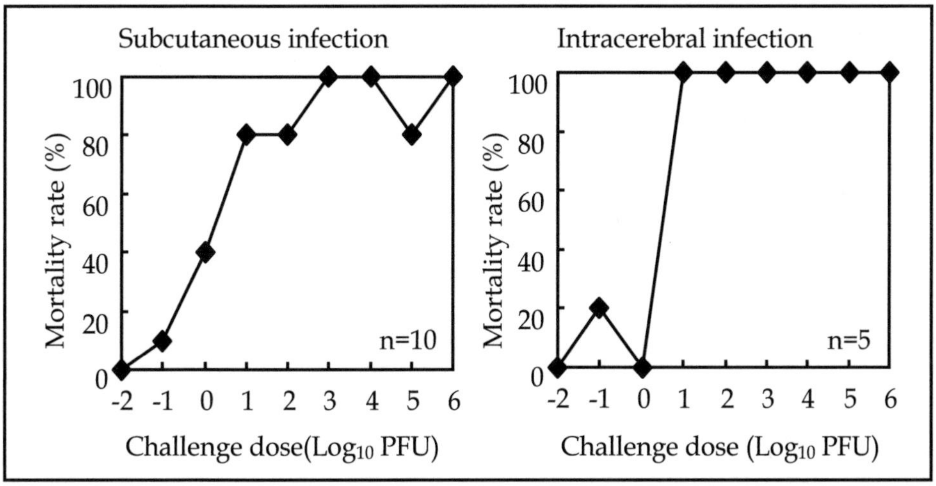

Fig. 1. Mortality rates following subcutaneous and intracerebral inoculation with serial challenge doses of TBEV IR strain

Two patterns of dose-independent mortality are suggested based on our studies. In the first pattern, no increase in mortality rate was observed for low dose challenges, e.g. around 50% mortality between 10^2 to 10^6 PFU inoculations (Hayasaka et al., 2009). This phenomenon was observed following peripheral infection with the Oshima, KH and VL strains (Chiba et al., 1999a; Hayasaka et al., 2001a; Hayasaka et al., 2001b; Hayasaka et al., 1999). All of the mice tested positive for TBEV-specific antibody in those challenge doses, indicating an infectious rate of 100% (Hayasaka, unpublished data). Furthermore, viral load in the CNS was not significantly different between 10^2 to 10^6 PFU challenge doses, and the level of infectious viruses detected in the CNS of recovering mice were similar to dying mice (Hayasaka et al., 2009). From these observations, we hypothesize that neuroinvasion following peripheral infection does not simply determine mortality, and dose independence is attributable to the outcome of viral infection and host response in peripheral and/or CNS tissues. Thus, elucidation of CNS pathology relating to disease severity and mortality could be an important approach to understand this pattern of dose-independent mortality.

Another pattern of dose-independent mortality is characterized by a reduction in mortality rate (<100%) using challenge doses higher than 100% lethal dose. For example, subcutaneous infection with 10^3 PFU of IR strain induced 100% mortality, but 10^5 PFU challenge dose exhibited 80% mortality rate (Fig. 1). Interestingly, the surviving mice did not have apparent clinical signs such as weight reduction, suggesting that peripheral infection and/or viral invasion in the CNS might not have occurred. We speculate that at early stage of infection, several factors involving innate immunity contribute to this pattern of dose-independent mortality.

2.4.2 Dose-dependent mortality

Dose-dependent mortality, on the other hand, is typically observed in intracerebral infection with any TBEV strain. For example, intracerebral inoculation with the Oshima or IR strain resulted to dose-dependent mortality, with 100% mortality attainable using more than 10^1 PFU (Hayasaka et al., 2010) (Fig. 1).

Furthermore, peripheral infection with some strains such as Sofjin, IR and Hochosterviz showed essentially dose-dependent mortality, and LD_{50} could be determined (Chiba et al., 1999a; Hayasaka et al., 2001a), although some dose-independent mortality was observed in challenge doses higher than 100%lethal dose, as described above (Fig. 1).

3. Two distinct features of early and late mortality

We recently showed that mice died either at early or late stages of infection after peripheral infection with the Oshima strain of TBEV (Hayasaka et al., 2009). Whether mice show early or late mortality is determined by the infectious route, virus strain and inoculation dose. Importantly, dose-dependent or dose-independent mortality is closely associated with early or late mortality, respectively. Thus, in order to understand dose-independent mortality, elucidating the mechanism of late mortality in particular is important.

3.1 Early mortality

3.1.1 Intracerebral inoculation

Intracerebral inoculation of the Oshima strain in mice caused death starting at 7 days p.i., and most died within 10 days p.i. regardless of the challenge dose (Hayasaka et al., 2010). Early death was also observed following intracerebral inoculation with the IR strain (Fig. 2). Infected mice remained asymptomatic for 4 to 5 days, after which they acutely exhibited clinical signs including weight loss, slowness in movement, ataxia, piloerection and anorexia. Mice exhibited neurological signs of paralysis such as rigidity and flaccid paralysis from 7 days p.i., although some mice did not have apparent paralysis before death (Hayasaka et al., 2010). Survivals challenged with less than 10^1 PFU were IgG negative for TBEV antigen, indicating that only positively infected mice eventually die (Hayasaka et al., unpublished data). These results suggest that intracerebral infection directly correlates with mortality, and is characterized by early death.

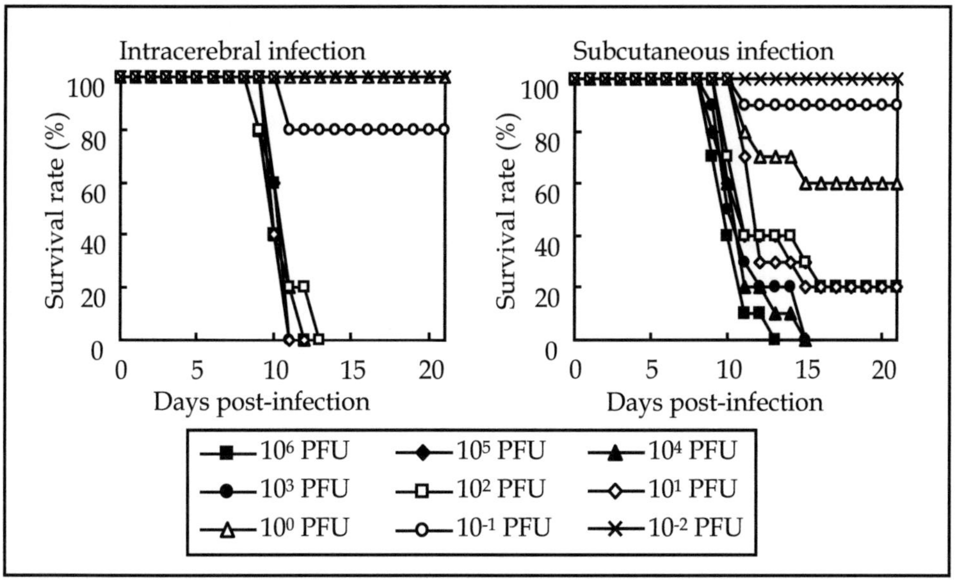

Fig. 2. Daily survival rates following intracerebral and subcutaneous inoculation with serial challenge doses of TBEV IR strain

3.1.2 Peripheral inoculation with highly virulent strains

Following intraperitoneal inoculation with Sofjin and Hochosterwitz strains, which exhibit dose-dependent mortality, mice died early at 8-10 days (Chiba et al., 1999b). Subcutaneous infection with the IR strain also exhibited early death; mice began to die at 8 days p.i., and most died within 11 days p.i. (Fig. 2). These observations suggest that peripheral inoculation with these TBEV strains cause early mortality like intracerebral infection.

3.1.3 Peripheral inoculation with high virus challenge dose

Subcutaneous inoculation with high challenge dose (>10^7 PFU) of the Oshima strain resulted in early mortality at a rate of more than 80% (Hayasaka et al., 2009). Mice started to die at 8 days p.i. and most mice died by 13-14 days p.i.. These infections elicited early onset of weight loss, with acute weight reduction from 5-6 days p.i. (Hayasaka et al., 2009). These observations suggest that high challenge dose of peripheral infection also induce early mortality like intracerebral infection and subcutaneous infection with highly virulent strains.

3.1.4 Severe CNS infection contributes to early mortality

Early mortality strongly correlates with acute and widespread neuronal degeneration due to viral cytopathic effects in the CNS (Hayasaka et al., 2009; Hayasaka et al., 2010). Following intracerebral infection with the Oshima strain, virus replication occurred almost simultaneously in peripheral and CNS organs. At day 6 p.i., viral load was significantly increased to more than 10^8 PFU/g of tissue in all regions of the CNS including the brain cortex, thalamus, cerebellum, brain stem and spinal cord (Hayasaka et al., 2010). Histopathological analysis corresponded well with the viral load, demonstrating acutely necrotic neurons and mild inflammation throughout the CNS, particularly in the brain cortex, thalamus, cerebellum and lumber spinal cord. All degenerated cells examined were TBEV antigen-positive (Hayasaka et al., 2010).

Subcutaneous infection with a high challenge dose of Oshima strain also showed early CNS infection at 1 day p.i., almost simultaneously with peripheral organ replication (Hayasaka et al., 2009). The viral load peaked in the CNS at 7 days p.i., and mice started to die at around the same period. Consistent with the viral load, histopathological examination showed acute necrotic neurons with TBEV antigens and inflammatory reactions throughout the CNS involving the brain cortex, thalamus, cerebellum, brainstem and spinal cord (Hayasaka et al., 2009). Furthermore, we showed that subcutaneous infection with low challenge dose of the Sofjin and IR strains also exhibited severe CNS infection in mice, indicating that even low dose challenges with these strains rapidly reach a lethal level (Hayasaka et al., unpublished data).

These results strongly suggest that early death primarily results from acute neurological dysfunction throughout the CNS due to viral cytopathic effects, and mice showing clinical signs of illness subsequently die. Thus, CNS pathology is directly linked to lethality, and mortality rate is dose-dependent in TBEV infections with early mortality.

3.2 Late mortality

3.2.1 Peripheral inoculation with low virulent strain

We previously showed that subcutaneous infection with a lower virus challenge dose (10^2 - 10^6 PFU) of the TBEV Oshima strain resulted in 40 to 60% mortality without obvious difference in mortality rates at any of the challenge doses. Mice started to die after 11 days p.i. and the average of survival times were around 15-16 days p.i., irrespective of the challenge dose (Hayasaka et al., 2009).

Interestingly, all low challenge doses (10^2 - 10^6 PFU) induced 100% morbidity and 100% infectivity as determined by weight loss and by TBEV-specific antibody positivity, respectively (Hayasaka et al., unpublished data). Furthermore, all brains infected with low challenge doses contained infectious virus at 9 to 11 days p.i., the period when mice exhibited weight loss (Hayasaka et al., 2009). These observations suggest that CNS pathology is not directly linked to lethality in TBEV infections with late mortality, and whether mice die or survive is determined at late stage of infection, independent of the challenge dose.

3.2.2 Complex mechanism of CNS infection and immune response contribute to late mortality

To examine the mechanism of late mortality in detail, we distinguished dying and recovering/surviving mice by their degree of weight loss following subcutaneous infection with low virus challenge doses of the Oshima strain (Hayasaka et al., 2009). Viral load in the CNS was not as high as intracerebral infection. Interestingly, viral load in the CNS was not significantly different between dying and recovering mice. Histopathological examination showed inflammatory reactions with focal proliferation of microglial rod cells in the brain cortex, thalamus, cerebellum, brainstem and spinal cord in both dying and recovering mice (Hayasaka et al., 2009). These observations suggest that following low challenge dose, mice develop encephalitis but also show features of virus clearance from the CNS. Furthermore, viral infection alone is not a critical determinant of late death, unlike that of early death (Hayasaka et al., 2009).

Inflammatory responses were assessed by measuring cell infiltration and inflammatory cytokine levels in brains (Hayasaka et al., 2009). Infiltrating leukocyte levels including $CD8^+$ T cells, $CD4^+$ T cells, neutrophils, natural killer cell and macrophages were significantly increased in TBEV-infected mice compared with mock-infected mice, but there were no significant differences between dying and recovering mice. Although the levels of inflammatory cytokines involving IFN-γ, IL-2, IL-5 and IL-10 in the brain were increased compared with mock-infected mice, there were no significant differences between dying and surviving mice either (Hayasaka et al., 2009). On the other hand, TNF-α levels were higher in dying mice than in recovering mice, suggesting that TNF-α response in the CNS correlates with severity.

Thymocytes and splenocytes were dramatically decreased in dying mice compared with mock-infected and surviving mice. In addition, corticosterone was most significantly increased in dying mice. These observations suggest that dying mice exhibited a severe stress response.

Serum levels of IFN-γ, RANTES and TNF-α were increased in both dying and recovering mice compared with mock-infected mice (Hayasaka et al., 2009). Interestingly, only serum TNF-α had significantly elevated levels in dying mice compared with surviving mice. Furthermore, among various cytokines examined, IL-10 expression was significantly increased in the spleen of dying mice compared with surviving and mock-infected mice (Hayasaka et al., unpublished data).

These results suggest that fatality is determined by a complex mechanism of CNS pathology and systemic response that involve stress response and increased levels of TNF-α and IL-10.

4. Conclusions

The laboratory mouse model is commonly employed to study the CNS pathology of TBEV *in vivo* because mice develop neurological symptoms and relatively comparable neurological dysfunction similar to that observed in humans (Chiba et al., 1999a; Pogodina and Savinov, 1964; Sokol, Libikova, and Zemla, 1959; Vince and Grcevic, 1969). However, in the mouse model of encephalitic flavivirus infection, dose-independent mortality has been an unresolved problem since the 1940's (King et al., 2007; Lennette, 1944). To explain its mechanism, we recently reported two distinct features of early and late mortality. Late death following low virus challenge doses appears to be a key feature of dose-independent mortality. Furthermore, we have shown that lethal levels of CNS infection cause early mortality, whereas immune and stress responses in addition to CNS infection contribute to late mortality (Hayasaka et al., 2009; Hayasaka et al., 2010). Importantly, whether mice show early or late mortality is associated with the infectious route, virus strain and inoculation dose (Fig. 3).

It is generally believed that human cases succumb to acute and critical neuronal dysfunction following direct viral infection of the neurons, suggesting that early death, as shown in this mouse study, possibly relates to the mechanism of mortality in human cases. Thus, TBEV strains that induce early mortality following peripheral inoculation in mice can be considered as highly virulent and can cause severe disease in humans. Since far-eastern subtypes of TBEV cause more severe disease with up to 20-40% fatality rate in humans, they can be predicted to exhibit early mortality. Contradictory to this however, Oshima, KH and VL strains of Far-eastern subtype exhibit late mortality: infected mice had mild CNS infection and some of them recovered. On the other hand, Sofjin (Far-eastern subtype), Hochosterwitz (European-subtype) and IR strain (Siberian subtype) strains induce early mortality following peripheral infection, indicating that these strains are potentially more virulent than Oshima, KH and VL strains. Thus, virulence is inconsistent with the TBEV subtype; rather, highly virulent types are more likely to be randomly distributed in endemic areas. In fact, recent studies suggest that seroprevalence rates differ in Europe (1–20%) and in Russia (30–100%), and thus the morbidity and mortality rates may be due to selective severe cases (Lindquist and Vapalahti, 2008).

Our results showed that in addition to CNS infection, systemic stress and inflammatory responses in late phases potentially contribute to the severity and lethality of TBE in human cases. Further elucidation of this mechanism using the mouse model is an important priority to enable the development of effective treatment strategies for human TBE.

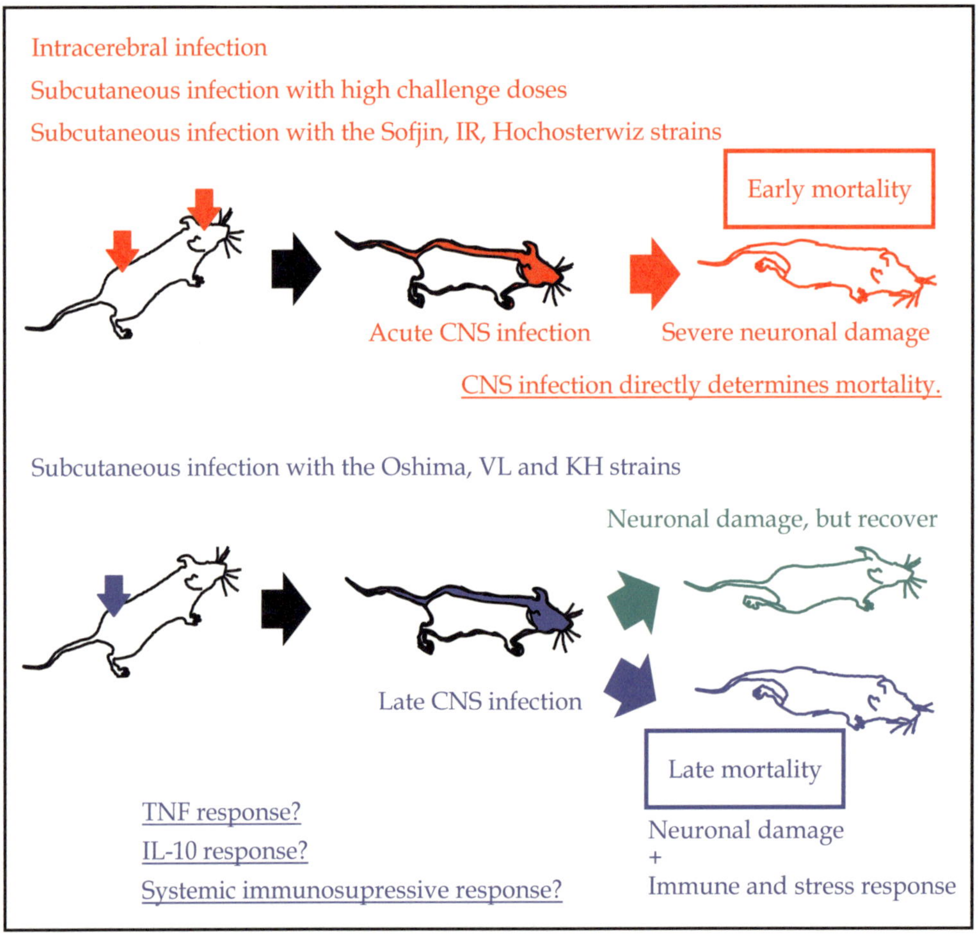

Fig. 3. Summary of early and late mortality observed following TBEV infection in mice

5. Acknowledgement

This work was supported by KAKENHI [Grant-in-Aid for Young Scientists (B)] from the Ministry of Education, Culture, Sports, Science, and Technology, Japan, and Health Grants for Research on Emerging and Re-emerging Infectious Diseases from the Ministry of Health.

6. References

Albrecht, P. (1968). Pathogenesis of neurotropic arbovirus infections. *Curr Top Microbiol Immunol* 43, 44-91.

Burke, S. D., and Monath, P. T. (2001). Flaviviruses. *In* "Fields virology" (D. M. Knipe, P. M. Howley, D. E. Griffin, R. A. Lamb, M. A. Martin, B. Roizman, and S. E. Straus, Eds.), pp. 991-1041. Lippincott Williams & Wilkins, Philadelphia, PA.

Byrne, S. N., Halliday, G. M., Johnston, L. J., and King, N. J. (2001). Interleukin-1beta but not tumor necrosis factor is involved in West Nile virus-induced Langerhans cell migration from the skin in C57BL/6 mice. *J Invest Dermatol* 117(3), 702-9.

Charrel, R. N., Attoui, H., Butenko, A. M., Clegg, J. C., Deubel, V., Frolova, T. V., Gould, E. A., Gritsun, T. S., Heinz, F. X., Labuda, M., Lashkevich, V. A., Loktev, V., Lundkvist, A., Lvov, D. V., Mandl, C. W., Niedrig, M., Papa, A., Petrov, V. S., Plyusnin, A., Randolph, S., Suss, J., Zlobin, V. I., and de Lamballerie, X. (2004). Tick-borne virus diseases of human interest in Europe. *Clin. Microbiol. Infect.* 10(12), 1040-55.

Chiba, N., Iwasaki, T., Mizutani, T., Kariwa, H., Kurata, T., and Takashima, I. (1999a). Pathogenicity of tick-borne encephalitis virus isolated in Hokkaido, Japan in mouse model. *Vaccine* 17(7-8), 779-87.

Chiba, N., Osada, M., Komoro, K., Mizutani, T., Kariwa, H., and Takashima, I. (1999b). Protection against tick-borne encephalitis virus isolated in Japan by active and passive immunization. *Vaccine* 17(11-12), 1532-9.

Couderc, T., Guivel-Benhassine, F., Calaora, V., Gosselin, A. S., and Blondel, B. (2002). An ex vivo murine model to study poliovirus-induced apoptosis in nerve cells. *J. Gen. Virol.* 83(Pt 8), 1925-30.

Dumpis, U., Crook, D., and Oksi, J. (1999). Tick-borne encephalitis. *Clin. Infect. Dis.* 28(4), 882-90.

Ecker, M., Allison, S. L., Meixner, T., and Heinz, F. X. (1999). Sequence analysis and genetic classification of tick-borne encephalitis viruses from Europe and Asia. *J. Gen. Virol.* 80, 179-85.

Garcia-Tapia, D., Hassett, D. E., Mitchell, W. J., Jr., Johnson, G. C., and Kleiboeker, S. B. (2007). West Nile virus encephalitis: sequential histopathological and immunological events in a murine model of infection. *J Neurovirol* 13(2), 130-8.

Hayasaka, D., Goto, A., Yoshii, K., Mizutani, T., Kariwa, H., and Takashima, I. (2001a). Evaluation of European tick-borne encephalitis virus vaccine against recent Siberian and far-eastern subtype strains. *Vaccine* 19(32), 4774-9.

Hayasaka, D., Ivanov, L., Leonova, G. N., Goto, A., Yoshii, K., Mizutani, T., Kariwa, H., and Takashima, I. (2001b). Distribution and characterization of tick-borne encephalitis viruses from Siberia and far-eastern Asia. *J. Gen. Virol.* 82(Pt 6), 1319-28.

Hayasaka, D., Nagata, N., Fujii, Y., Hasegawa, H., Sata, T., Suzuki, R., Gould, E. A., Takashima, I., and Koike, S. (2009). Mortality following peripheral infection with Tick-borne encephalitis virus results from a combination of central nervous system pathology, systemic inflammatory and stress responses. *Virology* 390(1), 139-50.

Hayasaka, D., Nagata, N., Hasegawa, H., Sata, T., Takashima, I., and Koike, S. (2010). Early mortality following intracerebral infection with the Oshima strain of tick-borne encephalitis virus in a mouse model. *J Vet Med Sci* 72(4), 391-6.

Hayasaka, D., Suzuki, Y., Kariwa, H., Ivanov, L., Volkov, V., Demenev, V., Mizutani, T., Gojobori, T., and Takashima, I. (1999). Phylogenetic and virulence analysis of tick-borne encephalitis viruses from Japan and far-Eastern Russia. *J Gen Virol* 80 (Pt 12), 3127-35.

Holzmann, H. (2003). Diagnosis of tick-borne encephalitis. *Vaccine* 21, S36-40.

King, N. J., Getts, D. R., Getts, M. T., Rana, S., Shrestha, B., and Kesson, A. M. (2007). Immunopathology of flavivirus infections. *Immunol. Cell Biol.* 85(1), 33-42.

Lennette, E. H. (1944). Influence of age on the susceptibility of mice to infection with certain neurotropic viruses. *J. Immunol.* 49, 175-91.

Liao, Y., Tang, Z. Y., Liu, K. D., Ye, S. L., and Huang, Z. (1997). Apoptosis of human BEL-7402 hepatocellular carcinoma cells released by antisense H-ras DNA--in vitro and in vivo studies. *J. Cancer Res. Clin. Oncol.* 123(1), 25-33.

Lindquist, L., and Vapalahti, O. (2008). Tick-borne encephalitis. *Lancet* 371(9627), 1861-71.

Mandl, C. W. (2005). Steps of the tick-borne encephalitis virus replication cycle that affect neuropathogenesis. *Virus Res.* 111(2), 161-74.

Monath, T. P. (1986). Pathology of the flaviviruses. *In* "The Togaviridae and Flaviviridae" (S. Schlesinger, and M. J. Schlesinger, Eds.), pp. 375-440. Plenum Press, New York.

Monath, T. P., Cropp, C. B., Bowen, G. S., Kemp, G. E., Mitchell, C. J., and Gardner, J. J. (1980). Variation in virulence for mice and rhesus monkeys among St. Louis encephalitis virus strains of different origin. *Am J Trop Med Hyg* 29(5), 948-62.

Pogodina, V. V., and Savinov, A. P. (1964). Variation in the pathogenicity of viruses of the Tick-borne encephalitis complex for different animal species. I. experimental infection of mice and hamsters. *Acta. Virol.* 8, 424-34.

Prikhod'ko, G. G., Prikhod'ko, E. A., Cohen, J. I., and Pletnev, A. G. (2001). Infection with Langat Flavivirus or expression of the envelope protein induces apoptotic cell death. *Virology* 286(2), 328-35.

Reed, L. J., and Muench, H. (1938). A simple method of estimating fifty per cent endpoints. *American Journal of Epidemiology* 27(3), 493-497.

Robertson, S. J., Mitzel, D. N., Taylor, R. T., Best, S. M., and Bloom, M. E. (2009). Tick-borne flaviviruses: dissecting host immune responses and virus countermeasures. *Immunol Res* 43(1-3), 172-86.

Ruzek, D., Salat, J., Palus, M., Gritsun, T. S., Gould, E. A., Dykova, I., Skallova, A., Jelinek, J., Kopecky, J., and Grubhoffer, L. (2009). CD8+ T-cells mediate immunopathology in tick-borne encephalitis. *Virology* 384(1), 1-6.

Samuel, M. A., and Diamond, M. S. (2006). Pathogenesis of West Nile Virus infection: a balance between virulence, innate and adaptive immunity, and viral evasion. *J Virol* 80(19), 9349-60.

Shrestha, B., Gottlieb, D., and Diamond, M. S. (2003). Infection and injury of neurons by West Nile encephalitis virus. *J. Virol.* 77(24), 13203-13.

Sokol, F., Libikova, H., and Zemla, J. (1959). Infectious ribonucleic acid from mouse brains infected with tick-borne encephalitis virus. *Nature* 184, 1581.

Vince, V., and Grcevic, N. (1969). Development of morphological changes in experimental tick-borne meningoencephalitis induced in white mice by different virus doses. *J. Neurol. Sci.* 9(1), 109-30.

Wang, T., Scully, E., Yin, Z., Kim, J. H., Wang, S., Yan, J., Mamula, M., Anderson, J. F., Craft, J., and Fikrig, E. (2003). IFN-gamma-producing gamma delta T cells help control murine West Nile virus infection. *J Immunol* 171(5), 2524-31.

9

The Cells of Innate Systems in Tick-Borne Encephalitis

Natalia G. Plekhova[1,2], Larisa M. Somova[1], Irina N. Lyapun[1,2], Nadejda M. Kondrashova[2], Natalia V. Krylova[1], Galina N. Leonova[1] and Euvgenii V. Pustovalov[2]

[1]*Lab. Pathomorphlogy and Electron Microscopy, Institute of Epidemiology and Microbiology, Siberian Branch of the Russian Academy of Medical Sciences, Vladivostok,*
[2]*Lab. Electronic Microscopy and Processing of Images, Far Eastern Federal University, Vladivostok*
Russia

1. Introduction

The immune system belongs to the protective basic system of an organism which is capable of identifying and destroying pathogens. There are two forms of the immune response of an organism: innate and adaptive ones. The innate response occurs within minutes of infection, providing the first wave of defense against the invading pathogen. The concept of innate or nonspecific immunity includes many factors of protection of an organism: biomechanical barriers, physiological, physical, chemical and biochemical factors, etc. The phagocyte (neutrophils, monocytes/macrophages, basophil cells, eosinophils and corpulent cells), into epithelium subpopulations of lymphocyte Tγδ-cells, killer cells - natural (NK-cells), lymphokine activity killer cells (LAK-cells) and so-called Pit-cells - a subpopulation of NK-cells with phenotype CD56/CD16 belong to cellular elements of innate immunity (Litvitskij & Sinelnikov, 2009). Functional properties of these cells are so diverse, that their inferiority as the consequence or the reason of pathological process, in due course inevitably forms the system defeat of an organism accompanied by immune insufficiency. Following virus infection, the host cell deploys the rapid response to limit virus replication in both the infected cell and in neighboring ones.

The family of Flaviviridae includes three genius: Flavivirus, Pestivirus and Hepacivirus. The tick-borne encephalitis (TBE) serocomplex comprises viruses belonging to the genus *Flavivirus* of the family *Flaviviridae* and includes TBE virus (TBEV), Powassan (POWV), Omsk hemorrhagic fever virus (OHFV), and Kyasanur Forest disease virus (KFDV). These viruses cause encephalitis, meningitis, and/or hemorrhagic fevers and represent a serious public health threat due to high morbidity and mortality rates following the infection. The TBEV species include 3 subtypes, Far Eastern (previously RSSE), Siberian (previously West-Siberian), and Western European (previously Central European encephalitis [CEE]) viruses. Recently, taxonomic improvements were proposed, and TBEV were divided into 4 types: Western, Eastern, Turkish sheep, and Louping ill (Grard et al., 2007). Eleven thousand TBE cases annually occur in Russia, but only ≈150 cases are registered in Primorsky District, Russia (Leonova et al., 2006). The Far Eastern subtype is considered to be the most pathogenic for humans, with a mortality rate of >20%. The Western European subtype is less virulent and lethal (Leonova et al., 2006). In addition to the tick-borne viruses, the flaviviruses include mosquito-borne dengue virus (DEN, serotypes 1 through 4), yellow fever virus (YFV), Japanese encephalitis virus (JEV), and West Nile virus (WNV).

All flaviviruses are virions uniform in shape; spheroidal; enveloped; 40-60 nm in diameter. An isometric nucleocapsid (composed of a single protein designated C) contains the positive-stranded RNA genome of about 11 000 nt, which has of single open reading frame (ORF) flanked by non-coding regions at its 5'- and 3'- noncoding ends regions. Following translation, the single polyprotein is cleaved by viral and cellular proteases into three structural proteins, C (capsid), prM/M (membrane and its precursor), and E (envelope), and seven nonstructural (NS) proteins (NS1, NS2A, NS2B, NS3, NS4A, NS4B, and NS5) (Murray et al., 2007). The C protein binds viral RNA to form the spherical nucleocapsid, which is enclosed within a host-derived lipid bilayer studded with viral prM and E proteins.

The transmission of flaviviruses to humans basically occurs following the bite of infected insects - tick, mosquito and so on. When the skin tissue is damaged during the sting of insects, the soluble mediators and cells contribute to the response. Soluble mediators released by injured cells activate polymorphonuclear neutrophils and other types of cells that accumulate at the site of injury. Concurrent with neutrophil accumulation, other cells migrate from both the epidermis [Langerhans cells (LC), dendritic cells (DC) and γδ T cells] and blood (granulocytes, monocytes, natural killer cells, and CD4/CD8 T cells). Following their recruitment, these cells play important roles in the early signaling that activates and orchestrates the immune response. It's establish that upon inoculation of dengue virus into the skin, initial infection and replication occurs in dendritic cells (DCs) localized in the skin and neutrophils (Wu et al., 2000). The macrophages and dendritic cells (DCs) are critical early responders in host defense against West Nile virus infections infection, not just because of their role in orchestrating the immune response, but also because of their importance as sites of early peripheral viral replication (Schneider et al., 2010). The research also showed that cutaneous West Nile virus (WNV) infection leads to a decrease in LC density in the epidermis with a concomitant increase in LC concentration in draining lymph nodes. DCs are thought to transport virus to nearby lymph nodes. Virus replication at this site leads to viremia and spread to peripheral organs including the central nervous system (CNS). The primary cellular targets of infection in the CNS are neurons. However, the mechanisms by which the virus enters and damages the CNS are not defined. Although critical for controlling virus infection in the CNS, the host immune response has been implicated in contributing to neuropathology (Chen et al., 2002). Recently, genetic analysis of TBE patients in Lithuania suggested that a deletion within the chemokine receptor CCR5 is a host genetic factor associated with severe TBE (Rios et al., 2006). Similarly, a mutation in the CCR5 gene was shown to correlate with severe disease in West Nile virus infections (Cologna & Rico-Hesse, 2003).

2. The role of neutrophils (polymorphonuclear cells) in Tick-Borne Encephalitis

The immune function of neutrophils (polymorphonuclear cells, PMNs) at infectious diseases, mainly, associates with phagocytoses and production of cytokines, including nitric oxide and oxygen radicals. The process of output neutrophils from blood in tissue occurs within the first minutes after infection for some stages: a stage of primary adhesion and rolling of leukocyte on endothelium surface; activation and a stop of cells on the certain site of endothelium; the adhesion to a surface and diapedesis of leukocyte with movement in loci of inflammation. The rolling and adhesion are necessary stages for transformation of neutrophils and monocytes in more mature cells and in this process the selecting receptors and integrins take part. The two kinds of selectin receptors: L (CD 62L) and E (CD 62E) and the 5 kinds of integrins to which concern three of heterodimers, consisting from the general β-chain (CD 18) and three α- chain (CD 11a, CD 11b, CD 11c) are identified (Holzer et al., 2010).

Leukocyte chemoattractants induce a series of metabolic changes including activation of trimeric G-proteins followed by enhancing intracellular calcium levels, lipid remodeling, and protein kinase activations. These events culminate in fusion of granule membranes with phagosomes or with the plasma membrane (Smolen & Boxer, 2001). Leukocyte chemoattractants stimulate signaling pathways that are evolved in Rho GTPases, including Rac-dependent NADPH oxidase activation, Rac- and Rho-dependent phospholipase D activity, and Racand CDC-42 regulate p21-activated protein kinases (Bokoch, 1996). The studies by Bokoch have illuminated the role of the GTPases especially the necessary requirement for Rac-dependent and NADPH oxidase activation.

Recruitment and activation of neutrophil is among the principal defensise mechanisms of innate immunity. However, neutrophil-derived proteinases and reactive oxygen species, which are required for the elimination of microorganisms, are also capable of inflicting tissue damage (Klebanoff, 1992). Myeloperoxidase (MPO), a heme protein abundantly expressed in the azurophilic granules, plays a central role in these events. MPO catalyzes the formation of hypochlorous acid, a potent oxidant that has been implicated in killing infects and tissue destruction through induction of necrosis and apoptosis. MPO, through formation of secondary oxidants and nitration of protein tyrosine residues, could modulate intercellular signaling in the vasculature and affect the activation state of neutrophils.

Neutrophil trafficking into inflamed tissues is intimately linked to prolonged survival. Mature neutrophils have the shortest half-life (7 hours) among leukocytes and die rapidly via apoptosis (Kebir & Filep, 2010). This constitutively expressed cell death program renders neutrophils unresponsive to proinflammatory stimuli and promotes their removal from inflamed areas by scavenger macrophages with minimal damage to the surrounding tissue, thereby facilitating the resolution of inflammation (Kennedy & DeLeo, 2009; Fox et al., 2010). Neutrophil survival is contingent on rescue from apoptosis bysignals, such as lipopolysaccharide or proinflammatory cytokines, from the inflammatory microenvironment.

Upon contact with their bacterial targets, neutrophils fire a barrage of antimicrobial peptides, sometimes releasing structures called neutrophil-associated extracellular traps, or NETs. In releasing their NETs, they commit suicide—unleashing their entire antibacterial arsenal via a specialized form of programmed cell death called NETosis (Hakkim et al. 2010). It is established, that NET release is a marker of disease progression in Feline leukemia virus infection in domestic cats (Wardini et al., 2010).

Neutrophils are key in innate immunity, but their role in viral pathogenesis is incompletely understood. In Flavivirus infection the protective role of neutrophils was researched in Japanese encephalitis, West Nile and Denge viruses infections. After entry into the host, these viruses generate a rapid inflammatory response, including peripheral neutrophil leucocytosis and infiltration of neutrophils into extraneural tissue (Khanna et al., 1994). In Japanese encephalitis virus (JEV) the inflammation results in an increased level of cytokines such as macrophage-derived chemotactic factor (MDF), tumour necrosis factor alpha (TNF-α) and interleukin 8 (IL-8) in the serum and cerebrospinal fluid (CSF) (Winter et al., 2004). JEV-stimulated neutrophils released reactive oxygen metabolites with maximum activity between days 7 and 9 (Chen & Wang, 2002). The increased levels of inflammatory mediators appear to play a protective role or to initiate an irreversible immune response leading to cell death. In West Nile virus (WNV) disease the neutrophils are rapidly recruited to the loci of infection and support efficient replication of virus. Thus the expression of neutrophil attracting chemokines, Cxcl1 and Cxcl2, was rapidly and dramatically elevated in macrophages. Mice depleted of neutrophils after West Nile virus inoculation developed higher viremia and experienced earlier death, compared with the control group, which suggest a protective role for this cells. These data suggest that neutrophils have a biphasic response to WNV infection, serving as a reservoir for replication and dissemination in early infection and later contributing to viral clearance (Bai et al., 2010).

Defensins product of neutrophils are antimicrobial peptides important to innate host defense. In addition to their direct antimicrobial effect, defensins modulate immune responses. Increasing evidence indicates that defensins exhibit complex functions by positively or negatively modulating infections of both enveloped and non-enveloped viruses (Ding et al., 2009). The effects of defensins on viral infections appear to be specific to the defensin, virus and target cell. Regulation of viral infection by defensins is achieved by multiple mechanisms. In virus infection: defensins bactericidal/permeability-increasing proteins - DEF1A and DEF4A are neutrophil-associated defensins with antiviral activity (Hartshorn et al., 2006; Hazrati et al., 2006; Furci et al., 2007). Dengue is a pantropic public health problem. It is established that in dengue shock syndrome (DSS) at children plasma concentrations of several canonical proteins associated with neutrophil degranulation (bactericidal/permeability-increasing protein, elastase 2, and defensin 1 alpha). Elevated levels of neutrophil-associated transcripts were independent of the neutrophil count and also of the genotype of the infecting virus, as genome-length sequences of dengue virus serotype 1 and serotype 2 sampled from DSS patients were phylogenetically indistinguishable from those sampled from uncomplicated dengue patients. Collectively, these data suggest a hitherto unrecognized association between neutrophil activation, pathogenesis, and the development of DSS and point to future strategies for guiding prognosis of diseases (Hoang et al., 2010).

We study the morphofunctional characteristic of neutrophils in TBEV infections. The TBEV strain Primorye-73 isolated from the brain of a person who died from TBE and these was the virulent for newborn white mice. TBEV was propagated in pig embryo kidney (PEK) cell line was grown at 37 ^{0}C in Eagle's minimal essential medium (MEM) that was supplemented with 8% fetal calf serum and L-glutamine and 100 U of penicillin/ml, and 10 μg of streptomycin/ml. The specific-pathogen free male mice (6 to 8 weeks old) peritoneal neutrophils were elicited by intraperitoneal injection of 5 mL of peptone water with meat extract (10%). Neutrophils 18 h after injection were collected by washing the peritoneal cavity of mouse once with 3 ml of cold minimal essential medium 199 (Sigma) containing preservative-free heparin (5 IU/ml). The cells were isolated by 3%dextran sedimentation and were placed in glass vials ($2X10^6$ /ml) in 2 mL medium for the following neutrophils

adherence for 45 min at 37 ^{0}C in 95% air ± 5% CO^2. Non-adherent cells were removed by washings and the cell monolayer were kept in tissue culture medium 199 containing 10% heat-inactivated fetal bovine serum (FBS) and 1000 U/mL penicillin and 1 mg/mL streptomycin (Invitrogen). For infection of neutrophils we used the virus containing culture liquid of PEK cells (2 units of the titer of cytopathogenic virus action on 50% of the cell culture; TCA50; multiplicity of infection [MOI]=1). The time of the contact of the neutrophils with TBEV was 15, 30, 45, and 60 min, 2, 3, 5, 6, 8, 24 and 48 h.
The cells were washed twice in PBS containing 1% FBS and stained for 30 min at -4 ^{0}C with antibodies for antigen of TBEV and then were fixed in gas of formalin for 15 min. After several washes, the bound antibodies were detected with Alexafluore 546 conjugated with IgG1 of mice (Molecular Probes) After incubation, slides were washed several times, and stored at -4 ^{0}C. The cells were examined by a LSM510META multiphoton confocal laser scanning microscope (Carl Zeiss, Germany). Fluorescence from the Alexafluore-546 dye was excited by 633 nm light and collected after passing through an HQ660LP emission filter. The lasers were programmed to scan over successive focal planes (0.25–0.5 μm intervals) at 50 lines per second. Lasersharp software was used to control the confocal system and to reconstruct individual focal planes into three-dimensional renderings.
The activity of enzymes ATPase, 5' nucleotidase, succinate and lactate dehydrogenases and myeloperoxidase were determined in infected neutrophils by F.G. Hayhoe and D. Quaglino's (1983) methods with our updating (Plekhova et al., 2007). The absorption of the product of cytochemistry reaction was measured by using a Multiscan Titertek Plus spectrophotometer (Flow lab, Finland) at lengths of waves corresponding to each reaction. Samples containing the reagent without cells and uninfected cells were used as controls.
The results of experiments were calculated using the equation: $T = [(N_0 - N_k)/N_k]*100\%$, where T is the index of stimulation of the phagocytes, N_k is the average absorption of the cytochemistry reaction product of uninfected cells, N_0 is the average absorption of this product of infected cells.
For determination of apoptosis neutrophils the method of staining by Hoechst 333258 (Sigma, USA) was used. Preparations investigated in system LSM510META, at excitation of 405 nm counted up 100 cells, and from them, on presence of a specific luminescence, defined a share of the apoptoses changed cells which expressed in the form of an index apoptoses (IA).
After 15 min of the contact of TBEV with the neutrophils, specific fluorescence of the cytoplasm was detected using the indirect fluorescent antibody method (Fig. 1). The fluorescence was mainly of diffuse character, and its intensity reached 42,6±5,6 standard units and the individual antigen-positive cells exhibited a localized fluorescence. The maximum intensity was determined in 4 h post infection made 234,56±15,7 standard units and then remained constant within 8 h of observation. After the first day of post infection the cells degraded.
The plasma membrane of cells is known to transform spatially during chemotaxis, and this directly depends on activities of its ectoenzymes 5′ nucleotidase and ATPase. In order to differentiate activated and resting cells, the intracellular contents of these enzymes were determined [Plekhova et al., 2007]. We found that an increase of the number of antigen positive cells was associated with a decrease of the activity of its enzymes (Fig. 2a). The parameters were significantly different from of the control ones in 2 hours post infection with TBEV. The values of stimulation index have made for 5′ nucleotidase 12.3±1.2 and for ATPase 11.4±1.1 %.

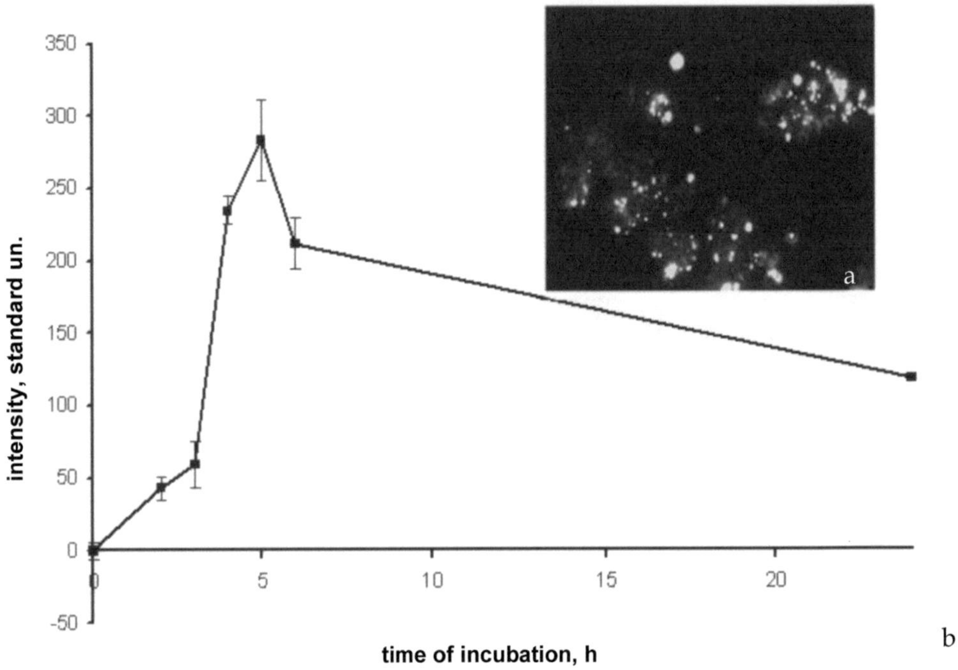

Fig. 1. Micrograph shows the neutrophils staining on TBEV by methods of indirect fluorescent antibody and analyzed by confocal laser scanning microscope, 5 hours post infection, original magnification, X 120 (a), intensity of fluorescence antigen-positive cells (b)

In terms of biochemical characteristics, phagocytes do not differ significantly from other cells. Nevertheless, the characteristic feature of their metabolism is the ability to generate various oxygen radicals under the influence of different factors. This phenomenon is called "respiratory burst". The formation of these short-lived, but reactive oxygen metabolites, which include superoxide anion, hydrogen peroxide, hydroxyl radical and others, is catalyzed in leukocytes by the membrane-associated enzyme, NADPH oxidase. This multi-component enzyme consists of both membrane-bound components (Nox2, p22 ^{phox}) and cytosolic regulatory proteins (p40 ^{phox} , p47 ^{phox} , p67 ^{phox} and Rac2 GTPase) (Klebanoff, 2005). Besides the pathway when the oxygen molecule accepts electrons, reactive oxygen species in phagocytes can be formed due to the hydrogen transfer from a substrate being oxidized (hydrogen donor) to another substrate (hydrogen acceptor). This reaction is catalyzed by dehydrogenases, participating in hydrogen transfer to substrates is specific for both the hydrogen donor and the hydrogen acceptor. The succinate dehydrogenases (SDH) is a flavoproteid dehydrogenase and belongs to the succinate oxidase enzyme complex that forms the membrane respiratory chain. The flavin group of this enzyme contains four iron atoms and is bound covalently to the protein. The SDH activity depends on the SH groups of the enzyme (Hayhoe & Quaglino, 1980). Investigation of the intracellular content of SDH in neutrophils infected with TBEV demonstrated a significant increase of its activity (18.2±1.6%, Fig. 2b) in 5 h post infection. The maximal value of the stimulation index for this enzyme was observed in 8 h post infection (27.95±2.4%).

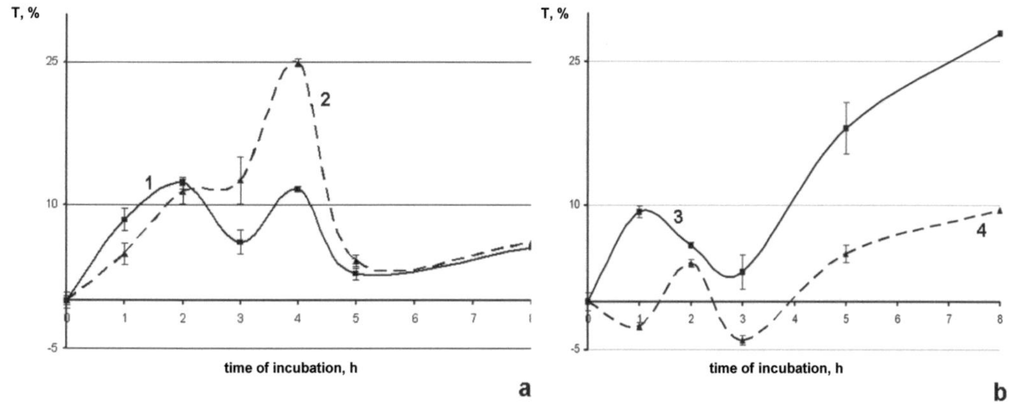

Fig. 2. The enzyme activity in infected TBEV neutrophils: a) 5′ nucleotidase (1) and ATPase (2); b) succinate dehydrogenases (3) and lactate dehydrogenases (4)

The lactate dehydrogenases (LDH) is a coenzyme dependent dehydrogenase and catalyzes the transfer of a reduced equivalent (hydrogen) from lactate to NAD+ or from NADPH to pyruvate. Usually, NAD+ is the coenzyme of LDH, but NADPH also can function as the coenzyme. LDH acts at the last step of hydrolysis that occurs under anaerobic conditions and results in the reduction of pyruvate yielding lactate and NAD+. Most of the enzyme in the cell is weakly bound to the cell structure and localized in the cytoplasm, a smaller part being attached firmly to mitochondrial membranes (Loida et al., 1982). Histochemical analysis can result in the enzyme diffusion into the incubation media. The spectrophotometric analysis used in the present work provided more precise determination of LDH activity in the cells. We determined a slight change in the activity of its enzyme in the neutrophils infected by TBEV that did not differ significantly from the value obtained for the intact cells during the experiment. Thus, in contrast to LDH, a significant increase in the intracellular content of SDH in neutrophils was observed at the later period of TBEV infection.

Among the antimicrobial systems formed in the phagosome is one consisting of myeloperoxidase (MPO), released into the phagosome during the degranulation process, hydrogen peroxide (H_2O_2), formed by the respiratory burst and a halide, particularly chloride. The initial product of the MPO-H_2O_2-chloride system is hypochlorous acid, and subsequent formation of chlorine, chloramines, hydroxyl radicals, singlet oxygen, and ozone has been proposed. These same toxic agents can be released to the outside of the cell, where they may attack normal tissue and thus contribute to the pathogenesis of the disease. The MPO-H_2O_2-halide system is strongly toxic to human immunodeficiency virus type 1, as measured by the inability of the virus to replicate in the lymphocyte cell line CEM (Klebanoff & Coombs, 1991). Investigation of the intracellular content of MPO in neutrophils infected by TBEV demonstrated a significant decrease of its activity (Fig. 3a). The minimal value of the stimulation index for this enzyme was observed in 3 h post infection (-34.4±2.8%). These data specified in TBEV infection cells the deficits of activity of protective system at the formation of oxygen radicals in them.

A variety of cationic peptides and proteins present in leukocyte granules has been implicated in the microbicidal activity of phagocytes. These include defensins, seprocidins, bactericidal/permeability-increasing protein, lysozyme, cathelicidins, phospholipase A_2, and lactoferrin. Defensins are antimicrobial peptides important to innate host defense. In addition to their direct antimicrobial effect, defensins modulate immune responses. Defensins are classified into two subfamilies, α and β, which differ in their three disulfide bond paring. Neutrophil α-defensins are mainly synthesized as prepropeptides in promyelocytes, neutrophil precursor cells in the bone marrow, and the mature peptide is stored in primary granules of neutrophils (Ganz, 2003). In studies of enveloped viruses, defensins α have been shown to have a potent direct inhibitory effect on herpes simplex viruses, a moderate direct effect on vesicular stomatitis virus, and little effect on cytomegalovirus (Daher et al., 1986). We researched the activity of cationic peptides in neutrophils infected by TBEV and found that intracellular included its enzymes decreased in reply to infection by TBEV. It specified on exocytose by infected TBEV cells of cationic peptides, which can influence on neutrophils in intracellular environment. The inhibition of its cell function can partially suppress of organism immune response. Recent evidence indicates that defensins modulate viral infection through multiple mechanisms (Ding et al., 2009).

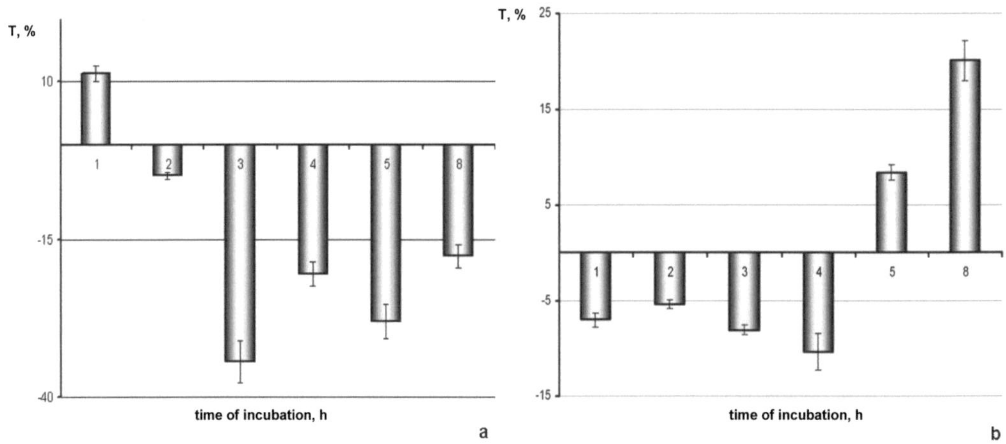

Fig. 3. The activity of myeloperoxidase (a) and cationic peptides (b) in infected TBEV neutrophils

Apoptosis, a programmed cell death that occurs to conserve toxic neutrophil contents, is one of such mechanisms. The benefits of apoptotic neutrophils are twofold as they also stimulate macrophages into a proresolution phenotype, reducing the inappropriate inflammatory response further (Fox et al., 2010). The increase of apoptosis these cells has been reported in chronically Simian Immunodeficiency Virus infected patients, and shown that degradation of neutrophils function is the consequence of upregulation apoptoses (Elbim et al., 2008). Morphologically the apoptosis of neutrophils is characterized the reduction of cytoplasm granules quantity, a rounding of nucleus and the condensation of chromatin, that is accompanied by depression of cells functions, especially their antiinfect abilities (Kennedy & DeLeo, 2009).

We researched the degradation of neutrophils infected by TBEV. Early display of the programmed destruction of neutrophils is sharply outlined of nucleus in the form of homogeneous substances with a uniform green luminescence (fig. 4a). At this stage apoptosis can be stopped by the action of inhibitors and it is designated as preapoptosis (Wilkie et al., 2007). The intermediate stage of apoptosis destructions of cell is accompanied by reduction of the sizes of nucleus and at the final stage it breaks up to discrete fragments the quantity of which are 3-5 and more (fig. 4b). Hoechst 33342 is used by us contacts with damaged sites of DNA cells at the final stage of apoptosis. We established the increase of quantity of apoptosis changed neutrophils, infected by TBEV (fig. 4c). This quantity accrued with the increase of time post infection, and reached the maximal value in 8 hours - 48±7.3 %. The decrease of apoptosis index in 18-24 hours of incubation was connected with degradation of cells.

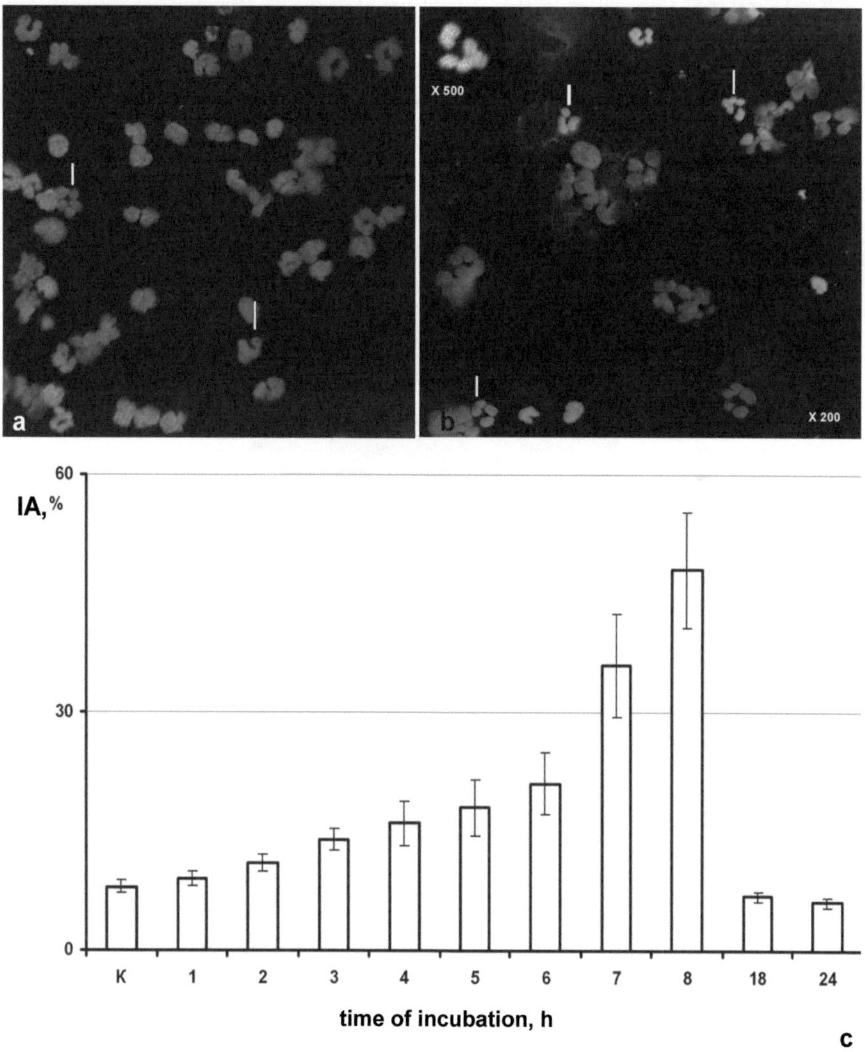

Fig. 4. The apoptosis of neutrophils infected by TBEV. a) preapoptosis (arrows) of cells – 2 hours post infection; b) apoptosis (arrows) of cells – 8 hours post infection; c) the quantity of apoptotic cells, AI – apoptotic index. The method of staining by Hoechst 333258, slides investigated in system LSM510META, at excitation of 405 nm counted up to 100 cells

Recently, a new microbicidal mechanism named NETosis was described in human, bovine and fish neutrophils, (Brinkmann et al., 2004; Palic et al., 2007). In this mechanism, neutrophils die after releasing neutrophil extracellular traps (NETs), threads composed of DNA, histones and granular proteins that not only ensnare microorganisms but also provide a high local concentration of antimicrobial molecules (Brinkmann et al., 2004; Lippolis et al., 2006). The release of NETs is dependent on reactive oxygen species (ROS) production and can be stimulated by bacteria, fungi, protozoa and some soluble molecules (e.g. interleukin-8, lipopolysaccharide, b-glucan and phorbol esters) (Brinkmann et al., 2004). NET formation requires a specialized form of cell death that is distinct from apoptosis and which is dependent on NADPH oxidase activity. It is show that a late phase of Nox2-mediated ROS production is sensitive to DNase treatment and suggest a role for myeloperoxidase-derived ROS in NET-dependent extracellular killing. In TBEV virus infection we have found in neutrophils the increase of activity enzymes which take part in reproduction of reactive oxygen species 8 h post infection (fig. 2a). The formation of NETs was determined in 6 h post infection (fig. 5). Their quantity was the small nearby 5 per 100 cells, but with the increase of time incubation it has made 8-10 per 100 cells. In our opinion the formation of NETs really occurs to participation of ROS which was produced at TBEV infection and the protective MPO-H_2O_2-chloride system of cells does not work (fig. 3).

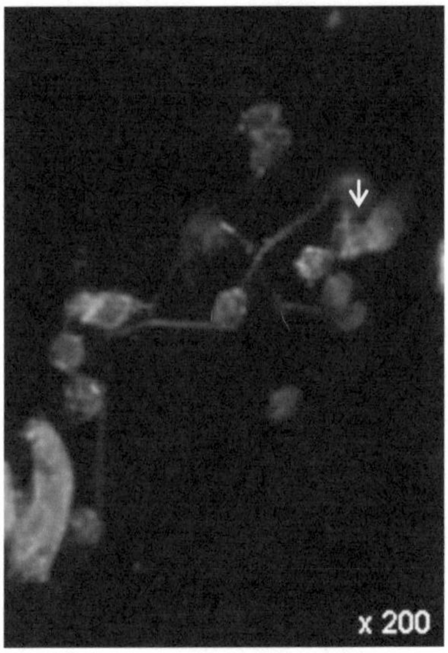

Fig. 5. Micrograph show the neutrophils staining on TBEV (arrow) and DAPI fluorescence shows NET analyzed by confocal laser scanning microscope 6 hours post infection. Cells were fixed with paraformaldehyde and stained with DAPI (5 ng ml^{-1})

Thus in TBEV infection the neutrophils activity of plasmalemma enzymes and degidrogenese increased. It is known, that neutrophils belong to cells with mainly aerobic type of an exchange (Walmsley et al., 2008). In these cells SDG has the important metabolic value as the increase of its activity does not give accumulation of lactate and the full oxidation of glucose occurs through a cycle of threecarbon acids with production of a plenty of energy (Arruda & Barja-Fidalgo, 2009). In this case the increase of an energy potential of a cell is the display of adaptive reaction neutrophils on TBEV infection. In its turn, the increase of LDG activity is connected with changes of glycolyses intensity the biological value of which consists in formation of phosphoric connections rich with energy that testifies an intensification of power supply neutrophils due to inclusion anaerobic glycolys (Koolman & Rohm, 1998). This way of oxidation can be regarded as compensated the mechanism of adaptive reaction neutrophils on TBEV infection. Thus, the moderate increase of SDG activity presence evidences about direction to anaerobic ways of production energy - the activity of glycolys in TBEV infected neutrophils testify the relative stability of a homeostasis of cells. Finally it brings to killing of neutrophils mainly by apoptoses as it is known, that necroses is accompanied with acid bioenergy hypoxia of cells at full inhibition of enzymes activity of a respiratory circuit (Arruda & Barja-Fidalgo, 2009).

3. The monocytes/macrophages in Tick-Borne Encephalitis

The existence of different populations of monocytes in the blood of a man and mammalian homologues of these populations is established (Geissmann et al., 2003). In addition to the classical monocytes, which are strongly positive for the CD14 cell surface molecule ($CD14^{++}$ $CD16^{-}$ monocytes), a population of monocytes was discovered, which coexpresses CD16 and low levels of CD14 antigens. These cells have some characteristic patterns of cell surface molecules when compared with the classical monocytes, and this includes high HLA-DR, epidermal growth factor module-containing mucinlike receptor 2 (EMR2), Ig-like transcript 4 (ILT-4), CD43, and CD45RA expression and expression of MDC8 on a fraction of $CD14^{+}$ $CD16^{+}$ monocytes (Ziegler-Heitbrock, 2007). The $CD14^{+}$ $CD16^{+}$ monocytes and their mammalian homologues are potent producers of TNF but show no-to-low IL-10 production supports the concept that they are proinflammatory cells. Also, these cells and their derived cells show a higher antigen-presenting capacity. The process of differentiation monocytes in macrophages accompanies the rises of adhesion receptors CD11c/CD18, and an activation of cells - the parity of receptors CD11a/CD18 (Ammon et al., 2000). The basis functions of monocytes and tissue macrophages are phagocytosis and intracellular killing of microorganisms. In addition, macrophages are capable of extracellular killing of infected or altered self target cells. In response to such a stimulus, monocytes adhere to activated endothelial cells on the blood vessel wall and extravasate into the adjacent tissue. While residing in the tissue, they differentiate to monocyte-derived macrophages. One of the most immediate responses of monocytes to a variety of activating stimuli is the production of the potent oxygen free radical, superoxide anion. Furthermore, macrophages contribute to tissue repair and act as antigen presenting cells, which are required for the induction of specific immune responses.

The applicability of monocytes/macrophages in virus infection is determined by their participation in the production of antibodies and interferon, cooperation with lymphocytes and maintenance of more perfect antibodies presentation for stimulation of B-lymphocytes. These cells can accept direct participation in elimination of infect agents by phagocytosis of the cells-targets infected by a virus and their fragments or adsorbing directly on the plasmalemma a virus with its subsequent ingesting. At present anti-virus activity of monocytes/macrophages subdivide on direct and mediated (Baskin, 1997). Both intrinsic and extrinsic antiviral mechanisms of macrophages have been described. Intrinsic antiviral activity is defined as the ability of macrophages to restrict virus replication in macrophages per se and thus to serve as nonpermissive targets for virus replication. Extrinsic antiviral activity is defined as the ability of macrophages to influence extracellular virus and to interfere with virus replication in surrounding permissive cells. Also it is marked, that during the development of some virus infections the activated macrophage gets an ability to distinguish infected and intact cells (Silva et al., 2007). Thus, the value of monocytes/macrophages in virus infections is defined by their functional condition. On the one hand, infected by virus monocytes as host cells at their maturation in macrophages can be a source of this virus in an organism. On the other hand, for viruses, inactivated by macrophages, these cells are the biological barrier interfering these distribution from the primary loci inflammation. It protects the high-sensitivity cells of the central nervous system and parenchymal bodies from the further infection. It is especially value able to studying influences on monocytes/macrophages at the first hour and day of the organism infection by virus. It is necessary to consider, that the concrete mechanisms of activation of these cells in various virus infections are not identical and are not clearly defined yet.

After contact with virus, the macrophages were considered as activated macrophages. In the resident macrophages, the activity of most lysosomal enzymes is in a latent state, being associated with glycolipid membrane complexes. As in resting primary human monocytes the enzyme complex nicotinamide adenine dinucleotide phosphate oxidase (NADPH) for the production of highly reactive oxygen species is unassembled and its components are located in the cytosol and the membrane. After activation, the cytosolic components translocate to the membrane and associate with the membrane components, and the newly formed enzyme complex actively catalyzes the production of superoxide anion. The membrane components include the cytochrome b558, consisting of gp91phox and p22phox (Babior, 1999). Cytosolic components include p47phox, p67phox, and Rac1 - Rho family member of small G-proteins (Abo et al., 1991). Also in contrast to resident macrophages the activated macrophages have a larger size, higher content of protein and RNA and exhibit a high enzymatic activity. While carrying out phagocytosis, pinocytosis, and exocytosis, macrophages constantly consume (interiorize) the plasma membrane, which is compensated by the constant synthesis of its components (Ballinger et al., 2010). The degree of macrophage stimulation can be estimated by the activity of their membrane ectoenzymes (ATPase, 5' nucleotidase, leucine aminopeptidase, D amino acid oxidase, serine esterase, alkaline phosphodiesterase) (Nathan & Shiloh, 2000). Numerous primary lysosomes of macrophages contain acid hydrolases (β-D-glucuronidase, N-acetyl-β-glucosaminidase, β-glycerophosphatase, α mannosidase, acid phosphatase, α naphthylesterase, esterase, RNase, arylsulfatase, lipase, β- galactosidase, naphthylamidase, cathepsins B, D, and G, and elastase) and antibacterial enzymes (lysozyme, neutral proteases, and B_{12} binding protein) (Cathcart et al., 2004). Secondary lysosomes (phagolysosomes) are formed by the fusion of the primary lysosomes with pinocytic and phagocytic vacuoles. Many lysosomal enzymes demonstrate combined and cumulative action (Williams & Burgo, 2009).

We researched the macrophages infected by TBEV. The patterns of peritoneal exudates were obtained by washing the peritoneal cavity of specific-pathogen free male mice (6 to 8 weeks old) once with 3 ml of cold minimal essential medium (RPMI) containing preservative-free heparin (5 IU/ml). Cell suspensions were placed in a glass vials ($4X10^6$ /ml) for 60 min at 37 ^{0}C in 95 % air ± 5% CO^2 to allow macrophages adherence. Non-adherent cells were removed by washings and the cell monolayer was kept in tissue culture medium RPMI containing 5% heat-inactivated fetal bovine serum (Sigma) for 72 h before infection. Thus we received the completely functionally mature population of cells.

The high-virulent for newborn white mice Primorye-73 TBEV strain was isolated from the brain of a person who died from tick borne encephalitis and two avirulent strains 202 and

69, isolated from blood of patient's disease of TBE subclinical form were used in this study. The monolayer of cells was washed once in serum-free RPMI, followed by suspension in 0.2 mL of virus (73, 69 and 202) giving the multiplicity of infection 0.3 plaque-forming units on cells (PFU/cell). For adsorbing the viruses were left with cells for 60 min at 37 ^{0}C. After 1 h at 37 ^{0}C the non-adsorbed viral particles were removed by serial washing of serum-free RPMI and monolayer of cells in medium RPMI containing 5 % heat-inactivated fetal bovine serum was incubated within 4 days. The supernatant medium was collected and frozen at - 70 $^\circ$ at 1, 5, 9, 24, 48, 72 and 96 h post infection time periods. The virus titers were determined by plaque assay on porcine kidney stable (PS) cell monolayers by A.T. De Madrid's method (1969). The tenfold dilutions of virus were placed in 24-well tissue culture plates to which a suspension of PS cells was added (0.5 - 1.5 x 10 ^{5} cells per well). After an incubation for 4 h, the suspension was overlaid with carboxymethylcellulose (1.5% in L-15 medium). After incubating at 37 $^\circ$ and 0.5% CO 2 for 5 - 6 days, the infected plates were washed with saline, and cell monolayers were stained with naphthalene black. Infectivity was expressed as PFU/ml.

The cells were stained with indicated antibodies to viral proteins conjugated secondary antibodies with followed by Alexafluore 546 (Molecular Probes). In brief, the monolayer of cells was fixed in gas of formalin for 15 min. Cells were then washed with PBS, labeled with either polyclonal mice anti-TBEV antibodies. After several washes, the bound antibodies were detected with rabbit anti-mouse antibodies directly labeled with Alexafluore. After incubation, the slides were washed several times, and stored at -4 ^{0}C until viral antigen was assessed. Caveolin-1 (CAV 1) were visualized by staining of anti-Caveolin-1 antibody produced in rabbit IgG fraction of antiserum (Molecular Probes) with Alexafluore 488 conjugated with IgG1 of mice. The revealing activity of inducible nitric oxide synthase (iNOS) was revealed by staining of monoclonal anti-iNOS antibody produced in mouse IgG fraction of antiserum (1:50; Sigma) with Alexafluore 586 conjugated with IgG1 of mice.

The slides were examined by a LSM510META multiphoton confocal laser scanning microscope (Carl Zeiss, Germany). Alexa-488 immunostain was excited using 488 nm light from a Krypton-Argon laser and the emitted light passed through an HQ515/30 filter. Fluorescence from the Alexa-546 dye was excited by 633 nm light and collected after passing through an HQ660LP emission filter. The lasers were programmed to scan over successive focal planes (0.25–0.5 μm intervals) at 50 lines per second. Lasersharp software was used to control the confocal system and to reconstruct individual focal planes into three-dimensional renderings.

For NO metabolite assays (nitrite ions) the infected monolayer of cells and the culture liquid were frozen and stored at -20°C. The suspension of destroyed cells was treated with 100 μl of Griess reagent (Schulz et al., 1999). The activity of enzymes ATPase, 5' nucleotidase, succinate and lactate dehydrogenases and myeloperoxidase were determined in infected neutrophils by methods of F.G. Hayhoe and D. Quaglino (1983) with our updating (Plekhova et al., 2007). The absorption of the product of cytochemistry reaction was measured by using a Multiscan Titertek Plus spectrophotometer (Flow lab, Finland) at lengths of waves corresponding to each reaction. Samples containing the reagent without cells and uninfected cells were used as controls.

The results of experiments were calculated using the equation: $T = [(N_0 - N_k)/N_k]*100\%$, where T is the index of stimulation of the phagocytes, N_k is the average absorption of the cytochemistry reaction product of uninfected cells, N_0 is the average absorption of this product of infected cells.

Electron Microscopy. The monolayer of macrophages was prefixed in 1 % glutaraldehyde in 0,1 mol/L cacodylate buffer for 18 hours at room temperature, then it was postfixed for an hour in 1 % OsO4 in the same buffer, dehydrated in a graded series of ethanols and embedded in epon-araldite medium. Thin sections unstained or stained with lead citrate were examined in Jeol 100S electron microscope. The control patterns consisted of macrophages without TBEV. To elucidate the role of nitric oxide (NO) in TBEV infected macrophages, the ultrastructural localization of the enzyme NO synthase (NOS), based on the cytochemical NADPH-diaphorase staining was studied in a cell. For the localization of NADPH-diaphorase activity a special tetrazolium salt (BSPT, Sigma) was applied (Faber-Zuschratter, 1994).

After 60 min of the contact of, specific fluorescence of the cytoplasm was detected using the indirect fluorescent antibody method. The fluorescence of TBEV in the macrophages was mainly of diffuse character, and 20 ± 0.9% of the antigen-positive cells exhibited a localized lumpy fluorescence (Fig. 6b,c). After 4 and 5 h of incubation, the number of such cells increased to 35±1.4 and 87±5.3%, respectively, and then remained constant within 24 h of observation. After 4 days of observation, the number of the antigen-positive macrophages was minimal, constituting 17.5 ± 0.8%.

The adhesion and reproduction of TBEV in the macrophages was confirmed by the titration method (Fig. 6d). After 60 min of incubation, the original virus titer decreased by 2.0 log units. After 24 h, this value increased in the cell monolayer by 1.0 log, decreasing to the end of the experiment (4 days). In the supernatant, the virus titer increased to 2.0 log on the second day. These data indicate the adsorption and subsequent reproduction of TBEV in the primary macrophage culture, and then its liberation from the cells 2 days after the infection.

Microscopic investigation of the preparations stained 60 min after the contact with TBEV revealed mainly activated macrophages with large nucleus occupying 1/3 of the cell area and numerous vacuoles on the periphery of the phagocyte cytoplasm. The intact cells were lengthened forms with 2 pseudopodials (Fig. 7a). After infected by TBEV the macrophages were stimulated and accepted the approximated form (fig. 7b). In infected by virulent strains TBEV, 15.0 ± 0.8% of cells with chemotactic activity were detected (fig. 7c). These cells acquired lengthened forms due to the formation of two pseudopodias on the opposite sides, and the number of such cells significantly increased in 7 h after the contact of the virus with macrophages, constituting 25.0 ± 2.1%. Then contacting phagocytes were observed, and 18 h later, symplast-like conglomerates composed (Fig. 7d), where the maximal specific fluorescence of the viral antigen was detected. In this period, macrophages with destroyed nucleus were detected (10.0 ± 1.3%), as well as apoptotic cells (5.0 ± 0.46%) with 2-3 nuclear fragments and a reduced cytoplasm area. After 24 h of incubation, the intensive vacuolization of the peripheral part of the phagocytes was observed, this indicating the beginning of degradation of the cell culture Further, the number of degrading cells increased, and at the end of the observation (the fourth day) all cells were destroyed.

To reveal the activated cells, investigators use the test for intracellular 5′ nucleotidase or adenosine 5′ phosphatase (EC.1.3.5), the enzyme bound to the external side of the plasma membrane through the glycosylphosphatidyl residue. We determined a slight change in the activity of 5′ nucleotidase in the macrophages infected by virulent strains TBEV that did not differ significantly from the value obtained for the intact macrophages during the experiment (fig. 8a). Whereas in cells infected by avirulent strains TBEV the parameters of enzyme activity increased it due to the activation of cells.

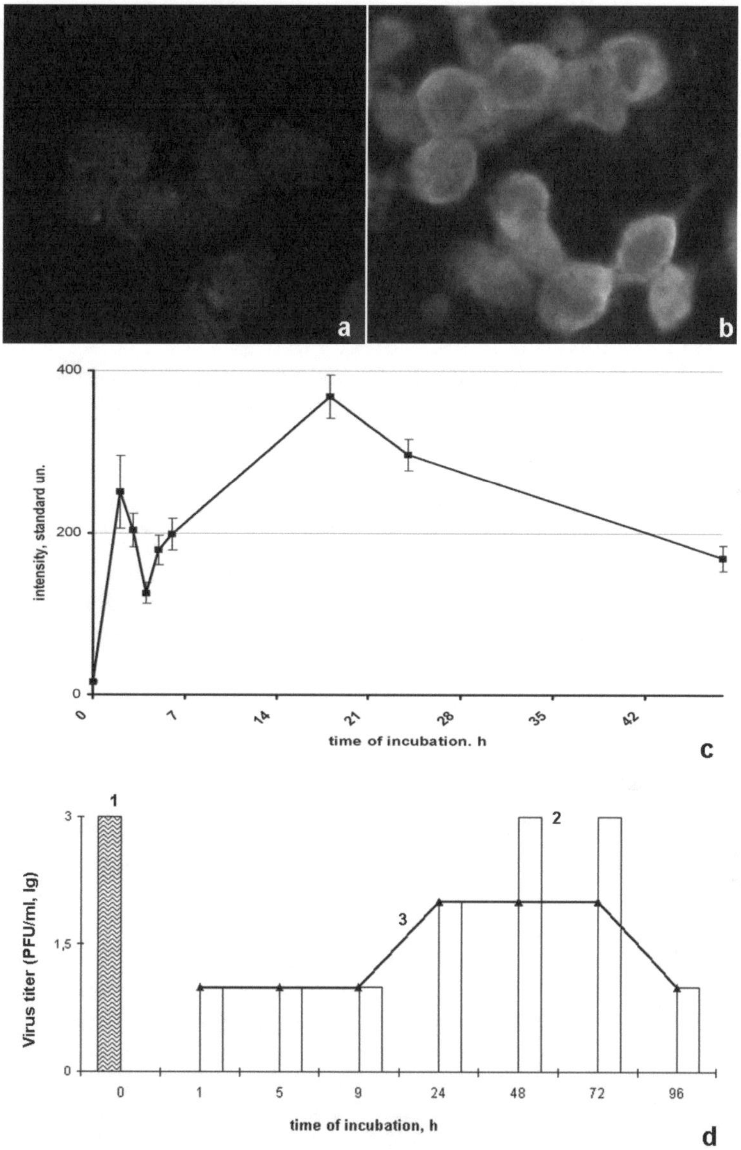

Fig. 6. Accumulation and visualization of TBEV antigen in macrophages. Uninfected macrophages (a) or cells (b) infected with virus were stained for presence of TBEV proteins. After infection, cells were fixed to spot slides and stained for TBEV proteins, followed by Alexafluor 546–conjugated antibodies. The bar represents 10 mkm. Data points show the mean of fluorescent intensity of antigen-positive cells (c); d) The growth of the high-virulence TBEV strain (73) in cultured mouse macrophages. The viral titers were quite stable after 2-day infection. In the case of the low-virulence strain (69 and 202), the virus was detected only at 18 h after infection; at later time point intervals, the virus titer was under the detection limit. These results are representative of 3 experiments of similar design. reproduction of TBEV in macrophages: 1) quantity of introduced TBEV; 2) TBEV in culture liquid; 3) TBEV in cells

Adenosine triphosphatase (ATPase, EC 3.6.1.3) of cell membranes is activated by potassium and sodium ions. This enzyme catalyzes hydrolysis of the high energy phosphate bonds, and the changes in its activity reflect the activation of cell metabolism. Investigation of the ATPase activity in avirulent strains of TBEV infected macrophages revealed a significant change in the intracellular content of this enzyme (fig. 8b). The ATPase activity decreased by 12.2 ± 1.5% compared to the control value 0.5 h post infection for the cells infected by strain 69 of TBEV, remaining constant for 8 h of incubation. Then the activity decreased until the end of the experiment (the third day). Thus, the data on the ATPase activity indicate pronounced stimulation of the macrophages infected by avirulent strains of TBEV.
The pathway when the oxygen molecule accepts electrons, reactive oxygen species in macrophages can be formed due to the hydrogen transfer from a substrate being oxidized (hydrogen donor) to another substrate (hydrogen acceptor). This reaction is catalyzed by dehydrogenases, besides, cytochrome oxidases can also be involved in the oxidation, acting as the additional substrates of the respiratory chain. To evaluate the activity of oxygen metabolism of the resident macrophages infected with TBEV, the intracellular content of SDH, LDH, and cytochrome oxidase was determined and the total activity of the respiratory chain enzymes was evaluated in the NBT test. Among the known methods for determination of the oxygen dependent activity of phagocytes, the cytochemical test for reduction of nitroblue tetrazolium (NBT test) is the simplest and the most reproducible method. The NBT test allows evaluation of the total activity of NADPH dependent enzymes of the respiratory chain. The activated macrophages consume tetrazolium and their enzymes convert it into insoluble diformazan. The formation of NBT into diformazan is attributed mainly to the powerful redox agent superoxide anion (Babior, 1999). Significant increase in the index in NBT test (91.6 ± 6.5%) was observed in macrophages after 15 min post infection (Fig. 9a). During 3 h of the experiment, the index decreased to 17.3 ± 0.9%, and then increased again, reaching its maximal value after 6 h of incubation (130 ± 11.6%). This value exceeded slightly the value obtained for macrophages treated with the bacterium *Staphylococcus aureus* as the stimulating agent (129.8 ± 7.8%). The parameters in NBT test of cells infected by avirulent strains 69 and 202 of TBEV statistically authentically did not differ from those of high virulent strain infected macrophages.
Dehydrogenases catalyzing hydrogen transfer to substrates are specific for both the hydrogen donor and the hydrogen acceptor. The investigation of the intracellular content of SDH in macrophages infected by avirulent strains 69 and 202 of TBEV demonstrated a significant increase in the enzyme content compared to the intact cells (Fig. 9b). As seen from the figure, 30 min after the contact of the cells with the strains 69 and 202, the stimulation index for SDH was 22.5 ± 1.9% and 28.5 ± 2.1% accordingly. Then the index decreased to the level of intact cells, and again increased during the observation time. The activity of LDH in macrophages infected by high-virulence strain 73 of TBEV decreased significantly (-13.4 ± 1.6%, Fig. 8c) after 30 min post infection. The maximal value of the stimulation index for this enzyme was observed after 2 h post infection in cell infected by avirulance strain 202 (11.8 ± 0.7%). Thus, in contrast to SDH, a significant decrease in the intracellular content of LDH in the macrophages was observed.
The level of oxygen radicals in the cells is regulated by the highly specific antioxidant enzyme superoxide dismutase (SOD, EC 1.15.1.11) with molecular weight of 31 kD (Allen et al., 1997). The scavenging of the oxygen radicals by SOD proceeds in the presence of $O_2^{\cdot}$ at pH > 4.8 (Webb et al., 2001). It is known that in an inflammation area, 80% of H_2O_2 is generated by phagocytes due to this reaction. The activity of SOD can be evaluated as the

amount of enzyme required for 50% inhibition of the superoxide anion formation in the presence of xanthine oxidase and NBT. An increase in SOD activity in macrophages infected by high virulent strain of TBEV was detected after 1 h of incubation (41.6 ± 3.4%, Fig. 9d). During the observation, the activity remained constant, exceeding significantly the value for the intact macrophages. The SOD activity was maximal after 72 h of incubation and constituted 26.4 ± 1.8%. In macrophages infected by avirulent strains 69 and 202 the SOD activity slightly differed from parameters for high virulent strain of TBEV infected cell.

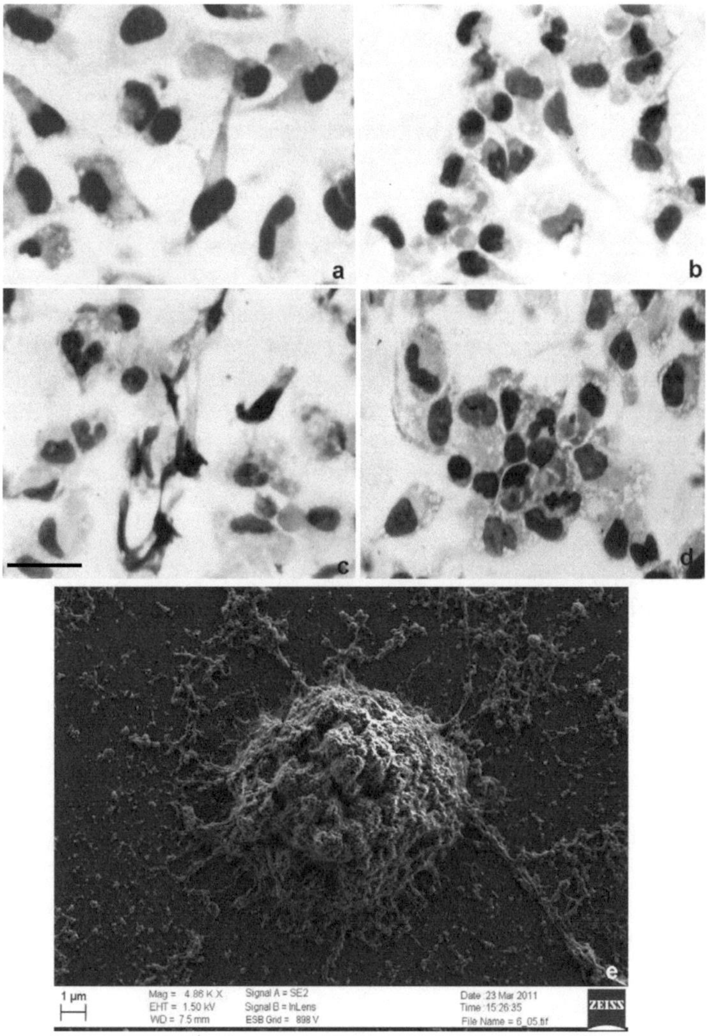

Fig. 7. Cytological investigation of infected by TBEV: a) intact cells; b) the stimulated cells in infected avirulant strain of TBEV; c) the chemotactic cells in infected virulant strain of TBEV (7 h); c) symplast (24 h); d) apoptotic macrophages with fragmentation of the nucleus. The cells were stained by method of Nocht-Maksimov (bar represents 8 mkm). e) micrograph show the stimulated macrophages infected by avirulent strain TBEV (69) with numerous long pseudopodia, scanning electronic microscopy

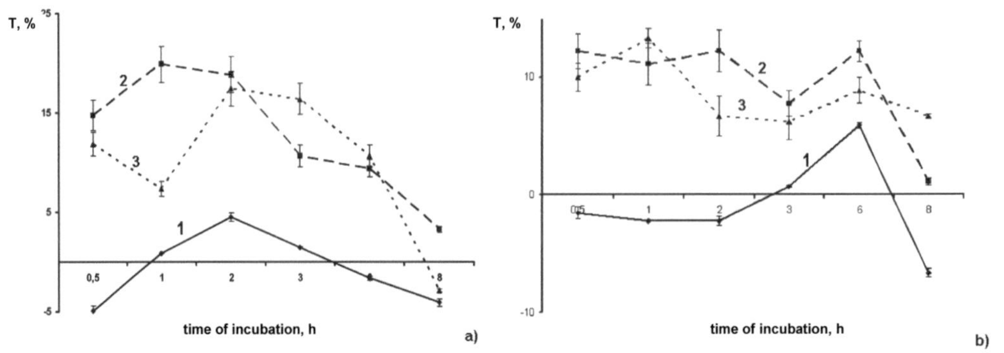

Fig. 8. The enzyme activity in infected by high-virulence strain 73 (1), avirulence strain 69 (2) and 202 (3) of TBEV macrophages: a) 5′ nucleotidase and b) ATPase

Thus, the research of metabolic activity of TBEV infected macrophages established the stimulation of cellular oxygen metabolism; the increase of NADPH-oxidase complex activity, as well as the mitochondrial enzymes lactate dehydrogenase, succinate dehydrogenase, and cytochrome oxidase. A wave-like change of these enzymes activity in the macrophages reflected the reaction of the cells in the first period (within 3 h) on virus penetration and in the second period (from 5 to 48 h) on the synthesis of the viral components and exit of virus into the extracellular space. The activity of these enzymes in cells depended on virulent property of TBEV strains which were infected macrophages. In infected cells high virulent strain 73 of TBEV the activity of enzymes was less than in macrophages infected by avirulens strains.

Nitric oxide (NO) is a free radical gaseous molecule that is produced in cell from molecular oxygen and a guanidino nitrogen from l-arginine, which is converted to citrulline l (Nathan & Shiloh, 1992). In activated macrophages this is exerted through the induction of expression of the inducible isoform of nitric oxide synthase (iNOS) gene, which encodes this enzyme. In recent years, much interest has been paid to NO as an important mediator of vital physiological functions, including host defense against virus (Kreil & Eibl, 1996). Unlike neutrophils, macrophages generally lack sub-stantial MPO activity, but have the capacity to induce a highly active inducible isoform of nitric oxide synthase (iNOS) with following activation by bacterial lipopolysaccharide and inflammatory cytokines. It is determinated that the stimulating influence of flavivirus on NO production activity of monocytes/macrophages, and in phagocytes NO-mediated inhibit action on replication these viruses was established (Chen & Wang, 2002; Chaturvedi et al., 2006). On model of the resident mouse macrophages infected by Denge virus, it is revealed, that for high-grade anti-virus action of phagocytes is necessary activity of oxygen depending enzymes system too. In this case at one-stage production of active oxygen metabolites and NO there is a formation of peroxynitrites which strengthens cytotoxicity of these cells concerning a virus. Thus, studying NO dependence activity of macrophages in infected by flaviviruses represents the certain interest and in this connection, the purpose of our research was the definition of production NO in resident macrophages in their infection by TBEV.

Cytochrome oxidase and SDH are the main components of the normal aerobic oxidative system of the tissue cells that are also known as the succinate dehydrogenase complex, where SDH is the first component and cytochrome oxidase is the second. Cytochromes are subdivided into three groups according to their chemical structure and spectrum: cytochromes a, b, and c. Oxidized cytochrome oxidase is reduced by cytochrome c catalyzing the transfer of four electrons to the oxygen molecule. Thus, cytochrome oxidase is a representative of the third group of oxidases. The cytochrome oxidase activity in the macrophages reflects the level of oxidative metabolism (Koolman & Rohm 1998). This enzyme contains cytogemmin with which molecule of NO communicates. In this case, the peroxynitrites of super oxygen anion with NO are formed at interaction - the powerful oxidizer capable of inhibiting activity of mitochondrial enzymes cell. The definition of this enzyme activity allows indirectly to estimating the ability of cells to produce NO on nitrite reductase ways.

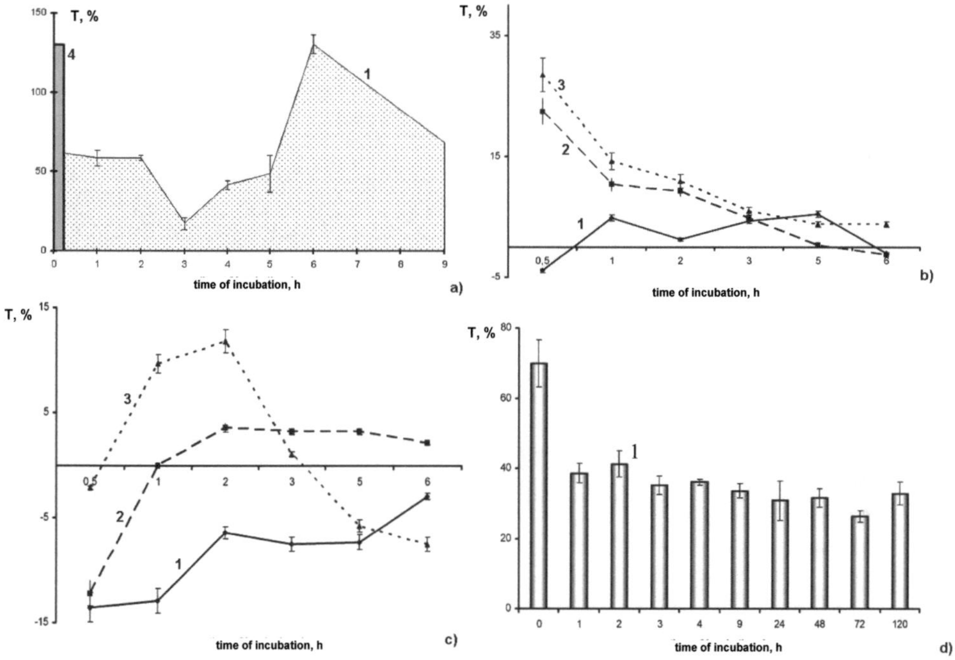

Fig. 9. The enzyme activity of oxygen dependent system in infected by high-virulence strain 73 (1), avirulence strain 69 (2) and 202 (3) of TBEV macrophages: a) NBT test; b) succinate dehydrogenases; c) lactate dehydrogenases; d) superoxide dismutase. 4 - NBT test, macrophages after 45 min of incubation with S. aureus

It was shown that the activity of cytochrome oxidase in the macrophages increased after 30 min post infection (10.6 ± 0.9%, Fig. 10b). A decrease in the cytochrome oxidase activity was observed during the period from 1 to 4 h post infection. After 6 h, the activity increased and reached 27.6 ± 1.8%, and then decreased again. It is necessary to emphasize the opposite direction in the changes of the activities of cytochrome oxidase and SDH in the macrophages infected with TBEV (the increase in the activity of one enzyme while decreasing the activity of the second).

At studying activity iNOS by methods of indirect immunofluorescent in the macrophages infected TBEV (fig. 10a), the greatest quantity of cells with a activity of this enzymes is marked after 1 h of incubation and has made 65±6,5%. Then in 5 h it decreased to a level of intact cells - 5±0,6% and in 7 h it increased up to 25±1,6%, going down to the end of experiment time. It is necessary to note the difference in the direction of iNOS activity changes and cytochrome oxidase in the macrophages infected by TBEV. It was shown in the increase of percentage of cells with positive reaction on iNOS whereas at this time the activity of cytochrome oxidase decreased, and the parameters of the NO metabolites quality in cells remained at a high level (fig. 10b).

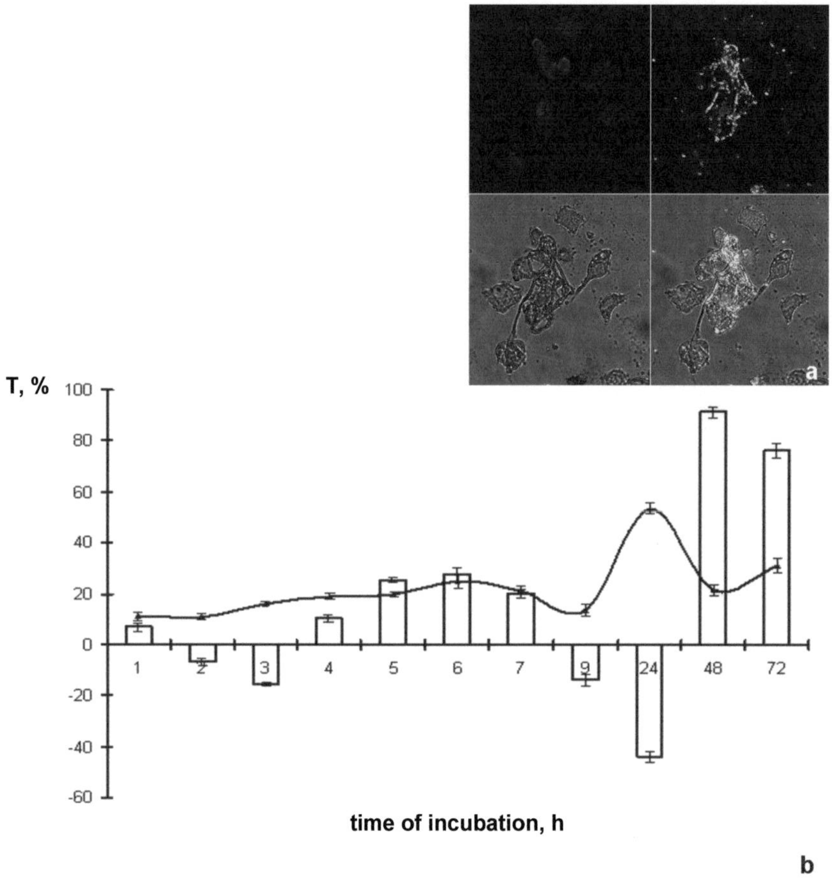

Fig. 10. a) the localization of iNOS in the infected TBEV macrophages, methods of indirect immunofluorescent, X 200. b) the quality of NO metabolites in cells (curve); the activity of cytochrome oxidase in the macrophages (columns). T - an index of stimulation

The ultrastructural research showed, that localization of NADPH diaphorase in the TBEV infected macrophages, it was mainly observed in intracellular vesicles (fig. 11a). BSPT-formazan, the product of the osmiophilic reaction, was found to be attached to intocellular membranes, predominantly the endoplasmic reticulum. Quantitative studies of TBEV infected macrophages revealed that the quantity of cells with similar granules was about 25 % in 10 min after inoculation and 15 % in 2 h and remained in these limits up to the end of experiment time. In parallel preparations which incubated in the environment without the addition of NADPH, the osmiophilic granules with positive reaction on NADPH diaphorase it was not revealed. It is necessary also to note the presence of NADPH diaphorase positive reaction at 7 % of intact cells which have been not infected with TBEV. These data confirm the known fact of enzymes of monocytes/macrophages of activation in the response on adhesion (Reutov, 2002).

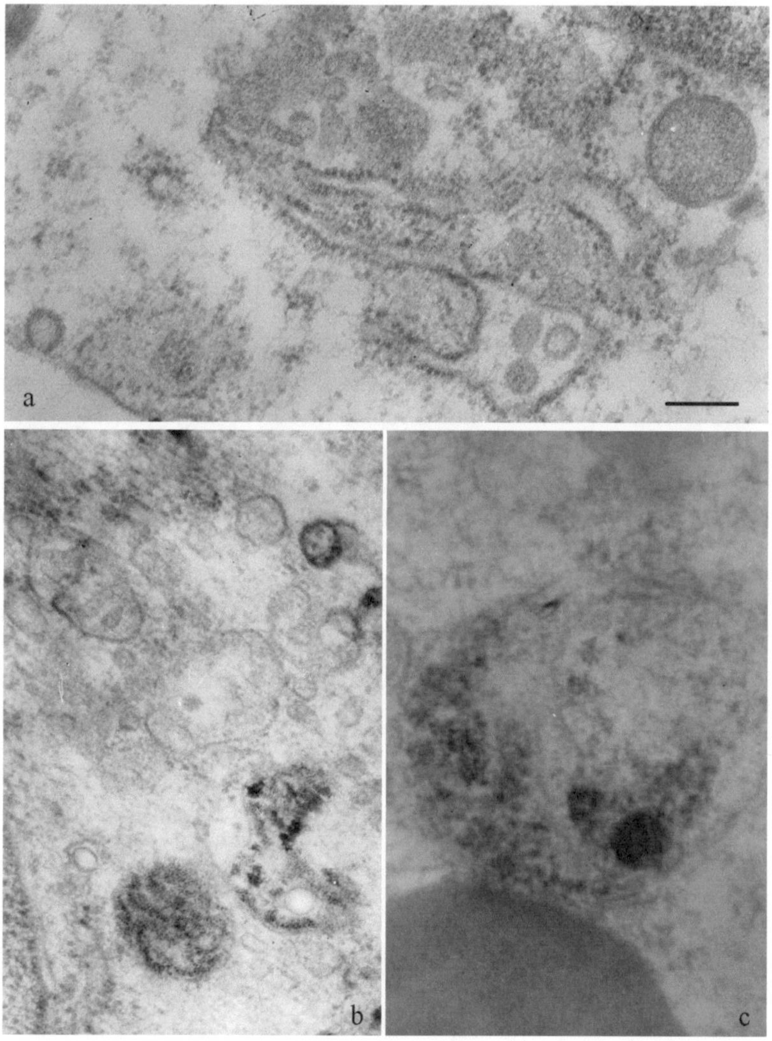

Fig. 11. The localization of TBEV in macrophages cytoplasm (a), the osmiophilic granules with positive reaction on NADPH diaphorase in the TBEV infected macrophages (b, c). Bar represents 100 nm

Now the monocytes/macrophages at virus infections are considered as the basic significance defined by their ability at stimulation to produce of reactivity metabolites oxygen and nitric oxide. These metabolites may influence on the synthesis of γ-interferon and tumor necrosis factor. In the researche by R. Kreil et al. (1996) it has been shown, that the macrophages from TBEV-infected mice, but not from control mice, spontaneously produced NO upon culture in vitro. In contrast to the inhibitory effect of NO on replication of several poxviruses and herpes simplex virus, high levels of NO production did not display an inhibitory influence on TBEV replication in vitro. And finally, in vivo administration of a competitive inhibitor of NO production, aminoguanidine, to TBEV-infected mice significantly increased their mean survival time. Thus the antiviral activity of NO in vitro may be confined to certain viruses, whereas others remain unaffected. Also, other researchers at infection of populations of monocytes/macrophages by the viruses of the Western Nile, Denge and Japanese encephalitis revealed the increase of NO metabolic production by cells in reply to their infection (Chaturvedi et al., 2006). Alongside with the increase in vitro a level of NO metabolic, produced by monocytes of the blood of the patients infected by virus Dehge, in the same cells it has been established the expression of iNOS (Chen et al., 2002) and it is proved, that activation of oxygen depended enzymes system is necessary for high-grade anti-virus action of macrophages.

With the help of different research methods we established the stimulation of NO production activity of TBEV infected macrophages. On the background of active production cells of NO metabolites during all observable time the activity of NADPH diaphorase and iNOS was determined. And the parameters of these enzymes activity in TBEV infected phagocytes were not always combined with the dynamics of activity of heme including enzymes of mitochondria - cytochrome oxidase. In our opinion, during this moment the generation of NO in cells can be carried out on nitrite reductase ways. It was shown the data the increase of cytochrome oxidase activity in TBEV infected macrophages. At the same time at the initial stage of infection the cells produce the NO metabolites in nitric oxide synthase way of the participation as the catalyst of this enzyme.

The activity of TNF α cytokine and nitric oxide production in TBEV infected macrophages depended on strains of virus. The avirulent strain considerably enhanced the production of TNF α cytokine and nitric oxide by phagocytes during an early period of infection (Fig. 12). On the contrary, the cells infected by highly virulent strain TBEV generated the small quantity of these components. Thus, the early increase in the activity of the cell enzymes indicates the activation of the macrophages, and the subsequent increase in their activity corresponds to the enhanced synthetic activity of the macrophages.

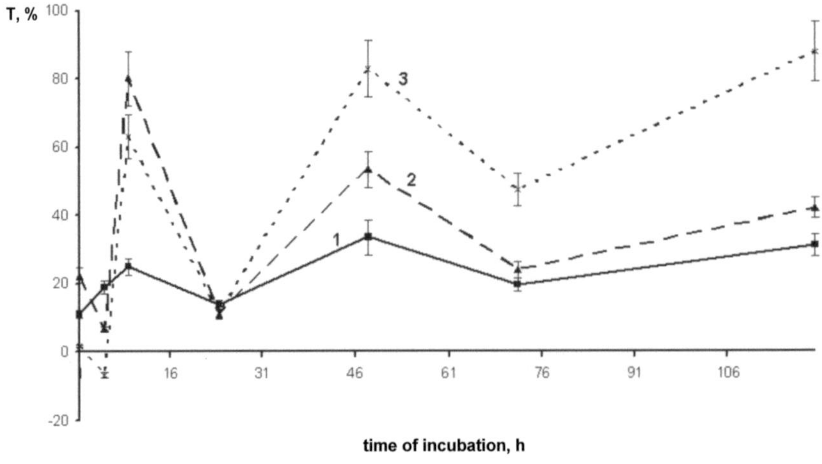

Fig. 12. The quality of NO metabolites in infected by high-virulence strain 73 (1), avirulence strain 69 (2) and 202 (3) of TBEV macrophages

4. Conclusion

So, for understanding the mechanisms of immunity reactions of an organism and their role in pathology of TBE infections it is necessary to estimate the role of phagocytoses, interferon, antibodies and local factors of immunity where the key cellular elements are neutrophils and monocytes/macrophages. As the data cited above specify, the functional expressiveness of these cells in TBE infections is various. So, alongside with that neutrophils and macrophages can carry out positive anti-viruses effect by absorption, neutralization and elimination of viruses and the cells infected by them, thus, becoming more active and producing in foci inflammation cytokines. As well, these cells can possess the negative influence during in the primary immune response in reproduction of ingesting viruses and them dissemination in various peripheral bodies. In that case, the given phagocytes act as the so-called "Troian horse", mediating a new formation of the foci inflammation. Thus, both depression of functional activity cells, and the display of undesirable consequences of similar change, namely, that they can destroy healthy cells in the place of an inflammation, excessively producing reactive radicals of oxygen and NO, arise. These metabolites are capable besides anti-virus to initiate actions process of apoptosis cells and to increase the permeability of capillaries. Thus, neutrophils and monocytes/macrophages in TBEV infection of an organism does not always prove as a protective barrier. At the same time, the activation of these cells at a reproduction in them of a virus allows them to carry out the antigen representing function for stimulation B-and T-lymphocytes and activation of cytotoxic T lymphocytes for destruction of the infected cells at the development of the specific immune response.

It was established by us that in TBEV infection of neutrophils the activity of plasmalemma enzymes and degidrogenese increased. The increase of succinate dehydrogenases activity is the display of adaptive reaction of neutrophils on TBEV infection. In its turn, the increase of LDG activity is connected with the changes of glycolyses intensity which consists of the formation of phosphoric connections rich with energy that testifies the an intensification of power supply neutrophils due to the inclusion of anaerobic glycolys (Koolman & Rohm, 1998). This way of oxidation can be regarded as a compensating mechanism of adaptive reaction neutrophils in TBEV infection. Finally it brings to killing neutrophils mainly by apoptoses as it is known, that necroses is accompanied by acid bioenergy hypoxia of cells at full inhibition of enzymes activity of a respiratory circuit.

We have demonstrated that TBEV is able to adhere from the virus containing liquid to the surface of the neutrophils and resident macrophages, penetrate into the cells, and reproduce in these cells. Similar data on selective adsorption to monocytes/macrophages were obtained while studying the interaction of these cells with TBEV (Ahantarig et al., 2009). Morphological examination of the cell culture infected by virulent strains TBEV revealed the features of the cytopathic action of this virus on the macrophages in contrast with the cells infected by avirulent strains. The virulent strains infected cells exhibited a granular cytoplasm, enhanced eosinophilicity of the cytoplasm, which characterizes the increase of the RNA and protein content, and karyopyknosis in some cells. Apoptotic neutrophils and macrophages were also observed.

It is established by us that the activation of oxygen metabolism in the cells depended from virulence strains of TBEV. Under physiological conditions, in contrast to other cells of the organism, superoxide anion is not produced in phagocytes or produced in small amounts. NADPH oxidases and oxidases of D-amino acids on the internal surface of the membranes also virtually do not function. After the infection of cells by TBEV, the activity of the primary NADPH oxidase complex (plasma membranes) increased according to the results of the NBT test. The activities of the mitochondrial enzymes of the third level (LDH, SDH, and cytochrome oxidase) also increased. These data indicate the stimulating effect of TBEV on the neutrophils and macrophages. It is known that redox molecules, active metabolites of oxygen, take part in the transmission of external signals arising on the plasma membrane. Further intracellular transfer of the signal can also be connected with the activation of the redox molecules of certain cytoplasm elements and transcriptional factors (Kliubin & Gamalei, 1998). Our results have revealed an instant reaction of the phagocytes in response to the infection by TBEV, since within the first 15-30 min of incubation a sharp increase of the activity of the enzymes involved in the generation of superoxide radicals was detected. In our opinion, the observed recurrence in the dynamics of the activity of the investigated enzymes in the neutrophils and macrophages infected by TBEV reflect the cell reaction to the penetration of the virus into the cell in the first period (within 3 h), and the replication and emission of the virus particles in extracellular space in the second period (18-48 h). The subsequent (after 48 h) decrease in the activity of the indicated enzymes of oxygen metabolism can be accounted by the beginning of degradation of the cell culture under the influence of TBEV.

It is necessary to mention the enzymes defending the macrophages from the excess of peroxide products. Although the cell culture infected with TBEV exhibited characteristic features of cell degradation in the late period of the observation (1-4 days), the activity of SOD (the enzyme scavenging excessive amounts of reactive oxygen species) Thus, complex evaluation of enzymatic changes in macrophages is a highly sensitive method of the indication of the virus reproductive activity in the cell cytoplasm allowing differentiation of the types of its cytopathogenic action.

5. Acknowledgment

This investigation was supported by a grant (16.740.11.0182) from The Ministry of Education and sciences Russian Federation.

6. References

Abo, A., Pick, E., Hall, A. Totty, N., Teahan, C.G., Segal, A.W. 1991. Activation of the NADPH oxidase involves the small GTP-binding protein p21rac1, *Nature*, Vol. 353, pp. 668-670, 0028-0836.

Ahantarig, A., Růzek, D., Vancová, M., Janowitz, A., St'astná, H., Tesarová, M., Grubhoffer, L. 2009. Tick-borne encephalitis virus infection of cultured mouse macrophages, *Intervirology*, Vol. 52, N 5, pp. 283-290, 0300-5526.

Allen, R.G., Keogh, B.P., Tresini, M., Gerhard, G.S., Volker, C., Pignolo, R.J., Horton, J., Cristofalo, V.J. 1997. Development and age-associated differences in electron transport potential and consequences for oxidant generation, *J. Biol. Chem.*, Vol. 272, N 40, Oct 3, pp. 24805-24812, 1864-6158.

Ammon, C., Meyer, S.P., Schwarzfischer, L., Krause, S.W., Andreesen, R., Kreutz, M. 2000. Comparative analysis of integrin expression on monocyte-derived macrophages and monocyte-derived dendritic cells, *Immunol.*, Vol. 100, N 3, pp. 364-389, 0019-2805.

Arruda, M.A., Barja-Fidalgo, C. 2009. NADPH oxidase activity: In the crossroad of neutrophil life and death, *Front. Biosci.*, Vol.14, pp. 4546-4556, 1945-0494.

Babior, B. M. 1999. NADPH Oxidase: An Update, *Blood*, Vol. 93, N 5, pp. 1464-1476, 0268-960X.

Ballinger, M.N., Welliver, T., Straight, S., Peters-Golden, M., Swanson, J.A. 2010. Transient increase in cyclic AMP localized to macrophage phagosomes, *PLoS One*, Vol. 5, N 11, Nov 11, pp. e13962, 1932-6203.

Baskin, H.S. 1997. Herpes simplex virus type 2 synergizes with interferon-γ in the induction of nitric oxide production in mouse macrophages through autocrin secretion of tumour necrosis factor α, *Gen. Virol.*, Vol. 78, pp. 195-203, 0022-1317.

Bokoch, G.M. 1996. Chemoattractant signaling and leukocyte activation, *Blood*, Vol. 86, pp. 1649-1660, 0268-960X.

Brinkmann, V., Reichard, U., Goosmann, C., Fauler, B., Uhlemann, Y., Weiss, D. S., Weinrauch, Y., Zychlinsky, A. 2004. Neutrophil extracellular traps kill bacteria, *Science*, Vol. 303, pp. 1532–1535, 0193-4511.

Cathcart, M.K. 2004. Regulation of superoxide anion production by NADPH oxidase in monocytes/macrophages: contributions to atherosclerosis, *Arterioscler. Thromb. Vasc. Biol.* Vol. 24, N 1, pp. 23-28, 1079-5642.

Chen, C.-J., Raung, S.-L., Kuo, M.-D., Wang, Y.-M. 2002. Suppression of Japanese encephalitis virus infection by non-steroidal anti-inflammatory drugs, *J. Gen.Virol.*, Vol. 83, pp. 1897-1905, 0022-1317.

Chen, Y.-C., Wang, S.-Y. 2002. Activation of terminally differentiated human monocytes/macrophages by Dengue virus: productive infection, hierarchical production of innate cytokines and chemokines, and the synergistic effect of lipopolysaccharide, *J. Virol.*, Vol. 76, pp. 9877–9887, 1816-4900.

Chaturvedi, U. C., Mathur, A., Tandon, P., Natu, S. M., Rajvanshi, S. & Tandon, H. O. 1979. Variable effect on peripheral blood leucocytes during JE virus infection of man, *Clin. Exp. Immunol.*, Vol. 38, pp. 492-498, 0009-9104.

Chaturvedi, U.C., Nagar, R., Shrivastava, R. 2006. Macrophage & dengue virus: Friend or foe? *Indian J. Med. Res.*, Vol. 124, pp. 23-40, 0022-4286.

Cologna, R., Rico-Hesse, R. 2003. American genotype structures decrease dengue virus output from human monocytes and dendritic cells, *J. Virol.*, Vol. 77, pp. 3929-3938, 1816-4900.

De Madrid, A.T., Porterfield, J.S. 1969. A simple microculture method for the study of group B arboviruses, *Bull. WHO*, Vol. 40, pp. 113–121, 0042-9686.

Daher, K.A., Selsted, M.E., Lehrer R.I. 1986. Direct inactivation of viruses by human granulocyte defensins, *J. Virol.*, Vol. 60, pp. 1068–1074, 1816-4900.

Dale, D.C., Boxer, L., Liles, W.C. 2008. The phagocytes: neutrophils and monocytes, *Blood*, Vol. 112, N 4, Aug., pp. 15935-15945, 0268-960X.

Ding, J., Chou, Y.-Y., Chang, T.L. 2009. Defensins in viral infections, *J. Innate Immun.*, Vol. 1, pp. 413–420, 1662-811X.

Elbim, C., Monceaux, V., Mueller, Y.M., Lewis, M.G., François, S., Diop, O., Akarid, K., Hurtrel, B., Gougerot-Pocidalo, M.A., Lévy, Y., Katsikis, P.D., Estaquier, J. 2008. Early divergence in neutrophil apoptosis between pathogenic and nonpathogenic simian immunodeficiency virus infections of nonhuman primates, *J. Immunol.*, Vol. 181., pp. 8613-8623, 1754-1441.

Faber-Zuschratter, H. 1994. Ultrastructural distribution of NADPH-diaphorase in cortical synapses, *Neuroreport*, Vol. 27, N 5, pp. 2029-2032, 0959-4965.

Fox, S., Leitch, A.E., Duffin, R., Haslett, C., Rossi, A.G. 2010. Neutrophil apoptosis: relevance to the innate immune response and inflammatory disease, *J. Innate. Immun.*, Vol. 2, pp. 216–227, 1662-811X.

Furci, L., Sironi, F., Tolazzi, M., Vassena, L., Lusso, P. 2007. Alphadefensins block the early steps of HIV-1 infection: interference with the binding of gp120 to CD4, *Blood*, Vol. 109, pp. 2928–2935, 0268-960X.

Ganz, T. 2003. Defensins: antimicrobial peptides of innate immunity, *Nat. Rev. Immunol.*, Vol. 3, pp. 710–720, 1474-1733.

Geissmann, F., Jung, S., Littman, D. R. 2003. Blood monocytes consist of two principal subsets with distinct migratory properties, *Immunity*, Vol. 19, pp. 71–82, 1074-7613.

Grard, G., Moureau, G., Charrel, R.N., Lemasson, J.J., Gonzalez, J.P., Gallian, P. 2007. Genetic characterization of tickborne fl aviviruses: new insights into evolution, pathogenetic determinants and taxonomy, *Virology*, Vol. 361, pp. 80–92, 0042-6822.

Hartshorn, K. L., White, M. R., Tecle, T., Holmskov, U., Crouch, E. C. 2006. Innate defense against influenza A virus: activity of human neutrophil defensins and interactions of defensins with surfactant protein D. *J. Immunol.*, Vol. 176, pp. 6962–6972, 1754-1441.

Hakkim, A., Fürnrohr, B.G., Amann, K., Laube, B., Abu Abed, U., Brinkmann, V., Herrmann, M., Voll, R.E., Zychlinskya, A. 2010. Impairment of neutrophil extracellular trap degradation is associated with lupus nephritis, *PNAS*, Vol. 107, N 21, May 25, pp. 9813–9818, 0027-8424.

Hazrati, E., Galen, B., Lu, W., Wang, W., Ouyang, Y., Keller, M. J., Lehrer, R. I., Herold. B.C. 2006. Human alpha- and beta-defensins block multiple steps in herpes simplex virus infection, *J. Immunol.*, Vol. 177, pp. 8658–8666, 1754-1441.

Hoang, L.T., Lynn, D.J., Henn, M., Birren. B.W., Lennon, N.J., Le, P.T., Duong, K.T., Nguyen, T.T., Mai, L.N., Farrar, J.J., Hibberd, M.L., Simmons, C.P. 2010. The early whole-blood transcriptional signature of dengue virus and features associated with progression to dengue shock syndrome in Vietnamese children and young adults, *J. Virol.*, Vol. 84, N 24, Dec., pp. 12982-12994, 1816-4900.

Kebir, E.l.D., Filep, J.G. 2010. Role of neutrophil apoptosis in the resolution of inflammation, *Scientific. World Journal*, Vol. 1, N 10, Sep., pp. 1731-1748, 1537-744X.

Kennedy, A.D., DeLeo, F.R. 2009. Neutrophil apoptosis and the resolution of infection. *Immunol. Res.*, Vol. 43, N 1-3, pp. 25-61, 0257-277X.

Khanna, N., Mathur, A., Chaturvedi, U.C. 1994. Regulation of vascular permeability by macrophage-derived chemotactic factor produced in Japanese encephalitis, *Immunol. Cell. Biol.*, Vol. 72, N 3, Jun., pp. 200-204, 0818-9641.

Klebanoff, S.J., Coombs, R.W. 1991. Viricidal effect of Lactobacillus acidophilus on human immunodeficiency virus type 1: possible role in heterosexual transmission, *J. Exp. Med.*, Vol. 174, pp. 289-292, 0022-099X.

Klebanoff, S.J. 1992. Oxygen metabolites from phagocytes. In: Gallin J.I., ed. Inflammation. New York: Raven Press.

Klebanoff, S.J. 2005. Myeloperoxidase: friend and foe, *J. Leukocyte biology*, Vol. 77, pp. 598-625, 0741-5400.

Kliubin, I.V., Gamalei, I.A. 1997. NADPH oxidase a specialized enzyme complex for the formation of active oxygen metabolites, *Tsitologiia,* Vol. 39, N 4-5, pp. 320-340, 0564-3783.

Koolman, J., Rohm, K.-H. 1998. Taschenatlas der Biochemie. New York: Georg Thieme Verlag Stuttgart.

Kreil, T.R., Eibl, M.M. 1996. Nitric oxide and viral infection: NO antiviral activity against a flavivirus in vitro, and evidence for contribution to pathogenesis in experimental infection in vivo, *Virology,* Vol. 219, N 1, May 1, pp. 304-306, 0042-6822.

Leonova, G.N., Pavlenko, E.V., Krylova, N.V. 2006. Prophylactic of the tickborne encephalitis with vaccines [in Russian]. Vladivostok: Dal'nauka.

Lippolis, J.D., Reinhardt, T.A., Goff, J.P., Horst, R.L. 2006. Neutrophil extracellular trap formation by bovine neutrophils is not inhibited by milk. *Vet. Immunol. Immunopathol.,* Vol. 113, pp. 248–255, 0165-2427.

Litvitskij, P.F., Sinelnikov, T.G. 2009. The innate immunity: mechanisms of realization and pathological syndromes, *Ques. Mod. Pediatrics.* Vol. 8, № 1, 2, 3, 4.

Loida, Z., Gossrau, R., Schiebler, T. 1982. Enzymes Histochemistry. A laboratory Manual, Springer-Verlag, Berlin, Heidelberg, New York, 272 p.

Murray, C.L., Jones, C.T., Rice, C.M. 2008. Architects of assembly: roles of Flaviviridae non-structural proteins in virion morphogenesis, Nat. Rev. Microbiol., Vol. 6, pp. 699–708,

Nathan, C., Shiloh, M. 2000. Reactive oxygen and nitrogen intermediates in the relationship between mammalian hosts and microbial pathogens. *Proc. Natl. Acad. Sci. USA.,* Vol. 97, N 16, pp. 8841-8848, 0027-8424.

Palic, D., Ostojic, J., Andreasenc, C. B. & Roth, J. A. 2007. Fish cast NETs: neutrophil extracellular traps are released from fish neutrophils. *Dev. Comp. Immunol.,* Vol. 31, pp. 805–816, 0145-305X.

Plekhova, N.G. , Somova, L.M., Drobot, E.I., Krylova, N.V., Leonova G.N. 2007. Changes in the metabolic activity of macrophages under the influence of Tick Borne Encephalitis virus, *Biochemistry (Moscow),* Vol. 72, N 2, pp. 199-207, 0006-2979.

Reutov, V.P. 2002. Nitric oxide cycle in mammals and the cyclicity principle, *Biochemistry (Mosc*), Vol. 67, N 3, Mar., pp. 293-311, 0006-2979.

Rios, M., Zhang, M. J., Grinev, A., Srinivasan, K., Daniel, S., Wood, O., Hewlett, I.K., Dayton, A.I. 2006. Monocytes-macrophages are a potential target in human infection with West Nile virus through blood transfusion *Transfusion,* Vol. 46, pp. 659-662, 0041-1132.

Schneider, B.S., Soong, L., Coffey, L.L., Stevenson, H.L., McGee, C.E., Higgs, S. 2010. Aedes aegypti saliva alters leukocyte recruitment and cytokine signaling by antigen-presenting cells during West Nile virus infection, *PLoS One,* Vol. 22, N 5(7), Jul., pp. e11704, 1932-6203.

Schulz, K., Kerber, S., Kelm, M. 1999. Reevaluation of the Griess method for determining NO/NO2- in aqueous and protein-containing samples, *Nitric Oxide,* Vol. 3, N 3), Jun., pp. 225-234, 1089-8603.

Silva, M.C., Guerrero-Plata, A., Gilfoy, F.D., Garofalo, R.P., Mason, P.W. 2007. Differential activation of human monocyte-derived and plasmacytoid dendritic cells by West nile virus generated in different host cells, *J. Virology,* Vol. 81, N 24, Dec., pp. 13640–13648, 0022-538X.

Smolen, J.E., Boxer, L.A. 2001. *Function of neutrophils.* (In: Beutler, E., Lichtman, M.A., Coller, B.S., Kipps, T.J., Seligsohn, U., eds. Williams Hematology. 6th ed.), NY: McGraw Hill pp. 761-784, ISBN

Walmsley, S.R., McGovern, N.N., Whyte, M.K., Chilvers, E.R. 2008. The HIF/VHL pathway: from oxygen sensing to innate immunity. *Am. J. Respir. Cell. Mol. Biol.*, Vol. 38, N 3, Mar., pp. 251-255, 1044-1549.

Wardini, A.B., Guimarães-Costa, A.B., Nascimento, M.T., Nadaes, N.R., Danelli, M.G., Mazur, C., Benjamim, C.F., Saraiva, E.M., Pinto-da-Silva, L.H. 2010. Characterization of neutrophil extracellular traps in cats naturally infected with feline leukemia virus, *J. Gen. Virol.*, Vol. 91, N Pt 1, Jan., pp. 259-264, 0022-1317.

Webb, J.L, Harvey, M.W., Holden, D.W., Evans, T.J. 2001. Macrophage nitric oxide synthase associates with cortical actin but is not recruited to phagosomes, *Infect. Immun.* , Vol. 69, N 10, Oct, pp. 6391-400, 0019-9567.

Wilkie, R.P., Vissers, M.C., Dragunow, M., Hampton, M.B. 2007. A functional NADPH oxidase prevents caspase involvement in the clearance of phagocytic neutrophils, *Infect. Immun.*, Vol. 75, N 7, Jul., pp. 3256-3263, 0019-9567.

Williams, K.C., Burdo, T.H. 2009. HIV and SIV infection: the role of cellular restriction and immune responses in viral replication and pathogenesis, *APMIS*, Vol. 117, N 5-6, May, pp. 400-412, 0903-4641.

Winter, P.M., Dung, N.M., Loan, H.T., Kneen, R., Wills, B., Thu le, T., House, D., White, N.J., Farrar, J.J., Hart, C.A., Solomon, T. 2004. Proinflammatory cytokines and chemokines in humans with Japanese encephalitis, *J. Infect. Dis.*, Vol. 190, N 9, Nov. 1, pp. 1618-1626, 0022-1899.

Wu, S.J., Grouard-Vogel, G., Sun, W., Mascola, J.R., Brachtel, E., Putvatana, R., Louder, M.K., Filgueira, L., Marovich, M.A., Wong, H.K., Blauvelt, A., Murphy, G.S., Robb, M.L., Innes, B.L., Birx, D.L., Hayes, C.G., Frankel, S,S. 2000. Human skin Langerhans cells are targets of dengue virus infection, *Nat Med.*, Vol. 6, N 7, Jul., pp. 816-820, 1078-8956.

Ziegler-Heitbrock, L. 2007. The CD14+ CD16+ blood monocytes: their role in infection and inflammation, *J. Leukoc. Biol.*, Vol. 81, N 3. pp. 584-592, 0741-5400.

10

Evaluation of Immunological Efficiency Among Patients Vaccinated Against Tick-Borne Encephalitis

Leonova G.N.
Institute of Epidemiology and Microbiology, Siberian Branch of the Russian Academy of Medical Sciences, Vladivostok, Russia

1. Introduction

Tick-borne encephalitis virus (TBEV) widespread in the Eurasian continent is a member of the genus *Flavivirus,* family *Flaviviridae.* Human TBE cases are registered in more than 30 countries of the world [*Charrel RN et al.,* 2004]. TBEV is subdivided into three main subtypes according to its genetic structure and antigen specificity: European, Siberian, and Far Eastern ones [*Holzmann H, et al.1992; Ecker M. et al.* 1999]. Differences in nucleotide sequences of TBEV genome of these subtypes may reach about 20% [*Loktev VB* et al. 2007]. Probably, a high TBEV genetic diversity provides its differences in human pathogenicity. Human pathogenicity of European subtype TBEV is less marked; however, towards the east, a severity of infection increases as well as lethality [*Loktev VB* et al. 2007; *Pogodina VV et al. 2007*]. In the Russian Far East, the lethality caused by this infection remains at the highest levels [Pavlenko et al. 2010]; for the last 40 years it has reached, on average, 17,5% [*Leonova et al., 2006; Leonova, 2009*]. A vaccination is known to provide the most reliable and effective protection from many virus infections. Tick-borne encephalitis (TBE) as a very danger infection for humans is not the exception as well. Practical application of different vaccines against tick-borne diseases shows that vaccination of the population is a key link in terms of mass TBE prevention in highly endemic territories [*Kunz C., 2003; Onishchenko G.G., et al. 2007*].

Tick-borne encephalitis is considered to be the international health issue, because the number of risk areas and reported cases across Europe, Russia, and parts of Asia is increasing. The incidence of TBE has fluctuated considerably from year to year in many countries, but in the past decade the number of TBE cases has significantly increased in the Baltic states, the Czech Republic, and Germany, in addition to the countries previously considered to be free from TBE, such as Denmark (specifically the main island of Zealand), France, and Italy. A number of factors have been suggested to explain the growth of incidence including climate changes, extended travelling, and outdoor pursuits increasingly placing people in contact with infected ticks [Eckhardt Petri et al., 2010].

Development of vaccine against TBE has started since the discovery of causative agent in 1937. A group of discoverers, headed by already well known virologist prof. L.A. Zilber, understood that only vaccine can become a reliable protection from this dangerous disease.

As early as in 1938 a group of young virologists headed by E.N. Levkovich started working on a vaccine against tick-borne disease; they obtained the first formalin-inactivated brain vaccine from the Far Eastern TBEV strain Sofjin [*Vanda Pogodina*. 2001].

In 1939, the study aimed to investigate the vaccine effectiveness was conducted in Oborsk forestry (Khabarovsk Region). Lethality was not registered among the vaccinated patients. Despite the obvious epidemiological effectiveness of this vaccine, it caused serious side effects in vaccinated patients. In some years, number of postvaccinal encephalitis reached 1:20000 of vaccinated patients. Reduction of concentration of brain tissue from white mice in the vaccine up to 2.5% did not make it better [3]. Thus, a search for safer approaches to the development of new vaccine was necessary. In 1960, development of the vaccine against TBE using chick-embryo cell culture for the virus reproduction was a significant step to improve quality of the vaccine preparation. TBE strain Sofjin was reproduced in a cell culture of chick fibroblasts, inactivated by formaldehyde in a concentration of 1:2000, and virus antigen was absorbed on aluminium hydroxide. However, vaccination of patients showed that not only reactogenicity, but also protective characteristics of this vaccine were lower in comparison with formolated brain vaccine [*Vorobyova MS et al., 2007*].

At the same time, at the Tomsk Scientific Research Institute of Vaccines and Sera, a cultural vaccine was developed using western TBEV subtype. It's immunological activity and protective characteristics were also insufficient [*Leonova GN, 1997; Vorobyova MS et al., 2007*]. From 1964, this vaccine was introduced in the Far East. It's immunologic effectiveness in hemagglutination-inhibition reaction (HAIR) was 70% with low immunity stress in HAIR (GTM 1:15). Soon, on the Primorye Territory, single TBE cases were reported among the patients vaccinated three times and revaccinated [*Dorokhova V.S. & Tatarinova L.G, 1969*]. In 1967, rate of vaccinated persons didn't exceed 1.8% of urban population and 13.2% of villagers. A cumbersome vaccination protocol and short-term humoral immunity in the patients vaccinated with a formalin-inactivated liquid tissue culture vaccine constantly initiated research work on production immunologically more active vaccines.

In the middle of 1980s at the Institute of Poliomyelitis and Viral Encephalitides, Academy of Medical Sciences of the USSR, a group of scientists headed by L.B. Elbert developed a new preparation technique of concentrated vaccine based on the TBE strain Sofjin of Far Eastern subtype. A specific activity of the obtained vaccine considerably exceeded activity of non concentrated preparation [*Vorobyova MS et al., 2007*]. Nowadays, this vaccine is widely used on endemic territories of the Russian Federation as a dry concentrated vaccine produced by M.P. Chumakov Institute of Poliomyelitis and Viral Encephalitides (IPVE) of Russian Academy of Medical Sciences (RAMS). The TBE strain 205 isolated in 1973 from ticks I.persulcatus on Khabarovsk Territory [*Vereta et al., 1990*] is now used as a master seed virus for Tomsk vaccine. From 1984, liquid tissue culture vaccine against TBE has being manufactured by scientific production association (SPA) "Virion" (affiliated with Federal State Unitary Enterprise (FSUE) SPA "MicroGen") on the base of this strain which is a typical representative of Far Eastern subtype of TBE. From 2003 it has being produced as liquid tissue culture inactivated, purified, concentrated, and absorbed vaccine "EnceVir".

Additionally, in 1970s, the development of live vaccine based on the attenuated strain TP-21 of the Langat virus and antigenically similar naturally attenuated Elantsev strain, isolated from human blood on the territory of Siberia, provoked a great response in scientific world [*Smorodintsev A.A.& Doubov A.V* , 1986]. Although these developments did not have any practical application, the authors outlined scientific approaches to creation of such vaccines.

According to these authors, the prime advantage of such vaccines consisted in absence of clinical and pathomorphological signs of central nervous system damage after intracerebral administration to monkeys.

In 1971, the first foreign inactivated tissue culture vaccine against TBE was developed in Austria on the base of the Neudorfl strain (western subtype of TBE) isolated from ticks I. ricinus. In 1980s, a new technique was implemented; this enabled to obtain a preparation up to 99% free of heterologous protein and to concentrate TBEV antigen. The vaccine was called "FSME-Immun-Inject" [*Kunz et al. 1980*]. In 1993, this vaccine produced by "Baxter Vaccines" (Austria - USA) was registered in Russia for adults (0.5 mL), and in 2006-2007 - for children 1-16 years old at half the volume (0.25 mL) [*Vorobyova MS et al., 2007*].

In 1998, another TBE vaccine manufactured by the German company "Chiron Behring" (currently "Novartis Vaccines and Diagnostics GmbH & Co KG") was registered in Russia. This vaccine was based on the strain K-23 (western subtype of TBE) isolated from ticks I. ricinus. In Russia, the vaccine is used in two variants: "Encepur® Adults" and "Encepur® Children". This high-purity vaccine, free of homologous and heterologous proteins, is practically a non-reactogenic preparation which is very important for evaluation of its safety [*Zent et al.* 2003]. The vaccine variants for adults and children differ only by the concentration of the virus antigen (1.5 mg/0.5 mL and 0.75mg/0.25 mL, respectively). So far, there have not been registered any TBE cases both in European countries and the Russian Federation among those vaccinated with this vaccine, unlike the other ones described above.

Availability of the above TBEV strains for vaccine preparations to protect from the current virus population including different subtypes of TBEV was reported in several papers [*Holzmann H et al., 1992; Leonova GN, et al., 2006; Leonova GN et al., 2007*]. On the other hand, new genetically different variants within the Far Eastern subtype of TBEV were found. They were Oshima, Senzhang, Glubinnoe/2004-like strains, and the strain of hemorrhagic form of TBE [*Loktev VB* et al. 2007; *Leonova GN & Pavlenko EV*, 2009]. Genetic diversity of TBEV was detected, when all three main TBEV genotypes could circulate simultaneously on the same territory [*Pogodina VV. et al., 2007*]. Thereupon, it is often a problem for public health in geographically different Eurasian regions to decide what vaccine among those consisting of different genovariant strains would be the most effective for protection of the population against TBE.

2. Characterization of the immune response to Encepur® Adult vaccine

Vaccine Encepur® Adult is produced using strain K23, which belongs to European subtype of TBEV (Bock HL, et al. 1990). Nucleotide sequences of Far Eastern and European TBEV subtypes have only 78–82% similarity. This naturally raises the question whether the vaccine based on the European subtype of TBEV is protective against the Far Eastern subtype of the virus. We sought to evaluate specific humoral immune response in volunteers immunized with vaccine Encepur® in relation to Far East strains TBEV.

We characterized genetic and antigenic variation among TBEV strains P-73, P-202 and P-69, isolated in Far Eastern region of Russia. Locations, dates and sources of isolation Far Eastern strains used in this study are presented in Table 1. Genotyping of strains P-73, P-202, and P-69 unambiguously demonstrated that they belong to Far Eastern subtype of TBEV (Leonova G. et al. 2007).

TBEV strain	Year of isolation	Source of isolation	Place of isolation	Reference
Primorye-73 (P-73)	1973	Human brain (lethal case)	Dal'nerechensk region, Primorsky krai	Leonova GN et al. 2004
Primorye-202 (P-202)	1997	Leukocytes of healthy human after tick bite	Ussuriisk region, Primorsky krai	Leonova GN et al. 2004
Primorye-69 (P-69)	2000	Leukocytes of healthy human after tick bite	Nadezhdinsk region, Primorsky krai	Leonova GN et al. 2004

Table 1. TBEV strains used in the study

The strains P-73, P-202, and P-69 are highly virulent for suckling mice. The invasivity index for these strains (the difference between log10 LD50 for intracerebral and subcutaneous challenge) were found to be 2.0, 1.4, and 0.7, respectively. Strains P-73 and P-69 were replicating efficiently in PEK cells (7.5 and 6.0 log TCID50/0.1 ml, respectively). However, strain P-202 was not able to replicate effectively in PEK cells—the titer did not exceed 4.75±0.25 log TCID50/0.1 ml. An attempt to adapt P-202 to cell culture by several passages in PEK cells was unsuccessful.

We also measured humoral immune response against these strains after complete vaccination of volunteers with Encepur® Adult. We have shown significant differences in levels of antibodies and the number of NT-positive sera against strains P-73, P-202, and P-69 1 year after the second immunization (Table 2). After the third immunization, key parameters of the immune response increased considerably and the number of sera positive in NT with strain P-202 reached 95.5±3.1 and 97.6±2.3% with strain P-73. The strain P-69 behaved differently, as the number of sera positive in NT was only 63.9±7.2%, which is statistically different from the corresponding data for the other strains.

TBEV strain	No. of positive human sera (%)		Maximal titer		Average titer[a]	
	Before	After	Before	After	Before	After
P-73 (a)	56.8	95.5	80	640	19.7	128
P-202 (b)	52.3	97.6	40	320	15	34
P-69 (c)	27.3	63.9	20	80	11.3	28

[a] Mean geometric titers of neutralizing antibodies.

Table 2. Titers of neutralizing antibodies to TBEV strains P-73, P-202, and P-69 in volunteer's sera before and after the third immunization with the vaccine Encepur® Adult ($n = 44$)
Note: Reverse titer values are shown. Statistical significance: before immunization for (a–b) $P < 0.05$; for (a–c) and (b–c) $P < 0.01$, after immunization for (a–b) and (a–c) $P < 0.001$; for (b–c) $P < 0.01$.

The most complete immune response to immunization with the German vaccine Encepur® Adult was achieved against highly virulent Far Eastern strain P-73. The volunteers were also seemed to be protected against the two other TBEV strains. Induction of neutralizing antibodies at titers considerably exceeding the minimal protection level was demonstrated after both double and triple immunizations.

3. Comparative evaluation of immunologic activity of vaccines against TBE used in the Russian Federation

In Russia, the following vaccines are certified and widely used: "FSME-IMMUN-Inject" (Austria), "Encepur® Adults" (Germany), and two local vaccines - the TBE vaccine manufactured by M.P. Chumakov Institute of Poliomyelitis and Viral Encephalitides (Moscow, Russia) and "EnceVir" manufactured by SPA "MicroGen" (Tomsk, Russia) [*Vorobyova MS*, 2007].

We have performed cohort and simultaneous study of immunologic effectiveness of the four vaccines against TBE in relation to several contemporary Far Eastern TBEV strains on 290 volunteers [*Leonova GN & Pavlenko EV*, 2009]. We evaluated immunologic activity of the vaccines against TBE according to the intensity of antibody response one and two years later after full course of immunization with the vaccines. Postvaccinal antibody response was evaluated by a level of virus neutralizing antibodies, total antivirus antibodies, and their avidity regarding different TBEV strains.

All volunteers were vaccinated three times during one year according to application instructions of the vaccines. The exception was made for a combined vaccination which consisted of alternate use of the Russian and foreign vaccines.

The mean age of the vaccinated patients was almost the same, and in the first period of study it varied from 32.6 to 47.3 years, in the second one - from 34.7 to 47.4 years. Blood sera of the volunteers vaccinated against TBE were studied by enzyme-linked immunosorbent assay (ELISA) and neutralization test (NT) with the strain Primorye-73 (P-73) of Far Eastern TBE subtype.

We have concluded that all studied vaccines are able to induce neutralizing antibodies against contemporary TBEV strains [*Leonova GN & Pavlenko EV*, 2009]. Levels of seroconversion for the vaccine "FSME-IMMUN-Inject" (Austria) were 88.2% in the year after full course of immunization and 78.1% of cases - two years later, "Encepur® Adults" (Germany) - 100% and 100%, the vaccine manufactured by IPVE RAMS (Moscow) - 100% and 94.1%, "EnceVir" (Tomsk) - 88.2% and 83.9%, and during the combined vaccination - 100% and 92.7% of cases, respectively. Use of different types of vaccines during the combined vaccination of a patient provided a high and stable level of seroconversion according to NT, which is important for revaccination with different vaccines available in order not to interfere with the recommended vaccination protocols (Table 3).

As a rule, antibodies with high affinity and avidity to surface proteins of TBEV virions are necessary for manifestation of neutralizing antibody activity. Only these antibodies do not allow the virus to interact with receptors and enter the cell. We have shown a variability of common and avid antibodies to different TBEV strains in vaccinated patients in the year of vaccination and two years later. Not all sera of those vaccinated with different vaccines had high-avid antibodies to the studied TBEV strains even in the year of vaccination.

Moreover, not only the proportion of patients having antibodies and the general GMT of antibodies, but also GMT of avid antibodies to all TBE strains decreased at remote observation time (two years later after the vaccination course). It has been shown using

ELISA (Fig. 1) that in the year of vaccination, GTM of antibodies to TBEV reached 6.5 log_2; two years later, GMT decreased up to 5.5 log_2.

Vaccine	Observation time point	Number of examined vaccinated persons	Mean age		ELISA (IgG %)	NT (Ab %)
			years	p		
FSME-Immune Inject («Baxter Vaccine», Austria)	After the primary vaccination course	51	32.6 ± 2.3	0.592	86.3	88.2
	2 years after vaccination	32	34.7 ± 3.3		75	78.1
Encepur® Adults («Novartis Vaccines», Germany)	After the primary vaccination course	6	36.8 ± 6.0	0.128	83.3	100
	2 years after vaccination	11	46.4 ± 3.0		100	100
Vaccine by Chumakov Institute of Poliomyelitis (Moscow, Russia)	After the primary vaccination course	30	41.2 ± 3.3	0.274	90	100
	2 years after vaccination	17	47.4 ± 4.7		94.1	94.1
EnceVir («Microgen» Tomsk, Russia)	After the primary vaccination course	17	45.8 ± 4.5	0.971	76.5	88.2
	2 years after vaccination	56	45.6 ± 2.7		66.1	83.9
Combined vaccination*	After the primary vaccination course	29	43.2 ± 3.9	0.596	100	100
	2 years after vaccination	41	45.6 ± 2.6		92.7	92.7

* The first two inoculations have been made by foreign vaccines consisting of the TBEV strains of European subtype, the subsequent booster vaccination – by the Russian vaccines consisting of the TBEV strains of Far Eastern subtype.

Table 3. Comparative assessment of the immune response in patients vaccinated with different TBE vaccines after the primary vaccination course and the two years later after the primary vaccination course.
Note: NT, neutralization test; Ab, the antibodies to TBEV strain p-73; *p*, significance at the confidence interval of 95%

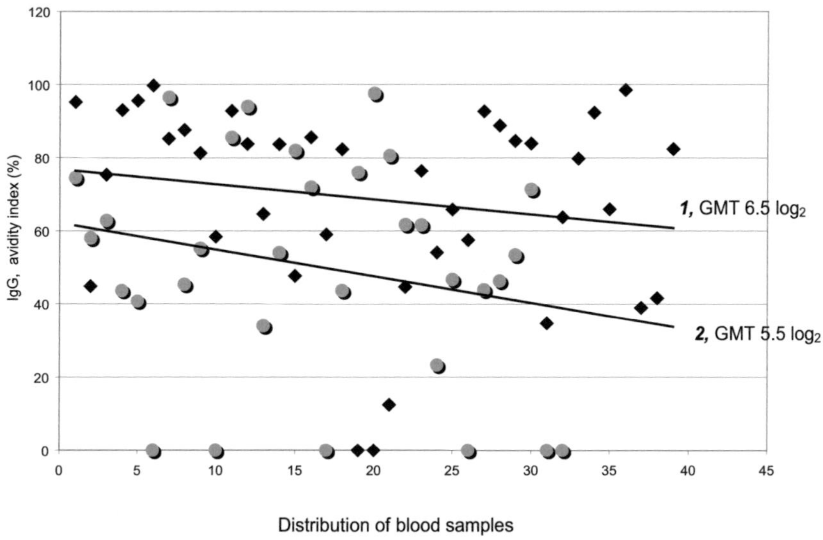

Fig. 1. Distribution of IgG avidity index in the patients vaccinated against TBE after the primary vaccination course and two years later after vaccination: ♦, blood samples after the primary vaccination course; ○, blood samples two years later after vaccination; trend line *1*, after the primary vaccination course; and trend line *2*, two years later after vaccination

Immune response of the patients vaccinated against TBE to different strains is known to vary [Holzmann al, 1992; Klockmann U. Et al,, 1999]. Figure 2 depicts comparative data on blood sera of the patients vaccinated against TBE in the first and second year after full course of vaccination studied by ELISA and indirect immunofluorescence assay (IFA). It is obvious that during both observation periods, antibodies of the vaccinated patients showed a closer immune relation to the strain P-73 in comparison with the other strains (P-202 and P-69) isolated from blood of the patients with inapparent TBE form. These data gave evidence that vaccinated patients had immunoprotection not only to pathogenic TBEV strain associated with focal form of infection with fatal outcome, but also to all other TBEV strains widely circulating on the territory of the Far Eastern region.
Therefore, all four vaccines against TBE can be recommended for wide use in the Russian Far East (possibly in China and Japan as well), where the most pathogenic TBEV strains circulate. Virus-specific antibody avidity test have a special significance for more adequate evaluation of a stress of postvaccinal immune response. Avidity of specific IgG antibodies characterizes immune response of the vaccinated patients more precisely. It is also important to study functional antibody activity of the vaccinated patients for evaluation of their protection, when it is necessary to determine immunity stress of these patients regarding TBEV, for example, after tick bite. Indeed, such studies are necessary for determination of immunity duration in vaccinated patients and time of remote revaccinations. Use of different types of vaccines for immunity formation in a patient also provided a high and stable seroconversion according to NT. These data have a practical importance to determine time of remote revaccinations using another type of vaccine against TBE and consider interchangeability of all four types of vaccines without any interference with recommended vaccination protocol. Such approach can also provide

formation of a more diverse immunity against the strains of western and Far Eastern subtypes of TBEV.

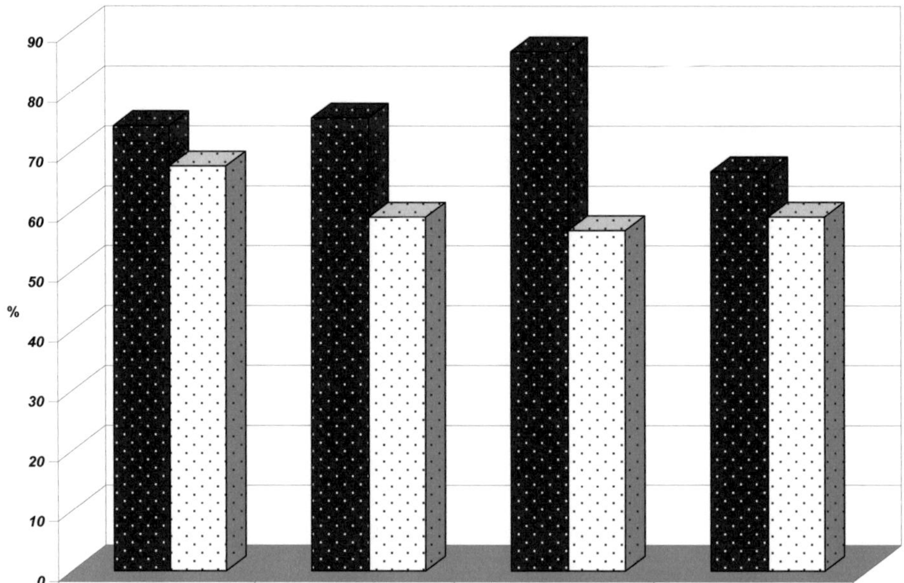

	IgG	P-73	P-202	P-69
■ A	74,3	75,6	86,7	66,7
□ B	67,6	59,1	56,8	59,1

Fig. 2. Rate of avid antibodies in patients vaccinated against tick-borne encephalitis after the primary vaccination course and two years later: IgG according to ELISA and the antibodies to P-73, P-202, and P-69 strains according to IFA; *A* – percentage of avid antibodies after the primary vaccination course; *B* – percentage of avid antibodies two years later after vaccination

4. Protective antibody titer and level of immunological memory in patients vaccinated against TBE

The notion of protective antibody titer appeared during the studies on evaluation of vaccinal immunological activity. Preventive effectiveness of vaccines against some infections was considered to be evaluated by a protective level of immunological characteristics [Briko NI. 2004]. In 1980 Kunz et al. [1980] suggested that the protective titer of hemagglutinating antibodies for TBEV vaccine is above 1:10. At present time the most of diagnostic laboratories use ELISA as the main standard detection method of specific IgG antibodies.

In the course of time, despite the decrease in characteristics of immune response, some vaccinated patients showed the ability to preserve antibodies for a long time [*Kunz C. et al.. 2003; Heinz FX, et al,. 2008*]. To determine a revaccination time, we have obtained the experimental evidence of protective effect of different antibody titers in patients vaccinated against TBE. Immunological characteristics obtained during examination of the vaccinated patients, allowed us to indirectly judge a possible epidemiological effectiveness of vaccinal prevention.

4.1 Experimental studies (experiment №1)

We performed the set of experiments using the specific anti-TBE immunoglobulin (titer from 1:6400 in ELISA, 1:160 – in IFA, and 1:320 – in NT). To find an optimum alternative of experimentation, we ranged experimental components by IFA: different dilutions of immunoglobulin containing antibodies of IgG class, different TBEV doses and time parameters. Fig. 3 (*A, B, C*) shows influence of different TBEV doses (1, 2, 3 lg TCID) on the specific antibodies with titers ranging from 1:160 to 1:10 (via IFA) at 5, 15 and 30 min. In experimental samples, virus titers had from two- to four-fold decrease depending on virus dose employed in experiment. The most convincing data on the decrease of virus titer can be observed in Fig.3 *C*. With the virus dose 3 lg $TCID_{50}$, the characteristics decreased significantly at all exposition times (5 - 30 min).

Further studies were carried out with samples containing different dilutions of immunoglobulin and only a virus dose of 3 lg $TCID_{50}$. Similar results were observed in ELISA and neutralization test (NT). While observing the antibody contact at different dilutions (antibody titers from 1:6400 to 1:12.5) with TBEV (3 lg $TCID_{50}$), we singled out the sample containing IgG with a titer of 1:400, in this sample the antibodies completely bounded to the virus antigen (Tabl. 4).

Virus antigen in this sample decreased to minimal values (K = 0.4). During the experiment, K values of virus antigen were ambiguous: with high titre values (1:6400 and 1:1600) K antigen was positive (3.9 and 1.6, respectively), then K antigen decreased up to 0.4. However, the further decrease of IgG titers led to the increase of K antigen up to the positive value (1.0). RT-PCR data were positive in all samples. Occurrence of free infective virus of 0.9 and 1.0 lg $TCID_{50}$ was an evidence of unfavourable conditions for a specific protection in samples with IgG titer less than 1:100. Similar results were observed in neutralization test, when the minimal protective threshold having the starting titer was analysed with that of 1:20.

ELISA		Neutralization test		Antigen K via ELISA	TBEV titration on PEK cells	RT-PCR
Initial IgG titer	Residual IgG titer	Initial IgG titer	Residual IgG titer			
6400	1600	320	80	3,8	0	+
3200	800	160	80	1,6	0	+
1600	400	80	80	0,8	0	+
800	200	40	40	0,5	0	+
400	**0**	**20**	**20**	**0,4**	**0**	**+**
200	0	10	0	1.0	0	+
100	0	5	0	0,8	0	+
50	0	2,5	0	**0,7**	**0,9**	**+**
0	0	**1,22**	0	**0,9**	**1,0**	**+**

Table 4. Experimental substantiation of protective IgG titer threshold under the influence of TBEV exposure (3 lg $TCID_{50}$) based on ELISA, Nt, virus titration, RT-PCR, and antigen detection via ELISA

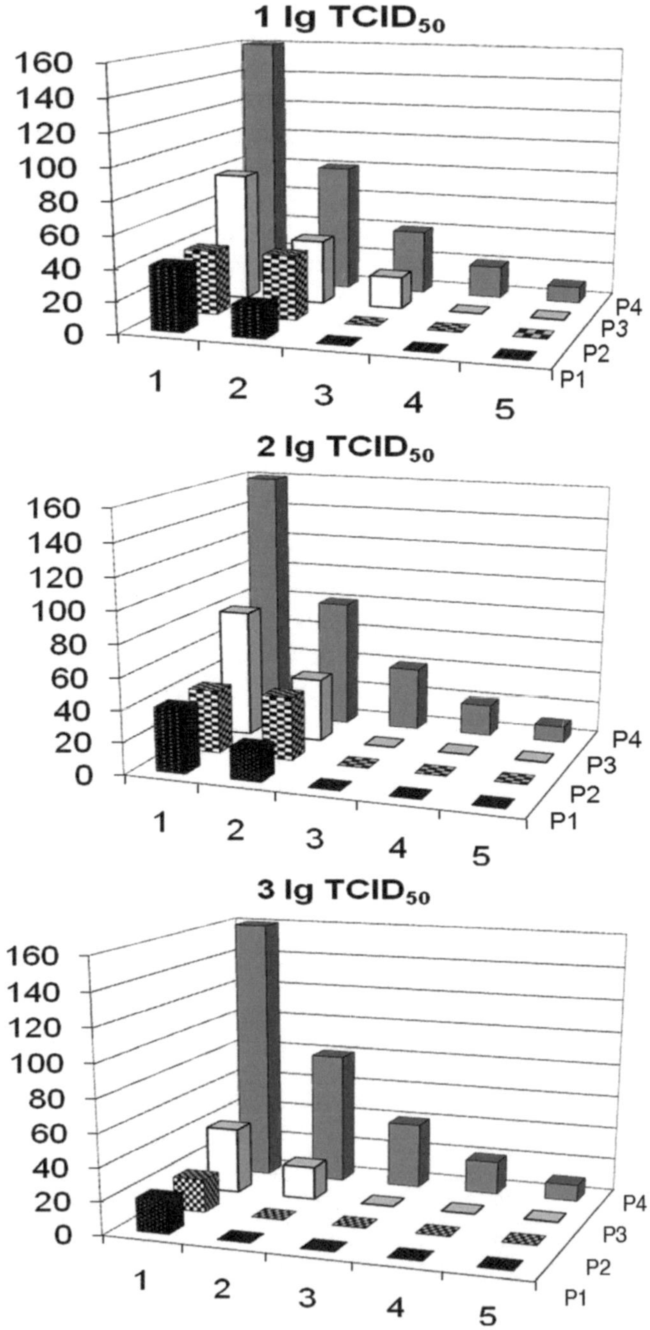

Fig. 3. Influence of different TBEV doses (*A*- 1 lg, *B*- 2 lg, *C*- 3 lg $TCID_{50}$) on IgG titer in 30 min (P1), 15 min (P2) and 5 min (P3), (P4 – control two-fold IgG dilutions 1:160-1:10) via IFA X-axis – sample number; Y-axis (left) – IgG titer via IFA TBEV vaccine was above 1:10. At present, most of diagnostic laboratories use ELISA as the main standard method of specific IgG antibodies detection

Fig. 4 depicts two-fold decrease of specific IgG *(2)* titers under the TBEV influence at a dose of 3 lg $TCID_{50}$. In addition, via IFA, it shows a gradual decrease in antigens *(3)* from the sample with IgG titer of 1:3200 to the one of 1:400 under the TBEV influence (3 lg $TCID_{50}$).

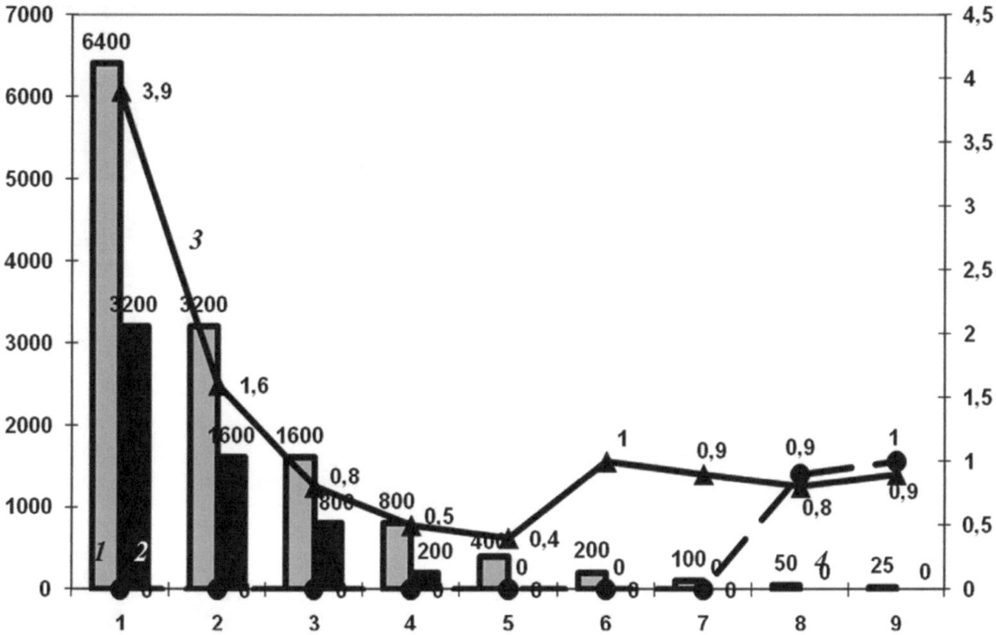

Fig. 4. Initial IgG titer (*1*), decrease of IgG titer (*2*), decrease of antigen titer (*3*), neutralization of TBEV
3 lg $TCID_{50}$ (*4*) in samples with serial two-fold IgG dilutions.
X-axis – sample number
Y1-axis (left) – IgG titer via ELISA, Y2-axis (right) – antigen titre via ELISA

There is also the virus neutralization from the sample with IgG titer of 1:3200 to the one of 1:100. With the further antibody dilution (1:50 and 1:25) on the monolayer of the pig embryo kidney (PEK) cell culture, a cytopathic effect of non-neutralized virus with a titer of 0.9 and 1.0 lg $TCID_{50}$ was detected in the samples.

4.2 Experimental studies (experiment №2)

To confirm the obtained data, we performed the second set of experiments (in vivo and in vitro). TBEV doses from 1 to 8 $TCID_{50}$ were compared via neutralization by immunoglobulin (titers 1:3200 and 1:400). Titration in PEK cells (Fig. 5 *A*) showed that IgG (titer 1:400) entirely neutralized 3 lg $TCID_{50}$ of TBEV as in the first set of experiments, and IgG (titer 1:3200) neutralized 4 lg $TCID_{50}$. Moreover, after IgG treatment (titer 1:3200), initial virus titer (5-6 lg $TCID_{50}$ or 7-8 lg $TCID_{50}$) was reduced by 3-4 lg $TCID_{50}$ or 1-2 lg $TCID_{50}$, respectively. Titration on mice (Fig. 5 *B*) showed that IgG (1:400) entirely neutralized TBEV at 3 lg LD_{50} and decreased TBEV titer by 3-4 lg LD50 in comparison with the initial 4, 5, 6 lg LD50, but was unable to neutralize 7 and 8 lg LD_{50}. IgG with titer of 1:3200 entirely neutralized 5 lg LD_{50} and decreased TBEV titer of 6, 7 and 8 lg LD_{50} by 5.5 lg LD_{50}, 3 lg LD_{50}, and 2 lg LD_{50} of TBEV, respectively.

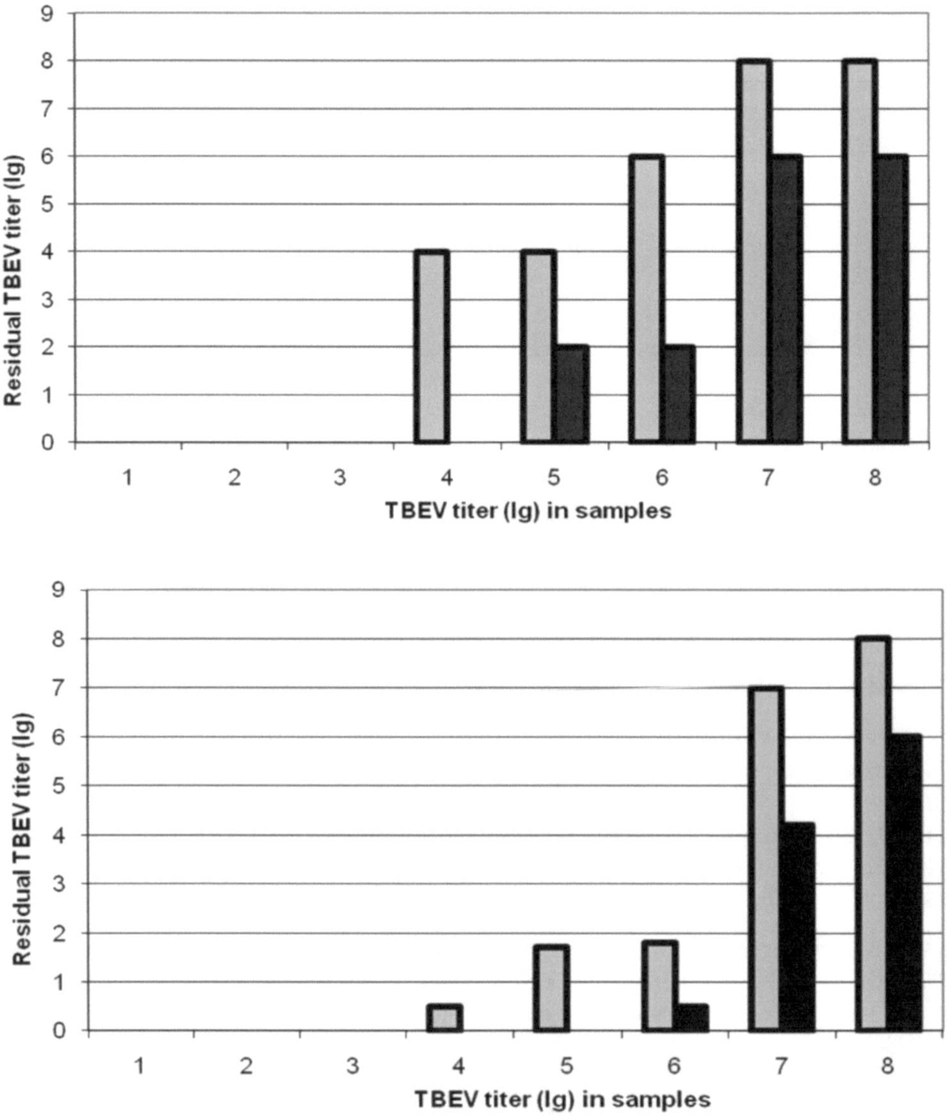

Fig. 5. IgG protective effect with titers of 1:400 (1) and 1:3200 (2) against TBEV (1-8 lg $TCID_{50}$ (A) & 1-8 lg LD_{50}(B)
A - PKE cells (*in vitro*); *B* - white mice (*in vivo*);
X-axis - sample number

According to our data on neutralization of different IgG antibody titers with one dose of TBEV (3 lg $TCID_{50}$), we considered a lower threshold of antibody protective level to be 1:400 in ELISA and 1:20 in NT. The second set of experiments confirmed that in ELISA IgG titer of 1:400 should be considered as the lower threshold of antibody protective level, and this threshold can be used for evaluation of immunological effectiveness of vaccines used for TBEV prevention.

Therefore, the set of experiments on neutralization of different antibody titers of IgG class with one TBEV dose (3 lg $TCID_{50}$) allowed us to consider a minimal protective antibody threshold level to be at 1:400 via IFA and 1:20 via NT. Additional evidence was obtained during neutralization of TBEV with different titers using immunoglobulin having maximal (1:3200) and minimal (1:400) antibody titers. These experiments confirmed the suggestion that IgG titer of 1:400 for IFA should be considered the minimal protective antibody threshold level. It can be used for evaluation of immunologic effectiveness of vaccines used to prevent from TBE. Additionally, antibody titer of 1:100 can be considered as a lower threshold of immunological memory.

Here we used TBEV at suboptimal doses of 1, 2, 3 lg $TCID_{50}$ which are usual for tick bites on humans. As a rule, such doses occur in nature not only in ticks (*Ixodidae*), but also in Muridae rodents as their main hosts. The viremia in these rodents may overweight infectivity threshold (2.7 - 3.0 lg LD_{50} of TBEV) and, thus, ensure the virus transfer to ticks, as well as the stable virus circulation in environment [*Chunikhin et al.* 1985]. Nevertheless, cases of tick infection with TBEV over the mentioned threshold, if compare with theoretical possibility, are rather rare. It is, in turn, a protective factor which provides a relatively low number of TBE cases.

Thus, at epidemiologically crucial virus dose of 3 lg $TCID_{50}$, IgG protective effect was observed in experimental samples from the titer of 1:6400 to 1:100. Hence, we consider that the antibody titer of 1:100 not as a protective threshold level according to Sanitary and epidemiologic rules and regulations of the Russian Federation [Sanitary and epidemiologic rules and regulations SP 3.1.3.2352-07. 2008], but a lower threshold of immunological memory which allows a vaccination course to be continued. At the same time, patients vaccinated against TBE and having antibody titer of 1:100 in their blood can not to fall ill, provided that after a tick bite, the virus titer penetrated into blood was very low. However, a possibility of TBE disease still remains. Moreover, in the group of vaccinated patients, there are tick bite cases followed not only by febrile TBE form, but also sometimes by a clinical picture of brain damage. In addition, it has been shown that high IgG titers (1:3200) actively neutralized TBEV and, obviously, were able to provide a reliable protection from this disease. In the second set of comparative experiments on neutralization of different TBEV doses (from 1 to 8 lg) with immunoglobulin and antibody titers of 1:400 and 1:3200, we obtained additional evidence that the IgG titer of 1:400 is a minimal protective antibody threshold level. The obtained data can be used at any postvaccinal time for observation on immunological effectiveness of vaccinal prevention. Antibody titers of 1:400 and below indicate that revaccination is necessary.

4.3 Evaluation of immunological effectiveness of vaccine Encepur® Adults

In our earlier studies [Leonova et al. 2006; Leonova, 2009], we noticed that during the whole course of three-fold vaccination, antibodies of IgG class were observed in all blood samples, in 100% of cases, when the patients had specific antibodies (seropositive group) before undergoing full course of immunization. In seronegative group, antibodies of IgG class increased dynamically during the whole course of vaccination. However, characteristics of immune response stress according to NT data were of special interest. In seropositive group, titers of the virus neutralizing antibodies after the third vaccine were significantly behind the ones in seronegative group (GTM 1:208). Such lag was evidence that the patients of this group had got an excessive antigen stress on the immune system which resulted in a considerable exhaustion and decrease in activity of immune response. This data should be taken into account when determining time of revaccinations.

We evaluated immunological effectiveness of vaccine Encepur® Adults in remote periods after the primary course of vaccination. We analyzed blood sera of the patients (n=10) three and five years later after the vaccination. ELISA data (Fig. 6) showed that IgG titers in the patients were high three years later after full course of vaccination: 1:3200 – six cases, 1:1600 – one case, 1:800 – one case and 1:400 – two cases. The avidity index of these antibodies was high or had a mean value. Five years later, characteristics of immune response decreased: IgG 1:3200 remained in three cases, 1:1600 – two cases, 1:800 – two cases, 1:400 – two cases, and 1:200 – one case. The avidity index also decreased: it had the mean value in five cases and was lower in another five cases.

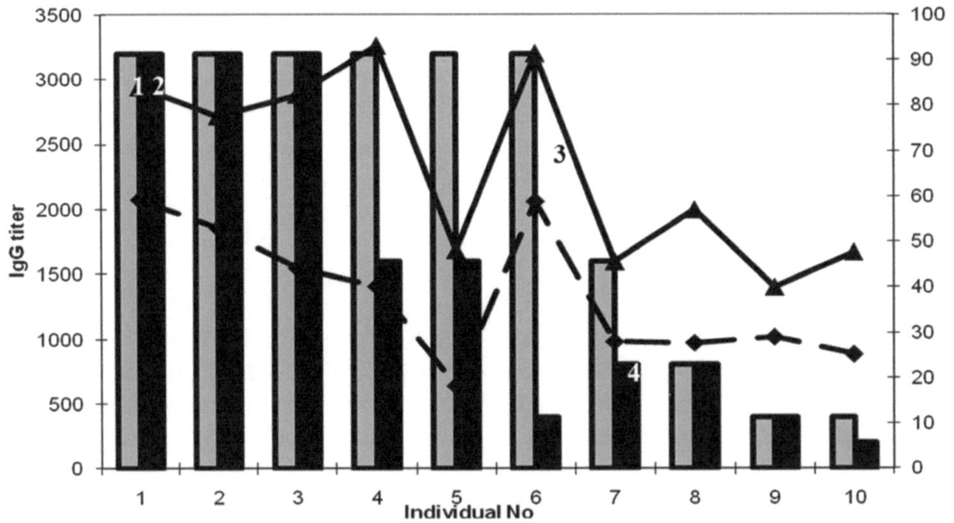

Fig. 6. The level of specific antibodies of patients immunized by Encepur® Adults
1 – IgG level three years later after immunization;
2 – IgG level five years later after immunization;
3 – antibody avidity later three years after immunization;
4 – antibody avidity five years after immunization
X-axis – sample number
Y-1 axis (left) – IgG titer via ELISA, Y-2 axis (right) – IgG titer via NT

Then, we continued studying immune response in this group of patients (n=15) in the last observation period, seven years later after full course of immunization, and one month later after the first revaccination (RV_1). It was determined that before RV_1, the percentage of patients with IgG antibodies according to IFA was 93.3% and GMT – 1:1120. Avid antibodies were found in 80% of the vaccinated patients, avidity index (AI) ranged from 45.2 to 91.4%, and was 69.6±4.5% at the mean. After RV_1, the values of immune response increased in these patients. We found specific antibodies in 100% of the patients. The stress of immune response was: IgG GMT – 1:3200 and AI – 83.6±4.8% (p=0,047).

The results of this study gave us evidence on reasonability of a selection of TBEV antigen stress in the vaccine Encepur® Adults having not only high values of immune response, but

also a long-term protective effect [*Zent et. al.* 2003; 2005; 2005]. Additionally, using IFA, we performed the comparative analysis of immunogenic activity of the vaccine Encepur® Adults to the TBEV strains P-73 (Far Eastern subtype) and Kolarovo (Siberian subtype) isolated from the ticks I. pavlovskiy. Before revaccination, the percentage of patients with antibodies to these strains was 100% while GMT to the strain P-73 was 1:91 and to the Kolarovo strain - 1:158. After revaccination, GMT to the strain P-73 was 1:239 and to the Kolarovo strain – 1:447. These data are evidence of a higher level of antibodies to the Siberian TBEV subtype in the vaccinated patients in comparison with that of the strain P-73 of Far eastern TBE subtype, thus, making a good reason to recommend using this vaccine not only in European countries and Far East, but also on the whole focal territory of Siberia.
For the first time, we obtained evidence for the lower threshold level of protective IgG titer in different experiments. Therefore, at the virus dose of 3 lg $TCID_{50}$, protective effect of IgG was detected with titers ranging from 1:6400 to 1:100. Cytopathic effect was not registered in the PEK cell culture infected with these samples. We considered a lower threshold of protective IgG activity to be 1:400 according to ELISA data, and 1:20 according to NT. Although this sample was positive according to RT-PCR, we did not identify virus antigen in ELISA, and antibodies in the examined sample eliminated completely. With the further decrease of antibody titer, we observed an increase in characteristics of K values via antigen-detection ELISA. Moreover, free infective virus up to 1lg TCD_{50} appeared in the samples with IgG titer lower than 1:100 (ELISA data). Due to this fact, we considered that antibody titer of 1:100 can not be called a threshold of protective level as it was reported by [*Leonova G.N.*, 2009], but a lower threshold of immunological memory enabling further vaccination. Patients vaccinated against TBE with antibody titer of 1:100 in blood cannot fall ill after a tick bite, if they receive a relatively low virus dose. However, the possibility of TBE infection still remains. In addition to febrile forms of disease, there are also some cases of severe damage of nervous system occurring among immunized patients. Moreover, high IgG titers (1:3200) actively neutralized TBEV and were probably capable of ensuring a safeguard against this disease. The second set of comparative experiments on neutralization of different TBEV doses (from 1 to 8 lg) with IgG titer of 1:400 and initial antibody titer of 1:3200 gave the additional evidence that IgG titer 1:400 is a minimal level of protective antibody activity. These data can be used at any time of observation after vaccination of the patients to evaluate the immunological effectiveness of vaccines used for TBEV prevention. Antibody titers of 1:400 and below indicate the necessity of revaccination.
Taking into account the experimental data, we analyzed the individual immune response of ten patients vaccinated with Encepur® Adults three and five years later after a course of three vaccine injections. We determined that this vaccine enables long-term production of antibodies which remains for up to seven years (observation time). As a rule, repeated vaccination contributes to formation of high-avidity antibodies [Leonova *GN & Pavlenko EV*, 2009] which usually have high affinity to specific antigen sites and are able to eliminate antigen actively. A considerable part of immune sera of vaccinated patients contained avid antibodies with high AI three years later after a full course of vaccination, and moderate AI five years later after vaccination. It reached the mean value in half of cases, and a lower value in the rest ones. In other words, patients with antigen titer of 1:400 and below, as well as those with low avidity should be revaccinated in five years after full course of vaccination. This approach to vaccination time was confirmed by the work of Heinz FX et al. [2008], who recommended revaccinations for all patients vaccinated against TBEV, and five

years later, revaccination was not recommended only to the aged patients. Therefore, the data obtained on the threshold level of antibody titer (1:400) and determination of a minimal level of their immunological memory (1:100) helps to determine an immunological protectiveness of the vaccinated patients and duration of postvaccinal protective immunity and, thus, specify revaccination schedule. To obtain the maximal immunological and epidemiological effectiveness of vaccinal prevention against TBEV, individual approach to each patient is appropriate. Moreover, it may have medical and economic importance.

5. Conclusion

The most important characteristics of a vaccine preparation are its immunogenic activity and capability of a long-term preservation of antibodies in vaccinated patients. These characteristics should be taken into account when determining time of revaccinations. Immunization course with different vaccines made from western and Far Eastern TBEV subtypes, as well as combined vaccination with different preparations provided the high and stable seroconversion according to IFA and NT. In accordance with the above experimental data, we have analysed an individual immune response in the patients vaccinated with Encepur® Adults three, five, and seven years later after the three-fold course of vaccination. It has been shown that this vaccine enables production of antibodies which are being preserved for a long time, up to seven years. As a rule, repeated vaccination contributed to formation of high-avidity antibodies [*Leonova G.N., 2009*] which usually had a high affinity level to specific antigen sites and were capable of active antigen elimination. Considerable part of immune sera from vaccinated patients contained avid antibodies which AI was still high three years later. Five and seven years later after full course of vaccination, AI decreased. High values of immune response after RV_1 seven years later after full course of vaccination gave us strong evidence that the obtained data on antibody avidity, protective antibody titer threshold (1:400) and minimal level of immunological memory (1:100) are considered to be the crucial parameters in detection of immunoprotection of vaccinated patients. Based on these data, we suggest that revaccination schedule should be individual for a vaccinated patient for obtaining the maximal immunological and epidemiological effect of vaccinal TBE prevention. Such approach to determination of revaccination time is of economic and medical importance.

6. Acknowledgements

Authors are grateful to Novartis GmbH. The work was supported by the ISTC grant No. 4006.

7. References

Bock HL, Klockmann U, Jungst C, Schindel-Kunzel F, Theobald K, Zerban R. (1990) A new vaccine against tick-borne encephalitis: initial trial in man including a dose-response study. *Vaccine* 8(1), pp. 22–4.

Briko NI. (2000). Criteria of vaccination effectiveness assessment, *Vaktsinatsiya*. 5, (11) http://medi.ru/doc/15b.1101.htm.

Charrel RN, Attoui H, Butenko AM, et al. (2004).Tick-borne virus diseases of human interest in Europe. *Clin Microbiol Infect*. 10, (12), pp. 1040-55.

Chunikhin SP. & Leonova GN. (1985). *Ecology and Geographic Distribution of Arboviruses.* Meditsina Publishers, Moscow, 126 p.

Dorokhova V.S. & Tatarinova L.G. (1969).Tick-Borne Encephalitis Morbidity in Primorye Territory. *Feral herd infections of Ural, Siberia and the Far East.* Sverdlovsk, pp. 56-57.

Ecker M, Allison SL, Meixner T, et al. (1999). Sequence analysis and genetic classification of tick-borne encephalitis viruses from Europe and Asia. *J Gen Virol.* 80, pp. 179–85.

Heinz FX, & Kunz C. (2004).Tick-borne encephalitis and the impact of vaccination. *Arch Virol.* 18, pp. 201-205.

Heinz FX, Holzmann H, Essl A, Kundt M. (2008). Analysis of the efficiency of tick-borne encephalitis vaccination in the population in the natural foci of Austria. *Vopr Virusol.* 53, (2).1, pp. 9-27.

Holzmann H, Vorobyova MS, Ladyzhenskaya I et al. (1992). Molecular epidemiology of tick-borne-encephalitis virus: cross-protection between European and Far Eastern subtypes. *Vaccine* 10, pp. 345–49.

Klockmann U., Krivanec K., Stephenson J.R., Hilfenhaus J. (1991). Protection against European isolates of tick-borne encephalitis virus after vaccination with a new tick-borne encephalitis. *Vaccine* 9, pp. 210-212.

Kunz CH., Heinz F, Hofmann H. (1980). Immunogenicity and Reactogenicity of a Highly Purified Vaccine against Tick-borne Encephalitis. *J. Med. Virol.* 6, pp.103-109.

Kunz C. (2003). TBE vaccination and Austrian experience. *Vaccine* 21, pp. S1/50–S1/55.

Leonova GN. (1997). *Tick-borne encephalitis in Primorsky krai.* ISBN 5-7442-0721-X, Vladivostok, 187 p.

Leonova GN, Belikov SI, Kulakova NV, Pavlenko EV, Borisevich VG. (2004) Molecular typing of tick-borne encephalitis
strains isolated from human cases differing in the degree of severity in the south of Russian Far East. *Mol Gen Mikrobiol Virusol* (2), pp.:32–37

Leonova GN, Pavlenko EV, Krylova NV. (2006). *Vaccine Prevention of Tick-Borne Encephalitis.* ISBM 5-9002274-32-2, Vladivostok, 100 p.

Leonova GN, Ternovoi VA, Pavlenko EV et al. (2007). Evaluation of vaccine Encepur® Adult for induction of human neutralizing antibodies against recent Far Eastern subtype strains of tick-borne encephalitis. *Vaccine* 25, pp. 895–901.

Leonova GN, & Pavlenko EV. (2009). Characterization of neutralizing antibodies to Far Eastern of tick-borne encephalitis virus subtype and the antibody avidity for four tick-borne encephalitis vaccines in human. *Vaccine* 27, (21). pp. 2899-2904.

Leonova G.N. (2009).*The tick-borne Encephalitis: actual aspects.* ISBM 978-5-91563-031-3, Moscow, 168 p.

Loktev VB, Ternovoi VA, Netesov SV. (2007). Molecular genetic characterization of tick-borne encephalitis virus. *Vopr Virusol* 5, pp. 10–16

Memoirs on Elizabeth Nikolaevna Levkovich (under V.V.Pogodinoj's edition) Moscow, 2001.

Onishchenko G.G., Fedorov Y.M., Pakskina N.D. (2007). Organization of supervision for tick-borne encephalitis and it's preventive maintenance in Russian Federation. *Vopr Virusol.* 5, pp. 8-10.

Pavlenko E.V., Leonova G.N., Radchenko L.P. (2010). Cliniko-epidemiological analyses of tick-borne encephalitis in Primorye Territory. *Des.delo* №1, pp. 27-30.

Petri E., Gniel D, Zent O. (2010). Tick-borne encephalitis (TBE) trends in epidemiology and current and future management. *Travel Medicine and Infectious Disease* 8, 233-245.

Pogodina VV, Karan' LS, Kolyasnikova NM, et al. (2007). The evolution of tick-borne encephalitis and the problem of the pathogen evolution. *Vopr Virusol.* 5, 16–26.

Prevention of tick-borne encephlitis. Sanitary and epidemiologic rules and regulations. SP 3.1.3.2352-07, 2008.

Smorodintsev A.A. & Doubov A.V. (1986). *Tick- borne encephalitis and its prevention.* Medicana, Moscow, 232 p.

Takashima I, Hayasaka D, Goto A, et al. (2001). Epidemiology of tick-borne encephalitis (TBE) and phylogenetic analysis of TBE viruses in Japan and Far Eastern Russia. *J Infect Dis.* 54, pp. 1–11.

Ternovoi VA, Protopopova EV, Chausov EV, et al. (2007). Novel variant of tick-borne encephalitis virus. *Emerg Infect Dis* 13 (10), pp. 1574–78.

Vereta LA, & Vorobyeva MS. (1990). *Natural heterogeneity and aim-directed selection of strains of the tick-borne encephalitis virus.* Moscow, 122 p.

Vorobyova MS, Rasshchepkina MN, Ladyzhenskaya IP. (2007). Vaccine, immunoglobulin, and test kits for prevention and diagnostics of tick-borne encephalitis. *Vopr Virusol.* 6, pp. 30-36.

Zent O, Beran J, Jilg W, Mach T, Banzhoff A. (2003). Clinical evaluation of a polygeline-free tick-borne encephalitis vaccine for adolescents and adults. *Vaccine.* 21(7-8), pp.738-41.

Zent O, & Bro¨ker M. (2005). Tick-borne encephalitis vaccines: past and present. *Expert Rev Vaccines.* 4(5), pp. 747-55.

Zent O, Hennig R, Banzhoff A, Bro¨ker M. (2005). Protection against tick-borne encephalitis with a new vaccine formulation free of protein-derived stabilizers. *J Travel Med.* 12(2), pp. 85-93.

11

Tick-Borne Encephalitis Virus Quasispecies Rearrangements in Ticks and Mammals

Bakhvalova V.N.[1], Panov V.V.[1] and Morozova O.V.[2]
[1]*Institute of Systematics and Ecology of Animals of Siberian Branch of the Russian Academy of Sciences, Novosibirsk,*
[2]*Institute of Chemical Biology and Fundamental Medicine of Siberian Branch of the Russian Academy of Sciences, Novosibirsk*
Russia

1. Introduction

Tick-borne encephalitis (TBE) is one of the most dangerous flavivirus infection of the central nervous system in Eurasia. The etiological agent, the TBE virus (TBEV) is transmitted to man by tick bytes. Geographic natural habitat of the TBEV appeared to be discontinuous and extended throughout southern part of Eurasian forest belt from Pacific to Atlantic ocean mainly within distribution areas of the virus vectors - ixodid ticks. TBE outbreaks have been registered in northern China and Japan in the east, through Russia to about 30 European countries including France, northern Italy and Norway in the west with the highest morbidity rates in Russia, Austria, Czech Republic, Slovenia and the Baltics (Latvia, Lithuania and Estonia) (Gritsun et al, 2003; Mansfield et al., 2009). In France, Italy, Greece, Norway and Denmark, TBE is of minor importance. In the United Kingdom, Ireland, Belgium, the Netherlands, Luxembourg, Spain and Portugal, TBE is not indigenous and no TBE cases have been reported yet. Detailed epidemiological statistics from 1990 onwards can be obtained from the website of the International Scientific Working Group on TBE [http://www.isw-tbe.info]. The TBE prevalence is increasing worldwide with spread of the virus to previously non-endemic countries in Europe (France) and Asia (China, Mongolia, Japan and South Korea). TBEV is listed as a category C agent on the Centers for Disease Control and Prevention (USA) list of select biological agents.
The TBEV persists in endemic regions or so-called natural foci, where it circulates among vertebrate hosts (mainly small rodents and insectivorous) and the arthropod vectors (ticks). Years of observations of the distribution of TBE incidences suggest that such natural foci are very stable. Formation, development and stability of the TBE natural foci are determined by the coincidence of several ecological factors including temperature, relative air humidity, soil humidity, biotope vegetation, population density and dynamics of ixodid ticks and their hosts, susceptibility of reservoir hosts to the TBEV, proportion of immune hosts as well as the virus prevalence among both ticks and vertebrate hosts (Hofmann, 1973; Plassmann, 1980; L'vov et al., 1989; Korotkov et al., 2007; Tick-Borne Encephalitis (TBE) and its Immunoprophylaxis, 1996 and references therein). Reservoir host species abundance, multiple transmission cycles and adaptation of the TBEV to different hosts cause long-term resistance of the parasitic system in endemic regions.

The TBEV as a typical member of the *Flaviviridae* family possesses a single-stranded, positive genomic RNA of approximately 11 kb in length, containing a 5′ cap and lacking a 3′-terminal polyadenylate tail (Gritsun et al., 2003; Mansfield et al., 2009 and references therein). Molecular typing of the TBEV using different methods (ELISA, molecular hybridization with radioactive oligonucleotide probes and RT-PCR with subsequent sequencing of E gene) revealed 3 main subtypes: Far Eastern, Siberian and European (Pogodina et al., 1981; Zlobin et al., 1996; Ecker et al., 1999; Bakhvalova et al., 2000).

Currently, according to the International Committee for Taxonomy of Viruses, TBEV is classified as one species with three subtypes, namely the Far Eastern subtype (mainly isolates from far-eastern Russia, China and Japan), currently widely spread Siberian subtype (earlier isolates from Eastern and Western Siberia, Urals and far-eastern Russia and at present dominant subtype in many TBE endemic regions of Russia and surrounding countries, gradually replacing 2 other TBEV subtype (Pogodina et al., 2007) and the European subtype (which comprises almost all known isolates from Europe) (Gritsun et al., 2003; Mantke et al., 2008; Mansfield et al., 2009 and references therein). The 3 TBEV subtypes are associated with varying degrees of disease severity. Human infections with Far Eastern subtype viruses are usually severe, frequently with encephalitic symptoms (focal meningoencephalitis or polyencephalitis), with an associated fatality rate between 5 and 35% (earlier 20-60%). This type does not cause chronic disease. In contrast, infection with the TBEV Siberian subtype cause a less severe disease (fatality rate between 1 and 3% (earlier 6-8%)), with a tendency for patients to develop chronic or extremely prolonged infections accompanied by diverse neurological and/or neuropsychiatric symptoms. In contrast to these two forms, infections caused by European strains typically take a biphasic course: the first (viraemic) phase presents as an influenza-like illness lasting 1–8 days with fever, malaise, headache, myalgia, gastrointestinal symptoms, leukocytopenia, thrombocytopenia and elevated liver enzymes, often followed by a symptom-free interval of about 1–33 days and the second phase in 20–30% of infected patients with clinical features of different severity (meningitis, meningoencephalitis, meningoencephalomyelitis or meningoencephaloradiculitis), the appearance of specific antibodies in the serum and cerebrospinal fluid and the fatality rate less than 2% (Gritsun et al., 2003; Mantke et al., 2008; Mansfield et al., 2009 and references therein). Accordingly, ratio of different TBEV subtypes could influence on the TBE severity.

Recently, a new classification of the tick-borne flaviviruses based on phylogenetic analysis of complete coding sequences of their genomes had been proposed (Grard et al., 2007). According to the recommendation the tick-borne flaviviruses should be divided into 4 types (i.e. Western tick-borne encephalitis virus, Eastern tick-borne encephalitis virus, Turkish sheep tick-borne encephalitis virus and louping ill tick-borne encephalitis virus) (Grard et al., 2007). However, it has not yet been accepted by the International Committee on Taxonomy of Viruses.

Moreover, new phylogenetically distant variants of the TBEV isolated in Irkutsk endemic region, Eastern Siberia, Russia and Mongolia that do not belong to any known genetic subtype (Khasnatinov et al., 2010; GenBank accession numbers EF469662 and EF469661 for strains 886-84 and 178-79, respectively).

Ticks are known to be main carriers (so-called vectors) and reservoir hosts of the TBEV in nature. Their ability to feed on a variety of vertebrate animals, intracellular digestion of blood and their long life cycle for 3-6 years and feeding at each stage of development make them ideal vectors for many tick-borne infectious agents including the TBEV. Natural TBEV infection had been revealed for 16 species of ixodid ticks (Korenberg, 1989). Thus, in Central Europe TBEV was revealed in 8 species of "hard" ticks having a dorsal shield: *Ixodes persulcatus* Schulze, *Ixodes ricinus* L., *Ixodes hexagonus, Ixodes arboricola, Haemaphysalis punctata, Haemaphysalis concinna* Koch, *Dermacentor marginatus* Sulz. and *Dermacentor reticulatus* (Tick-Borne Encephalitis and references therein). In the Western Siberia population of ixodid ticks in the TBE endemic regions included *I. persulcatus* Sch., *I. ricinus* L., *Ixodes pavlovskyi* Pom., *D. reticulatus* Fabr., *D. marginatus* Sulz., *Dermacentor silvarum* Ol., *Dermacentor nuttalli* Ol., *H.concinna* Koch (Bogdanov, 2006).

The distribution of TBE may be determined by the occurrence of the respective tick vectors in certain regions. While *Ixodes ricinus* is the prevalent hard tick species across Europe and therefore the most important transmitter of the TBEV European subtype, *Ixodes persulcatus* inhabits in forest regions of the Urals, Siberia, far-eastern Russia and China and is the main vector of the other subtypes. Co-circulation of two or all three subtypes could be shown for Finland and the Baltic states where the distribution areas of the two main tick species overlap. The TBEV can be transmitted to vertebrate hosts or man by larvae, nymphs or adult ticks. Ticks provide the TBEV persistence during each stage of development, the virus amplification as well as both transovarial and transstadial transfer (Balashov, 2010). The TBEV was described to activate ticks in their host pursuit and to induce hormone of molt thus reducing a period of a tick development (Alekseev, 1990; Korotkov, Burencova, 2006).

The ixodid ticks parasitize more than 100 different species of mammals, birds, reptiles and amphibians thus providing the TBEV transmission and the vertebrate reservoir hosts involvement into epizootic process (Levkovich et al., 1967; Filippova, 1985). For most vertebrate natural hosts, TBEV is apathogenic without any infection manifestations but induces the virus-specific antibodies (Bakhvalova et al., 2006 and references therein). The TBEV is capable for lifelong persistence with reduced reproduction activity mainly within mammal cells to escape from extracellular specific antibodies (Bakhvalova et al., 2006 and references therein).

Transmission of the TBEV in the wild takes place in different interrelated ways. During feeding of ticks on animals, either viremic or nonviremic transmission can take place (Bakhvalova et al., 2006 and references therein). In addition, vertical transovarial, transstadial and horizontal sexual transmission may take place between both ticks and warm-blooded hosts (Bakhvalova et al., 2009 and references therein). TBEV maintenance mechanisms may differ in acute and persistent infection (Bakhvalova et al., 2006 and references therein).

Evolution of flaviviruses evidently depends on their hosts (Zanotto et al.1995, Gould et al. 1997). Arthtopod-borne viruses reproduce in distantly related hosts such as vertebrates and invertebrates. Essential differences of host organisms cause selection of certain genetic variants of flavivirus quasispecies. Tick-adapted variants of TBEV were shown to exhibit small-plaque phenotype and slower replication in mammal cells, decreased neuroinvasiveness in laboratory mice and higher yield in laboratory line of ticks caused by 15 nucleotide substitutions (Romanova et al., 2007). Mammal-adapted variants possess inherent inverse properties. Host switch induce changes in ratio of the host-adapted variants. Tick-adapted variants might have selective advantages during reproduction of the virus in ticks during diapause without involving mammal hosts. Similarly, during TBEV persistence in mammals with vertical transmission from parents to their progeny, the mammal-adapted variants could accumulate and prevail. However, the TBEV adaptation to different hosts in the wild under natural conditions remains unclear.

Our aim was to compare the TBEV infection of ticks and small mammals in an endemic region for 30 years of observation.

2. Ticks and tick-adapted variants of the TBEV

Study of the TBE parasitic system includes system analysis of dynamics and interrelationships of all 3 components: TBEV with detection, identification and viral load quantitation, population density and dynamics of both ticks and vertebrate hosts.

TBE epidemiology is closely related to the ecology and biology of ticks. Throughout the world about 850 tick species are classified into 2 families: The *Ixodidae* (ixodid or hard ticks) and the *Argasidae* (argasid or soft ticks). Ticks transmit viruses, bacteria, fungi, protozoa and nematodes. Approximately 25% of the viruses isolated from field-collected arthropods are from ticks. At least 14 from more than 70 known flaviviruses are transmitted by ticks, generally ixodid species. Digestive process is an unusual feature of ticks from other arthropods. Except for hemolysis of the blood cells in the midgut lumen, digestion in ticks is entirely intracellular, a process known as heterophagy. All digestion is accomplished within epithelial cells of midgut. Tick saliva apparently lacks hemolytic enzymes, and the erythrocytes and other cellular elements are ingested unchanged. Blood taken into the midgut of the tick remains largely undigested for long periods, therefore viruses and bacteria remain in nonhostile environment, favors virus entry as extracellular virions and via infected host cells. The undigested blood meal remains as a food reserve. Therefore, ticks are able to survive for extended periods of starvation (Nutall and Labuda, 2003). Ixodid ticks feed for periods ranging from a few days to several weeks. To concentrate the dilute blood meal, ticks use their salivary glands to periodically secrete excess water from the blood meal back into the host. All developmental stages (except males) consume many times their original body weight in blood and other fluid, mated females often imbibe more than 100 times their unfed body weight. The ability of ticks to produce thousands of eggs is important in their population dynamics. An *I. ricinus* or *I. persulcatus* females are capable of laying 350 to 5000 eggs, depending mostly on the amount of consumed blood. Immature stages of *I. ricinus* and *I. persulcatus* often feed on rodents and birds, whereas adults feed on goats and other ungulates (Nutall and Labuda, 2003). In nature, once infected ticks at each developmental stage remain permanently infected.

Our research was carried out in a recreation zone of Novosibirsk (54°49′ N, 83°05′ E), South-Western Siberia, Russia. For the area temperature is optimal but humidity is rather limited factor for ixodid ticks. Therefore, population density of ticks in Western Siberia is relatively low with high TBEV infection rate (Fig. 1). Since 1980 population density of the ixodid ticks varied from 4.4 to 51.8 ticks/km. One should note that earlier in the region *I. persulcatus* absolutely prevailed, however during the last years rate of *I. pavlovskyi Pom.* in urban and suburban biotopes was significantly grown up to 80% from total ixodid tick population in 2011. Whereas in distant forest areas located at 10-15 km from the city the ratio of *I. pavlovskyi* did not exceed 15%. Similar observations were previously described for other Western Siberian region [Romanenko and Kondratieva, 2010). The changes in ixodid tick fauna might be caused by anthropogenic pressure.

Until now, surveillance of the TBEV infection rate in different endemic regions of Eurasia is not uniform and may affect the prevalence estimates. Thus, currently available data from different countries are difficult to compare. Furthermore, little is known about the true TBEV prevalence in tick populations or about the circulation of new genetic subtypes and hemagglutination-deficient variants. TBEV prevalence in the tick population of endemic areas in Austria was revealed by bioassays to be 0.44-6.2%, in Czech Republic - 0.30-4.50%, in Finland - 0.07-2.56%, in Germany - 0.2-2.0%, in Italy - 0.05%, in Sweden 0.1-1.0%, in Switzerland - 0.1-1.36 and in Russian Federation 3.0-40.0% (Tick-Borne Encephalitis (TBE) and its Immunoprophylaxis, 1996 and references therein). Since discovery of the TBEV in 1937 various methods such as bioassays with infection of permissive tissue cultures or laboratory suckling mice, ELISA, direct and reverse molecular hybridization of nucleic acids (MHNA), reverse transcription (RT) with subsequent PCR and detection of their products by electrophoresis or by fluorescence measurements in real time were used for the virus detection. Currently, the European Network for Diagnostics of "Imported" Viral Diseases (ENIVD) suggests to improve the diagnostics and monitoring of encephalitis viruses in Europe (Mantke et al., 2008).

In Russia tick suspensions from pool (10 ticks in each one) were used for infection of newborn or 2-week-old mice with subsequent identification of the TBEV isolates in serological reactions. TBEV infection rate of adult ticks collected from vegetation varied from 3 to 31.1% of pools of ticks (or from 0.3 to 3.7% of individual ticks) (Beklemishev, 1963) (Fig. 1). Long-term dynamics of population density and TBEV prevalence in ticks were earlier supposed to have positive correlation (Neckiy, Bogdanov,1966). However, later on positive correlation between an abundance and TBEV infection rate of ticks was indeed registered only in natural foci with optimal conditions for tick development, particularly in Far East of Russia (Khabarovsk region) (Vereta, 1975; Vershinskyi, 1984; Okulova, 1986). For taiga endemic regions of Western Siberia correlation was tended to be rather negative (Katin and Pustovalov, 1983). Natural conditions of forest-steppe near Ob river are unfavourable for *I. persulcatus* (Dobrotvorskyi et al., 1994) with diapausa stage for essential part of nymphs. The correlation coefficient between the abundance and TBEV prevalence in ticks appeared to be $r = -0{,}45$, $p = 0{,}012$ during period 1980-2010. The negative correlation ($r = -0{,}75$) is especially evident during the last 6 years (Fig.1).

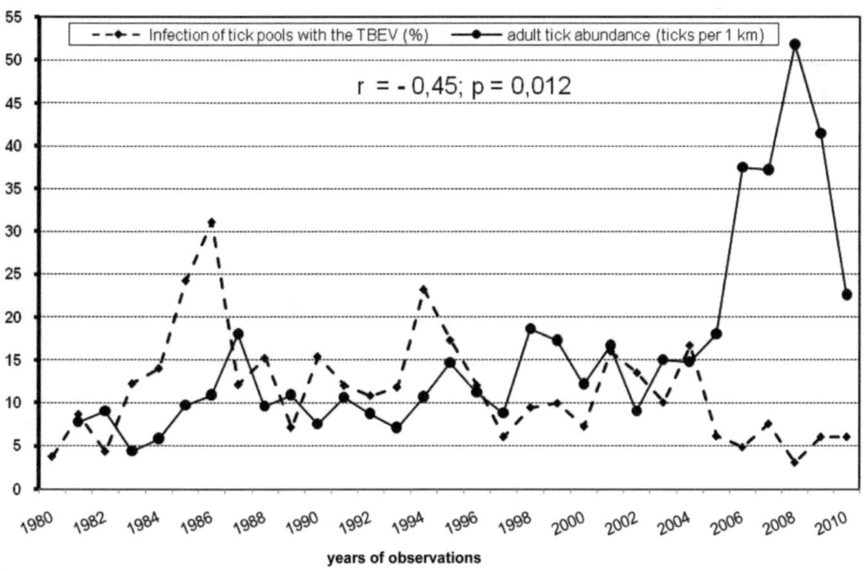

Fig. 1. Long-term dynamics of ixodid ticks abundance and the TBEV infection prevalence

TBEV is typically a hemagglutinating (HA) virus. Ability to agglutinate goose erythrocytes reflects the binding of the TBEV with host cell receptors with subsequent fusion activity and the virus penetration into cells. Whilst most strains of TBEV show HA activity, during the past 10 years atypical HA-deficient strains have been isolated with increasing frequencies in Europe from both ticks and patients. More than 40 HA-deficient strains are now recognized and all of them exhibit reduced pathogenicity for mice in comparison with HA-competent strains (Khasnatinov et al., 2009). The isolation of HA-lacking strains of TBEV from wild ticks from natural populations and from patients confirmed earlier described tick-adapted laboratory TBEV variants with decreased neuroinvasiveness in mice and absence of HA activity (Romanova et al., 2007). However, for laboratory tick-adapted variant of the TBEV Siberian strain EK-328 only 2 amino acid substitutions in the virion surface glycoprotein E - E122G and T426I were found (Romanova et al., 2007), whereas for wild TBEV HA-deficient isolates of European subtype – 3 mutations D67G, E122G and D277A in the envelope protein (Khasnatinov et al., 2009), with the only change E122G being common for all HA-deficient tick-adapted variants. Multiple alignment of amino acid sequences of the TBEV E glycoprotein revealed that mutation E122G is rare event and was not found in our collection of 255 TBEV strains isolated from ticks in Novosibirsk region, South-Western Siberia, Russia during 1980-2010. The one thing that is evident is the constancy of E122. If that amino acid is associated with the mammalian phenotype as described by (Romanova et al., 2007), then a single passage of the tick-adapted strain in mammalian cells may be sufficient to result in the emergence of the mammalian phenotype in most of the quasispecies.

For other tick-borne flavivirus Powassan despite quasispecies rearrangements with average frequency 0.0123% mutations/nucleotide all sequences derived directly from ticks without a passage in mammalian cells included E122 and V427 (427 corresponds to 426 in TBEV) (Ebel, 2009) as previously suggested to be associated with mammal-adapted variants (Romanova et al., 2007). Therefore, the host-induced alternations of amino acids at those positions could hardly cause tick- or mammalian cell-adapted TBEV phenotypes.

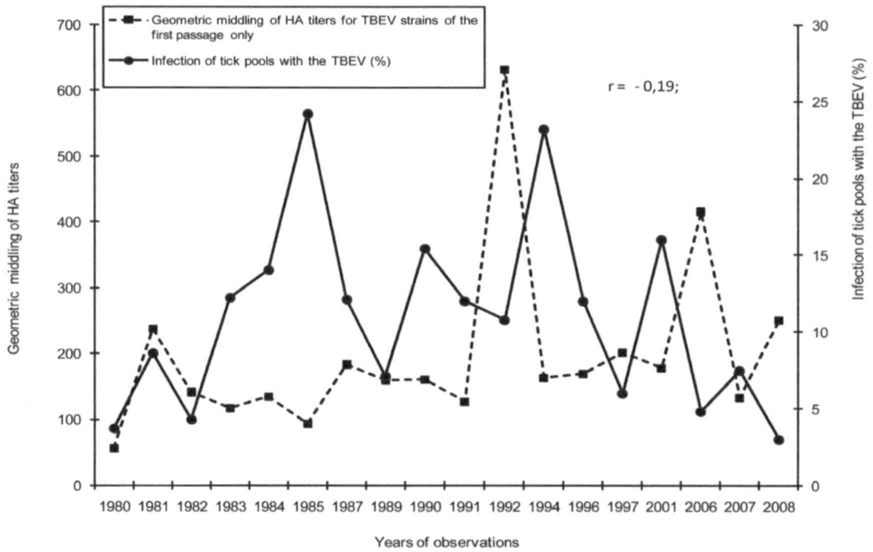

Fig. 2. Reverse correlation between the TBEV prevalence in ticks and hemagglutination (HA) of the TBEV strains for 1980-2008.

Note: geometric middling of HA titers for TBEV strains of the first passage only. For missing years HA titers were determined for other passages of the virus strains

Comparison of long-term dynamics of TBEV prevalence in ticks and HA of the virus strains isolated from the ticks demonstrated slightly negative correlation (r = - 0,19) (Fig. 2). Growth of TBEV-infected tick proportion might cause selection of tick-adapted variants with decreased HA (Romanova et al., 2007; Khasnatinov et al., 2009).

Since 2006 TBEV detection in ticks was performed by using independent methods of bioassays with laboratory white suckling mice, ELISA for the TBEV antigen detection E, reverse transcription with subsequent real-time PCR with primers and fluorescent hydrolysis probes corresponding to the TBEV NS1 or NS5 gene of Siberian or Far Eastern genetic subtype or nested PCR with primer pairs specific to gene E (Bakhvalova et al., 2006; 2009). Molecular methods always confirmed bioassay data but annually allowed us to reveal additional positive samples among tick pools containing apathogenic HA-lacking TBEV or its components - viral RNA and/or glycoprotein E (Fig. 3). Additional passages of the RT-PCR and/or ELISA positive samples using 2-3-days-old mice did not result in TBE symptoms and HA activity but accumulation of TBEV RNA and protein E was observed. The most statistically significant increase of ELISA- and/or RT-PCR-positive samples (p<0,001) was found in 2010 (Fig. 3) compared to steady pathogenic virus prevalence.

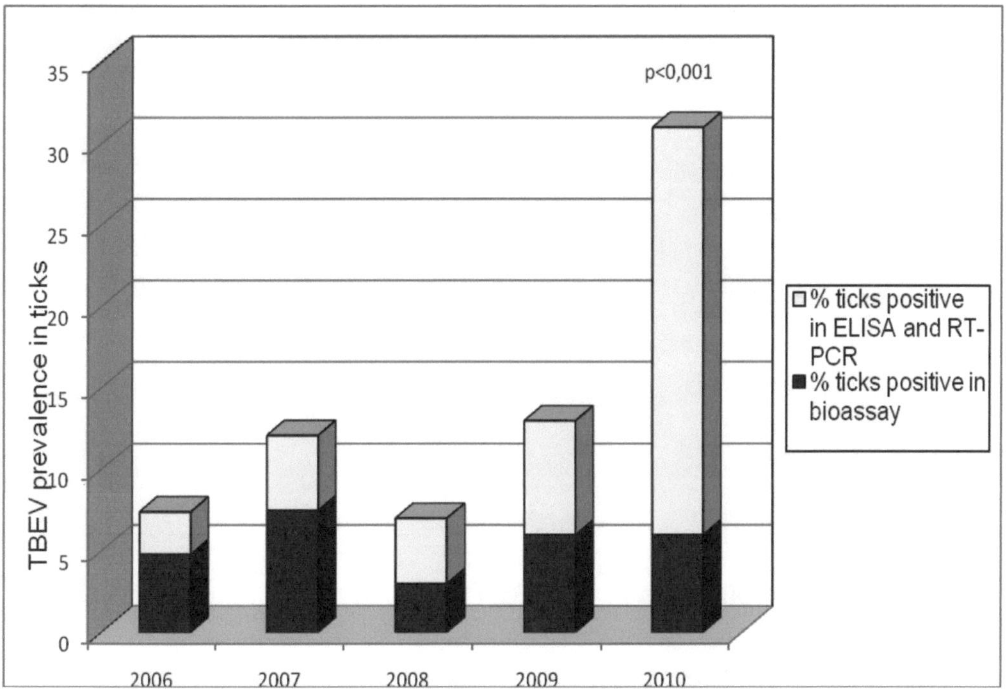

Fig. 3. TBEV detection in pools of unfed adult ticks from Novosibirsk endemic region, South-Western Siberia, Russia by using bioassays (black) and molecular approaches (grey)

During recent decades the epidemiology of the TBEV appears to have been changing, with Siberian genetic subtype gradually replacing Far Eastern and Western European subtypes (Pogodina et al., 2007; Khasnatinov et al., 2009 and references therein). Moreover, Siberian subtype is being isolated more frequently from patients with severe encephalitis. All the TBEV strains isolated for 1980-2010 from ticks in Novosibirsk region, South-Western Siberia,

Russia appeared to belong to Siberian genetic subtype (Morozova et al., 2007). However, real-time RT-PCR with subtype-specific fluorescent probes revealed both Far Eastern and Siberian subtypes with partly mixed infection directly in tick suspensions (Fig. 4).

Quantitation of TBEV RNA using reverse transcription with subsequent real-time PCR with fluorescent hydrolysis probes showed a variation of threshold cycles (Ct) within a range 21-33 for cDNA derived from infected ticks (Fig. 5). According to our calibration with purified plasmid DNA containing cloned full-length DNA copy of the TBEV RNA and taking into account the reverse transcription efficiency as 50% these Ct corresponded to 10^2 -10^7 RNA genome-equivalents per each tick. Analysis of chronological rows of TBEV strains can be performed after numerous passages in mice or tissue cultures with possible quasispecies rearrangements in various hosts.

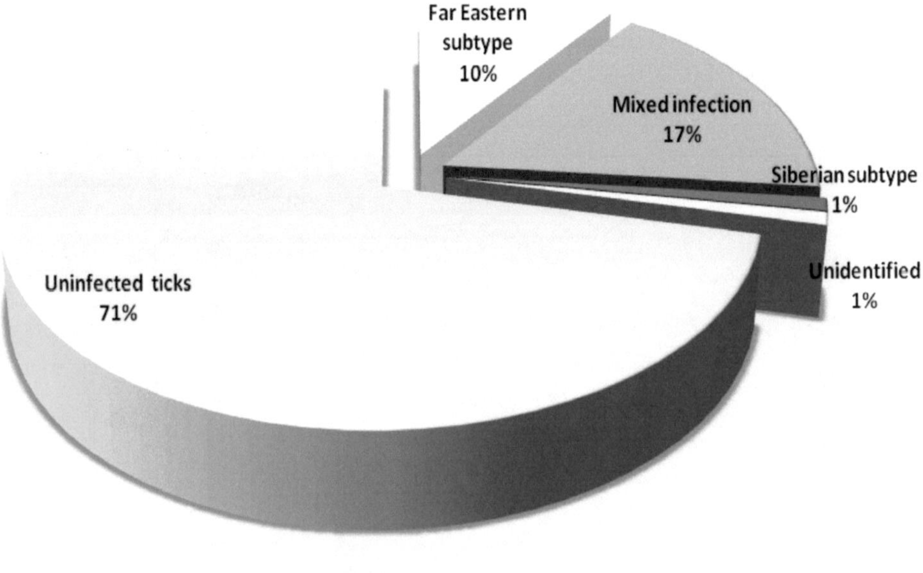

Fig. 4. Ratio of different TBEV subtypes in tick suspensions in 2010

3. Vertebrate reservoir hosts of the TBEV and mammal-adapted variants of the virus

Ixodid ticks feed on more than 100 species of vertebrate hosts including mammals, reptiles, amphibians and birds (Filippova, 1985). Coevolution of viruses with their hosts toward less deleterious infections ensures the survival of both host and virus. Therefore, most wild vertebrates are susceptible and resistant to both mosquito- and tick-borne flaviviruses. Resistance to flavivirus-induced diseases in wild mammals is conferred by the autosomal *Flv*-resistance gene recently identified as 2'-5' oligoadenylate synthetase 1b (*oas*1b) gene that expresses constitutively, does not require interferon induction and inhibits flavivirus replication (Brinton and Perelygin, 2003). Resistant animals are infected productively by flaviviruses but produce lower virus titers, especially in their brains.

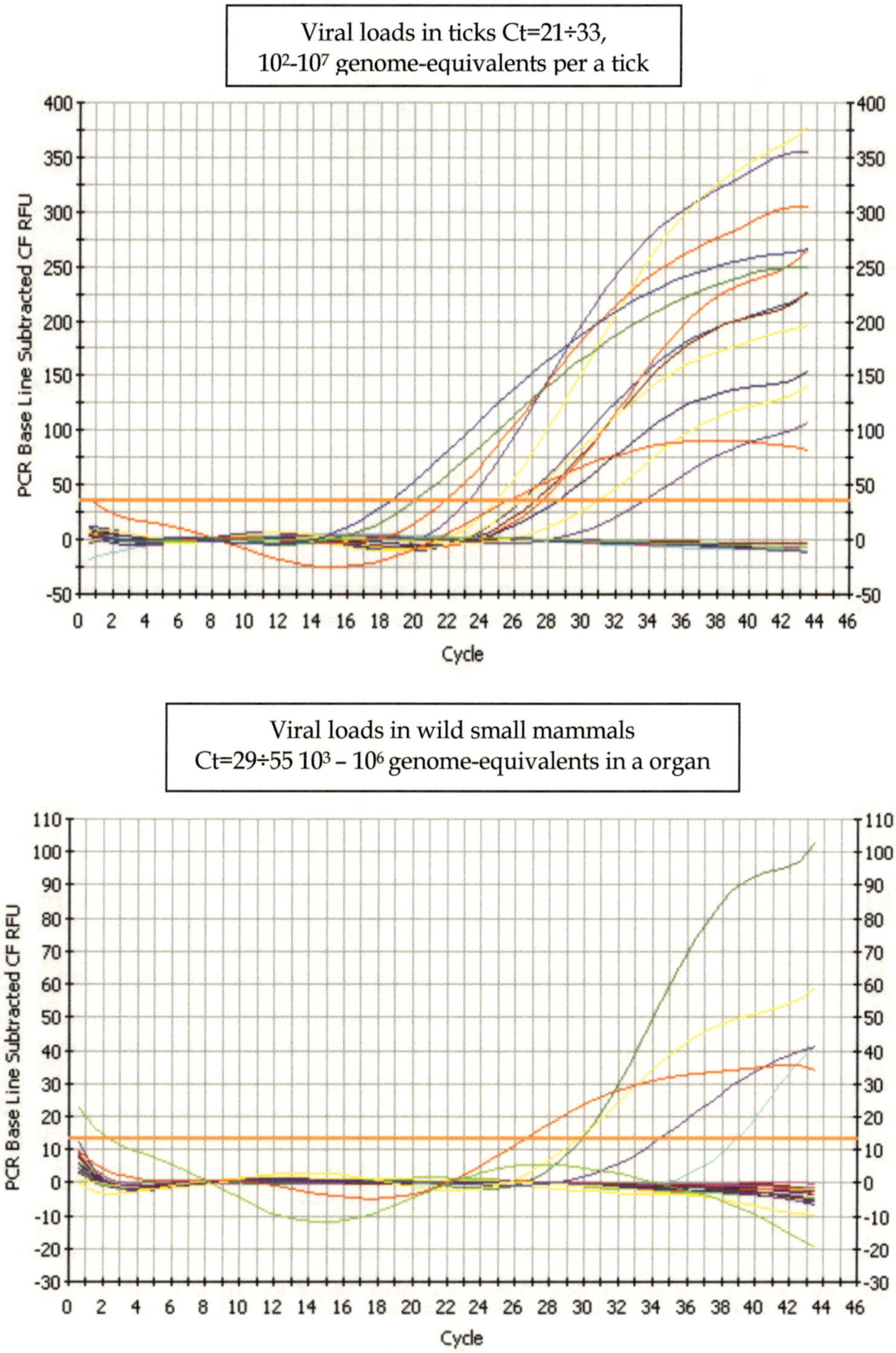

Fig. 5. Real-time PCR quantitation of the viral loads in ticks and small mammals from Novosibirsk endemic region, Western Siberia, Russia

Small mammals mainly rodents (*Rodentia)* and insectivorouses (*Insectivora*) with high reproduction rates and their life span even shorter than that of ixodid ticks are natural hosts for both immature ticks (mainly larvaes) and TBEV. Several small rodent species are highly competent in supporting the tick-borne transmission of TBEV, whereas avian species are not. Regardless the sensitivity of vertebrate hosts to the TBEV their susceptibility estimated by viraemia after infection essentially differs (Levkovich et al., 1967; Chunikhin et al., 1990). A long viraemic stage (2-8 days) along with a high virus titer was observed in small mammals such as field mice, red voles, common voles etc. The duration of viraemia is influenced by the environmental and body temperature with prolongation up to 8-14 days in cold seasons. In large mammals (roes, goats) viraemia is short-lived and only low virus titers were revealed. During the viraemic stage, milk from goats, cows and sheep contains the virus and may serve as the infection source for man. Birds only pass through a very short viraemic stage and play no role as reservoirs of TBEV. But often they serve as hosts for the immature stage of ticks and thus may contribute to the spread of infected ticks (Tick-Borne Encephalitis (TBE) and its Immunoprophylaxis, 1996 and references therein). Regardless of species variations and regional features life-long persistence of apathogenic TBEV in the presence of the virus-specific antibodies is typical for small rodents and insectivorous (Bakhvalova et al., 2006 and references therein).
Conventional estimations of the TBEV prevalence in small mammals are based on both virological and serological data with currently evident limitations. Despite the presence of specific antibodies serves as an evidence of TBEV infection in animals seronegative data may be consequences of immunocompromised or even immunodeficient individuals but not necessarily prove the absence of contacts with the virus. Isolation of the TBEV strains from wild adapted mammals is hardly possible because of the TBEV trace amounts and unpredictable viraemic period since the infection time remains uknown. Molecular approaches including RT-PCR permit to reveal a real infection rate. In our research both serological (ELISA and hemagglutination inhibition (HI) test), RT-nested PCR with subsequent sequencing and real-time PCR with fluorescent hydrolysis probes were used. In the endemic region studied wild small mammals include 9 species of insectivorous with dominant species of common shrew *(Sorex araneus* L.*)* and 12 species of wild small rodents excluding synanthropic rodent species associated with human societies. Rearrangements of dominance structure among rodents are unessential and total population remains stable (Litvinov et al., 2010). Analysis of long-term population dynamics of small rodents and insectivorous in the natural focus of Novosibirsk region, South-Western Siberia, Russia showed their similarity $r = 0{,}56$; $p = 0{,}001$ (Fig. 6), that might be explained by similar habitation abiotic and biotic (such as carnivoreses and epizootic infections) factors.
During last 30 years (1980-2010) population densities of small mammals periodically changed from 7.5 to 108.7 animals per 100 cylinder-days. On the average, among trapped small mammals 36% were rodents, 64% - insectivorous. In spite of relative minority, small rodents fed for approximately 90% of immature ixodid ticks, among them 45%-77% were found on red voles *Myodes rutilus* Pallas (earlier *Clethrionomys rutilus* Pallas) and field mice *Apodemus agrarius* Pallas. In many seasons of tick activity in Siberia lasting from May to August relative abundance of immature ticks was maximal for red voles with mean abundance up to 11.2 ticks per 1 animal (Bakhvalova et al., 2006).
TBEV-specific HI antibodies were also found mainly in small rodents and especially in red voles. For many years HI antibodies were not detected in insectivorous sera at all. For the last 4 years levels of seropositive small mammals were high with relative frequencies for red voles – up to 61.9±5.4% and for common shrews - 14.3±7.8%.

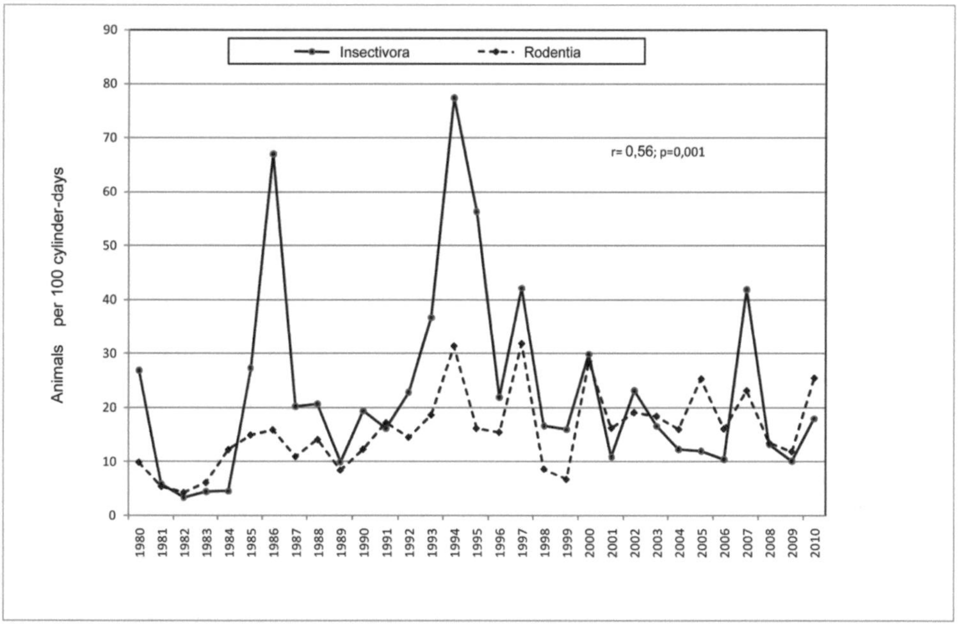

Fig. 6. Long-term population dynamics of small mammals of *Rodentia* and *Insectivora* in recreation zone of Novosibirsk endemic region, South-Western Siberia, Russia

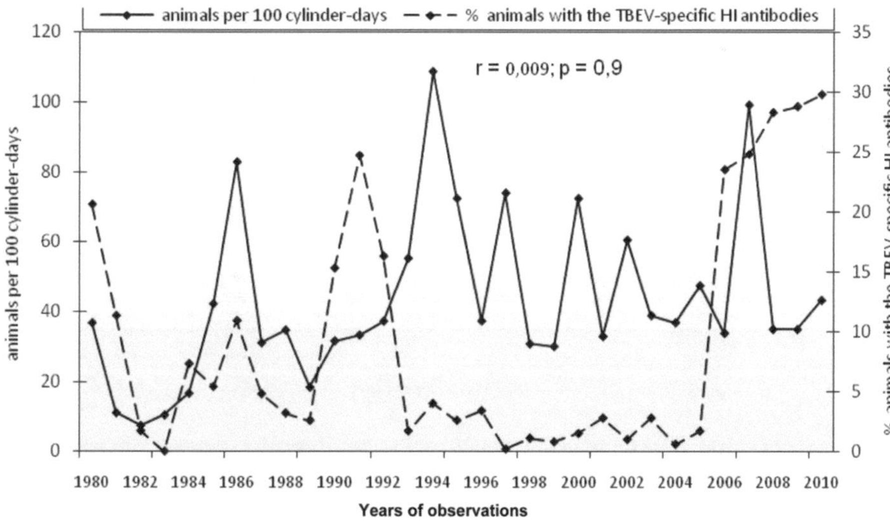

Fig. 7. Long-term dynamics of population density and HI antibody prevalence among small mammals in Novosibirsk endemic region, South-Western Siberia, Russia

Analysis revealed cyclic variations of both small mammals abundance and HI antibodies prevalence (Fig.7). For TBE parasitic system both short (less than 7 years) and middle (more than 12 years) cycles were described (Naumov et al., 1984).

For proportions of immune hosts short cycles lasted during 3-7 years whereas middle - 12-19 years with HI antibodies prevalence less 4% for short cycles and from 0 to 28.8±4.5 % for

middle ones (Fig.7). For animal abundance middle cycles lasted for less than 14 years. One should note that proportion of immune hosts did not significantly correlate with the abundance of all small mammals (r=0,009; p=0,9), insectivorous (r= -0,6; p=0,7) or rodents (r= -0,8; p=0,67). However, the calculated correlation coefficients (r) allowed us to reveal rather slightly negative correlation. At population depression stages with decreasing amounts of small mammals the growth of proportion of immune animals might be caused by elevated tick infestation and/or activation of endogenous persisting TBEV.
Prevalence of HI antibodies coincided with ELISA-detected IgM antibodies typical for the virus reproduction periods. But IgG levels were essentially higher and corresponded to natural TBEV infection among wild small mammals (data not shown).
TBEV persistence among wild small mammals was studied using bioassay, HI test, ELISA and RT-real-time PCR with subtype-specific fluorescent hydrolysis probes or nested PCR with subsequent sequencing. Average TBEV prevalence for common shrews was 82.6±3.3%, for red voles - 71.7±2.6% and but for field mice - significantly lower 36.8±3.8% ($p<0.001$) in organs (Fig. 8) and in blood samples from red voles 71.2±5.9% and from field mice 41.3±7.3%.

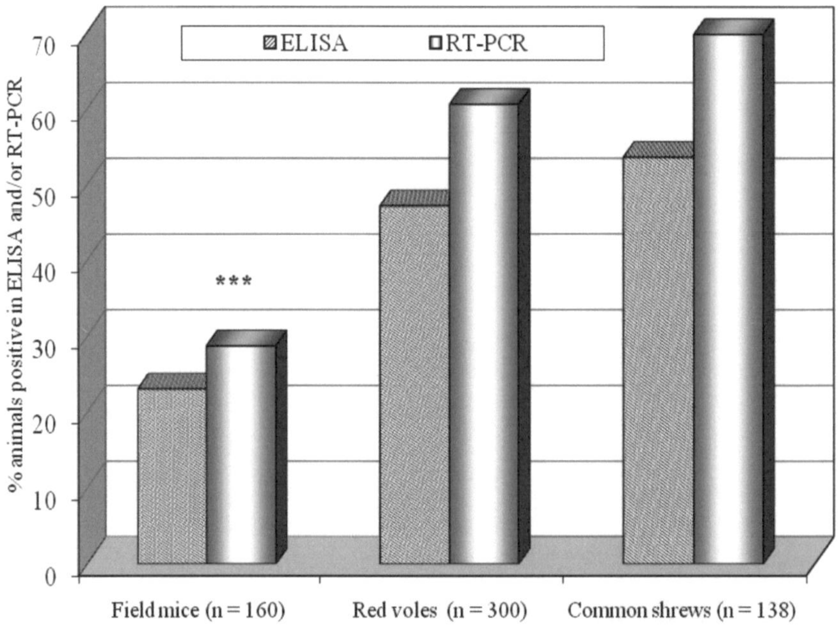

*** - p<0,001 - significance level for field mice compared to red voles and common shrews.

Fig. 8. Detection of TBEV RNA and glycoprotein E in organs of small mammals for 1998-2009

Despite high TBEV prevalence detected in ELISA and RT-PCR pathogenic in bioassay and hemagglutinating TBEV was found in a few samples of small mammal organs only. In 7-15 days postinfection of 1-2-day-old suckling mice with homogenates of organs from wild small mammals weak clinical manifestations of TBE such as languor, lack of appetite or refusal to eat, slight tremor of extremities were registered for mice of both first and second passages without subsequent death. Majority of TBEV strains isolated from wild small mammals were not stable in spite of detection of both TBEV RNA and protein E in organs of bioassay laboratory mice.

TBEV infection rate among wild animals were significantly lower (p<0.001 - p<0.01) at stages of their population growth and maximal density in comparison with periods of population decline and minimal density (Fig. 9).

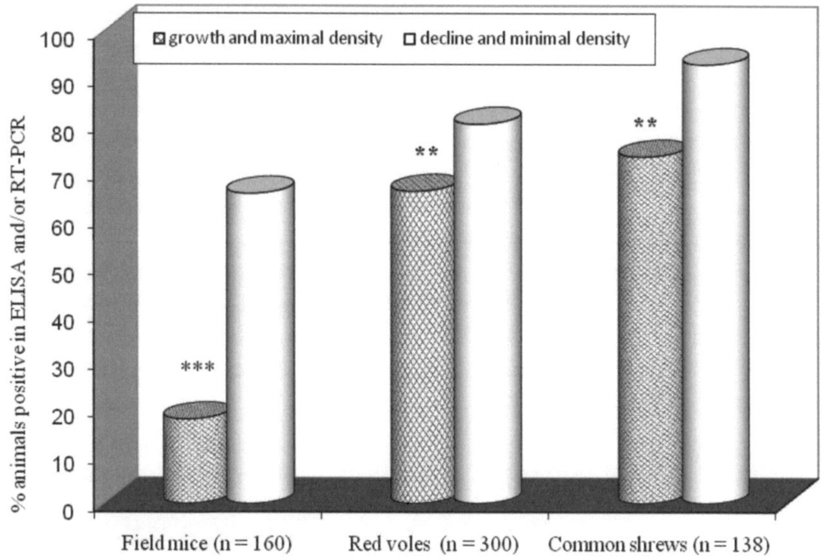

*** - p<0,001; ** - p<0,01 – significance levels for each species.

Fig. 9. Detection of TBEV RNA and/or glycoprotein E in organs of wild small mammals (average values for 1998-2009) versus their population cycles

During cold seasons (October 16 – April 15) average TBEV infection levels were significantly higher (p<0,001) compared to warm periods (April 16 - October 15) for all 3 species of small mammals studied. Relative abundance of TBEV infected red voles remained high in any seasons of year whereas for field mice and common shrews more essential prevalence (p< 0.01; p< 0.05, respectively) were noticed in winter time (Table 1). Dependence of the TBEV infection rate on the mammal species, a season of an year or a population cycle phase could be caused by the different innate unspecific resistance of species of wild animals to infections, cold immunosupression and/or hormonal influence during reproductive cycles.

Species of animals	TBEV detection (%)		Student's criterion and significance levels
	Autumn-winter period	Spring-summer period	
Red voles *Myodes rutilus*	71,9±3,8 (100/139)	71,6± 3,9 (96/134)	-
Field mice *Apodemus agrarius*	61.1± 8.2 (22/36)	22.3± 4.3 (21/94)	t = 4.3; p< 0.001
Common shrews *Sorex araneus*	83.1±4.7 (54/65)	54.7± 7.8 (23/42)	t = 3.1; p<0.01

Table 1. Detection of TBEV RNA and glycoprotein E in organs of wild small mammals trapped in different seasons of year (data pooled 1998-2008)

Molecular typing of TBEV from organs and blood cells of wild small mammals was performed by RT-nested PCR with subsequent sequencing and phylogenetic analysis as previously described (Bakhvalova et al., 2006) and by RT-real-time PCR with TBEV subtype-specific fluorescent probes. Both Far Eastern, Siberian and European genetic subtypes with predominance of the first as well as mixed infection up to 20% were revealed in organs and blood cells of small mammals in Western Siberia, Russia. Siberian subtype prevalence and corresponding viral loads in blood of small rodents of 2 species were significantly ($p<0.01$ - $P< 0.001$) lower in comparison with Far Eastern subtype. Siberian subtype was detected mainly as mixed infection with Far Eastern subtype. Viral loads were similar for 3 species of small mammals studied. Threshold cycles (Ct) of the TBEV in organs of wild small mammals varied from 29 to 55 and allowed us to estimate the TBEV RNA quantities as 10^3-10^6 copies per brain or spleen (Fig. 5). In cells of 100 μl of blood the viral loads varied from a few copies to 10^2 for Siberian subtype and up to 10^7 - for Far Eastern subtype but in sera the TBEV RNA was not detected (data not shown). Thus, for small mammals high levels of life-long persistent infection with the TBEV of Far Eastern, Siberian and rarely European subtypes were observed in the presence of the virus-specific antibodies including HI- and virus-neutralizing antibodies (Okulova, 1986).

4. TBEV quasispecies genetic rearrangements in ticks and mammals

RNA viruses commonly exist as a swarm of viruses with varying genomes. The variations are predominantly the result of the lack of proof-reading capability in the virally-encoded RNA-dependent RNA polymerases, the production of large numbers of viral genomes and the absence of RNA repair systems in both host eukaryotic cells and in virus. Eigen and colleagues introduced the concept that this genetic heterogeneity could be described as a quasispecies, a "complex self-perpetuating population of diverse related entities that act as a whole" (For review see Biebricher and Eigen, 2006). Survival of the fittest is replaced by survival of the fittest quasispecies. In a quasispecies, the wild type is not a specific sequence, but consists of the weighted average of nucleotides at each position. However, the interpretation that genetic variability in RNA viruses should invariably be attributed to quasispecies has been questioned (Holmes and Moya, 2002). Most authors reporting sequence heterogeneity ignore these theoretical considerations and label any genetic variation in the same specimen as evidence for quasispecies. By repeated sequencing of the same specimen, quasispecies in flaviviruses have been well documented for dengue virus types 1 (DENV-1) (Aaskov et al., 2006) and 3 (DENV-3) (Chao et al., 2005) as well as for West Nile virus (WNV)(Jerzak et al., 2005) and TBEV (Romanova et al., 2007).

Phylogenetic analysis of E gene nucleotide sequences for TBEV RNA isolated from brain, liver, spleen and blood cells of small mammals using 4 alternative algorithms of Mega 4.1 software revealed Far Eastern and Siberian subtypes with predominance of the first (Fig. 10) Despite of the different genetic subtypes TBEV isolates from wild small mammals were notable for their low pathogenicity, immunogenicity and reproduction activity.

Analysis of the TBEV 3'UTR nucleotide sequences of chronological row of the TBEV strains isolated in Novosibirsk endemic region, South-Western Siberia, Russia during 1980-2010 revealed the presence of large, variable deletions located near oligo(A) fragments within hypervariable region located downstream from termination codon of a single open reading frame and numerous nucleotide substitutions (Morozova et al., 2007; GenBank accession numbers DQ473396-DQ473404). Lengths of the TBEV 3'UTR for isolates from ticks were shorter than those from mouse brain suspensions after infection with corresponding tick homogenates. Large deletions did not arise only during serial passages with high multiplicity of infection as previously supposed but could be also found in primary isolates. The deletions were found in the 5′-terminal region of the 3′UTR, a region considered to be variable and, at least under laboratory conditions, not necessary for virus viability. Deletions may also occur in the 3′ end of the 3′UTR, a region that contains sequences and calculated structures essential for viral propagation. One of these is the cyclization sequence CGGUUCUUGUUCUCC. Another is a calculated long stable hairpin (3'LSH).

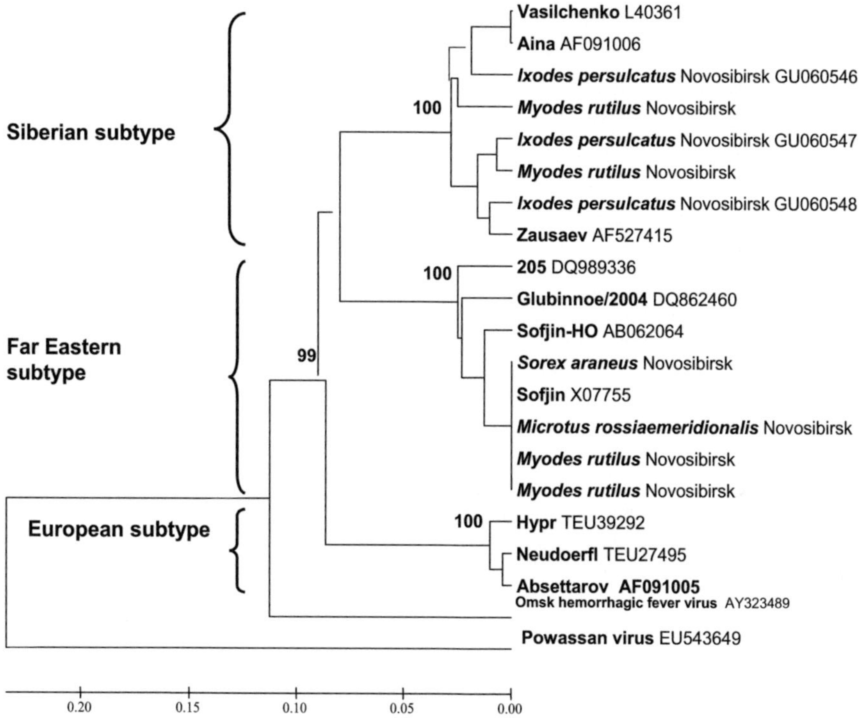

Fig. 10. Phylogenetic tree using UPGMA algorithm of Mega 4.1 software of nucleotide sequences of the TBEV E gene for the viral RNA isolated from ticks and wild small mammals from Novosibirsk endemic region, Western Siberia, Russia

Manual multiple alignment starting at the 3′ end of 3′UTR sequences of the TBEV strains from our collection revealed that the sequences could be divided into 3 groups. The first contained 712-730 nucleotides corresponding to full length 3′UTR. The second group contained deletions, principally in the 5′ end, but occasionally in the 3′ end that did not include deletions in the predicted cyclization sequence and usually not in the calculated 3'LSH. The third group contained deletions that included both the cyclization sequence and the entire 3'LSH. According to current concepts members of the second group might be viable, but the third group should not be. These findings suggest that viability in the third group that had characteristically been passaged multiple times was maintained by dual infection with fully viable virus. The results suggest the presence of sequence variability sometimes referred to as quasispecies. One should note that 3′UTR sequences obtained from small rodents and insectivorous naturally-infected with TBEV indicate a multiplicity of electrophoretic bands, a finding that also supports the presence of quasispecies in TBEV. Perhaps, the variable fragment of 3'UTR might be responsible for binding with host cell replication factors thus permitting to select tick- or mammal-adapted variants of the virus quasispecies.

5. Periodic variations of TBE morbidity rate

In endemic regions TBEV transmission has been found to occur in one of about 200 tick bites. Moreover, tick bites are not often noticed and in the case histories references to tick bites are mentioned in 10-85% (Tick-Borne Encephalitis (TBE) and its Immunoprophylaxis, 1996). Maximal TBE morbidity rate had been registered in 1956 (5,163 cases) and 1964 (5,205 incidences). Then until 1974 TBE prevalence gradually declined to 1,119 cases. During 1976-1989 an average annual morbidity level in Europe and Russia was 2,755 and between 1990 and 2007 - an average of 8,755 reported cases of TBE per year (Mansfield et al., 2009). In 1999 11,356 cases of TBE in Eurasia (www.tbe-info.com) (and among them 9,955 – in Russia alone) render the highest sickness level in all endemic regions. However, these underestimations of TBE rate are based on confirmed hospitalized cases of severe encephalitis or meningoencephalitis and comprise nearly 20-30% of real TBEV infection prevalence among populations from endemic regions. The figures are second only to those for Japanese encephalitis (Mansfield et al., 2009 and references therein). An annual TBE vaccination campaign was introduced in Austria in 1981. Despite once having the highest incidence rate in Europe (up to 700 hospitalised cases annually), this campaign caused a steady decline in the number of cases of TBE in Austria alone. In surrounding European countries under similar climate conditions vaccination have had varying degrees of success, since the vaccines are expensive and must have repeated administrations in order to maintain protective immunity. For example, the Czech Republic still has one of the highest incidence rates in Europe, with 400–1000 clinical cases reported annually (Ruzek et al., 2008). In Russia TBE morbidity rate during last decade gradually decreased but it could not be attributed to vaccination with an average rate 5-7%.

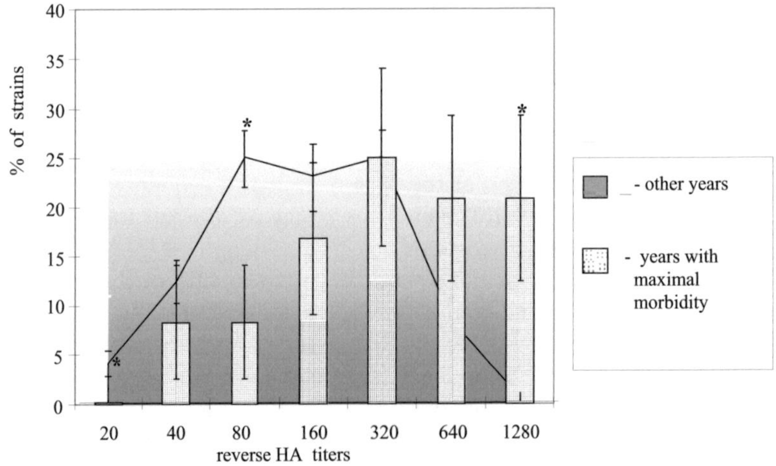

Fig. 11. HA titers of the TBEV strains during periods with different TBE rate in humans (* -P<0.05)

One of the striking epidemiological features of TBE is periodic variation in the occurrence and severity of TBEV infections in different endemic regions from Far Eastern Russia to Europe. Peak values last 1-2 years and trough values last for 6-7 years separated by intervals of gradual transition over 1-5 years. Three such cycles have been observed in the Novosibirsk region, South-Western Siberia, Russia spanning a period of 30 years of observations beginning from 1980. The TBE morbidity in Novosibirsk region periodically changed with maximal sickness rate in 1981 (47.7 incidences per 100,000 population), 1992 (60.7 incidences per 100,000) and 1999 (32.9 incidences per 100,000). The TBEV infection rate of the main arthropod vectors-ixodid ticks was previously shown to vary from 0.3 to 3.1 % according to bioassays (Fig. 1) and up to 46% based on RT-PCR. The TBEV strains isolated from ixodid ticks during period between 1980 and 2010 years in the same endemic region of Siberia, Russia were analyzed after 1-15 passages in susceptible laboratory suckling mice. Changes in TBE incidence in patients paralleled the viral hemagglutination titers and neuroinvasiveness indexes for the TBEV strains isolated from unfed ticks. The 3'UTR turned out to be one of the most variable parts of the genome. Sequencing revealed numerous 3'UTR rearrangements including microdeletions of 1-5 nucleotides located near oligo (A)-tracts 2-6 nucleotides long. The first group of the TBEV strains included the high-virulent strains isolated in 1982 and 1992 with high morbidity among people in Novosibirsk region whereas all the TBEV strains from the second group have been isolated during periods with relatively low sickness rate in the endemic region (1984, 1988 and 2006). Diversity observed for the 3'UTR sequences appeared to be not essential for the viability of the TBEV strains. Longer incubation period for more than 5 days in suckling mice observed for the TBEV strains with shorter 3'UTR fragment sequences (less than 200 nucleotides) in comparison with strains with longer (more than 300 bp) sequences (4 days incubation period) might be probably caused by slower rate of RNA replication. However, reduced neuroinvasiveness could not also be excluded as the reason for different incubation periods. Thus, structural rearrangements in the TBEV 3'UTR presumably did not significantly affect translation but probably could compromise RNA synthesis.

Hemagglutination titers varied from 1:20 to 1:1280 for the TBEV strains and did not correlate with length of 3'UTR fragment. However, cyclic variations of the TBEV HA titers coincided very well with periodic changes of the disease rate in humans (Fig. 11). Neuroinvasiveness indexes for 40 TBEV strains varied in a range 0.3 -4.3 (titers 5.8-8.5 lgLD50 after intracerebral infection and 2.7-7.0 lgLD50 after subcutaneous administration). It is interesting to note that in years with peak sickness rate in human's neuroinvasiveness indexes of the TBEV strains studied were higher than in other years.

Periodic variations in the incidence and severity of TBE have been shown to be inversely correlated with both adult tick abundance (A) and TBEV prevalence in ticks (B) (Fig. 12). At least three possibilities should be taken into consideration to explain the inverse association of these two parameters. One is that the changes are the result of differences in the proportion of infections caused by the three phylogenetically defined subtypes (Far Eastern, Siberian and European). A second possibility is that cyclic alterations in TBEV loads in arthropod vectors might be involved. Finally, TBEV quasispecies rearrangements including variable ratio of both tick-adapted and mammal-adapted variants cannot be exluded . The 3 possibilities could be interrelated.

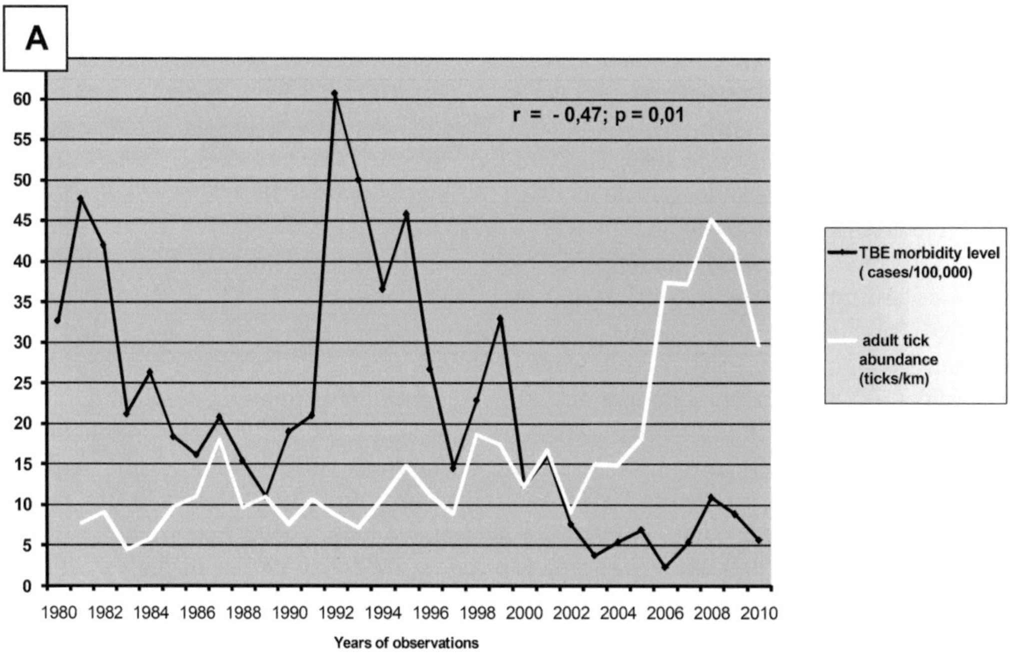

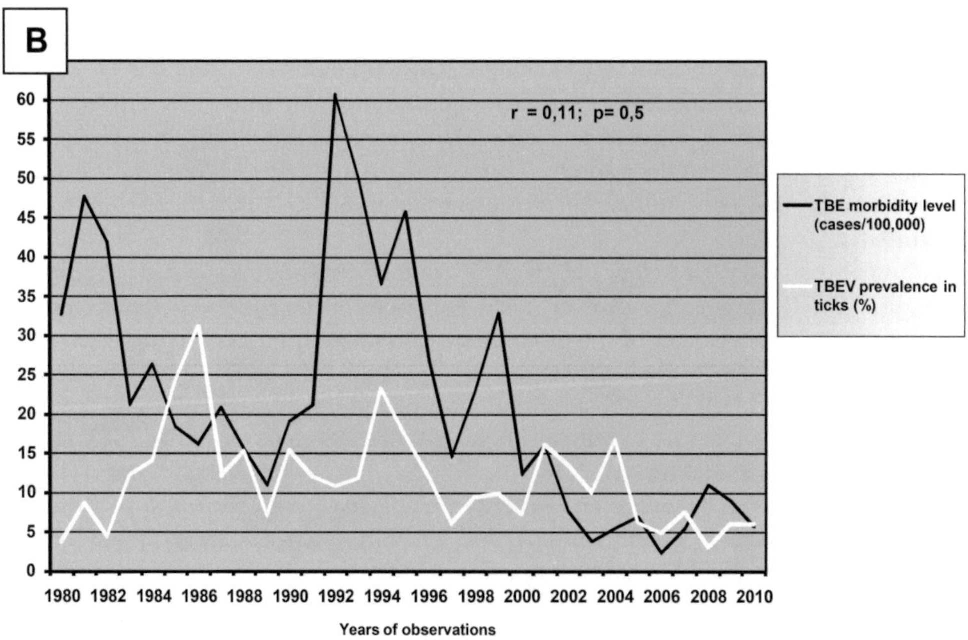

Fig. 12. Reverse correlation between TBE morbidity rate, adult tick abundance (part A) and TBEV prevalence in ticks (part B) in Novosibirsk endemic region, South-Western Siberia, Russia

6. Conclusion

Taken together, our long-term observations of the TBEV in its natural hosts in the endemic region of Western Siberia, Russia revealed the followings.

1. Essential differences of the TBEV infection rate and the viral loads were observed between different reservoir hosts (Fig. 2, 5, 7-9, table 1). The TBEV prevalence among ixodid ticks was significantly lower compared to the corresponding infection rate among vertebrate hosts, whereas the viral loads in a tick was in 10-100 times higher than in organs and blood cells of mammals. However, pathogenic TBEV could be easily isolated from ticks but hardly only in a few cases from mammals. Both Far Eastern, Siberian and European genetic subtypes were identified in the virus isolates from reservoir hosts but in different proportions. One should note the selection of Siberian genetic subtype in brains of laboratory suckling mice used for bioassay that might distort a real structure of the TBEV quasispecies in wild hosts. Specific features of the TBEV in different reservoir hosts might be the consequences of a long adaptation resulting in the resistance of the whole parasitary system.
2. The TBEV natural population (Fig. 2, 11) together with the reservoir hosts of the virus (Fig. 1 and 6) periodically changed as the whole system. For periods of isolation of the TBEV strains with high hemagglutination (HA) titers (≥1:320) (Fig. 11) and elevated geometric middling (Fig. 2) the TBE morbidity rate in the endemic region was also maximal (Fig. 11, $r=0,63$, $p\leq 0,05$). The changes of the TBEV HA activity in ticks correlated with dynamics of small mammals with HI antibodies ($r=0,69$; $p\leq 0,01$) with interval of 1 year required for transstadial transmission of the TBEV from immature ticks to adults and, consequently, with the viral encephalitis rate ($r=0,49$; $p\leq 0,001$).
3. Cyclic changes of the TBEV infection rate in ticks as well as tick abundance (Fig. 12) did not correlate with TBE morbidity rate in the same endemic region.

7. Acknowledgments

Current work was supported in part by integration projects №19, №83 of Siberian Branch of the Russian Academy of Sciences.

8. References

[1] Aaskov J., Buzacott K., Thu H.M., Lowry K., and Holmes E.C. (2006) Long-term transmission of defective RNA viruses in humans and Aedes mosquitoes. *Science, V.* 311, P. 236-238.

[2] Alekseev A.N. (1990) Transmissive diseases agents homeostatic mechanisms (vector behavior changes, transmission ways multiformity. *Bull. soc. fr. parasitol.* V. 8, N2, P. 1168.

[3] Bakhvalova V.N., Dobrotvorsky A.K., Panov V.V., Matveeva V.A., Tkachev S.E., Morozova O.V. (2006) Natural tick-borne encephalitis virus infection among wild small mammals in the southeastern part of western Siberia, Russia. *Vector Borne Zoonotic Dis.* V. 6(1), P. 32-41.

[4] Bakhvalova V.N., Potapova O.F., Panov V.V., Morozova O.V. (2009) Vertical transmission of tick-borne encephalitis virus between generations of adapted reservoir small rodents. *Virus Res.* V. 140(1-2), P. 172-178.

[5] Bakhvalova V.N., Rar V.A., Tkachev S.E., Matveeva V.A., Matveev L.E., Karavanov A.S., Dobrotvorsky A.K. and Morozova O.V. (2000) Tick-borne encephalitis virus strains of Western Siberia. - *Virus Research,* V. 70 , № 1-2, P. 1-12.

[6] Balashov Yu.S. (2010) Meaning of population structure of ixodid ticks (*Parasitiformes, Ixodidae*) for the infection natural foci support. *Zoological Journal,* V. 89, №1, P. 18-25 (In Russian).

[7] Beklemishev V.N. (1963) Study of tick-borne encephalitis prevalence in ticks using bioassays. *Voprosi virusologii,* №2. P. 240 - 242 (In Russian).

[8] Biebricher C.K. and Eigen M. (2006). What is a quasispecies? *Curr. Top. Microbiol. Immunol.,* V. 299, P. 1-31.

[9] Bogdanov I.I. (2006) *Ixodid ticks of the Western Siberia.* Report VII. Types of populations of ixodid ticks. "Vestnik Omskogo pedagogicheskogo universiteta", www.omsk.edu.

[10] Brinton M.A. and Perelygin A.A. (2003) Genetic resistance to flaviviruses. *Advances in Virus Research,* Elsevier Inc., V. 60, P. 43-85.

[11] Chao D.Y., King C.C., Wang W.K., Chen W.J., Wu H.L. and Chang G.J. (2005) Strategically examining the full-genome of dengue virus type 3 in clinical isolates reveals its mutation spectra. *Virol. J.,* V. 2, P. 72.

[12] Chunikhin S.P. (1990) Experimental study of tick-borne encephalitis virus ecology. *Vopr. Virusol.* V. 3, P. 183-188 (In Russian).

[13] Dobrotvorsky A.K., Bakhvalova V.N., Charytonova N.N., Sapegina V.F. (1994) Dynamics of tick-borne encephalitis virus parasitic system under conditions of Northern forest-steppe of Priobye. *Siberian Ecological Journal,* V.1, №4, P. 369-375 (In Russian).

[14] Ebel G. (2009)"Analysis of genetic diversity within a stable focus of Powassan virus in Northern Wisconsin. *American Society for Tropical Medicine and Hygiene Meetings in New Orleans* Nov. 18-22, p. 27.

[15] Ecker M., Allison S.L., Meixner T., and Heinz F.X. (1999). Sequence analysis and genetic classification of tick-borne encephalitis viruses from Europe and Asia. *J. Gen. Virol.* 80 (Pt 1), P. 179-185.

[16] Filippova N.A. (1985) Taiga tick *Ixodes persulcatus* Schulze (*Acarina, Ixodidae*). Leningrad, *Nauka,* 416 pp.

[17] Gould A.E., Zanotto P.M., Holmes E.C. (1997) The genetic evolution of flaviviruses. In: *Factors in the Emergence of Arbovirus Diseases.* (J.F.Saluzzo, B.Dobet, eds.), P. 51-62. Elsevier, Paris.

[18] Grard G., Moureau G., Charrel R.N., Lemasson J.J., Gonzalez J.P., Gallian P., Gritsun T.S., Holmes E.C., Gould E.A., and de Lamballerie X. (2007). Genetic characterization of tick-borne flaviviruses: new insights into evolution, pathogenetic determinants and taxonomy. *Virology* 361, P. 80-92.

[19] Gritsun T.S., Lashkevich V.A., and Gould E.A. (2003). Tick-borne encephalitis. *Antiviral Res. 57,* 129-146.

[20] Hofmann H. (1973) Die unspezifische Abwehr bei neurotropen Arbovirusinfektionen. *Zbl. Bakt. Hyg. I. Abt. Orig.* A223, P.143-163.

[21] Holmes E.C. and Moya A. (2002). Is the quasispecies concept relevant to RNA viruses? *J. Virol.* V. 76, P. 460-465.

[22] Jerzak G., Bernard K.A., Kramer L.D. and Ebel G.D. (2005). Genetic variation in West Nile virus from naturally infected mosquitoes and birds suggests quasispecies structure and strong purifying selection. *J. Gen. Virol.*, V. 86, P. 2175-2183.

[23] Katin A. A., Pustovalov I.N. (1983) Pattern of relationships between tick and virla populations in tick-borne encephalitis natural foci in connection with prediction questions. Natural focus infections in regions of economic reclamation of Siberia and Far East. Republic collection of scientific articles. Omsk, P. 41-47 (In Russian).

[24] Khasnatinov M.A., Danchinova G.A., Kulakova N.V., Tungalag K., Arbatskaia E.V., Mironova L.V., Tserennorov D., Bolormaa G., Otgonbaatar D., Zlobin V.I. (2010) Genetic characteristics of the causative agent of tick-borne encephalitis in Mongolia]. *Vopr Virusol.* V. 55 (3), P. 27-32 (In Russian).

[25] Khasnatinov M.A., Ustanikova K., Frolova T.V., Pogodina V.V., Bochkova N.G., Levina L.S., Slovak M., Kazimirova M., Labuda M., Klempa B., Eleckova E., Gould E.A., Gritsun T.S. (2009) Non-hemagglutinating flaviviruses: molecular mechanisms for the emergence of new strains via adaptation to European ticks. *PLoS One.* V. 4, Issue 10, e7295.

[26] Korotkov Yu.S., Burencova L.A. (2006) Influence of the tick-borne encephalitis virus to the process of metamorphosis of engorged larvae and nymphs of the ticks *Ixodes ricinus. Bulletin of Siberian Medicine,* V. 5, Supplement 1, P. 36-41 (In Russian).

[27] Korotkov Yu.S., Nikitin A.N., Antonova A.M., (2007) Role of climatic factors in long-term dynamics of the tick-borne encephalitis morbidity rate in Irkutsk. *Bulleten of VSNC SO RAMN,* №3 (55), P.121-125 (In Russian).

[28] Korenberg E.I. (1989) Tick-borne encephalitis. In: L'vov D.K., Klimenko S.M., Gaidamovich S.Ya. Arboviruses and arboviral infections. Moscow, "Medicine". P. 256 -264 (In Russian).

[29] Levkovich, E.N., Pogodina, V.V., Zasukhina, G.D., Karpovich, L.G., (1967) Viruses of tick-borne encephalitis complex [in Russian]. Leningrad, Meditsina Publishers; 1-243.

[30] Litvinov Yu.N., Abramov S.A., Panov V.V. (2010) Dynamics of structure of rodent populations of model landscapes in connection with problems of stability and resistance. Communities and populations of animals: ecological and morphological analysis. Proceeding of Institute of Systematics and ecology of Animals of Siberian Branch of the Russian Academy of Sciences. Ed. Bolshakov V.N., Novosibirsk-Moscow, Association of scientific publishers KMK, P. 66 -92.

[31] Mansfield K.L., Johnson N., Phipps L.P., Stephenson J.R., Fooks A.R., Solomon T. (2009) Tick-borne encephalitis virus - a review of an emerging zoonosis. *J. Gen. Virol.* 90(Pt 8), P. 1781-1794.

[32] Mantke O.D., Schädler R., Niedrig M. (2008) A survey on cases of tick-borne encephalitis in European countries. Eurosurveillance, Volume 13, Issue 17, Article 5. http://www.eurosurveillance.org/ViewArticle.aspx?ArticleId=18916)

[33] Morozova O.V., Bakhvalova V.N., Morozov I.V. (2007) Heterogeneity of 3'-untranslated region of genome RNA of the tick-borne encephalitis virus (TBEV) strains isolated from ticks in the Western Siberia, Russia. *International Journal of Biomedical Science,* V. 3(3), P. 206-209.

[34] Naumov R.L., Labzin V.V., Gutova V.P. (1984) Cyclic variations in elements of parasite system of tick-borne encephalitis. *Parasitology collection.* Leningrad, Nauka, V.32, P.139 -160.

[35] Neckiy, G.I., Bogdanov I.I. (1966). Indicator of potential epidemiological significance of natural fociTick-borne encephalitis and Omsk hemorrhagic fever. Medical parazitology and parazit. diseases. V.3. P. 290-292. (In Russian)

[36] Nutall P.A. and Labuda M. (2003) Dynamics of infection in tick vectors and at the tick-host interface. *Advances in Virus Research,* V. 60, pp. 233-272.

[37] Okulova N.M. (1986) Biological relationships in forest ecosystems (natural foci of tick-borne encephalitis as an example) Moscow, *Nauka,* P.1-246 (In Russian).

[38] Plassmann E. (1980) Zecken-Enzephalitis auch durch infizierte Milch. *Arztl. Praxis,* V. 32. P. 2025-2026.

[39] Pogodina V.V., Bochkova N.G., Koreshkova G.V. (1981) Properties of the tick-borne encephalitis virus strains of serotype Aina/1448. *Vopr. Virusol.,* N 6, P. 741-746.

[40] Pogodina V.V., Karan' L.S., Koliasnikova N.M., Levina L.S., Malenko G.V., Gamova E.G., Lesnikova M.V., Kiliachina A.S., Esiunina M.S., Bochkova N.G., Shopenskaia T.A., Frolova T.V., Andaev E.I. and Trukhina A.G. (2007) Evolution of tick-borne encephalitis and a problem of evolution of its causative agent. *Vopr. Virusol.* V. 52, P. 16-21.

[41] Romanova L.Iu., Gmyl A.P., Dzhivanian T.I., Bakhmutov D.V., Lukashev A.N., Gmyl L.V., Rumyantsev A.A., Burenkova L.A., Lashkevich V.A., Karganova G.G. (2007) Microevolution of tick-borne encephalitis virus in course of host alternation. *Virology.* V. 362(1), P. 75-84.

[42] Romanenko V.N., Kondratieva L.M. (2010) Infection of ticks (*Ixodidae*) with the tick-borne encephalitis virus in Tomsk and surrounding regions. Proceedings of 8th Meeting of entomologists of Siberia and Far East "Entomological research in Northern Asia", Novosibirsk, P. 354-356.
ttp://www.eco.nsc.ru/science/conferenceisea.html (In Russian).

[43] Ruzek D., Gritsun T.S., Forrester N.L., Gould E.A., Kopecky J., Golovchenko M., Rudenko N. and Grubhoffer L. (2008) Mutations in the NS2B and NS3 genes affect mouse neuroinvasiveness of a Western European field strain of tick-borne encephalitis virus. *Virology,* V. 374, P. 249–255.

[44] Tick-Borne Encephalitis (TBE) and its Immunoprophylaxis. Immuno AG, Vienna, Austria, 1996.

[45] Vereta L.A. (1975) Principles of prognosis of tick-borne encephalitis incidence rate. Moscow, *Medicine,* 135 pp. (In Russian).

[46] Vershinsky B.V. (1984) Paleogeographic factors of formation of of natural foci of tick-borne encephalitis and the present structure of nosoarea // Parasitology (collected articles). Leningrad, *Nauka,* V. 32. P.124 – 138 (In Russian).

[47] Zanotto P.M., Gao G.F., Gritsum T., Marin M.S., Jiang W.R., Venugopal K., Reid H.W., Gould E.A (1995). An arbovirus cline across the Northern Hemisphere. *Virology,* V. 210, P. 152-159.

[48] Zlobin V.I., Mamaev L.V., Djioev Yu.P., Kozlova I.V. (1996) Genetic types of the tick-borne encephalitis virus. *Journal of infectious pathology,* V. 3, № 4, P. 13-17 (In Russian).

12

Genetic Studies of Tick-Borne Encephalitis Virus Strains from Western and Eastern Siberia

S. E. Tkachev et al.*
Institute of Chemical Biology and Fundamental Medicine SB RAS, Novosibirsk
Russia

1. Introduction

Tick-borne encephalitis is a zoonotic infection of a central nervous system whose clinical course is often severe, even fatal, and complications (such as paralysis) are frequent [Zlobin and Lvov, 2008]. It is caused by tick-borne encephalitis virus (TBEV) belonging to the mammalian tick-borne flaviviruses group in the genus Flavivirus (Flaviviridae). The group includes several species found in geographically distant regions of Eurasia and North America. Evolutionary and genetic relationships among these viruses as well as among TBEV strains proper are not clear, which results in the contradiction of classification schemes suggested by different authors. There is a widely shared opinion that three antigenic TBEV subtypes correspond to three major TBEV genotypes, the Far Eastern (TBEV-FE, with Sofjin strain as a prototype), European (TBEV-Eu, prototype Neudoerfl strain), and Siberian or Ural-Siberian (TBEV-Sib, prototypes Vasilchenko and Zausaev strains) (Fig. 1) [Ecker et al., 1999; Hayasaka et al., 1999, 2001; Zlobin et al., 2001a, 2003; Pogodina et al., 2002, 2004].

In 2001 as a result of studying TBEV genetic variability the existence of six genotypes of the virus was supposed on the basis of homology analysis of a small part of the E gene (160 nt) of 34 strains [Zlobin et al., 2001a,b]. Three of them were accepted as the main ones [Zlobin et al., 2003]. The Turkish strain described earlier as a separate strain in the TBEV virus subgroup [Gao et al., 1993] was included in the genotype 6 together with the strain Vergina [described as a strain of TBEV by Pogodina et al., 1993] and classified as the variant of Louping ill virus (LIV, the Scottish sheep encephalomyelitis virus) [Heinz et al., 2000]. Genotypes 4 and 5 were represented by single strains, 178-79 and 886-84. These strains were isolated in the Irkutsk region and met the criteria for classification into independent genotypes according to the degree of genomic differences [Zlobin et al., 2001a]. Then, the complete genome sequences of 178-79 and 886-84 strains have been determined [Karan' et al., 2007a,b]. Phylogenetic analysis has revealed that strain 178-79 to the greater degree and

---

*T.V. Demina[1], Yu.P. Dzhioev[2], I.V. Kozlova[1,2], M.M. Verkhozina[3], E.K. Doroshchenko[2], O.V. Lisak[2], V.N. Bakhvalova[4], A.I. Paramonov[2] and V.I. Zlobin[1]
[1]*Irkutsk State Medical University of Russian Ministry of Health, Irkutsk, Russia;*
[2]*Institute of Epidemiology and Microbiology, Scientific Center of Family Health and Human Reproduction Problems, SB RAMS, Irkutsk, Russia;*
[3]*Center of Hygiene and Epidemiology in Irkutsk Region, Irkutsk, Russia;*
[4]*Institute of Systematics and Ecology of Animals SB RAS, Novosibirsk, Russia*

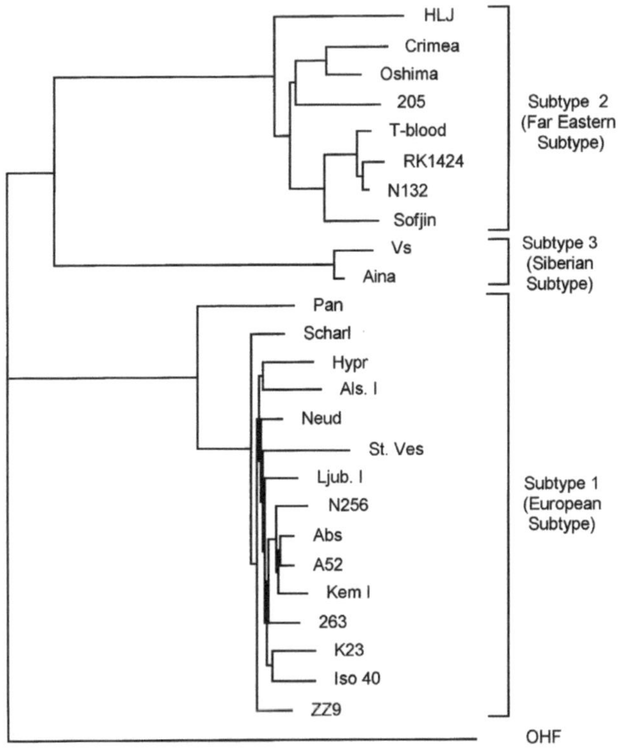

Fig. 1. Phylogenetic tree illustrating the genetic relationship of TBE virus isolates (generated by the DNADIST/FITCH program). The tree was rooted using Omsk haemmorrhagic fever (OHF) virus as the outgroup virus [Ecker et al., 1999]

Differences in coding genome region (10,242 nt)				
	Genotype 1	Genotype 2	Genotype 3	178-79
Genotype 1	5,2			
Genotype 2	16,5	2,6		
Genotype 3	14,6	15,4	6,6	
178-79	11,2	16,2	14,3	
886-84	12,6	15,6	13,7	11,8
Differences in full-length polyprotein sequences (3,414 aa)				
Genotype 1	1,5			
Genotype 2	6,8	1,2		
Genotype 3	5,0	5,9	1,7	
178-79	3,2	6,3	4,6	
886-84	3,8	6,2	4,3	3,2

Five strains of genotype 1 (DQ989336, AB062064, AB062063, AY182009, DQ862460) and three for genotype 2 (U27495, U27491, U39292) and 3 (L40361, AF527415, DQ486861) were used for analysis. The substitutions levels within the genotypes are marked with gray background.

Table 1. The Differences in Level of Nucleotide and Amino Acid Sequences for 13 TBEV Strains According to Karan' et al. [2007b] (%)

strain 886-84 to the lesser degree adjoined the TBEV-FE genotype and amino acids alternation observed in the polyprotein structure were typical for two and three genotypes within one gene (Table 1).

The last attempt of re-classification of TBEV was suggested by Grard et al. [2007]. During the analysis of full-length genomes of Spanish and Turkish sheep encephalitis viruses they made the conclusion that it could be possible to divide TBEV into four genotypes: Western, Eastern, Turkish sheep encephalitis and Scottish sheep encephalitis (Fig.2). According to the proposed classification TBEV-Sib was included into the Eastern genotype. However, genotype 3 (TBEV-Sib) widely spread in Russia demonstrates the high level of genetic differences from genotypes 1 (TBEV-FE) and 2 (TBEV-Eu) including some type-specific markers possessed by a large number of circulating variants.

Siberia is the part of Russia located between European part and Far-Eastern part and can be divided to Western Siberia and Eastern Siberia (Fig. 3). The aim of the study was the molecular-genetic investigations and genotyping of TBEV strains and isolates samples collected at different regions of Western and Eastern Siberia.

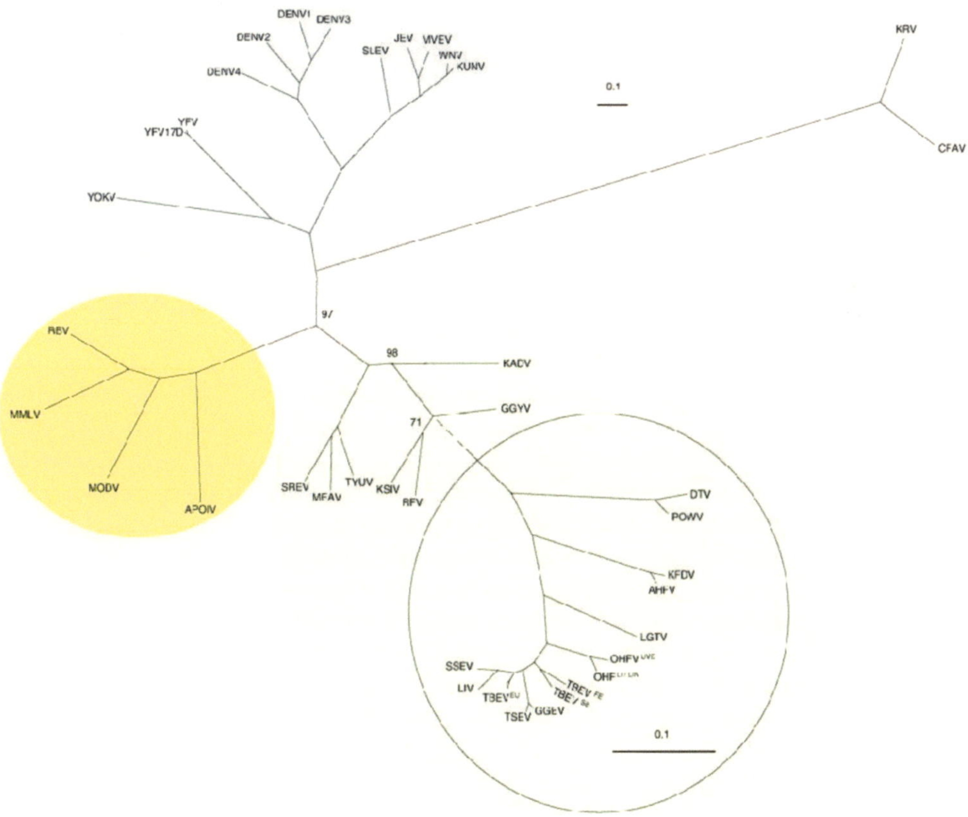

Fig. 2. Phylogenetic analysis based on complete polyprotein sequences [Grard et al., 2007] Phylogenetic reconstruction was performed using the maximum likelihood method. The tick-borne flavivirus group is highlighted in green, the mosquito-borne flavivirus group in blue and the no-known vector flavivirus group in yellow

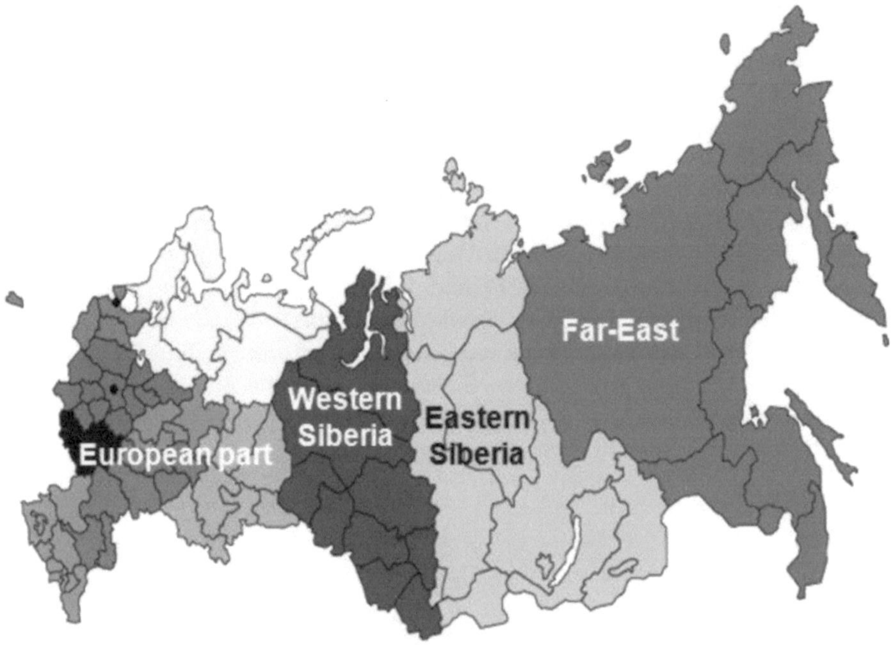

Fig. 3. Location of different parts of the Russia territory

2. Genotyping by molecular hybridization of nucleic acids test with genotype-specific deoxyoligonucleotide probes

2.1 Design of genotype-specific deoxyoligonucleotide probes

The experiments with TBEV genotype-specific probes performed earlier [Zlobin et al., 2001c] revealed the following important points: 1) the differentiation of TBEV strains by using three genotype-specific probes yields an absolute answer and thus does not allow to type strains that have mutation(s) within the annealing sites; 2) an overlapping region of eight conserved nucleotides shared by all TBEV genotypes presented in the probes can cause nonspecific hybridization; and 3) the annealing temperatures of probes varying from 51 to 67°C may cause inconveniences in performing serial experiments. Thus, the following conclusions have been made. Firstly, simultaneous use of genotype-specific probes targeting all TBEV genes (instead of one) will allow to eliminate the influence of single mutations on the result of genotyping and to perform more detailed genetic analysis of each strain. Secondly, the structure in which the target nucleotides are located evenly (the distances that are not more than seven nucleotides are preferable) will react more reliably as a genotype-specific probe. Thirdly, for simultaneous analysis of a large number of TBEV strains the probes with annealing temperatures of 45–47°C should be selected to achieve a highly specific reaction of each probe.

2.2 Viruses

In this study 189 TBEV strains from the collection of Institute of Epidemiology and Microbiology, SCFHHRP ESD RAMS (Irkutsk, Russia) were used. The collection contained

165 strains from Eastern Siberia (Chita region: 8, Buryatiya Republic: 54, Irkutsk region: 88, Krasnoyarsk region and Khakassia Republic: 15) and 24 strains from Western Siberia. The strains were isolated from different biological sources: from Ixodes genus ticks: 148, Dermacentor genus ticks: 2, rodents: 24, insectivorous: 1, birds: 1, from cow milk: 2 and 11 strains were isolated from clinical samples, blood, and medullispinal fluid of patients with tick-borne encephalitis (Table 2). Strains were isolated and cultivated by intracerebral infection of 2-day newborn laboratory mice and then preserved in freeze-dried state. The most strains were lyophilized on 3–7 passages. To accumulate the virus the suspension of freeze-dried strains was prepared with dilution 10^{-3} in Eagle's medium, 2% bovine serum, and antibiotics (200 U/ml). Then suckling nonlinear mice (30 µl intracerebrally) or transplantable cell culture (porcine embryo kidney cells) was infected. The gathering of the virus culture was followed by cell lysis. Mouse autopsies were carried out 5–7 days after infection at the peak of disease. Cultural fluid was centrifuged for detritus removal (3,000 rpm/min for 30 min) and then virus was precipitated with polyethylene glycol according to Mahy [1985].

2.3 Isolation of total RNA and hybridization

RNA from cultivated virus and total cellular RNA from cerebral suspensions were isolated by the method of phenol extraction [Herrington and McGee, 1992]. RNA was spotted on kapron or cellulose nitrate filters (2 mkg/dot of total RNA from mice brain tissue or 1 ng/dot of RNA isolated from the cell culture). Radioactive labeling, hybridization, and detection of hybridized probes were carried out as described [Herrington and McGee, 1992]. Hybridization with all probes was carried out at 45–47°C.

2.4 Probe selection

The TBEV genome sites most suitable for genotyping were selected on the basis of the analysis of TBEV sequences taking into account the requirements for primer design [Innis and Gelfand, 1990] and the previously obtained experience on molecular hybridization [Zlobin et al., 1992, 2001c]. Twelve regions were selected for each of the three genotypes. The probes were targeted to all 10 genes of TBEV: one probe for genes M, C, NS1, NS2A, NS2B, NS3, NS4A, NS4B and two probes for genes E and NS5 (Fig. 4).

There were also probes targeting the E protein-encoding sequences for two subgenotypes of Siberian genotype ("Vasilchenko" and "Zausaev") and the E protein-encoding sequence of strain 178-79. Notably, the targets for three last probes are localized on the E gene since it was best studied and the largest number of sequences was known for this gene. For example, the target sequence specific for the isolate 178-79 was selected based on the 160 nt long region (encoding aa residues 190–242) of 90 TBEV strains. The majority of probes were designed on the basis of the comparison of 10 full-length TBEV genomes. The TBEV species-specific probe sh5 (specific for TBEV) has been described earlier [Shamanin et al., 1990]. The proposed panel includes 40 probes targeting all 10 genes of TBEV (Table 3). Among them, 1 probe (sh5) is species specific, 36 probes are genotype specific (12 probes for each of the three main genotypes), 2 probes (designated as 3a and 3b) are subgenotype specific, differentiating subgenotypes "Vasilchenko" and "Zausaev" of Siberian genotype, and 1 probe, based on the TBEV strain 178-79, is strain specific (for genotype 4).

Region	Isolation source	Isolation year/amount of strains	Strains total	Genotype				
				1	2	3	4	5
Eastern Siberia, Russia	Clinical samples	1963/1, 1979/2, 1982/1, 1986/1, 1998/1, 2003/1, 2004/2, 2005/1	**10**	**1**	**1**	**8**	**-**	**-**
	Cow milk	1971/1, 1979/1	**2**	**1**	**-**	**1**	**-**	**-**
	Rodents	1971/2, 1975/1, 1981/5, 1984/5, 1987/4, 1995/5, 2002/1, 2006/1	**24**	**9**	**4**	**8**	**-**	**3**
	Common shrew	1995/1	**1**	**1**	**-**	**-**	**-**	**-**
	Hazelhen	1982/1	**1**	**1**	**-**	**-**	**-**	**-**
	I. persulcatus	1976/1, 1979/1, 1980/5, 1983/3, 1986/14, 1987/7, 1988/26, 1989/5, 1990/34, 1991/12, 1992/11, 1993/5, 2002/2, 2005/1	**126**	**6**	**-**	**112**	**1**	**7**
	D. nuttalli	1986/1	**1**	**-**	**-**	**1**	**-**	**-**
Total			**165**	**19**	**5**	**130**	**1**	**10**
Western Siberia, Russia	Clinical samples	1961/1	**1**	**-**	**-**	**1**	**-**	**-**
	I. persulcatus	1985/1, 1986/21	**22**	**3**	**5**	**14**	**-**	**-**
	D. pictus	1986/1	**1**	**-**	**-**	**1**	**-**	**-**
Total			**24**	**3**	**5**	**16**	**-**	**-**

Table 2. Summary of TBEV isolates and strains From Western and Eastern Siberia

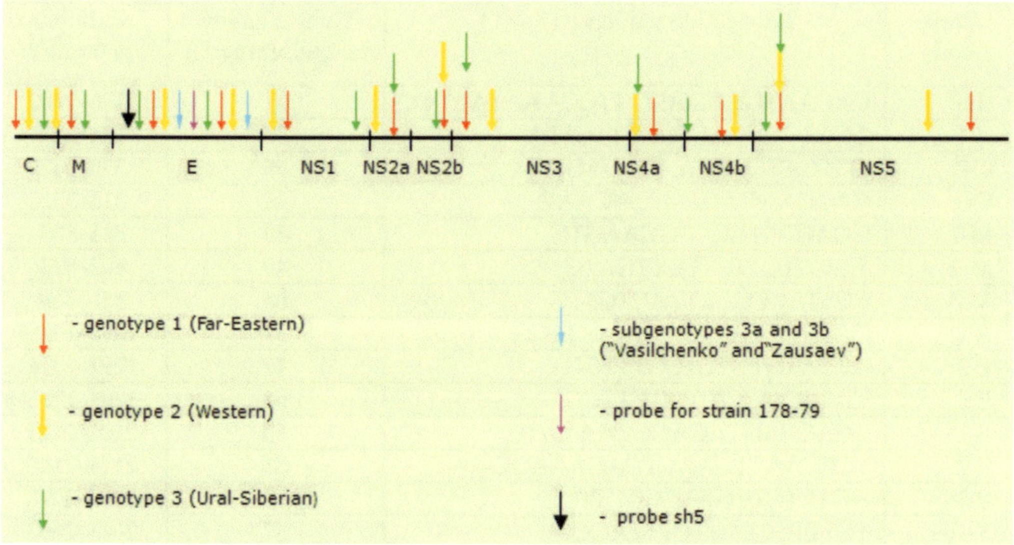

Fig. 4. The arrangement of desoxyoligonucleotide probes on TBEV genome

2.5 Testing of the probes

In the course of testing all 189 TBEV isolates have been divided into five groups corresponding to five genotypes (Tables 2 and 4). It was stated that at the territory of Eastern Siberia (165 strains) 19 strains (11.5%) belong to genotype 1 (Far Eastern), 5 strains (3.0%) belong to genotype 2 (European), and 130 strains (78.8%) belong to genotype 3 (Ural-Siberian or Siberian). The fourth group (genotype 4) included only one strain, 178-79 (0.6%). The fifth group (''group 886''or genotype 5) consisted of 10 strains (6.1%), and one of them (886-84 strain) characterized earlier [Zlobin et al., 2001a,b] was considered to be unique. As for Western Siberia territory (24 tested strains) it was demonstrated that 3 strains belong to Far-Eastern genotype (12.5%), 5 strains - to European genotype (20.8%) and 16 strains - to Siberian genotype (66.7%). None of the strains of 4th or 5th genotypes were found.

Analysis of the efficiency of the genotype-specific probes (Table 4) revealed that (i) with rare exceptions, these probes interacted only with the strains of the same name genotype and (ii) the probes specific to two different subgenotypes within genotype 3 reacted only with the strains of this genotype. All the strains of genotype 3 were further divided into three groups: subgenotype 3a (that reacted with the corresponding subgenotype-specific probe); subgenotype 3b (reacting with the corresponding probe); and ''neither 3a nor 3b'' strains reacting with neither of the subgenotype-specific probes. (iii) The probe intended for recognizing the strain 178-79 was strain specific. Constant interaction of some genotype 1 probes with RNA of genotypes 4 and 5 strains is explained by the fact that the structures of these reacting probes are complementary to the corresponding sites on the genome of these two strain groups. These cross-reactions could be avoided by means of selecting probes specific for genotype 1 only. C-1 probe reacted nonspecifically. This fact may be explained by the difference between its theoretical annealing temperature (57°C) and the temperature used in the experiments (47°C). Specific interaction of the probe NS5-2′ with TBEV strain 178-79 confirmed that this strain is unique. Two probes, C-1 and M-2, cross-reacted with Omsk hemorrhagic fever virus (OHFV), most likely due to shared stretches of 8 and 14 nucleotides, respectively.

Probe code	Nucleotide sequence (5′->3′)	Hybridization temperature (°C)	Location on genome*
sh5**	CACAATGCTGCCTTTTCCAAATAATCC	71	1156–1182
C-1	GGGTGCTCACTGCCTTCTTA	57	234–253
C-2	CGTCATCCCCAACAGAGTAA	55	323–342
C-3	CAGCAAGACAGTGACAAC	49	316–333
M-1	GCACTGTGGCTGCAAGTG	53	341–358
M-2	AGGCTCTTCTCCTTGATC	49	508–525
M-3	CCTTCCCGCCTTACTGTTG	55	350–368
E-1	GAGTCTCATTAGCAGCGACG	57	1290–1309
E-2	ACTATGTGTCTCGTTTGC	47	1297–1314
E-3	CAGTGGCCTTCTTCTTCG	51	1208–1225
E-1'	CCACCAGTAGAGCCAAAATC	55	2104–2123
E-2'	TCCCAATTGAACTCAGAAAGC	55	2123–2143
E-3'	AGTCTCTCGATGCCCTTCC	55	2060–2078
NS1-1	TCTTTCCCCTTCTTTAGC	47	2643–2660
NS1-2	TAGTCAGTGGGGTCAAAC	49	2604–2621
NS1-3	AAGAACCACAACGCCTC	47	3497–3513
NS2A-1	CCTCGAATCAGTTTCCAG	49	3939–3956
NS2A-2	CTGGAGTAGCATCAAGG	47	3614–3630
NS2A-3	TCCCCTGATCAATCTCC	47	3941–3957
NS2B-1	ATCTTCGAGCCGTTCTC	47	4452–4468
NS2B-2	TCAGACCTTCGGGATGA	47	4456–4472
NS2B-3	CAAGCCCAGCAAGTAAC	47	4368–4384
NS3-1	CACTGCCCCTATCCTCCTA	55	4836–4854
NS3-2	TTTTAGGCCATTTCCGTATAGC	57	4920–4941
NS3-3	GTATTGCTCCCATCTTTCTCC	57	4835–4855
NS4A-1	ACCAAACGACGCCAAGAG	51	6521–6538
NS4A-2	CATCTCAACCATAGTCAG	47	6484–6501
NS4A-3	TCACCTCCACCATCGTGAG	55	6484–6502
NS4B-1	TCCCTCTCCAAATGGATTG	51	7242–7260
NS4B-2	ATGAGGCACAACACTGTG	49	7308–7325
NS4B-3	CTCTCAAGGAACCCCATC	51	6783–6800
NS5-1	CTCTCCTGAGGAGTTCC	49	7656–7672
NS5-2	TCCTCTTCTGAGCAACTC	49	7657–7674
NS5-3	CCTTCCTTAGCAGCTCT	47	7656–7672
NS5-1'	TTCGAGAAGCCAACCGAATG	55	9622–9641
NS5-2'	GTGGTTGCCAATTGTTTG	47	9219–9236
NS5-3'	CAGCTGTTCAGTCTCTGT	49	7572–7589
E-3a	ACAATCCGCAGTGATTGC	49	1145–1162
E-3б	AAGGCGCCACCGAGAAC	53	2158–2174
E-4	TACCCCTTCGTGTCTCC	49	1520–1536

*Numeration is done for the coding region. **Probe sh5 is described earlier [Shamanin et al., 1990].

Table 3. Genotype-specific deoxyoligonucleotide probes and their respective targets on TBEV genome

Probe code	Strains of genotype 1 (Far Eastern subtype)		genotype 4 178-79		genotype 5 "Group 886"		Strains of genotype 2 (European subtype)		Strains of genotype 3 (Siberian subtype)	
	P/N*	%**	P/N	%	P/N	%	P/N	%	P/N*	%
sh5	17/22	77	1/1	100	6/10	60	8/10	80	137/144	95
C-1	20/22	91	1/1	100	10/10	100	0/10	0	89/146	61
M-1	20/22	91	1/1	100	0/10	0	0/10	0	1/146	1
E-1	19/22	86	1/1	100	0/10	0	0/10	0	2/146	1
E-1'	20/22	91	0/1	0	0/10	0	0/10	0	1/146	1
NS1-1	6/22	32	1/1	100	10/10	100	0/10	0	3/146	2
NS2A-1	20/22	91	0/1	0	0/10	0	0/10	0	1/146	1
NS2B-1	20/22	91	1/1	100	0/10	0	0/10	0	4/146	3
NS3-1	21/22	95	1/1	100	10/10	100	0/10	0	22/146	15
NS4A-1	16/22	72	0/1	0	0/10	0	0/10	0	0/146	0
NS4B-1	19/22	86	0/1	0	0/10	0	0/10	0	2/146	1
NS5-1	9/22	41	0/1	0	0/10	0	0/10	0	1/146	1
NS5-1'	15/22	68	0/1	0	0/10	0	1/10	10	11/146	8
C-2	0/22	0	0/1	0	0/10	0	10/10	100	0/146	0
M-2	0/22	0	0/1	0	0/10	0	10/10	100	12/146	8
E-2	0/22	0	0/1	0	0/10	0	10/10	100	0/146	0
E-2'	0/22	0	0/1	0	0/10	0	5/10	50	0/146	0
NS1-2	0/22	0	0/1	0	0/10	0	7/10	70	1/146	0
NS2A-2	0/22	0	0/1	0	0/10	0	9/10	90	2/146	1
NS2B-2	0/22	0	0/1	0	0/10	0	1/10	10	1/146	1
NS3-2	0/22	0	0/1	0	0/10	0	10/10	100	0/146	0
NS4A-2	1/22	5	0/1	0	0/10	0	5/10	50	1/146	1
NS4B-2	1/22	5	0/1	0	0/10	0	3/10	30	1/146	1
NS5-2	0/22	0	0/1	0	0/10	0	10/10	100	0/146	0
NS5-2'	0/22	0	1/1	100	0/10	0	10/10	100	7/146	5
C-3	0/22	0	0/1	0	0/10	0	0/10	0	15/146	10
M-3	0/22	0	0/1	0	0/10	0	0/10	0	38/146	26
E-3	0/22	0	0/1	0	0/10	0	0/10	0	96/146	66
E-3'	0/22	0	0/1	0	0/10	0	0/10	0	44/146	99
NS1-3	0/22	0	0/1	0	0/10	0	0/10	0	112/146	77
NS2A-3	1/22	5	0/1	0	0/10	0	0/10	0	80/146	55

Probe code	Strains of genotype 1 (Far Eastern subtype)		genotype 4 178-79		genotype 5 "Group 886"		Strains of genotype 2 (European subtype)		Strains of genotype 3 (Siberian subtype)	
	P/N*	%**	P/N	%	P/N	%	P/N	%	P/N*	%
NS2B-3	1/22	5	0/1	0	0/10	0	0/10	0	60/146	41
NS3-3	1/22	5	0/1	0	0/10	0	0/10	0	131/146	90
NS4A-3	0/22	0	0/1	0	0/10	0	0/10	0	71/146	49
NS4B-3	2/19	9	0/1	0	0/10	0	0/10	0	105/146	72
NS5-3	0/22	0	0/1	0	0/10	0	0/10	0	114/146	78
NS5-3'	1/22	5	0/1	0	0/10	0	1/10	10	85/146	58
E-3a	0/22	0	0/1	0	0/10	0	0/10	0	34/146	23
E-3b	0/22	0	0/1	0	0/10	0	0/10	0	30/146	21
E-4	0/22	0	1/1	100	0/10	0	0/10	0	0/146	0

1′,2′,3′ – Probes targeting the gene of the same TBEV genotype.
*Number of positive reactions/number of tested samples. **Hybridization efficiency (%).

Table 4. Effect of hybridization of genotype-specific deoxyoligonucleotide probes with investigated TBEV strains

3. Genotyping by phylogenetic analysis approach

3.1 Viruses

In this study 1) 70 TBEV strains from the collection of Institute of Systematics and Ecology of Animals SB RAS (Novosibirsk, Russia) and 2) 54 strains from the collection of Institute of Epidemiology and Microbiology, SCFHHRP ESD RAMS (Irkutsk, Russia) were used. The first ones were isolated by bioassay method from *Ixodes persulcatus* ticks collected at the territory of Novosibirsk scientific center and its suburbs in 1981-2001 and cultivated for 2–16 passages in laboratory mice. The second ones were isolated from different source at the territory of Western and Eastern Siberia (see part 2 of the Chapter) and cultivated by intracerebral infection of 2-day newborn laboratory mice and then preserved in freeze-dried state.

3.2 Isolation of total RNA, reverse transcription (RT)-PCR and sequencing

RNA from cultivated virus and total cellular RNA from cerebral suspensions were isolated by the method of phenol extraction [Herrington and McGee, 1992]. The reverse transcription was performed with the kit "RevertaL-100" contained random hexanucleotides (Amplisence, Moscow, Russia). Amplification was done with primers corresponding to specific regions of the E gene (positions 1089–1108 and 2367–2386 the genome of TBEV Sofjin-HO strain (AB062064)) or fragments of E and NS1 genes (positions 2216–2236 and 3364–3383 or 2199-2219 and 2517-2539 on the genome of TBEV Sofjin-HO strain). The primers were synthesized in the Institute of Chemical Biology and Fundamental Medicine of the Siberian Branch of the Russian Academy of Science (Novosibirsk, Russia). These primers were selected on the basis of sequences of highly conservative sections of three TBEV genotypes (strains Sofjin, Neudoerfl, Vasilchenko, and Zausaev). One- or two-round PCR was carried out using these oligonucleotides as primers following the manufacturer's recommendations (Biosan, Novosibirsk, Russia). The direct sequencing of PCR products corresponded to E or E and NS1 genes was performed with BigDye Terminators Cycle Sequencing Kit v.3.1 (Applied Biosystems, Foster City, CA, USA) in the Center of DNA sequencing of the Siberian Branch of the Russian Academy of Science (Novosibirsk, Russia).

3.3 Molecular-genetic analysis

The alignment of obtained sequences was performed with ClustalW program [Larkin et al., 2007]. Homology search with known TBEV genome fragments sequences was made with BLAST program (http://www.ncbi.nlm.nih.gov/blast/). The sequences of the strains of different TBEV genotypes from GenBank database (http://www.ncbi.nlm.nih.gov/Genbank/index.html) were used for comparison. Evaluation of phylogenetic interactions of TBEV based on the full-length genomes or genome fragments was implemented using programs Mega 4.0 [Tamura et al., 2007] and TreeCon [Van de Peer and De Wachter, 1994]. Sequences of the following strains were used: Sofjin [Pletnev et al., 1990], Sofjin-HO (AB062064), 205 (DQ989336), Oshima-10 (AB062063), Senzhang (AY182009), MDJ-01 (AY217093), Glubinnoe (DQ862460), Prymorye-69 (EU816453), Prymorye-86 (EU816455), Prymorye-94 (EU816454), Prymorye-212 (EU816450), Prymorye-253 (EU816451), 178-79 (EF469661), 886-84 (EF469662), Prymorye-270 (EU816452), Neudoerfl (TEU27495), 263 (TEU27491), Hypr (TEU39292), K23 (AM600965), Salem (FJ572210), Vasilchenko (L40361), Zausaev (AF527415), Ek-328 (DQ486861), and Omsk hemorrhagic fever virus (NC_005062)).

3.4 TBEV strains genotyping

The nucleotide sequences of genomes fragments with length 518 bp (207-724 nr from the beginning of E gene) obtained by RT-PCR followed by sequencing were determined for 70 TBEV strains isolated at the territory of Novosibirsk scientific center (58 strains) and Novosibirsk city suburbs (12 strains) in 1981-2001. According to the different structure models this E protein region encoded by the appropriate gene region was shown to contain I and II domains fragments [Rey et al., 1995] or E1 an E2 functionally significant domains fragments [Tsekhanovskaya et al., 1993], or A and C antigenic domains fragments [Mandl et al., 1989]. The obtained sequences were submitted into GenBank database (accession numbers EF467840-EF467846, EF469738-EF469741, EF469743, EF469744, EF469746-EF469748, EF469750, EF469751, EF469754, EF469755, EF469757, EF469760-EF469762, EF469764, EF470568-EF470575, EF470577, EF470578, EU443258-EU443260, EU443263-EU443271, EU443274, EU443275, EU443277-EU443279, EU443281-EU443284, EU836250).

For the further comparative analysis the sequences of TBEV prototype strains of Far-Eastern (Sofjin strain), Siberian (Zausaev and Vasilchenko strains) and European (Neudoerfl strain) genotypes were used. The analysis of obtained data and homology search revealed high homology level of investigated sequences with Siberian genotype TBEV strains (>92% of homology with Zausaev subgenotype and >93% of homology with Vasilchenko subgenotype) and reliable differences from TBEV strains of European and Far-Eastern genotypes (<87% and 85% of homology, respectively). But one should note that 100% homology level wasn't found between obtained sequences and sequences of flavivirus genome fragments from Genbank database.

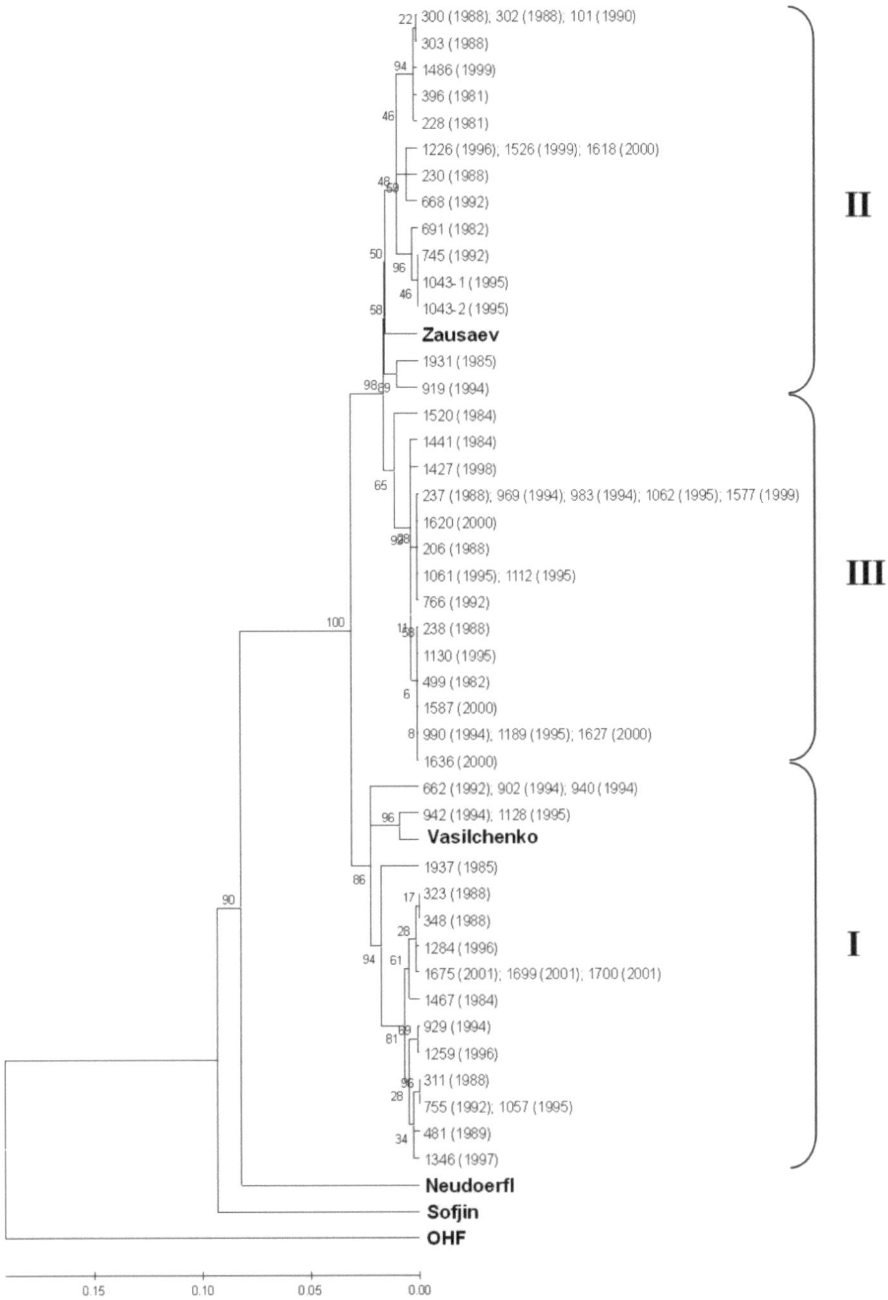

Fig. 5. Dendrogram based on TBEV E gene fragment sequences built by UPGMA method. In brackets - year of strain isolation; Prototype strains marked with bold. I -Vasilchenko subgenotype group; II -Zausaev subgenotype group; III - possible subgenotype non-described earlier

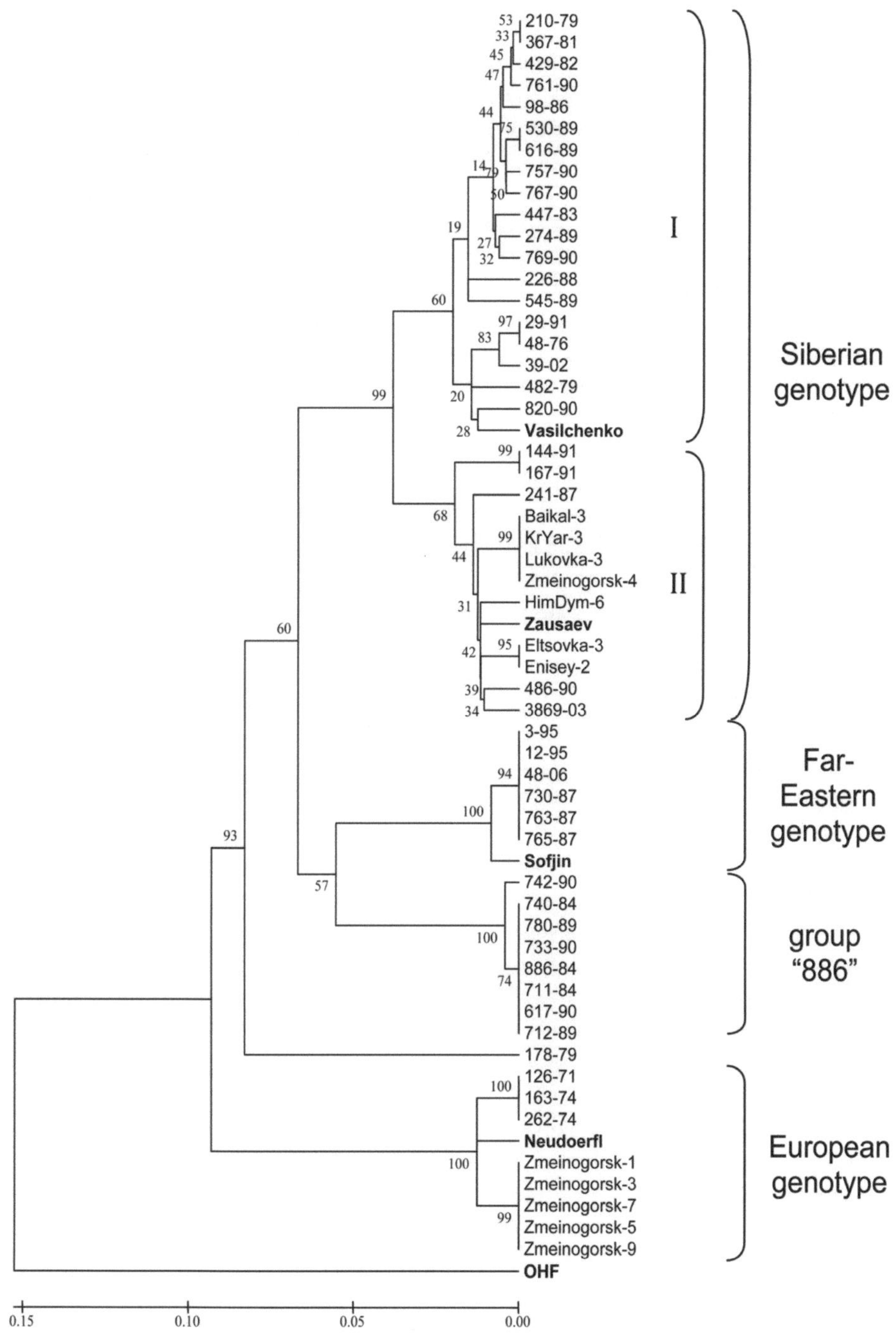

Fig. 6. Dendrogram based on TBEV E-NS1 gene fragment sequences built by UPGMA method. Prototype strains marked with bold; I -Vasilchenko subgenotype group; II -Zausaev subgenotype group

Phylogenetic analysis was performed with Mega 4.0 program [Kumar et al., 2004]. The sequence of Omsk hemorrhagic fever virus genome fragment was used as outgroup. The analysis of dendrogram built by UPGMA method demonstrated that all investigated strains could be divided to three groups: the first one corresponded to Vasilchenko subgenotype TBEV strains (group I), the second one - to Zausaev subgenotype (group II) and for the group III the prototype strain wasn't found (Fig. 5).

For the phylogenetic analysis of TBEV strains from the collection of Institute of Epidemiology and Microbiology, SCFHHRP ESD RAMS (Irkutsk, Russia) 54 strains from the set used for molecular hybridization of nucleic acids test with genotype-specific deoxyoligonucleotide probes (see part 2 of the Chapter) were chosen. RT-PCR with the primers corresponded to E-NS1 gene fragment was performed followed by sequencing. It was demonstrated that methods of molecular hybridization of nucleic acids with genotype-specific probes and molecular-genetic analysis resulted in identical data. It was shown that TBEV strains from Eastern Siberia could be referred to European (3 strains), Far-Eastern (6 strains) and Siberian (31 strains) genotypes (Fig. 6). The last one was shown to divide only into Vasilchenko and Zausaev subgenotypes. Also five TBEV strains from Altai region (Western Siberia) were found to be European genotype. Also one should pay a special attention to the strain 178-79 and to the group of eight strains including 886-84 strain.

3.5 Sequence analysis of TBEV strains from "group 886" and phylogenetic analysis of strains 178-79 and 886-84

All the strains from "group 886" originated from four natural foci located in the Bichura and Barguzin districts of Buryatia; Krasnochikoisk district of Chita region; and Ekhirit-Bulagatsk district of Irkutsk region. The strains were typed preliminarily as Far-Eastern, albeit with unusual hybridization pattern: 3 of 12 genotype 1 specific probes react with these strains (athough all over the surveyed area the strains of genotype 1 with reactivity corresponding probes within the limits of 42–100% circulate). In addition to strain 886-84, this group included strains 740-84 and 711-84 originated from red vole (*Clethrionomys rufocanus*) and seven strains from ticks *I. persulcatus*: 418-90, 712-89, 608-90, 617-90, 636-90, 691-90, and 287-83 isolated in the period from 1983 to 1990.

For strains 617-90, 740-84, and 711-84, the sequences coding protein E (1,322 nt) and NS1 (872 nt) were obtained (EU878283, EU878282, EU878281). Comparison of these sequences with the corresponding genome region of the 886-84 strain (EF469662) revealed a high level of homology (99.3–99.8%) for all four sequences. Differences in the sequences between strains from "group 886" and strains belonging to three genotypes made up 12% (Fig. 7) which corresponds to the criteria of genotyping suggested by Zlobin et al. [2001a, b]. Thus, the genetic evidence of the circulation in Eastern Siberia of genotype 5 strains described earlier by Zlobin and coauthors was obtained.

Phylogenetic analyses confirmed the uniqueness of two East Siberian TBEV strains, 178-79 and 886-84. These strains were located on distinct branches and most often grouped with genotype 1 strains. Depending on the genome region analyzed, these strains adjoined with either genotype 2 or genotype 3 isolates. For example, the phylogenetic trees drawn up for three TBEV genes showed that both East Siberian isolates differed from other 21 TBEV strains, which formed three groups (Fig. 8). Phylogenetic trees drawn up for the other seven TBEV genes possessed the same branching pattern as the bottom tree ("all genome").

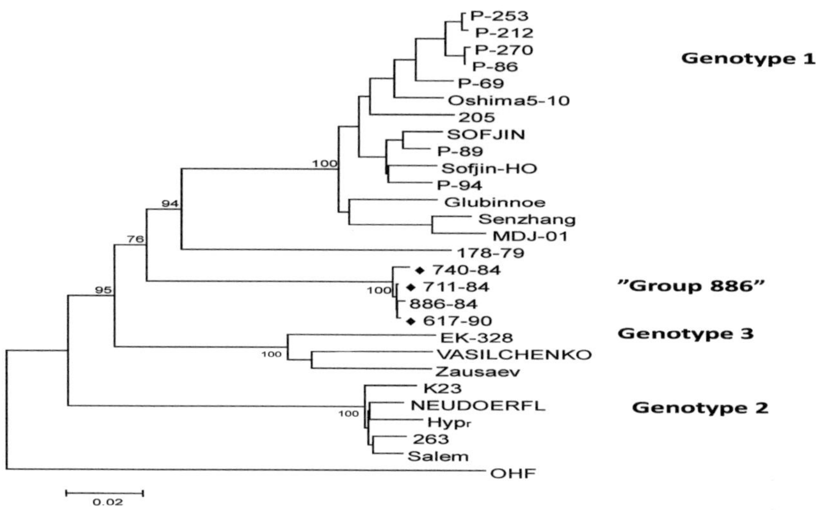

% of sequences (2194 nt) distinction among strains within groups and between groups

	genotype 1	178-79	«group 886»	genotype 2	genotype 3
genotype 1	4,7				
178-79	12,4				
«group 886»	12,8	13,0	0,85		
genotype 2	16,1	16,4	16,3	2,2	
genotype 3	14,8	14,3	13,1	15,6	6,7
OHF	19,9	20,6	19,6	19,1	20,0

Fig. 7. Phylogenetic tree (NJ, Kimura-2-parameter) and differences levels between TBEV strains according to analysis of the genome fragments coding the major part of E and NS1 genes

4. Discussion

Although TBEV strains had gone through several passages in laboratory animals the patterns of RNA hybridization for the strains isolated from the same natural focus for several years were similar. Thus, the results obtained with the panel of probes could be used for characterization of TBEV variants circulating in different natural foci.

The set of investigated in molecular hybridization of nucleic acids test TBEV strains based mostly on the local collection appeared to contain mainly Eastern Siberian variants. The geographic distribution of TBEV genotypes correlated well with the previously published data [Zlobin et al., 2003]. The genotype 2 (European) was found mostly at the territory of Altai (5 of 8 isolates in Western Siberia) (Table I and Fig. 3) and more rarely in Eastern Siberia (5 of 165 isolates). Genotype 1 (Far-Eastern) was found everywhere in minor cases. Genotype 3 (Siberian) was more common in Eastern and Western Siberia.

Four above-mentioned foci located in Eastern Siberia (Bichura and Barguzin districts of Buryatia, Krasnochikoisk district of the Chita region, and Ekhirit-Bulagatsk district of the Irkutsk region) are of special interest due to circulating strains of genotype 5. Notably, within the Ekhirit-Bulagatsk focus, in addition to 886-84 strain, the representatives of all three main genotypes were present but also strains of different subgenotypes and unique

178-79 strain were found. The strain 178-79 was the only one that was recognized by a specific probe E-4. The annealing site for this probe contains several single genotype 2- and genotype 3 specific nucleotide substitutions. From more than 600 TBEV sequences of this region known so far none resembles the sequence of 178-79 strain. The results of this study demonstrated the existence of a relatively stable set of TBEV genetic variants within a specific area, which were recorded for the last 70 years.

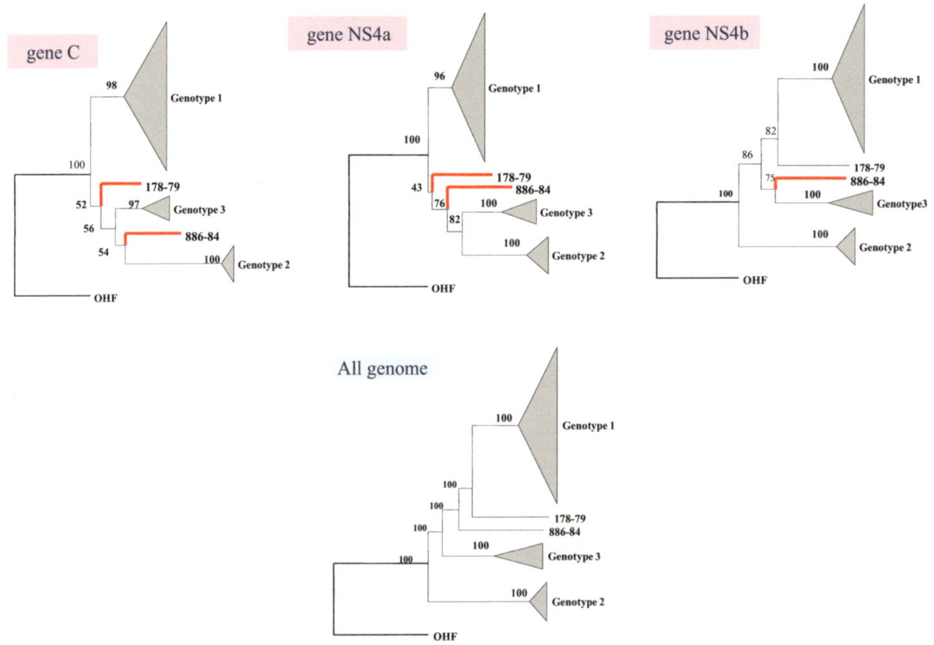

Fig. 8. Phylogenetic tree (NJ, Kimura-2-parameter) and differences levels between TBEV strains according to analysis of the genome fragments coding the major part of E and NS1 genes.
Genotype 1 claster: Sofjin, Sofin-HO, 205, Oshima5-10, Senzhang, MDJ-01, Glubinnoe, Primorye-69, Primorye-86, Primorye-94, Primorye-212, Primorye-253, Primorye-270 strains.
Genotype 2 - Neudoerfl, 263, Hypr, K23, Salem strains;
Genotype 3 - Vasilchenko, Zausaev, Eκ-328 strains

These TBEV strains, 178-79 and 886-84 originated from the same natural focus in Eastern Siberia, are of special interest. Their singularity was first observed in the study of serological properties and short E gene sequences [Trukhina et al., 1988; Zlobin et al., 1996, 2001a, b, 2002; Verkhozina et al., 2002]. These studies suggested that the 886-84 strain occupied an intermediate position between the East Siberian and Far Eastern serotypes of TBEV and possessed the properties of both serotypes [Trukhina et al., 1988]. This strain has an identical degree of similarity with all the three subtypes of TBEV in reaction of diffusion precipitation in agar (RDPA) with cross-adsorbed strain-specific sera [Verkhozina et al., 2002; Zlobin et al., 2002]. Pogodina et al. [1981] have included 178-79 strain in the Aina-like strain group (in modern classification – the Ural-Siberian or Siberian genotype). Zlobin et al. [1996] also have come to the conclusion that this strain is clearly differentiated from representatives of other antigen subtypes both in RDPA and in reaction of neutralization. According to the analysis

of E gene fragment sequences (160 nt in length) in 34 TBEV strains the 886-84 and 178-79 strains were not included in any of the known three genotypes, but the analysis of amino acid sequences derived from corresponding nucleotide sequences of the studied fragment has demonstrated that 886-84 strain belongs to genotype 3 and 178-79 strain to genotype 1 [Zlobin et al., 2003]. It should be noted that, according to Zlobin et al. [2001b], genotype 1 corresponded to the FE serotype while genotype 2 corresponded to the Western serotype. Genotype 3 included two antigenic variants, Ural-Siberian and Central Siberian trans-Baikal, or serotype Aina. Corresponding prototype strains for these two variants were Lesopark-11 [Zlobin et al., 1991] and Aina [Pogodina et al., 1981]. Nowadays, both variants belong to the same serotype, Ural-Siberian and Central Siberian trans-Baikal, with the prototype strain Vasilchenko. Uniqueness of isolates 178-79 and 886-84 was shown in the atypical (for genotype 1) hybridization pattern and was also apparent in the phylogenetic trees (Figs. 7 and 8). The existence of this so-called "group 886" showed that TBEV variants of the genotype 5 existed in nature and occupied a certain niche, since they were isolated from different species (rodents and ticks), within different regions in Eastern Siberia, and for several years (1983–1990). These findings raise the question whether the genotype 5 variants are health threatening. Severe TBE cases were observed in the natural foci where TBEV variants from "group 886" circulated [Demina et al., 2007]. These foci are located in Bichura area of Buryatia and Krasnochikoisk district of Chita region [Lohov and Blinnikova, 1986; Gorin et al., 1992]. Recently, TBEV sequences have been revealed by RT-PCR from a fatal TBE case in Bulgan aymack, Mongolia [Khasnatinov et al., 2009]. This district borders on the four known foci of "group 886" in the south of Eastern Siberia. When compared with the strain 886-84 the 281 nt long fragment of the E gene of this strain showed a high level of sequence homology (98.5%). So it should be important to reveal the origin of these unusual genetic variants of TBEV that remains unknown.
The analysis of existing sequence data of TBEV shows that the arrangement of specific oligonucleotide sequences suitable for genotyping does not always coincide with flashpoints of amino acid mutations and secondly, that genotypic differences are often revealed at the level of the third position in the codon. It means that genotypic differences are possibly connected not only with amino acid substitutions but also with the substitutions in the third positions of codons. So it is possible that natural selection takes place not only at the protein level but also at the RNA level.

5. Conclusions

It was shown that strains of three TBEV genotypes were found at the territories of both Western and Eastern Siberia that was confirmed by both molecular hybridization of nucleic acids test and sequencing followed by phylogenetic analysis. Based on phylogenetic analysis, all strains from Western Siberia corresponded to Siberian genotype were divided into three subgenotypes - Zausaev, Vasilchenko and subgenotype non-described earlier. On the contrary, the strains from Eastern Siberia were divided only into Zausaev and Vasilchenko subgenotypes. Also two groups of strains that could possibly be the new TBEV genotypes meeting the requirements of differences in genome sequences homology level with other genotypes were detected. The fourth possible genotype was presented by only one isolate, 178-79, originated from Irkutsk region, Russia. The fifth possible genotype included 10 isolates, one of them, 886-84, was described earlier. So, the existence of this so-called "group 886" showed that such TBEV variants existed in nature and occupied a certain niche, since they were isolated from different species (rodents and ticks), within different regions in Eastern Siberia and for several years (1983–1990). It is unknown whether "group 886" variants are health threatening because recently the comparison of genome fragment sequence of TBEV from clinical samples of fatal case in Mongolia revealed a high level of homology (98.5%) with the strain 886-84.

6. Acknowledgements

This work was supported in part by interdisciplinary integration projects of SB RAS №6 and 63.

7. References

Demina, T.V., Dzhioev, Yu.P., Verkhozina, M.M., Kozlova, I.V., Doroshenko, E.K., Lisak, O.V., Protasova, H.G. & Zlobin V.I. (2007). Investigation of tickborne encephalitis virus with genome probing. *Bulletin of ESSC SB RAMS,* № 36 pp. 94–98 (Russian).

Ecker, M., Allison, S.L., Meixner, T. & Heinz, F.X. (1999). Sequence analysis and genetic classification of TBEV from Europe and Asia. *J. Gen. Virol.* V. 80, pp. 179–185.

Gao, G.F., Hussain, M.H., Reid, H.W. & Gould, E.A. (1993). Classification of a new member of the TBE flavivirus subgroup by its immunological, pathogenetic and molecular characteristics: Identification of subgroup-specific pentapeptides. *Virus Res.* V. 30, pp. 129–144.

Gorin, O.Z., Mungalova, N.P., Leonov, V.A., Sozanskiy, B.E., Zharskaya, S.L., Arbatskaya, E.V., Trukhina, A.G. & Kovsharov, A.F. (1992). Situation on tick-borne encephalitis at the west of Chita region. In: *Ethiology, epidemiology and infectious diseases diagnostics of Eastern Siberia: Collection of scientific articles,* V.I. Zlobin, (ed.), 44–53, IEM ESD SB RAMS, Irkutsk (Russian).

Grard, G., Moureau, G., Charrel, R.N., Lemasson, J.J., Gonzalez, J.P., Gallian, P., Gritsun, T.S., Holmes, E.C., Gould, E.A. & de Lamballerie, X. (2007). Genetic characterization of tick-borne flaviviruses: New insights into evolution, pathogenetic determinants and taxonomy. *Virology.* V. 361, pp. 80–92.

Hayasaka, D., Suzuki, Y., Kariva, H., Ivanov, L., Volkov, V., Demenev, V., Mizutani, T., Gojobori, T. & Takashima, I. (1999). Phylogenetic and virulence analysis of tick-borne encephalitis viruses from Japan and far-eastern Russia. *J. Gen. Virol.* V. 80, pp. 3127–3135.

Hayasaka, D., Ivanov, L., Leonova, G.N., Goto, A., Yoshii, K., Mizutani, T., Kariwa, H. & Takashima, I. (2001). Distribution and characterization of tick-borne encephalitis viruses from Siberia and far-eastern Asia. *J. Gen. Virol.* V. 82, pp. 1319–1328.

Heinz, F.X., Collett, M.S., Purcell, R.H., Gould, E.A., Howard, C.R., Houghton, M., Moormann, R.J.M., Rice, C.M. & Thiel, H.J. (2000). Family Flaviviridae, In: *Virus taxonomy. Seventh Report of the International Committee on Taxonomy of Viruses,* M.H.V. Van Regenmortel, C.M. Fauquet, D.H.L. Bishop, E.B. Carstens, M.K. Estes, S.M. Lemon, D.J. McGeoch, J. Maniloff, M.A. Mayo, C.R. Pringle, R.B. Wickner, (Eds), 858–878, Academic Press, San Diego.

Herrington, C.S., McGee, J.O.D. (1992). *Diagnostic molecular pathology: A practical approach,* IRL Press at Oxford University Press, Oxford, New York, Tokyo.

Innis, M.A., Gelfand, D.H. (1990). Optimization of PCRs. In: *PCR protocols: A guide to methods and applications,* M.A. Innis, D.H. Gelfand, J.J. Sninsky, T.J. White, (Eds.), 3–12, Academic Press, San Diego.

Karan', L.S., Braslavskaya, S.I., Myazin, A.E. (2007a). Development of detection methods and genotyping of TBE virus in terms of amplification technologies. *Vopr. Virusol.* № 16, pp. 17–22 (Russian).

Karan', L.S., Malenko, G.V., Bochkova, N.G., Levina, L.S., Pivanova, G.P., Colyasnikova, N.M., Gamova, E.G., Trukhina, A.G., Zlobin, V.I., Verkhozina, M.M., Kozlova, I.V., Dzhioev, Yu.P., Demina, T.V. & Pogodina, V.V. (2007b). Application of molecular genetic methodic for examination of structure of strains of TBEvirus. *Bulletin of SB RAMS.* № 4, pp. 34–40 (Russian).

Khasnatinov, M.A., Danchinova, G.A., Unursaikhan, U., Tyngalag, K.H., Tserennorov, D., Undraa, B., Baigalmaa, B., Abmed, D., Mironova, L.V. & Otgonbaatar, D. (2009). Characterization of tick-borne encephalitis virus that caused the lethal meningoencephalitis human in Mongolia. In: *Zoonotic infectious diseases and tourism (reports). Inter. Conference.*, D. Otgonbaatar & B. Burmaa, (Eds.), 88–93, Ulaanbaatar.

Larkin, M.A., Blackshields, G., Brown, N.P., Chenna, R., McGettigan, P.A., McWilliam, H., Valentin, F., Wallace, I.M., Wilm, A., Lopez, R., Thompson, J.D., Gibson, T.J. & Higgins, D.G. (2007). Clustal W and Clustal X version 2.0. *Bioinformatics.* V. 23, pp. 2947-2948.

Lohov, M.G. & Blinnikova, I.A. (1986). Structural-functional characteristics of tick-borne encephalitis pestholes in Bichur region of Buryatiya Republic. In: *Annual of scientific articles*, M.A. Rybalko, (Ed.), 44–52, Medical Institute, Irkutsk.

Mandl, C.W., Guirakhoo, F., Holzmann, H., Heinz, F.X. & Kunz C. (1989). Antigenic structure of the flavivirus envelope protein E at the molecular level, using tick-borne encephalitis virus as a model. *J. of Virology.* V. 63, № 2, pp. 564-571.

Mahy B.W.J. (1985). *Virology: A practical approach*, IRL Press, Oxford, Washington, DC.

Pletnev, A.G., Yamshikov, V.F. & Blinov, V.M. (1990). Nucleotide sequence of the genome and complete amino acid sequence of the polyprotein of tick-borne encephalitis virus. *Virology.* V. 174, pp. 250–263.

Pogodina, V.V., Bochkova, N.G., Levina, L.S., Zhezmer, V.Yu. & Meerova, R.A. (1981). Immunological and etiological aspects of a study of the Aina/1448 serotype of the tick-borne encephalitis virus. *Vopr. Virusol.* № 6, pp. 735–741 (Russian).

Pogodina, V.V., Bochkova, N.G., Zlobin, V.I., Frolova, M.P., Drokin, D.A., Levina, L.S. & Dzhioev, Yu.P. (1993). Genetic characteristic of Vergina's serotype of TBEV, and its pathology features. *Vopr. Virusol.* № 14, pp. 158–163 (Russian).

Pogodina, V.V., Bochkova, L.S., Levina, L.S., Frolova, T.V., Trukhina, A.G., Frolova, M.P. & Malenko, G.V. (2002). Complex characteristics of Siberian subtype of tick-borne encephalitis virus. In: *Tick-borne encephalitis*, G.N. Leonova & L.M. Somova-Isachkova, (Eds.), 72–87, State Unitary Organization "Primorskiy poligraphkombinat", Vladivostok (Russian).

Pogodina, V.V., Bochkova, L.S., Karan, L.S., Frolova, T.V., Levina, L.S., Malenko, G.V. & Platonov, A.E. (2004). Monitoring of tick-borne encephalitis virus population in European and Asian regions of Russia. Practical aspects of the problem. *Biological Drugs.* № 2, pp. 7–13 (Russian).

Rey, F.A., Heinz, F.X., Mandl, C., Kunz, C. & Harrison S.C. (1995). The envelope glycoprotein from tick-borne encephalitis virus at 2 A resolution. *Nature.* V. 375, pp. 291-298.

Shamanin, V.A., Pletnev, A.G., Rubin, S.G. & Zlobin V.I. (1990). Differentiation of strains of tick-borne encephalitis virus by means of RNA-DNA hybridization. *J. Gen. Virol.* V. 71, pp. 1505–1515.

Tamura, K., Dudley, J., Nei, M. & Kumar, S. (2007). MEGA4: Molecular Evolutionary Genetics Analysis (MEGA) software version 4.0. *Mol. Biol. Evol.* V. 24, pp. 1596–1599.

Trukhina, A.G., Chipanin, V.I., Vasenin, A.A., Voronko, I.V., Arbatskaya, E.V. (1988). *Ecology peculiarities of combined pestholes of two serotypes of tick-borne encephalitis virus in Eastern Siberia deposit,* All-union Scientific-Research Institution of Medical and Medical-Technical Information, Russia (Russian).

Tsekhanovskaya, N.A., Matveev, L.E., Rubin, S.G., Karavanov, A.S. & Pressman, E.K. (1993). Epitope analysis of tick-borne encephalitis (TBE) complex viruses using monoclonal antibodies to envelope glycoprotein of TBE virus (persulcatus subtype). *Virus Research.* V. 30, pp. 1-16.

Van de Peer, Y. & De Wachter, R. (1994). TREECON for Windows: A software package for the construction and drawing of evolutionary trees for the Microsoft Windows environment. *Comput. Appl. Biosci.* V. 10, pp. 569–570.

Verkhozina, M.M., Zlobin, V.I., Kozlova, I.V., Belikov, S.I., Demina, T.V., Butina, T.V., Dzhioev, Yu.P., Adel'shin, R.V., Gazo, M. & Mamaev, L.V. (2002). Molecular-epidemiology characterization of tick-borne encephalitis virus regional population in Eastern Siberia. *Bulletin of ESSC SB RAMS.* № 2, pp. 46–49 (Russian).

Zlobin V.I. & Lvov D.K. (2008). Tick-borne encephalitis. In: *Medical virology: Manual,* D.K. Lvov, (Ed.), 548–552, Medical Informational Agency, Moscow (Russian).

Zlobin, V.I., Drokin, D.A., Mansurov, P.G., Kalmin, O.B. & Iakimenko, V.V. (1991). The typing of tick-borne encephalitis virus strains by the soluble antigen. *Vopr. Virusol.* № 36, pp. 24–27 (Russian).

Zlobin, V.I., Shamanin, V.A., Pletnev, A.G., Drokin, D.A., Dzhioev, Yu.P., Voronko, I.V., Mel'nikova, O.V. & Gusarova, N.A. (1992). The specific reactivity of cDNA- and deoxyoligonucleotide probes, complementary to the tick-borne encephalitis virus genome, with the RNA of strains of different geographical origins. *Vopr. Virusol.* № 5-6, pp. 248–252 (Russian).

Zlobin, V.I., Mamaev, L.V., Dzhioev, Yu.P., Kozlova, I.V. & Verkhozina, M.M. (1996). Molecular biological data confirmthe genetic independence of East Siberian subtype of TBE virus (prototype strain Aina/1448). In: *Abstract Book of International scientific conference "Tick-borne viral, rickettsial and bacterial infections."*, 58–59, IEM ESSC SB RAMS, Irkutsk.

Zlobin, V.I., Demina, T.V., Belikov, S.I., Butina, T.V., Gorin, O.Z., Adel'shin, R.V. & Grachev, M.A. (2001a). Genetic typing of TBEV strains in terms of homology analysis of an envelope protein's gene fragment. *Vopr. Virusol.* № 1, pp. 17–22 (Russian).

Zlobin, V.I., Demina, T.V., Mamaev, L.V., Butina, T.V., Belikov, S.I., Gorin, O.Z., Dzhioev, Yu.P., Verkhozina, M.M., Kozlova, I.V., Voronko, I.V., Adel'shin, R.V. & Grachev, M.A. (2001b). Analysis of genetic variability of TBEV strains on the primary structure of a cover protein's gene fragment. *Vopr. Virusol.* № 1, pp. 12–16 (Russian).

Zlobin, V.I., Gazo, M., Belikov, S.I., Dzhioev, Yu.P., Demina, T.V., Verkhozina, M.M., Kozlova, I.V., Adel'shin, R.V. & Doroshenko, E.K. (2001c). Molecular probes for genetic typing of tick-borne encephalitis virus. *Vopr. Virusol.* V. 4, pp. 43–47 (Russian).

Zlobin, V.I., Borisov, V.A., Verkhozina, M.M., Malov, I.V. & Kholmogorova, G.N. (2002). *TBE in Eastern Siberia.* RPD ESSC SB RAMS, Irkutsk (Russian).

Zlobin V.I., Belikov, S.I., Dzhioev, Yu.P., Demina, T.V. & Kozlova, I.V. (2003). *Molecular-epidemiology characterization of tick-borne encephalitis virus regional population in Eastern Siberia,* EPD ESSC SB RAMS, Irkutsk (Russian).

Analysis of the Incidence of Tick-Borne Encephalitis as an Occupational Disease and of the Costs of the Diagnosis and Treatment of Acute Tick-Borne Encephalitis in the Slovak Republic from 1989 to 2009

Viera Svihrova, Henrieta Hudeckova,
Janka Buchancova and Maria Avdicova
Jessenius Faculty of Medicine Comenius University in Martin,
Regional Authority of Public Health in Banska Bystrica
Slovak Republic

1. Introduction

Tick-borne encephalitis is a viral disease of the central nervous system that is caused by flaviviruses. The disease can be mild; however, in 35 to 58% of cases, the course of the disease includes long-lasting neurological problems, and the disease can be lethal in 1 to 5% of cases (WHO, 2011). The first symptoms appear about 7 days (incubation period 2 to 28 days) after an infected tick latches on to its host and may present as a flu-like illness. In some people, the second phase of the disease begins after 2 to 4 weeks and is characterised by violent headache, disorientation and high fever; eventually, the patient may lose consciousness, and in many cases, this stage is followed by a long convalescence.

Ixodes ricinus, the three-host tick species is parasitic on various stages of development in different hosts, is a disease vector. The larvae is parasitic on small mammals, lizards and birds searching for food on the ground; the nymph is parasitic on larger mammals (hedgehog, squirrel), birds and occasionally on rodents and the imago is parasitic on large mammals (rabbit, fox, deer, wild boar, goat, sheep, cattle, etc.). Imago's activity in nature is highest from March to October, usually with two peaks: the first peak occurs in June and July, and the second peak occurs in September and October (Grešíková, 1999). The virus is found in the saliva of the tick in all developmental stages but does not harm its host. Humans are infected when they are bitten by an infected female tick. Humans are also infected in alimentary ways, such as by goat, cow or sheep milk and cheese that are insufficiently thermally modified, but this happens less often (WHO, 2009).

During the last decade, a shift of infected ticks to the northern regions of Europe and to higher altitudes has been observed. As a result, an increase in the incidence of tick-borne encephalitis has occurred in new locations in Europe and in the Slovak Republic.

In the Slovak Republic, the employer is responsible for the damage that is caused to the professional staff by acute occupational poisoning, acute occupational infectious disease and occupational disease, according to the current legislation. The employer is obliged to provide compensation for loss of earnings, pain and suffering, and he must eventually compensate the employee for a loss of social status. The goal of this study was to evaluate the incidence of tick-borne encephalitis as an occupational disease in Slovakia and in the Czech Republic from 1989 to 2009 and to compare it with the incidence in the general population. We also analysed the average direct and indirect costs of the diagnosis and treatment of acute tick-borne encephalitis in Slovakia. We also wanted to point out the possible financial impact of the disease on employers for compensating workers for occupational disease, compared with the costs of active prevention of the infection of employees by vaccination.

2. Material and methods

We have analysed data that was obtained from the Epidemiological Information System of the Public Health Authority of the Slovak Republic, the National Health Information Centre of the Slovak Republic, the National Institute of Public Health of the Czech Republic and the Institute for Health Information and Statistics of the Czech Republic for the period from 1989 to 2009. Admission criteria for the detection of disease in the Epidemiological Information System of the Slovak Republic and the National Institute of Public Health of the Czech Republic, respectively, were infectious diseases, tick-borne encephalitis, diagnosed according to International Classification of Diseases ICD-10 A84.1 during the period from 1989 to 2009. Identification data were age, sex, and epidemiological data, which included the mechanism of transmission, the location and the period of infection. According to the entry criteria, the absolute and relative numbers of the disease, the location of disease and the incidence by sex and age group were assessed. From the Epidemiological Information System of the Slovak Republic data from 2009, we evaluated the clinical form of disease, the number of hospitalisation days, the locality of isolation and the subject's occupation.

When analysing the data on the occupational diseases from statistical surveys from the Slovak Republic and the Czech Republic, the Slovak Republic entry criterion for the disease was from file "26 - diseases transmissible from animals to humans either directly or through vector", and the Czech Republic identification was through registration code 5.02.12, specifically "V.02.12 viral encephalitis transmitted by ticks."

We based the analysis of occupations for the unification of the data for the Slovak Republic and the Czech Republic on the classification of economic activities. We included the building industry, manufacturing and electricity, gas and water and activity of social organisations in the group that was called "others."

A more detailed age professional analysis of reported occupational tick-borne encephalitis in the Slovak Republic was performed according to data that was obtained from four claiming departments: the Department of Occupational Medicine and Toxicology at the University Hospital in Martin, the Department of Occupational Medicine and Clinical Toxicology of Pavol Jozef Šafárik University in Košice, the Department of Occupational Medicine and Toxicology of Medical Faculty Comenius University in Bratislava and the Department of Occupational Medicine and Toxicology of Roosevelt Hospital in Banská Bystrica.

Furthermore, we performed a retrospective analysis of the direct and indirect costs for patients who were hospitalised with a diagnosis of tick-borne encephalitis in the Slovak

Republic in 2009. The data for each patient were received from the Epidemiological Information System of the Slovak Republic. According to the General Health Insurance Company (VšZP a.s.) data and the medical records of patients who were hospitalised at the University Hospital in Martin, we calculated the direct costs of diagnosis and treatment during hospitalisation in 2009. Direct costs include the cost of the total time in the hospital ("finished hospitalisation") and the cost of laboratory and imaging tests, which are common diagnostic and therapeutic components.

Indirect costs include the costs that were paid by employers in the form of wages, sickness benefits paid by social insurance and loss of productivity due to lower gross of domestic product during the hospitalisation of the patient. In the Slovak Republic, the employer pays income compensation for economically active patients during the first ten days of working disability: 25% of the daily earnings for the first three days and 55% for the remaining days (Act No. 461, 2003; Act No. 462, 2003). After the tenth day of working disability, the Social Insurance Company pays sickness benefits that are 55% of the daily earnings. We based the calculations of cost on the cost of the minimum monthly wage, which was 295.50 EUR for 2009 (Decree No. 422, 2008). To calculate the productivity loss, we used the amount of gross domestic product per citizen per day, which amounted to 32.03 EUR in 2009 (Statistical Office of the Slovak Republic, 2010).

Patients were divided into three age groups: up to 14 years of age, from 15 to 64 years of age and over 65 years of age. For the analysis, we included only economically active hospitalised patients who were over 15 years of age, excluding students and pensioners.

For the evaluation of the results, we used descriptive methods of statistical analysis (Microsoft Office Excel 2007 and statistical program SPSS version 11.0). Values of $p < 0.05$ were considered to be statistically significant.

3. Results

3.1 The incidence of tick-borne encephalitis reported by the Epidemiological Information System of the Slovak Republic and the National Institute of Public Health of the Czech Republic

For the designated period, there were 1,299 cases of tick-borne encephalitis reported in the Slovak Republic and 11,714 cases reported in the Czech Republic (table 1). The average incidence of tick-borne encephalitis in the last 21 years was 1.2 cases per 100,000 people in the Slovak Republic and 5.4 cases per 100,000 people in the Czech Republic.

The number of reported cases in the Slovak Republic and in the Czech Republic tends to have a slightly upward trend (figure 1).

3.2 Occurrence of occupational tick-borne encephalitis reported by the departments of Occupational Medicine and Toxicology in the Slovak Republic and departments of Occupational Diseases in the Czech Republic

In the Slovak Republic from 1989 to 2009, there were 22 cases of diagnosed occupational tick-borne encephalitis, and in the Czech Republic, there were 190 cases during the same period (table 2).

Of these reported cases of occupational tick-borne encephalitis, there was an equal proportion of men and women (50%) in the Slovak Republic. A statistically significant difference was found between genders in the Czech Republic, where the male sex represented 71.0% of the cases, and the women represented 29.0% of the cases.

	Slovak Republic		Czech Republic	
year	n	incidence/100,000	n	incidence/100,000
1989	18	0.3	166	1.3
1990	14	0.3	193	1.9
1991	24	0.5	356	3.5
1992	16	0.3	338	3.3
1993	51	1.0	629	6.1
1994	60	1.I	613	5.9
1995	89	1.6	744	7.2
1996	101	1,9	571	5.5
1997	73	1.4	415	4.0
1998	57	1.1	422	4.1
1999	63	1.2	490	4.8
2000	92	1.7	719	7.0
2001	75	1.4	633	6.2
2002	62	1.2	647	6.3
2003	74	1.4	606	5.9
2004	70	1.3	507	5.0
2005	50	0.9	643	6.3
2006	91	1.7	1,029	10.0
2007	58	1.1	546	5.3
2008	84	1.6	631	6.1
2009	77	1.4	816	7.8
Total	1,299	1.2	11,714	5.4

Table 1. Number of reported cases of tick-borne encephalitis in the Slovak Republic and the Czech Republic from 1989 to 2009 (source: Epidemiological Information System of the Slovak Republic, National Institute of Public Health of the Czech Republic)

The number of reported cases of occupational tick-borne encephalitis has demonstrated a slight downward trend in the Slovak Republic; a statistically significant downward trend in reported occupational diseases is present in the Czech Republic (figure 2).

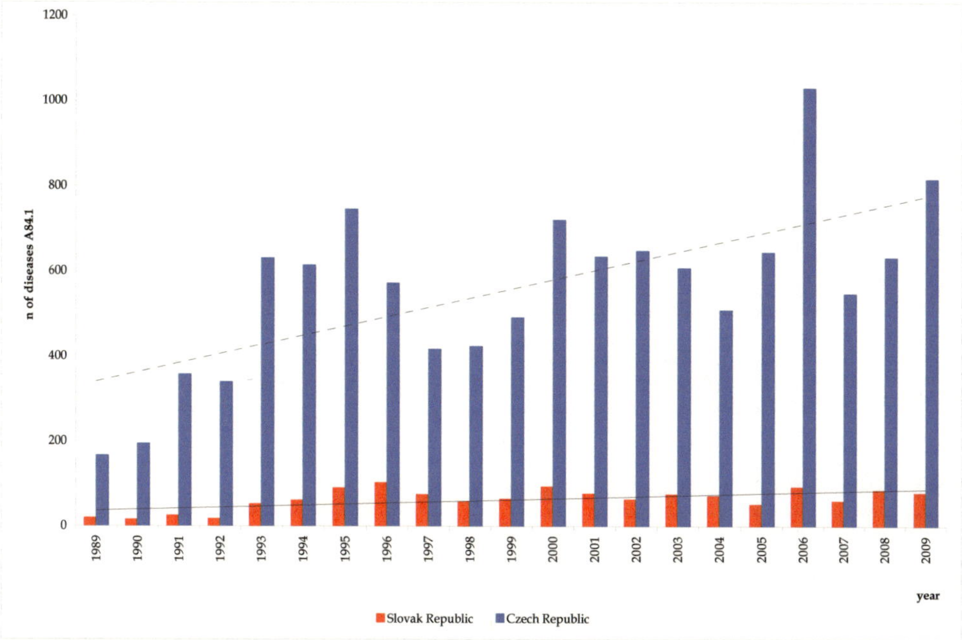

Fig. 1. Number of reported cases of tick-borne encephalitis in the Slovak Republic and the Czech Republic from 1989 to 2009 (source: Epidemiological Information System of the Slovak Republic, National Institute of Public Health of the Czech Republic)

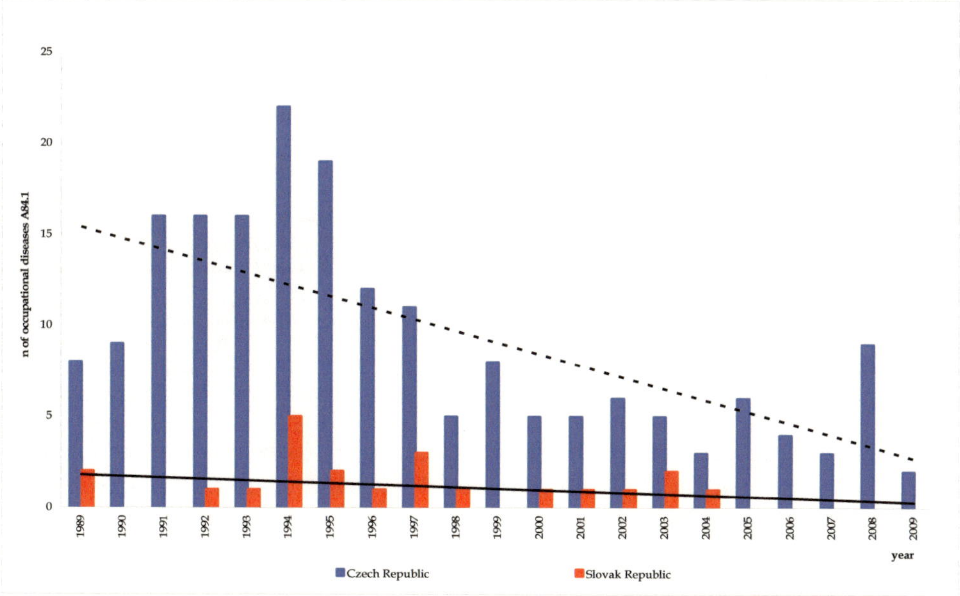

Fig. 2. Number of reported occupational diseases according to the diagnosis of tick-borne encephalitis A84.1 and according to sex (source: National Health Information Centre of the Slovak Republic, National Institute of Public Health of the Czech Republic)

	Slovak Republic					Czech Republic				
year	n total	n male	% male	n female	% female	n total	n male	% male	n female	% female
1989	2	1	50.0	1	50.0	8	5	62.5	3	37.5
1990	0	0	0.0	0	0.0	9	7	77.8	2	22.2
1991	0	0	0.0	0	0.0	16	13	81.2	3	18.8
1992	1	1	100.0	0	0.0	16	13	81.2	3	18.8
1993	1	0	0.0	1	100.0	16	11	68.8	5	31.2
1994	5	3	60.0	2	40.0	22	15	68.2	7	31.8
1995	2	1	50.0	1	50.0	19	14	73.7	5	26.3
1996	1	1	100.0	0	0.0	12	7	58.3	5	41.7
1997	3	2	66.7	1	33.3	11	9	81.8	2	18.2
1998	1	1	100.0	0	0.0	5	4	80.0	1	20.0
1999	0	0	0.0	0	0.0	8	5	62.5	3	37.5
2000	1	1	100.0	0	0.0	5	1	20.0	4	80.0
2001	1	0	0.0	1	100.0	5	5	100.0	0	0.0
2002	1	0	0.0	1	100.0	6	5	83.3	1	16.7
2003	2	0	0.0	2	100.0	5	3	60.0	2	40.0
2004	1	0	0.0	1	100.0	3	2	66.7	1	33.3
2005	0	0	0.0	0	0.0	6	5	83.3	1	16.7
2006	0	0	0.0	0	0.0	4	2	50.0	2	50.0
2007	0	0	0.0	0	0.0	3	2	66.7	1	33.3
2008	0	0	0.0	0	0.0	9	6	66.7	3	33.3
2009	0	0	0.0	0	0.0	2	1	50.0	1	50.0
Total	22	11	50.0	11	50.0	190	135	71.0	55	29.0

Table 2. Number of reported occupational diseases according to the diagnosis of tick-borne encephalitis A84.1 and according to sex (source: National Health Information Centre of the Slovak Republic, National Institute of Public Health of the Czech Republic)

The incidence of occupational tick-borne encephalitis in proportion to the total number of occupational diseases in the Slovak Republic and the Czech Republic is listed in table 3 and figure 3. These data are processed for the time period from 1993 to 2009; due to the reclassification of occupational diseases in miners in the period from 1990 to 1992 in both republics, an enormous increase in the number of reported occupational diseases occurred.

Using data for the period from 1989 to 1992 would result in a misrepresentation of the total number of cases of occupational tick-borne encephalitis. In the Slovak Republic, occupational tick-borne encephalitis represents, on average, only 0.2% of all annually reported occupational diseases during the designated time period and exhibits a downward trend. In the Czech Republic, the proportion is almost twice as high; occupational tick-borne encephalitis represents only 0.3% of the total number of reported occupational diseases, but the trend is also downward.

	Slovak Republic			Czech Republic		
	occupational diseases	professional disease of tick-borne encephalitis		occupational diseases	professional disease of tick-borne encephalitis	
year	n	n	%	n	n	%
1989	1,041	2	0.2	4,846	8	0.2
1990*	1,194	0	0.0	11,575	9	0.1
1991	1,311	0	0.0	8,697	16	0.2
1992	1,076	1	0.1	3,393	16	0.5
1993	939	1	0.1	2,983	16	0.5
1994	722	5	0.7	2,684	22	0.8
1995	601	2	0.3	2,852	19	0.7
1996	726	1	0.1	2,543	12	0.5
1997	697	3	0.4	2,376	11	0.5
1998	740	1	0.1	2,111	5	0.2
1999	673	0	0.0	1,886	8	0.4
2000	660	1	0.2	1,751	5	0.3
2001	577	1	0.2	1,677	5	0.3
2002	609	1	0.2	1,600	6	0.4
2003	551	2	0.4	1,558	5	0.3
2004	613	1	0.2	1,388	3	0.2
2005	413	0	0.0	1,400	6	0.4
2006	504	0	0.0	1,216	4	0.3
2007	575	0	0.0	1,291	3	0.2
2008	429	0	0.0	1,403	9	0.6
2009	483	0	0.0	1,313	2	0.2
SPOLU	15,134	22	0.2	60,543	190	0.3

* reclassification of occupational diseases in the Czech Republic

Table 3. Number of occupational tick-borne encephalitis cases in proportion to the total number of occupational diseases (source: National Health Information Centre of the Slovak Republic, National Institute of Public Health of the Czech Republic)

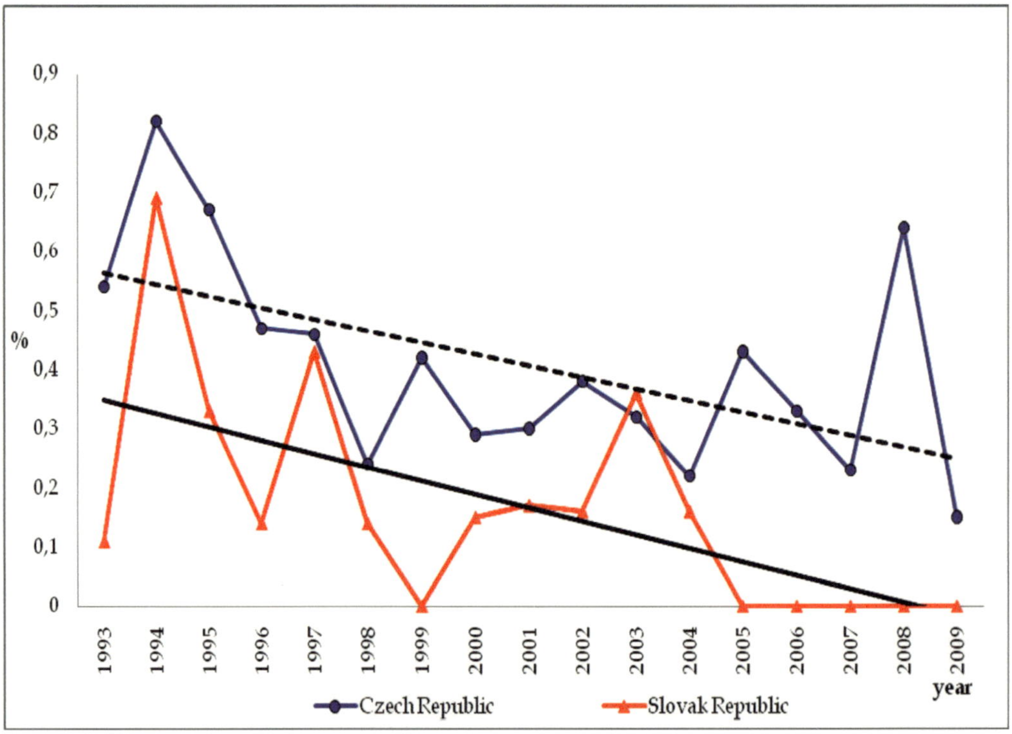

Fig. 3. Number of cases of occupational tick-borne encephalitis in proportion to the total number of occupational diseases (source: National Health Information Centre of the Slovak Republic, National Institute of Public Health of the Czech Republic)

3.3 Age-professional analysis of the incidence of tick-borne encephalitis as an occupational disease in the Slovak Republic

In table 4, the occurrence of occupational tick-borne encephalitis according to industrial classification is shown. In the Czech Republic, the highest number of cases was 117 in the forestry sector (62.2%); 15 cases (7.9%) occurred in both the agriculture and transport sectors.

A more detailed analysis by occupation, sex and age could be done for the Slovak Republic alone. Based on the analysis of the data from four workplaces in the Slovak Republic, there were 22 cases of occupational tick-borne encephalitis, and the highest incidence of the disease occurred in the group of 45 to 54 year-olds. The average age in the reported cases was 46.9 ± 7.8 years. Women were represented the most frequently in the 35 to 44 year-old and 45 to 54 year-old age groups, and men were represented most frequently in the 45 to 54 year-old age groups.

The most frequent occurrence of occupational tick-borne encephalitis was recorded in the forestry sector, which had 17 cases (77.2%); 11 of these cases were female forest workers, 4 were chainsaw operators, 1 was a forester and 1 was a forest management planner. The agriculture sector had 3 cases (13.6%), of which 2 were tractor drivers, and 1 was a nurse for sheep. One case was reported in the public sector administration and defence (a guard dog handler), and one case was classified in the "others" category (a technique of protective circuits).

	Slovak Republic						Czech Republic	
	n total	%	n male	% male	n female	% female	n total	%
agricultural	3	13.6	3	27.2	0	0.0	15	7.9
forestry	17	77.2	6	54.6	11	100.0	117	61.5
fishery	0	0.0	0	0.0	0	0.0	4	2.1
freight	0	0.0	0	0.0	0	0.0	15	7.9
public administration and defence	1	4.6	1	9.1	0	0.0	11	5.8
educational	0	0.0	0	0.0	0	0.0	11	5.8
health service	0	0.0	0	0.0	0	0.0	3	1.6
other activities	1	4.6	1	9.1	0	0.0	14	7.4
Total	22	100.0	11	100.0	11	100.0	190	100.0

Table 4. Number of reported occupational diseases according to the diagnosis of tick-borne encephalitis A84.1 and according to economic activities from 1989 to 2009 (source: National Health Information Centre of the Slovak Republic, National Institute of Public Health of the Czech Republic)

3.4 Direct and indirect costs of diagnosis and treatment of tick-borne encephalitis during hospitalisation in the Slovak Republic in 2009

During the observed period, 77 cases of tick-borne encephalitis were reported in the Slovak Republic. The disease did not require hospitalisation in 4 patients who were older than 15 years. Altogether, 73 patients were hospitalised, 50 (68.5%) males and 23 (31.5%) females. In subjects up to 14 years old, there were 5 patients, and in the group of subjects who were over 15 years old, there were 68 patients. There were 52 economically active hospitalised patients. Their average age was 41.6 years (18 to 62 years), their average length of hospital stay was 11.8 days (3 to 29 days), and together they accumulated 613 days of hospitalisation (table 5). When comparing the sexes, we did not find statistically significant differences in the age or in the length of hospitalisation in the economically active population of inpatients.

In 2009, VšZP a.s. spent 34,992.74 EUR for the diagnosis and treatment of patients who were diagnosed with tick-borne encephalitis. Expenses for the constitutional health care (inpatients) accounted for 57% of the expenses, the cost of laboratory and imaging diagnosis accounted for 32%, the cost of specialised ambulatory care (outpatients) accounted for 6% and drug costs accounted for 5% of the total expenses for this health insurance company (figure 4).

Average direct expenses for hospitalised patients in 2009, calculated from VšZP a.s. data and available medical records, equalled 901.37 EUR (511.98 EUR to 2,927.39 EUR). For 52 economically active hospitalised patients, the total direct expenditures of the health insurance company equalled 46,871.24 EUR.

	0 - 14	15 - 64	65+	total
number of inpatients	5 (6.9%)	61 (83.6%)	7 (9.6%)	73
age	8.4 ± 3.2	40.3 ± 13.8	72.4 ± 10.6	41.2 ± 18.2
length of hospitalization	14.6 ± 1.7*	11.5 ± 4.3	10.7 ± 2.8	11.6 ± 4.1
days of hospitalization	73	701	75	849
form	n (male + female)	n (male + female)	n (male + female)	
febrile	1 (0 + 1)	16 (11 + 5)	0	17 (23.39%)
meningeal	4 (1 + 3)	44 (32 + 12)	7 (5 + 2)	55 (75.3%)
neurological	0	1 (1 + 0)	0	1 (1.4%)

* $p < 0,05$

Table 5. Patients hospitalised with a diagnosis of tick-borne encephalitis in the Slovak Republic in 2009 (source: Epidemiological Information system of the Slovak Republic)

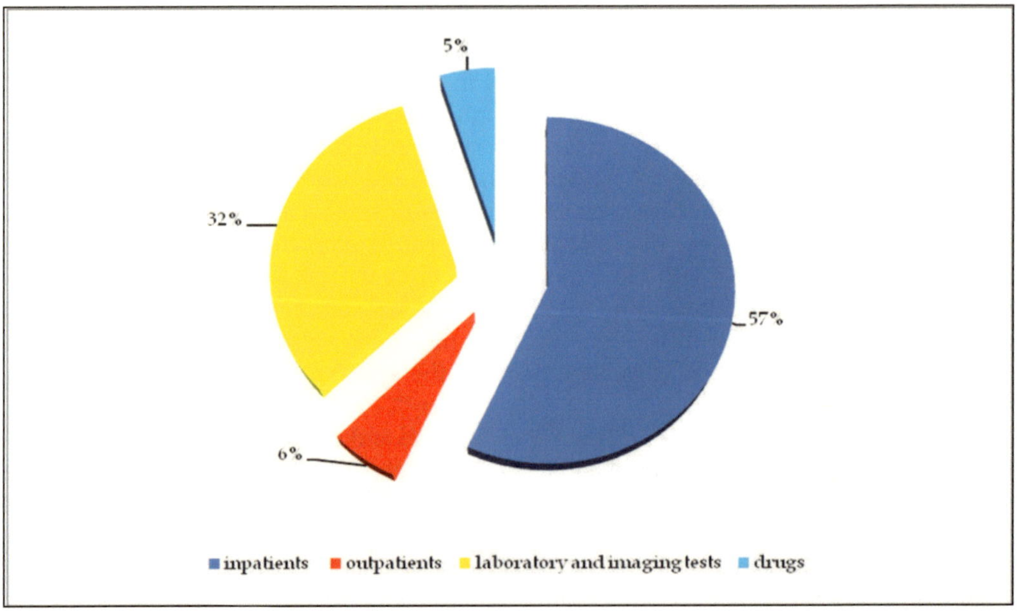

Fig. 4. The total direct costs of the VšZP a.s. for tick-borne encephalitis according to the type of healthcare in 2009 (source: VšZP a.s.)

The indirect costs for 52 economically active hospitalised patients at a minimum monthly salary would be 76.56 EUR (10.07 EUR to 202.15 EUR) for 12 days of working disability. The loss of earnings for a patient for 12 days of working disability was 84.57 EUR (30.22 EUR to 187.37 EUR). Indirect costs in the form of the loss of productivity at work and a decrease in gross domestic product would have reached 19,634.39 EUR at a minimum monthly salary. The total indirect cost for these patients was 23,534.32 EUR (table 6).

	for 12 day of hospitalization	**for 52 of hospitalized patients**
direct costs	**EUR**	**EUR**
expenditures during hospitalization	901.37	46,871.24
indirect costs		
loss for the state	460.92	23,534.32
income compensation, sickness benefit	76.56	3,899.93
loss of gross of domestic product	384.36	19,634.39
total direct and indirect costs	1,362.29	70,405.56
loss of income for empoyee	84.57	4,333.78

Table 6. Direct and indirect costs for 52 economically active patients who were hospitalised with a diagnosis of tick-borne encephalitis in the Slovak Republic in 2009

3.5 Occupational tick-borne encephalitis and financial compensation

By law, the employee has to be compensated for pain and possibly for difficulties in society that are a result of an occupational injury. A scoring system for pain is defined in Annex No. 1 in section III., and the scoring system for difficulties in society is defined in Annex No. 1 in section IV. of Act No.437/2004 (Act No. 437, 2004). The basic scores for pain that is related to occupational diseases for tick-borne encephalitis are, according to Annex No. 1, section III., item 41, "The acute forms of infectious and parasitic diseases," ranging from 30 to 150 points. The basic score for difficulty in society for the occupational diseases are, according to Annex No. 1, section IV., item 46, "The results of the TBE," ranging from 300 to 3000 points. The amount of compensation for pain and the amount of compensation for difficulties in society was set at 14.46 EUR per point for 2009 (Measure of Ministry of Health of the Slovak Republic, 2009).

In 2009 in the Slovak Republic, the average price of the tick-borne encephalitis vaccine FSME-IMMUN was 19.07 EUR; ENCEPUR ADULTS was 16.85 EUR. The median life expectancy in Slovakia being 71.3 years in men and 78.7 years in women (Statistical Office of the Slovak Republic, 2010). If the first vaccination was implemented at 18 years of age and was being implemented till death, about 15 doses of vaccine would be required (table 7).

The cost for the 15 doses of vaccine at the prices from 2009 would amount to 286.05 EUR (FSME-IMMUN), respectively 252.75 EUR (ENCEPUR ADULTS).

	EUR		
	min	max	average
rate for the pain on occupational diseases (30 – 150 points)	433.8	2,169.00	1,301.40
rate for difficulty in society (300 – 3000 points)	4,338.00	43,380.00	23,859.00
average direct and indirect costs for one inpatient	618.14	4,058.41	1,362.29
average prices for 15 doses of vaccine	252.75	286.05	269.40
utility costs	365.39	3,772.36	1,092.89

Table 7. Comparison of financial compensation and the price of vaccines at the minimum rates in the Slovak Republic in 2009

4. Discussion

The purpose of our study was to map the occurrence of tick-borne encephalitis in the Slovak Republic, since the statistics of the National Health Information Centre of the Slovak Republic are not currently tracked nor is tick-borne encephalitis analysed as a separate occupational infectious diseases problem. Occupational tick-borne encephalitis is reported in a group of diseases that are transmissible directly from animals to humans or transmissible by the carriers. Tick-borne encephalitis is separately mentioned only to indicate the patient's gender and the location of the medical facility. Similarly, in the Czech Republic, tick-borne encephalitis is separately monitored only to indicate the patient's gender and the area of the origin of the occupational diseases. Details regarding the age groups, the length of the exposure and the sections and classes of economic activities are reported in the Slovak Republic and Czech Republic together for all the diseases that can be transmitted from animals to humans.

Issues of the occurrence of tick-borne encephalitis and other diseases that are transmitted by ticks were addressed by other countries. In the Netherlands, for example, the foresters` antibody levels were monitored (Charante et al., 1998). At high exposure the prevalence odds ratios (with 95% CI between brackets) were for tick-borne encephalitis 1.0 (0.3 to 3.0), and for Lyme borreliosis 15 (5.5 to 42). Similarly, France has confirmed the presence of antibodies in workers who are at risk. Among the 2,975 subjects included in the study, the observed seroprevalence were 3.4% for tick-borne encephalitis and 14.1% for Lyme borreliosis (Thorin et al., 2008). In the Slovak Republic and the Czech Republic, we have confirmed the presence of occupational tick-borne encephalitis, particularly among forestry workers.

Despite the fact that the tick-borne encephalitis virus is transmitted by only about 1 to 2% of ticks (Máderová, 2005), it can be expected that with failure to provide preventive measures, the number of occupational cases of tick-borne encephalitis will increase. There are fields that demonstrate an increased number of the infected ticks in Europe, especially in Germany, the Czech Republic, Poland, Switzerland, Sweden, Finland, the Slovak Republic, Hungary, Slovenia and Austria (Suss, 2008).

In the Slovak Republic in the past, 33 endemic areas of tick-borne encephalitis were located in the districts of Nitra, Komarno, Bratislava and Rožňava (Máderová, 2005). Currently, 37 areas of endemic outbreaks have been identified, especially in Tribeč, Vtáčnik, Nitrianska pahorkatina, Pohronská pahorkatina and the Vah valley down to the Považská Bystrica district, Malé Karpaty, Záhorská nížina, Kováčske kopce, Krupinská planina, Slovenský Kras and Slánske vrchy (Slováková, 2008).

In the Slovak Republic, the risk of possible occupational health hazards due to tick-borne encephalitis is not publicized. In a study of the occupational disease Lyme borreliosis, anamnesis data of the patients indicated that during the past few years, there were significant increases in the number of seasonal tick bites, especially while working on slopes situated on the southern side and in the higher areas of Slovakia (Buchancová, 2009). The literature has described the movement of the tick into higher altitudes, exceeding 1,000 m altitude, of northern Slovakia (Peťko et al., 2008). A similar situation is also described in the Czech Republic (Danielová et al., 2008). Failure to provide preventive measures would mean an increase in the occupational cases of tick-borne encephalitis.

Apart from the primary protection, which is generally focused on the prevention of an infection that is transmitted by ticks, active immunisation is a possible protective measure against tick-borne encephalitis for workers who are working in endemic areas. Vaccination is one of the most effective forms of protection against tick-borne encephalitis. In some European countries such as Austria, Finland, Germany, Hungary, Lithuania, Slovenia, Russia and Switzerland, the vaccination is included in the national immunisation programme (Mantke et al., 2008).

In the Czech Republic, the health insurance companies contribute to the prevention of disease. In 2008, all health insurance companies contributed for vaccination and revaccination of children and adolescents, for vaccination of adults ages 19 to 55 years, except Military ("Vojenská zdravotní pojišťovna") and Union health insurance ("Oborová zdravotní pojišťovna"), and for vaccination of people over 55 years old (all with the exception of the Military health insurance) (Dolanský, 2008). According to the available data in the Czech Republic, 17% of the population received immunisation in 2007 (Kříž & Beneš, 2007).

Until August 31, 2009, there was a total of 17,093 vaccinated children under 15 years of age in the Slovak Republic; this means that 2% of this age group was immunised (Public Health Authority of the Slovak Republic, 2010). In Austria, the proportion of the population that is immunised rises up to 88% in places where there is a high occurrence of the disease, and the number of cases of the disease is only counted in tens (Suss, 2008). Currently in the Slovak Republic, two out of three health insurance companies contribute to the package of higher standards for vaccination against tick-borne encephalitis. Dovera Health Insurance Company a.s., for example, refunds only contributions that are made to vaccinate children and adults in the last of three doses of the vaccine (Dovera ZP a.s., 2011). Union Health Insurance Company a.s. currently pays 50% of the cost of three doses of the tick-borne encephalitis vaccine for its members (Union ZP a.s., 2011). There are not available data, which could determine the rate of re-vaccination for the professional workers in the Slovak

Republic and Czech Republic; these workers are at an increased risk of infection by a tick bite and of subsequent inflammation of the brain.

In the Slovak Republic, according to the Ordinance of Ministry of Health No. 585 in 2008, vaccination of the employees of virology laboratories, in which people work with the tick-borne encephalitis virus, is obligatory. In pursuance of doctors' recommendations, the vaccination of people who are professionally exposed to an increased risk of brain inflammation (Ordinance of Ministry of health No.585, 2008) is suggested. In such cases, the employer should pay for the vaccination. The employer and the self-employed should have access to information about the cost of prevention, treatment and, in the case of the employer, the amount financial compensation for employees who are exposed to acute infectious diseases in their occupation.

Tick-borne encephalitis is a disease that can be combated by both nonspecific preventive measures and by specific prevention in the form of vaccination. We calculated that the average direct and indirect cost per patient during hospitalisation for tick-borne encephalitis was 1,353.95 EUR. The average price for 15 doses of the vaccine was 252.75 EUR. The utility cost is 1,092.86 EUR for health insurance and country. For the employer, compensation for low levels of pain (a score of 30 points) would cost 433.80 EUR. It would be cheaper to pay for the employees' vaccination from 18 years of age until retirement than to pay compensation for pain and social difficulties because of an employee's occupational disease. Considering our results, it is important for Slovakia to consider reimbursement for vaccination as a form of primary prevention for employees, especially if the place of work is in the endemic area. While the economic benefit is obvious, the benefits to health and quality of life are difficult to quantify. After overcoming occupational tick-borne encephalitis, the employees may have permanent residual damage, which may result in the limitation of employment activity, may force a change in employment and may even result in permanent disability. In these cases, the financial costs are increased by the requirement of additional financial compensation for health damage. This compensation is an annuity, which is currently paid in the Slovak Republic through social insurance from accident insurance. The social insurance from accident insurance is paid by the employer and the amount paid is specified according to the security risks of economic activities with the employer (Act No. 461, 2003).

One problem in the forestry industry is that there is a significant group of self-employed workers, especially in the mining, wood processing and handling divisions. They often lack both the necessary information about the risk of infections that are transmitted by ticks and the opportunities to personally ensure the protection of their health through vaccination for tick-borne encephalitis. Also, due to the periodical variation of seasonal workers in the forestry sector, there are insufficient funds for employers to invest in primary prevention (vaccination).

To ensure the efficacy of vaccination, a conventional vaccination scheme requires vaccination three doses of the vaccine and a regular booster dose after three years. People who are 12 to 49 years old should be vaccinated at 5-year intervals after the first booster dose (ENCEPUR) and who are 16 to 60 years old should be vaccinated every 3 to 5 years. People who are older than 60 years should be vaccinated every three years (FSME IMMUN). For the accelerated vaccination scheme, first booster dose is recommended after 12 to 18 months and then every three years. Only among 12 to 49 years old is recommended every five years (ENCEPUR). For FSME IMMUN first booster dose is recommended after 5 to 12 months and then booster every 3 to 5 years among 16 to 60 years of age. For people who are older than 60 years the booster dose is recommended every three years (State Institute for Drug Control 2011a, 2011b).

5. Conclusion

For employers who are considering funding primary prevention by vaccination, it is important to know the risk of the workers' contraction of a disease in endemic areas, the associated treatment costs and the cost of a confirmed occupational disease.

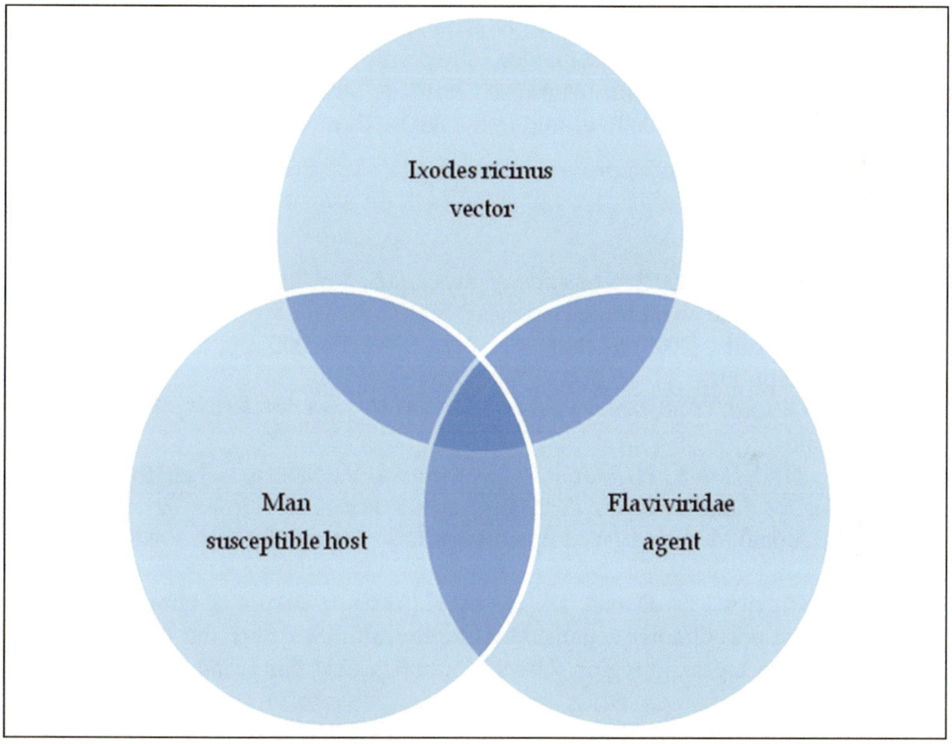

Fig. 5. Relationship between the agent, vector and the susceptible host

Figure 5 shows the relationship between ticks as the vector, the tick-borne encephalitis virus itself and the exposed man. The most common cause of morbidity is a bite by an infected tick and the subsequent development of the disease, which is shown as a result of penetration of the agent, vector and susceptible host in the diagrams. Less frequent morbidity is shown on the diagram as a result of penetration of the agent and a susceptible host, which occurs, for example, with the consumption of contaminated goat milk. An important fact is that, in endemic areas, the population is gradually infected, and after a number of evident and latent diseases, immunity develops at various stages. Non-native people who are visiting endemic areas for recreation or work and at-risk groups of the native population are most susceptible to the disease.

In the Slovak Republic in the past, virus prevalence in the tick populations in the endemic areas was 2.6%. Morbidity of population was 2.2% and the presence of antibodies in healthy people ranged from 15 to 27% (Grešíková, 1999). The Parasitological Institute of the Slovak Academy of Sciences attempted to assess the immune status of the workers who were working in at-risk professions between 2008 and 2009 by researching tick-borne diseases in hunters and forestry workers from the territory of the Slovak Republic (Parasitological Institute SAS, 2008). Mapping the areas where ticks are present, identifying the new endemic areas and detecting the immune status of the population is extremely important.

6. Acknowledgments

This work was supported by the Centre of Experimental and Clinical Respirology of the Jessenius Faculty of Medicine Comenius University in Martin. Our thanks for the cooperation of the General Health Insurance Company (VšZP a.s.) for making the costs of the medical treatment accessible to us and to the Baxter Company for providing the prices of vaccines in 2009.

7. References

Act No. 461/2003 Coll. (2003). *Collection of Acts*, 2003. Vol.200, pp. 3550-3703, Bratislava, Slovak Republic

Act No. 462/2003 Coll. (2003). *Collection of Acts*, 2003, Vol.200, pp. 3704-3708, Bratislava, Slovak Republic

Act No. 437/2004 Coll. *Collection of Acts*, 2004, Vol.185, pp. 3994-4032, Bratislava, Slovak Republic

Buchancová, J., Hudečková,. H, Murajda, L., Švihrová, V., Bátora, I., Legáth, Ľ., Osina, O., Vilček, R., Jakubovičová, E. (2009). Lyme borreliosis from the perspective of Occupational Medicine - a comparative study. *Pracov Lék*, 2009, Vol.61, No.2, pp.46-55

Danielová, V., Kliegrová, S., Daniel, M., Beneš, Č.(2008). Influence of climate warming on tick-borne encephalitis expansion to higher altitudes over the last decade (1997-2006) in the highland region (Czech Republic). *Cent Eur J Publ Health*, 2008, Vol.16, No.1, pp.4-11

Decree of Government of the Slovak Republic No. 422/2008 Coll. (2008). Collection of Acts, 2008, Vol.156, p.3655, Bratislava, Slovak Republic

Dolanský, H. (2008). Prevence onemocnění klíšťovou encefalitidou z pohledu zdravotní pojišťovny (Prevention of tick-borne encephalitis cases in terms of health insurance). *Praktický lékař*, 2008, Vol.89, No.2, pp.78-81

Dovera ZP, a.s. (2011). Nadštandard - produktové balíky- balík očkovania - kliešťová encefalitída (Nadstandard - Product packages - Package of vaccination - Tick-borne encephalitis) [on-line]. 2011 [cit. 2011-03-18] Available from: http://www.dovera.sk/sk/servis/vyhody-a-zlavy/prevencia/kliestova-encefalitida/

Grešíková, M. (1999). Kliešťová encefalitída - trvalý verejno-zdravotnícky problém (Tick-borne encephalitis - a permanent public-health problem). *VEDA*, 1999, 102 p., ISBN80-224-0627-9, Bratislava, Slovak Republic

Charante, A.W.M., Groen, J., Mulder, P.G.H., Rijpkema, S.G.T., Osterhaus, A.D.M.E. (1998). Occupational risks of zoonotic infectious in Dutch forestry workers and muskrat catchers. *Eur J Epidemiol*, 1998, Vol.14, No.2, pp.109-116

Kříž, B., Beneš, Č. (2007). *Klíšťová encefalitida – epidemiologická data (Tick-borne encephalitis – the epidemiological data).* [on-line]. 2007-06-13. [cit. 2009-04-04]. Available from: http://www.szu.cz/tema/prevence/klistova-encefalitida-epidemiologicka-data

Máderová, E. (2005). Kliešťová encefalitída na Slovensku (Tick-borne encephalitis in Slovakia). *Via pract.*, 2005, Vol.2, No.1, pp.51-54

Mantke, O.D., Schädler, R., Niedrig, M. (2008). A survey on cases of tick-borne encephalitis in European countries. *Eurosurveillance*, 2008, Vol.13, No.17, pii=18848

Measure of Ministry of Health of the Slovak Republic No. 12284/2009-OL z 12. mája 2009 na rok 2009. (2009). Obzor, 2009, Vol.57, No.22-24, p. 173, Bratislava, Slovak Republic

Ordinance of Ministry of Health of the Slovak Republic No. 585/2008 Coll. (2008). *Collection of Acts*, 2008, Vol.202, pp.5024–5041, Bratislava, Slovak Republic

Parasitological Institute of the Slovak Academy of Sciences. (2008). *Dobrovoľné vyšetrenie poľovníkov a lesníckych pracovníkov na kliešťami prenášané ochorenia (Voluntary testing of hunters and forestry workers on tick-borne diseases).* [on-line]. 2008 [cit. 2009-04-04]. Available from: http://www.spzba.sk/Dobrovolne_vysetrenie_BA.doc

Peťko, B., Stanko, M., Majláthová, V., Bullová, E., Vichová, B. (2008). Aktuálne problémy s výskytom kliešťov na Slovensku (Current problems with the occurence of ticks in Slovakia). *Zdravotnícke štúdie*, 2008, Vol.1, No.2 supp 1, p.26

Public Health Authority of the Slovak Republic. (2008). *Výročná správa o činnosti Úradu verejného zdravotníctva Slovenskej republiky rok 2009 (Annual report of the Public Health Authority of the Slovak republic year 2009).* PHA, 2010, pp.160-266, Bratislava, Slovak Republic

Slováková, A. (2008). *Kliešte už začínajú útočiť (Tick are already starting to attack).* [on-line]. 2008-04-28. [cit. 2009-02-28]. Available from: http://www.sme.sk/c/3845704/Klieste-uz-zacinaju-utocit.html

State Institute for drug control. (2011b). Príloha č.1 k rozhodnutiu o predĺžení registrácie lieku, ev. č. 2106/0464. *Súhrn charakteristických vlastností lieku FSME-IMMUN.* [online]. 2011-03-20. [cit. 2011-03-25]. Available from: http://www.sukl.sk/sk/pomocne-stranky/detail-lieku?lie_id=94989

State Institute for drug control. (2011a) Príloha k rozhodnutiu o zmene v registrácii ev. č. 2108/04246. *Súhrn charakteristických vlastností lieku ENCEPUR.* [on-line]. 2011-03-20. [cit. 2011-03-25]. Available from: http://www.sukl.sk/sk/pomocne-stranky/detail-lieku?lie_id=76041

Statistical Office of the Slovak Republic. (2010). *Slovenská republika v číslach, 2010 (Slovak republic in figures, 2010).* Štatistický úrad, 2010, 36 p. ISBN 978-80-89358-64-9. Bratislava, Slovak Republic

Suss, J. (2008). Tick-borne encephalitis in Europe and beyond – the epidemiological situation as of 2007. *Eurosurveillance*, 2008, Vol.13, No.26, pii=18916

Thorin, C., Rigaud, E., Capek, I., Andre-Fontaine, G., Oster, B., Gastinger, G., Abadia, G. (2008). Seroprevalence of Lyme Borreliosis and tick-borne encephalitis in workers at risk, in Eastern France. *Med Malad Infect*, 2008, Vol.38, No.10, pp.533-542

Union ZP a.s. (2011). *Pre poistencov – Výhody na rok 2011 – očkovanie proti kliešťovej encefalitíde (For policyholders. – Benefits for 2011 – Vaccination against tick-borne encephalitis)* [on-line]. 2011 [cit. 2011-03-18]. Available from: http://www.unionzp.sk/ockovanie-proti-kliestovej-encefalitide2.html

World Health Organization. (2009). *International travel and health.* WHO 2009: pp.77 - 78. ISBN 978 92 4 158042 7. Copenhagen, Denmark

World Health Organization. (2011). *Biologicals - Tick-borne encephalitis Vaccine.* [on-line]. 2009 [cit. 2011-03-18]. Available from: http://www.who.int/biologicals/areas/vaccines/tick_encephalitis/en/

14

Natural Focal Transmissible Infections with Neurological Manifestations in Ukraine

H. Biletska, I. Lozynskiy, O. Drul, O. Semenyshyn,
I. Ben, A. Shulgan and V. Fedoruk
Lviv Research Institute of Epidemiology and Hygiene
Ukraine

1. Introduction

Ukraine is a country in the East of Europe. It lies between latitudes 44° and 53° N, and longitudes 22° and 41° E. It has an area of 603,628 km^2, making it the largest contiguous country on the European continent. Ukraine borders the Russian Federation to the east and northeast, Belarus to the northwest, Poland, Slovakia and Hungary to the west, Romania and Moldova to the southwest, and the Black Sea and Sea of Azov to the south and southeast, respectively. Ukraine is subdivided into twenty-five oblasts (provinces) and one autonomous republic (AR), Crimea. Additionally, the cities of Kiev, the capital, and Sevastopol, both have a special legal status.

Forming of natural foci of transmissible zoonoses in Ukraine is related with the presence of three physical-geographical areas: mixed forests (Ukrainian Polissya), Forest-Steppe, Steppe and two, placed extrazonal physical-geographical areas (Carpathian and Crimean Mountains).

Largely forested area in the western region is 20% of Polesie - 25,7%, in Ukrainian Carpathians - over 60%. Prevails landscape of broadleaf forests, which grows about 120 trees and shrub species, including pine, oak, fir, beech, ash, hornbeam, linden, maple. Variety of natural-vegetable associations, favourable abiotic terms (temperature and humidity) are pre-conditions of existence of numerous representatives of vertebral and bloodsucking arthopods – potential reservoirs and vectors of various infections pathogenes. On territory of Ukraine existence of natural foci of transmissible infections of different etiology is well-proven long-term researches: viral (TBE, CCHF, WNF, HFPS, Kemerovo, Ukuniemi, Caliphornia serologic group and other), bacterial (tularemia, Lyme-borreliosis), ricketsial (Q-fever, HGA, Ixodo-Rickettsiosis Marseliensis). On the breadth of geographical distribution, weights of clinical manifestatons and remote consequences most actuality for the health protection of country is presented by a tick-borne encephalitis (TBE) and Lyme-borreliosis (LB).

2. Tick-borne encephalite in Ukraine

Tick-borne encephalitis (synonyms - taiga encephalitis, Russian spring–summer encephalitis, central european encephalite - further in the text referred to as TBE) - natural foci disease of viral etiology with primary lesions of central nervous system. Virus affects the tunics, white and grey substances of a brain and spinal cord, spinal and cranial roots, peripheral nerves.

TBE was first described in 1927 by Austrian scientist H. Schneider under the name of epidemiologic seasonal meningitis of unknown etiology' in suburbs of Vienna, a capital of Austria. In former Soviet Union, in Far East, TBE was first described in 1932. In 1937 L. Zilber with his team of scientists isolated the causative agent of this disease - virus and discovered the transmitting vector - ticks.

From modern times position TBE virus is a polytypical type of high prevalence, which is characterized by a significant geographical and intrapopulative variability due to the range of antigens and biological features. Its area constantly widens over the southern part of forest zone of extra-tropical Eurasia from the Atlantic to the Pacific Ocean [Votjakov V.,1978].

Studies of TBE molecular epidemiology conclude that there are 3 main genotypes of TBE virus in nature, which concur with antigens subtypes. It was shown proven that far-east genotype of TBE virus (genotype 1) prevails in the regions of Russian Far East and in Japan. In Eastern and Western Siberia, in Ural and European part of area on the territory of Russia absolutely prevails Ural-Siberian type (genotype 3). Westward, on the territory of Eastern European countries including Ukraine, in Central, Western and Northern Europe there prevail strains of western genotype (genotype 2).

Thus each genotype has its own areal. However some strains of a far-east genotype can be found with different detection rates in other regions as well, and, for example, make about 10 % of natural virus population in Eastern Siberia.

Within TBE areal there are significant distinctions among complication of the course of the disease, predominance of certain clinical forms, lethality. Thus, there is no form of total infection in terms of far-east TBE, while in terms of western TBE (Belarus) it makes 20,4%, meningeal - 32,2% and 50%, meningoencephalitic - 30,2% and 0%, polioencephalomyelitic - 21,5% and 0%, myeloradiculoneuritic - 10,9% and 2,7%[Votjakov V.,1978, Randolf SE.,2002]. Lethality in terms of western TBE is of a fraction of a percent, while in terms of far-east TBE the percent of lethality is very high: meningoencephalitic form - 13,3%, polioencephalomyelitic form - 62,5%. Apparently western TBE differs from far-east TBE by considerably milder course and favourable outcome. Feverous period is longer (11 days) than in terms of eastern nozogeographic form (8-9 days) and is often characterized by two-wave course. Constant symptoms of western nozogeographic form are radicular pains and distal type of paresis, lesions of nuclei of a brain stem and cervical part of spinal cord are uncommon. The course of an acute period is slighter: without comatosic condition with respiratory disorders and generalized convulsions. About 10 000 clinical cases of TBE are registered yearly. There is noted the increase in TBE morbidity in recent decade. In western European countries, where it has never been found any eastern subtype of TBE virus neither in patients' blood nor in ticks, the TBE mortality rates range from 0% to 3,9%, and paresis - from 3,0% to 23,5% [Kunz Ch.,1992, Gratz N.,2005].

2.1 Stages of TBE studing in Ukraine

TBE is one of the most common arbovirus infections in Ukraine. Human gets infected with TBE from ticks or by consuming raw, mostly goat's milk. In 1950 - 1960s a significant part of all TBE cases in European part of a former Soviet Union territory was caused by alimentary infection.

First in Ukraine TBE virus was isolated in 1960 from blood of the patient and ticks *I.ricinus* in Zkarpattia and Volyn oblasts.

Virological surveillance, that has been conducted by scientists of the laboratory of Transmissible Virus Infections (TVI) of Lviv Scientific Research Institute of Epidemiology and Hygiene of Ministry of Health of Ukraine, enabled detection of 38 strains of TBE virus. Most of them (26 strains) were isolated from *I.ricinus* ticks, whose rates of TBE infection in active natural foci are 19,5%, from mouse-like rodents (*Apodemus agrarius, Ap. sylaticus*) - 2 strains, from birds (*Fulica atra*) - 1 strain and from TBE patients - 9 strains (table 1).

Material name	Number of objects studied		Number of isolated arboviruses strains:							
	examples	pools	Total in strains:							
			no	%	TBE	WN	TAH	TRI	BAT	UUK
Clot of blood and cerebro-spinal fluid	198	237	14	11,1	5	7	2	0	0	0
Ticks (Ixodidae)	143000	3119	51	40,5	26	0	0	3	3	19
Mosquitoes (Culicidae)	218000	2906	37	29,4	0	13	4	0	18	2
Small mammals	8700	1745	6	4,7	6	0	0	0	0	0
Wild birds	1750	435	18	14,3	1	3	0	1	5	8
Totals	371648	8441	126	100	38	23	6	4	26	29

Table 1. Results of virological examination of biological objects and identification of isolated arboviruses in Ukraine during 1970-2007 years

Due to their antigen characteristics, strains of TBE virus isolated in Ukraine belong to ricinus serotype (genotype 2) and have almost same biological characteristics as causative agent of Central-European encephalitis of countries of Eastern and Western Europe [Vynograd I., 1996].

We found that the formation of arbovirus natural foci is closely connected to three physically-geographical zones in Ukraine - mixed forest zone (Ukrainian Polissya -1), forest - steppe zone (2), steppe zone (3) and two extra-zonal natural areas - Carpathian (4a) and Crimean mountains (5) (fig.1).

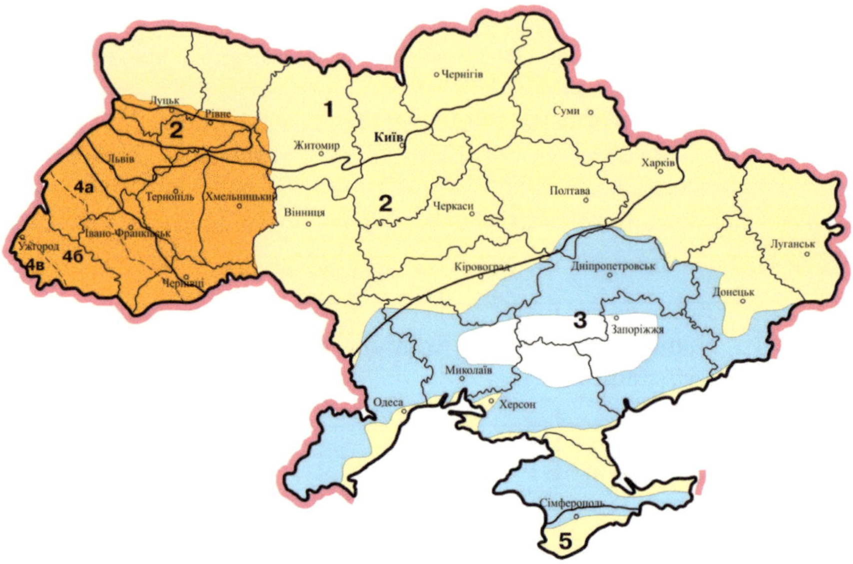

- territory with domination of *I. ricinus*
- territory of massive breed of *I. ricinus*
- territory without massive breed of *I.ricinus*
- separate foci of breed of *I.ricinus*

1 - mixed forest zone
2 - forest–steppe zone
3 - steppe zone
4 – Carpathian mountains
5 - Crimean mountains

Fig. 1. Prevalence of *I.ricinus* L. on the territory of Ukraine
(data from the Institute of Zoology, Academy of Science of Ukraine)

Thus on the territory of Ukrainian Polissya, in Carpathian and Crimean mountains there are favourable conditions for the formation of natural foci of mainly those types of arbovirus, which are transmitted by ticks - TBE, Tribech, Ukuniemi. In forest-steppe zone - both arbovirus transmitted by ticks and those by mosquito. In a steppe zone intensively circulate arboviruses associated with blood-sicking mosquitoes: West Nile, Sindbis, Californian serological group (Tahinja, Inko), Batai and others (fig.2).

2.2 TBE Epidemiology in Ukraine

Natural TBE foci in Ukraine are mainly associated with Polissya territories (Volyn, Rivne, Zhytomyr, Kyiv and Chernigiv oblasts), Pre-Carpathian and Trans–Carpathian regions [Vynograd I., 1996]. This predisposes different circulation intensity rates of TBE virus on different territories. Thus, immune layer of farm animals against TBE virus gets considerably thinner from west to east. We found 8,2% of seropositive farm animals in Zakarpattia (Trans-Carpathian), 9,4% - in Western forest-steppe zone territories, 6,3% - in pre-Dnister region (Kyiv, Vinnytsia and Cherkasy oblasts), and 3,5% in left-bank region (Poltava, Kirovograd and Dnipropetrovsk oblasts). The same tendencies are observed also in human population.

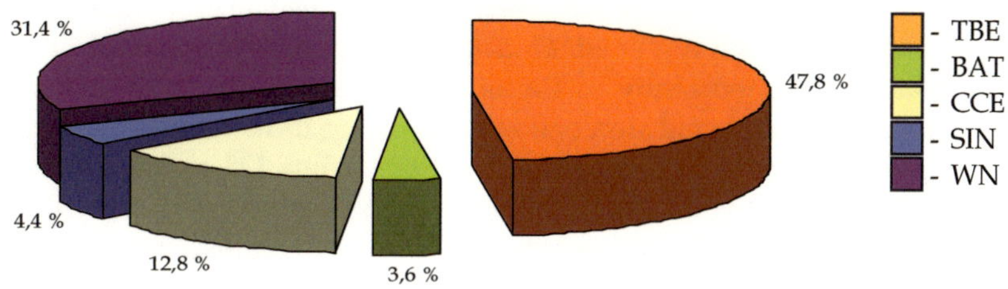

Fig. 2. Nosologic structure of arboviral infections in Ukraine

The percent of immune layer against TBE among healthy people (donors) in Zakarpattia was 6,8 %, in western oblasts 5,2 %, in right-bank- 3,8 % and in Eastern (from Dnipro) oblasts 1,6 - 2,4 %. In TBE natural focuses in the Volynska oblast and to Crimea percent seroprevalense among clinically healthy donors to virus TBE has been- 30,3 - 75,2 %.

2.2.1 Vectors and hosts

Intensive circulation of TBE virus was also detected among mouse-like rodents population. 15,8% of all observed samples of them have antibodies to TBE virus.

Implementation of ELISA method for detection of antigen and antibodies to TBE virus significantly contributed to our knowledge concerning the peculiarities of circulation of the mentioned virus in Ukraine. We detected the main reservoirs and carriers of the virus in nature. These are *I. ricinus* ticks (68,1% of all infected ticks) and *D. reticulatus* (30,6%). Apart from the main carriers, such species as *D. marginatus, H. plumbeum, H. marginatum, Rh. rossicus* also participate in virus circulation.

Among mouse-like rodents the main role is of Cl. glareolis (26,8%), A. agrarius (22,5%), M. arvalis A. sylvaticus and A. flavicollis, M. oeconomus, M. socialis, M. musculus, Sorex araneus.

For 2010 enzootic as to TBE territories, distinguished according to one or combination of such characteristics as natural infection (presence of antigen) of ixodic ticks and small mammals (potential carriers and reservoirs of pathogen) with causative agent, diagnosed cases of the disease with local infection, high degrees of population immunity, were registered in almost all administrative oblasts of Ukraine except some of eastern oblasts (Sumska, Luganska).

2.2.2 TBE morbidity

During the period of 2003-2010 we observed 223 cases of sero conversion in diagnostic titers of people from 14 oblasts of Ukraine: Polissya - Volyn oblast (77 cases), Rivne oblast (8), Zhytomyr (1), Sumy (23); forest-steppe zone - Lviv oblast (19), Khmelnytsk oblast (2), Vinnytsia oblast (1); steppe zone - Dnipropetrovsk (6), Donetsk (9), Zaporizhia (26), Mykolaiv (1), Kherson (13) oblasts; in Zakarpattia (36). We also observed highly intensive circulation of TBE virus in the Crimea.

For present moment local cases of TBE among people are registered yearly in 16 out of 25 oblasts of Ukraine, in cities Kyiv and Sevastopol. However the official data don't reflect the real state of things with the morbidity in Ukraine. The present condition can be explained basically due to the prices of import diagnostic systems which are not affordable for most of medical institutions and lack of Ukrainian diagnostic systems production. Due to this fact, the official data on TBE morbidity in Ukraine show the lowest rates compared to other countries of Eastern Europe and don't show a tendency to increase. During the period of 1955 to 2007 there were only 562 TBE cases registered, while 122 of them were registered in the period of 2000 - 2010 (fig. 3). And correspondingly, the indices of morbidity in Ukraine during the decade varied in the range 0,005 - 0.1/100 000 population, including per oblast from 0 - 1,5 and make only 0,02 (2010).

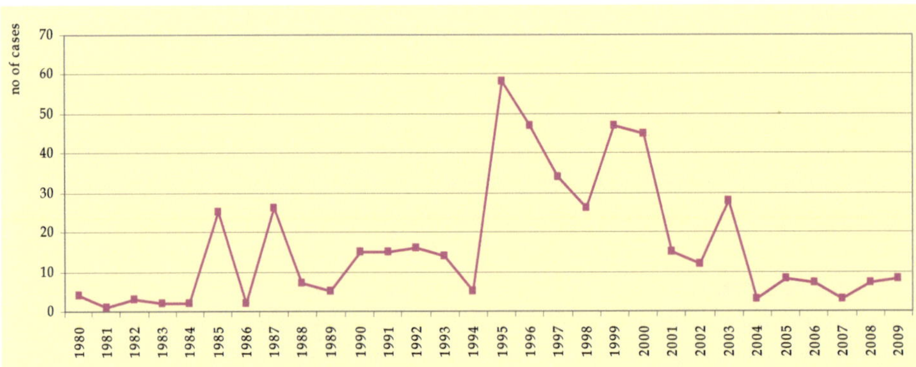

Fig. 3. Cases of TBE in Ukraine (1980-2009)

According to their clinical manifestations we distinguish three main basic forms of acute tick-borne encephalitis: feverous, meningeal and focal. Feverous form is characterized by the milder course and favorable prognosis. Its leading feature is a fever without any signs of meningitis and organs pathology. Meningeal form is characterized by presence of meningeal syndrome, which is accompanied by changes in liquor. The main manifestations of focal forms are symptoms of focal lesions of nervous system, which complicates the course of the disease. Due to its clinical manifestations the focal form of TBE is often separated according to the degree of lesions of different parts of nervous system: meningoencephalitic form, polio-encephalo-myelitic form, myeloradiculoneuritic form etc (table 2).

2.3 TBE in Ukrainian Polissja

The most active natural TBE foci in Ukraine are located on the territory of Volyn oblast (Ratniv, Kivertsi, Kamen–Kashyr raions) and Autonomous Republic of Crimea (Simferopol, Bilogiria, Bakhchisarai, Sudak raions and Great Yalta) [Vynograd I.,1983].

The activity of TBE natural foci in Volyn oblast was manifested by group infection of people in 1995. In the period of April-October central raion hospital of Ratniv raion hospitalized more than 80 people with fever and lesions of respiratory and central nervous system. Forty six of them were serologically diagnosed with TBE. The layer of seropositive as to TBE virus among healthy people ranged in different villages from 14,8% to 50% with the mean value of 33,3%. The presence of a natural TBE foci in Ratniv raion was also confirmed by isolating of a TBE virus strain from ticks I.ricinus and numerous cases of indication of TBE antigen in

I. ricinus and *D. reticulatus* ticks and in internals of *Apodemus agrarius*. Areal of TBE virus apart from the most active Ratniv and less active Lutsk raions includes also Kivertsi, Kovel, Rozhyshen and Liubomyl raions of Volyn oblast, which is indicated by yearly reporting of TBE cases and detections of a virus antigen in ixodic ticks and mouse-like rodents.

Years, Country	Quantity of patients	Total infection form, %	Meningeal form, %	Meningoencephalitic form, %	Polioencephalomyelitic form, %
1996, Germany	300		50,0	38,0	12,0
1998, Horvatia	92		9,8	85,9	4,3
1995, France	21	4,8	28,6	62,0	4,8
1987, Russia, Ural region	190	34,6	50,6	10,6	4,2
1984, Poland	215		58,1	28,4	6,9
1992, Austria	117		61,0	24,0	15
1994, Slovenia	1044		63,0	30,1	6,9
1975, Chechia	633	0,7	6,3	84,0	9,0
2002, Lytva	133		43,6	43,6	3,8
2002, Ukraine, Polissja	80	60,0	24,0	16,0	
1996, Ukraine, Forest-steppe	56	35,7	41,0	21,4	1,9
1989, Ukraine, AR Crimea	52	67,0	15,4	17,3	

Table 2. Clinical forms of TBE in countries of Europe and in Ukraine

The disease was registered in spring-autumn period, starting in May and ending in November, with the peak in July-August. The main means of infection was transmitting (68,0%). The cases of alimentary infection with TBE (32,0%) were due to a consumption of raw cow's milk and its products. The development of a serious and complicated clinical forms of a disease was more common in terms of the transmitting way of infection ($P<0,05$).

In general TBE in Volyn is characterized by one-wave feverous period, with predomination of feverous (60%) and meningeal (24%) forms of a disease with only 16% of focal form, coordination disorders, insignificant quantity of paralytic forms and cases of a development of a chronic disease.

Clinical manifestations are similar to the western type of this infection, but there predominated one-wave character of thermal curve, while two-wave type of fever and changes in hemogram were observed in half frequency. The temperature curve of part of the patients had three waves.

In terms of neurological complaints there predominated the vertigo, walk unsteadiness, bones and lips tremor. Sensitivity disorders in forms of paresthesia were common as well. From the side of vegetative nervous system during the acute period the leading symptoms were the following: bradycardia, growth of blood pressure, clearly manifested hyperhidrosis, stable diffuse dermographism. In the acute period of the disease some

patients developed thyroid enlargement, asymmetry of skin temperature. Highly notable were various 'pseudonevrasthenic' complaints which followed the course of the disease: memory decrease, irritability, obsessive fears and thoughts, emotional lability. The before-mentioned clinical form was called by author as 'attenuate TBE' [Morochkovski R., 2002].
Almost half of patients - (48,2%) - the initial stage of the disease was characterized by some prodromal indications, manifestation of which wasn't pathognomonic for the given disease. As a result of a transmissible form of infection ($P<0,05$), there were more complicated manifestations of it, when in terms of clearly manifested intoxication and general-cerebral syndrome, changes from the side of a nervous system there developed a disfunction of a vegetative nervous system which prevailed in different parts of it ($P<0,05$), there were observed pathologic indications in cardio-vascular system ($P<0,05$), liver enlargement ($P<0,001$). All disorders of a vegetative nervous system were of central genesis as a rule, and developed mainly as a result of more considerable lesions of a central nervous system. As a common indication there was observed a skin hyperhidrosis, especially of a local character, which developed in all patients with poliomyelitic -like form of a disease.
It has to be mentioned that the rates of TBE forms with the lesions of a central nervous system which followed the tick bites and those which followed the alimentary way of infection didn't differ significantly ($P>0,05$).

2.4 TBE in forest-steppe zone

In a forest-steppe zone of Ukraine, within the described natural foci, the TBE morbidity is of a sporadic character and the course of the disease is varied.
In Pre-Carpathian zone, forest-steppe and steppe zones TBE is characterized by a two-wave course of a feverous period accompanied by a meningoencephalitic syndrome and insignificant quantity of focal lesions of a central nervous system.
In terms of study of immunity structure of healthy population there was observed the decrease in immune layer against TBE virus from west to east. There was noted the same tendency - the specific gravity of TBE cases was falling from 9,2% in Zakarpattia (Transcarpathian) to 7,0% in western oblasts, 4,2% in pre-Dnister forest-steppe regions, and few cases (1,7%) in the left-bank Ukraine. This serves the evidence of a connection between TBE morbidity in a forest-steppe zone of Ukraine with natural foci of a virus of a right-bank part of a forest-steppe zone.
The TBE incidence rates among pediatric populations are considerably lower than those of adults: among age groups of 0 to 20 years old - 12,5% of total number of cases. The incidence rates of elderly population (60 years old and more) made 3,5%, and 83,9% of all cases are people of the most productive age (20-60 years old), who populate the forest-steppe zone of Ukraine (fig. 4). TBE virus caused 24,8% of cases of arbovirus etiology.
Most of observed TBE cases were characterized by central nervous system lesions, without any focal symptoms in their course. A syndrome of a general fever with the
body temperature of 39-40°C which remained steady for 4-6 day was common for all cases as well. The patients had severe headaches with a frontal-temporal localization, nausea, hypersensitivity to bright light, dryness and tickling in a throat. Meningeal syndrome was observed in 1/3 of all cases. Lesions of brain tunics were indicated by a vertigo, nausea, vomiting, rigidness of occiput muscles, positive syndromes of Curnig, Brudzinski, pain in Kerrer's points. Feverous period lasted for 9-17 days. Full recovery, without residual effects, was observed on 21-35 day of a disease.

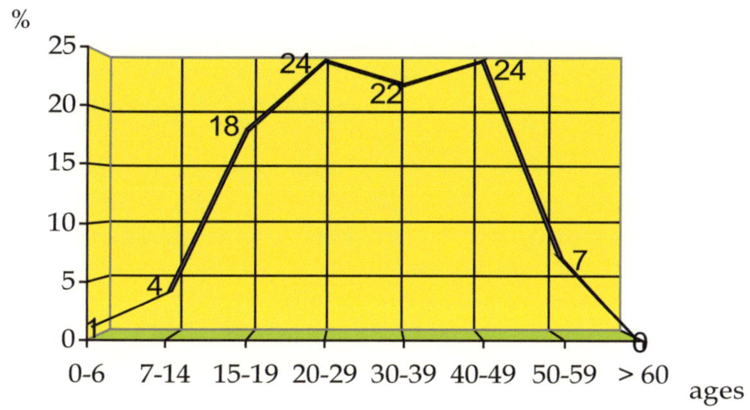

Fig. 4. Age morbidity structure of TBE

Focal form was observed in 21,4% of cases. It was characterized by a long-lasting hyperthermia with clearly manifested syndrome of total infection. Part of patients had a two-wave course of fever with the more complicated course of a second wave- it was characterized by encephalitic lesions. They were manifested by loss of consciousness, sometimes with psychomotor agitation. Among the indications of focal lesions there were observed hyperkinesis and hemiparesis. The disease lasted for 35-60 days. Three patients were released from hospital with signs of ataxia, slight signs of shoulder girdle muscles paresis. Three patients had muscle atrophy as residual effect.

It has to be mentioned that focal forms of TBE were detected by us only in western oblasts of Ukraine (Lviv, Ivano-Frankivsk and Zakarpattia oblasts). Lesions of peripheral nervous system were observed in one patient and were manifested by an exacerbation of a chronic polioradiculoneuritis which the patient had.

In 35,7% of TBE cases the course of a disease was complicated by lesions of respiratory system in terms of a syndrome of total infection. A feverous period had a one-wave course and lasted for 3-9 days. Nine patients were clinically diagnosed with pneumonia or bronchitis [Lozynski I., 1996].

2.5 TBE natural foci in the Crimea

The discovery of TBE natural foci in the Crimea is of a great importance because the territory is intensively exploited as a recreational zone. The discovery of TBE natural foci was preceded by the detection of antibodies against the virus in farm animals (sheep, cattle) and birds which inhabit forest landscapes. The rates of seropositive animal units were 18,1% and 19,8% respectively. The first patient with laboratory proved diagnosis of TBE was hospitalized in 1980 [Evstaf'ev I., 2001]. The following studies enabled isolation of TBE virus from ticks and rodents, it also led to the detection of number of serologically proved TBE cases.

The main carrier of TBE in the Crimea is *I. ricinus*, more than 95% of all isolated TBE strains were isolated from this species. According to the data obtained in studies of the Crimean Sanitary Station, the rates of ticks infection with TBE virus are low (the level of infection with virus is 0,5%). There was also detected the participation in pathogene circulation of *Hyalomma plumbeum, D. reticulatus Fab., D. marginatus Sulz* by isolating TBE viruses from them. The peculiarity of Crimean TBE natural foci is virus-carrying of *H.plumbeum* ticks (13,7%), which keep the intensity of virus circulation in nature. The main feeders of preimaginal stages of ixodic ticks and reservoirs of virus in nature are background small mammals: *S. uralensis, S. flavicollis, M. obscurs*, and *Crocidura suaveolens* [Omelchenko O., 1989].

The highest rates of *I. ricinus* ticks population were registered in Simferopol-Zui forests, with totals of morbidity for three years of surveillance (2,00-2,35 per 100 000 population) four times higher than in regions of periphery of the Crimean mountains, where there is the most numerous population of *H. plumbeum* ticks.

The study of antigene structure of strains, isolated from ticks which inhabit different foci of the Crimean peninsular, showed a significant polymorphism of a TBE virus population. Initially it was detected that there circulate both strains of a western variant ('Absetar'), which are common for European countries, and of an eastern variant ('Sofia'). The deeper study showed, that five strains isolated from *I. ricinus* had antigene differences from a reference strain 'Sofia' in one out of three domains of glycoprotein E. This epitope of Crimean strains was significantly different from that of a virus detected in the Far East of Russia (1 genotype).

Etiological diagnostic of yearly seasonal neuroinfections in the Crimea proved their connection with natural TBE foci. In 1985-1987 there were hospitalized 173 persons due to the tick bites and development of feverous diseases; 50 patients were laboratory diagnosed with TBE. The study of immune status showed a considerable level (12,0%-18,0%) of population immunity of almost all regions of a mountain-forest zone of the peninsular, which also indicates a potential epidemic hazard of this territory in respect of TBE. In Simferopol and Bilogiria regions, where there were detected the highest morbidity rates, 55,1%-75,2% of healthy population had antihemagglutinin to TBE virus.

Since 1985 premountain-mountain forest part of the Crimea has been defined as natural foci of TBE. After the outbreak of the disease there started the intensification of TBE studies in the Crimea. Since 1985 the number of registered TBE cases ranged from 2-3 to 33 cases yearly. Real state of things with morbidity is considerably higher, due to the fact that a lot of TBE cases are not diagnosed and not detected, which is connected to non-specific course of TBE and prevalence of feverous and not distinct forms.

Simferopol, Bilogiria, Bakhchisarai, Alushta, Kirov and Krasnogvardeisk regions as well as forest-park zones of Yalta, Alushta and Simferopol are defined as endemic TBE regions. According to the official statistic data for the recent ten years, the morbidity rates in the AR of the Crimea are from 0,05 to 1,5 per 100 000 population. In recent years we annually register from 2 500 to 4 500 reports from people, who suffered from tick bites.

3. Lyme-borreliosis in Ukraine

Among the infections which take stably high positions in the structure of infectious pathology of population and cause more considerable medically-social and economical damages in comparison to other zoonoic diseases, equally with a tick-borne encephalitis Lyme-borreliosis (LB) is of the highest topicality in Eurasian continent. LB is transmissible natural-focal zoonosis, caused by spirochaete of genus *Borrelia*. LB is characterized by the propensity to a chronic course, polysystemic lesions of skin, nervous and cardio-vascular system, liver, spleen, eyes and locomotor system. The disease has several stages of its development, apart from infection stage and primary manifestations. Immunity is unsterile, causative agent has a long-term persistence in an organism, with possible super- and reinfections. The first description of LB was given in 1977 in the US, and in 1982 they deciphered its etiology. The use of modern molecular-biological techniques enabled detecting of more than 10 (up to 15) genotypes of LB causative agent [Strube et al., 2010], which were consolidated in *Borrelia burgdorferi* sensu lato complex. Apart from known 'classical' pathogenic representatives - *Borrelia* (*B.*) *burgdorferi sensu stricto* (s. s.), *B. afzelii* и *B. garinii* [Baranton et al.,1992; Canica et al.,1993], the recent studies proved the role of *B. bavariensis* (a close relative of *B. afzelii*) *B. bissettii, B. lusitaniae, B. valaisiana, B. spielmanii* in infectious pathology. Genetical variety of causative agents determined the change of LB definition from «a monoinfection» to «a group of nosoologically independent infectious diseases» of human [Gratz, 2005]. There is some basement for assumption that genotype and antigenic differences of *Borrelia* determine peculiarities of pathogenesis and clinical manifestations of the disease in different regions. Intensive study of LB in the late twentieth century has established the pandemic spread of the disease. Lyme-borreliosis occurs on all continents except Antarctica. In the USA they annually report of 12 000 to 40 000 cases of LB [MMWR, 2007], incidence rates in Russia - up to 70 [Naumov, 2005], in Europe are - 70-130 in per 100 000 population [Gratz, 2005].

3.1 Stages of LB studing in Ukraine

First cases of LB in Ukraine were diagnosed later than in other, including neighbouring, countries - in 1989-1993 [Nebogatkin&Semenova,1994].. Since 1995 there have started studies on LB in Lviv Scientific Research Institute of Epidemiology and Hygiene, Ministry of Health of Ukraine. The official registration of a new nosologic form of LB has been held since 2000. In the course of implementation of clinical and laboratory diagnostics of LB the topicality of this disease came into light. Among the most important characteristics of current LB in Ukraine the following has to be mentioned: a) constant broadening of a nosoarea; b) rapid increase in population morbidity rates; c) prevalence of urban population among cases in total (70%-80%); d) increase in number of patients who were bitten by ticks under different social and behavioral conditions; e) prevalence of human infections in antropurgical foci; f) increase in number of infected ticks in nature; g) formation of urban foci; h) circulation of five pathogenic *Borrelia* genotypes; i) pathomorphism of the disease with the prevalence of neurological and rheumatological (arthritis) forms; j) existence of territorial and population-combined foci of LB-TBE and LB-HGA and cases of mixed infections.

3.2 LB natural foci

3.2.1 The vectors

LB areal in Ukraine coincides with the areal of European forest tick *I. ricinus,* which is the main vector of *B. burgdorferi* sensu lato in European countries. By method of dark-field microscopy we detected that on the average from 6,45% of *I. ricinus* in Carpathian mountains to 10,8% in Polissya with maximum of 25,0% in some biotopes are carriers of *Borrelia*. Out of *I. ricinus* ticks collected in western part of Lviv oblast we isolated 4 genotypes of *Borrelia*: *B. b. sensu stricto, B. afzelii, B. garinii* и *B. valaisiana* (atypic), in the southern part - *B. b. sensu stricto, B. afzelii, B. garinii* и *A14S*. Thus for present days in Ukraine we discovered 5 genotypes of *B. b.* sensu lato out of 7 genotypes existing and discovered in Europe. Currently in Ukraine natural infection with *Borrelia* has been proved also for *I. trianguliceps* [Akimov&Nebogatkin, 1997], and more than once, for *D. reticulatus* [Biletska et al., 2007], and in recent years - for *D. marginatus* in regions where these species prevail (Donetsk and Kharkiv oblasts) (fig. 5).

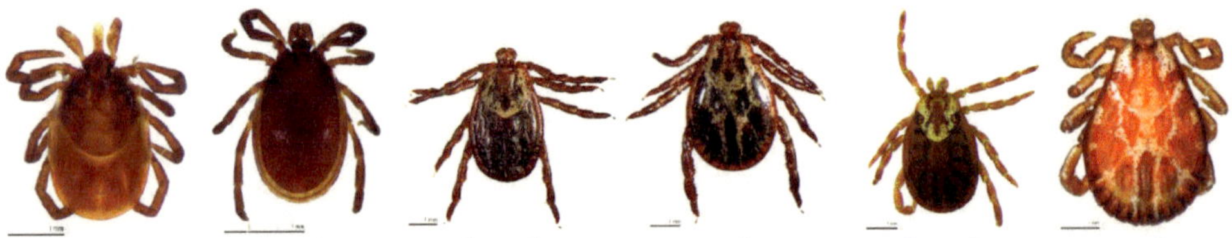

female male female male female male
I.ricinus Lin. *D. reticulates* *D. marginatus*

Fig. 5. Vector of *B. burgdorferi* sensu lato in Ukraine

According to Akimov, 5 more species can participate in *Borrelia* circulation - *I. crenulatus, I. kaiseri, I. redikorzevi, I. hexagonus, H. punctata*. .More frequent cases of *Borrelia* exposure in *D. reticulatus* and their infection rates in places of their prevalence (mixed forest zone), serve the evidence of their being secondary carriers of LB. The mean index of infection of *D. reticulatus* in Europe and in Russia is between 1,72% and 3,6% [Rudakova, 2005, Nijhof, 2007], while in Ukraine - 5,4% (8,0%-15,4%-2010). We got some evidences of existence on the territory of Volyn, Lviv and Sumy oblasts polivectorial (bivalent) natural LB foci, where Borrelia carriers are ticks of two background types - *I. ricinus* and *D. reticulatus,* which makes the risk of infection of population with LB considerably higher.

3.2.2 The hosts

It is known that in different natural LB foci borrelia can be kept during the long term and transmitted to ticks by 2-3 basic and up to 10-15 additional types of mammals and also birds, which get their feed from the earth [Gorelova et al., 2001; Peteny et al., 1996; Miyamoto et al., 1997; Humair et al., 1998; Humair, Gem, 1998; Pichon et al., 2000]. For 2002 terriofauna of Ukraine had 132 species, among them 53 species and 29 genders of micromammals [Zagorodniuk, 2002]. Reservoir role of certain species of these mammals which inhabit natural LB foci remains unstudied, except western region. Occurring everywhere in different landscape subzones of western part of Ukraine 5 species of small rodents of *Muridae* family are wide spread: 3 species of *Murinae* family (mice): *Apodemus agrarius*. (index of abundance - 20,22%), *Apodemus flavicollis* (6,61%) and *Apodemus sylvaticus* (7,81%), 2 species of *Microtinae* family (voles): *Clethrionomys glareolus* (26,52%) and *Microtus arvalis* Pal. (22,58%) and 1 species of *Insectivora* family - *Sorex araneus* (5,19 %). On the average 10,04% (5,77% - 13,14%) of these animals had antibodies against Borrelia detected, which corresponds to the showings from LB foci of high activity. Among vertebral of countries of Central and Western Europe the main role in circulation and reservation of LB causative agents belongs to (*A. flavicollis*) and (*Cl. glareolus*) [Stefancikova, 2004]. In different regions of Ukraine the indices of infection with borrelia of *Cl. glareolus* (14,1-14,3%), *A. silvaticus* (12,7%) and *A. flavicollis* (8,0%) were almost the same as findings of studies in other European countries (12,5% and 17,4% respectively), which serves the evidence of first-priority part of these species in borrelia reservation on the territory of western region of

Ukraine. Four more species of *Rodentia* were found seropositive: *A. agrarius, M. arvalis* и *Mus musculus* and *S. araneus* (table 3).

Landscape zones	No. exa-mi-ned	No. of serum-positive small mammals	Examined small mammals species:						
			A. agrarius Pal.	*A.flavicollis* Mart.	*M.arvalis*	*M. glareolus* Sch.	*Mus musculus* Linn.	*S.araneus* Sch.	*A.silvaticus* Linn.
Ukrainian Polissya	703	66 (9,4%)	19 (11,8%)	4 (3,8%)	10 (8,9%)	18 (14,1%)	11 (15,3%)	1 (2,3%)	3 (4,4%)
Forest-steppe	459	59 (12,9%)	12 (9,8%)	2 (8,0%)	38 (21,6%)	5 (7,9%)	2 (33,3%)	0	0
Carpathian region	365	32 (8,8%)	10 (7,0%)	0	10 (12,9%)	3 (14,3%)	0	0	9 (12,7%)
Total	1988	157 (7,9%)	41 (7,5%)	6 (3,2%)	58 (11,3%)	26 (10,8%)	13 (10,1%)	1 (1,8%)	12 (7,7)

Table 3. Prevalence of antibodies to *Borrelia burgdorferi s.l.* in small mammals

3.2.3 Epidemiology

Currently in Ukraine due to its morbidity rates LB has the first place among all tick-borne natural foci infections. In the period of 2000-2010 there were officially registered 4597 cases, the index of morbidity increased by 23,2 times: from 0,12 in 2000 up to 2,79 per 100 000 population in 2010 respectively (fig. 6).

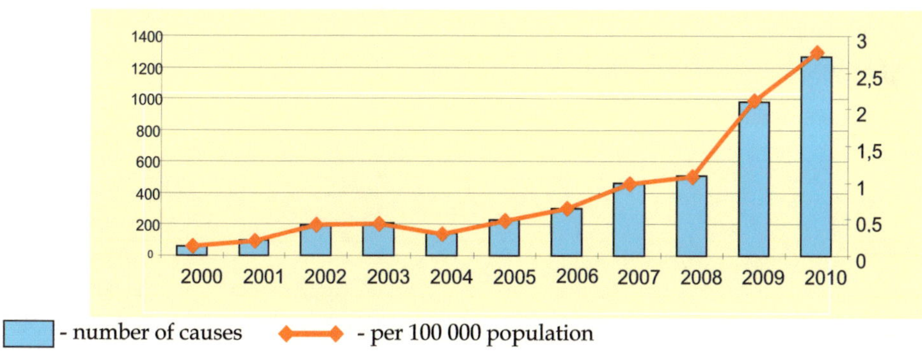

Fig. 6. Lyme-Borrelioses morbidity in Ukraine (2000-2010)

In some administrative regions of Lviv and Donetsk oblast and in Kyiv, where there have been formed special centers for LB surveillance, this index reaches 11,2–19,4 per 100 000 population, thus coming to proximity with these indices in other (neighbouring) European countries. Cases of LB have been registered in all regions of Ukraine: in 25 administrative oblasts and in Autonomous Republic of Crimea (fig. 7).

Number of enzootic as to LB territories is considerably increasing with every year and for 2010 makes 1809 populated areas in 477 administrative regions. According to the mean value of many years standing index of morbidity in different administrative territories of Ukraine amounts of 0,05 (AR Crimea) to 10,3 cases (Kiev) per 100 000 population. The development of the disease in most cases (85,7%) is connected to sticking of ixodic ticks, while in 5,6%-10% of cases it may be connected to bites of bloodsucking mosquito (*Culicidae*). Yearly dynamic of LB morbidity is characterized by notable seasonal prevalence, connected to period of activity of carriers (*I.ricinus).* The vast majority of new LB cases (81,7%-85,6%) is registered in May-September. First cases are reported in April (2,9%), last – in November (4,9%) with peak in May-June (70,8%). In the period of April-October there are 95% of tick attacks registered and almost 90,0% of new LB cases. As distinct from tick-borne encephalitis, 3,8% of LB cases for the first time clinically manifested in low-season period (December-February). In polivectorial (binary) LB foci epidemic season may be prolonged (up to 8-9 months) due to early (in March) appearance of *D.reticulatus* in nature (fig. 8).

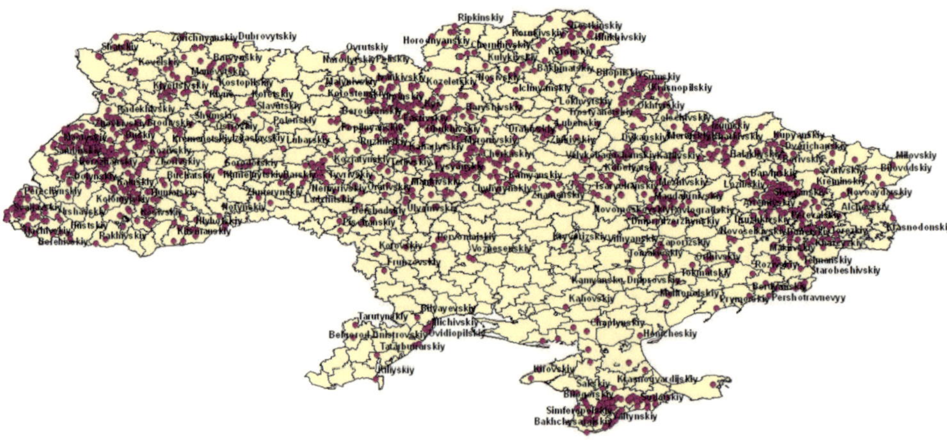

- cases of morbidity

Fig. 7. Map of Lyme-borrelioses morbidity in Ukraine

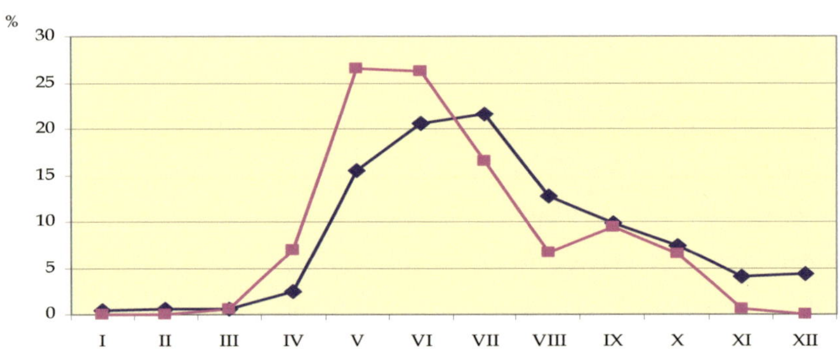

- Lyme borreliosis incidence   - tick bites incidence

Fig. 8. Dynamics of Lyme borreliosis incidence and tick bites incidence

Part of rural population among LB cases makes only 15,2%, while the main part of cases (84,8%) is urban population of Ukraine. The leading role of LB epidemiology is of antropurgical foci. Their number is increasing rapidly and currently in Ukraine 44,6% of cases of human infection occur within towns and small towns, 11,0%- on the territory of villages and only 34% - in terms of visits to forests with recreational purposes, gathering mushrooms,

berries and the like. There were also noted the cases of tick attacks in residential areas, in out-of-town recreational institutions, in parks and gardens, on the territories of cemeteries.
The rates of contact between population and *B.burgdorferi* are quite high: more than a third (34,3%) of healthy people and from 34,7% to 49,3% of persons, whose jobs are connected with forests, contain antiborrelia antibodies IgG, and from 9,1% to 15,2% of them are within the diagnostics titers. The highest rates of infection (up to 70%) the population with borrelia were detected in Ukrainian Polissya and forest-steppe zone. The results of epidemiological studies of 1104 LB cases, obtained in different random periods (from 2000 to 2010) differ insignificantly. Lyme-borreliosis affects all age groups (from 1,9 to 87), however the age groups of 30-49 (>30,0%) and 50-59 and older (>40,0%) are considered to be high-risk groups. The incidence rates of female population were higher than these of male (>60%). According to socially-professional distribution the groups of the highest risk (>70%) go as follows: employees and workers- 40,6%, retired and unemployed - 34,6%. Persons from the professional risk group (forestry workers, livestock breeders, tree and shrub planting workers) make the least numerous group (1,2% - 1,8%), thus there is no connection between LB and professional activity detected.

3.3 Clinical manifestation

According to the analysis of medical records of 1104 LB cases the main clinical manifestations of the disease are referred to as stages of early local (1) and disseminated infection (2) and only 1,7% - as a stage of a late chronic infection (3) (according to the conventional classification). The spectrum of clinical manifestations of LB in Ukraine includes most of symptoms described in literature. It is known that in Europe LB is mainly manifested by dermal and neurological manifestations [Stanek&Strle, 2009]. Among prevailing forms of LB in Ukraine there are erythematic forms as well (64,9%). Neuroborreliosis has the third position (21,4%) preceded by ME and locomotor apparatus pathologies [Biletska et al., 2001,2008] (fig. 9).

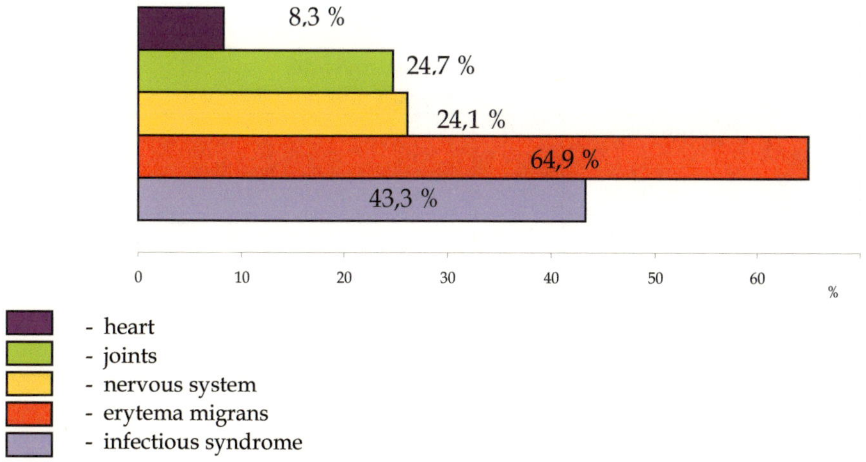

Fig. 9. The main clinical symptoms of LB at the patients

Quite often (60,6%) the erythematic form is accompanied with a fever (up to 38-39°C), asthenia, indisposition, headache, arthralgia, myalgia. On the initial stage of the disease

43,3% of patients were observed with general-infection syndrome. Secondary elements of erythema developed in 4,1% of cases, which is considerably rare in comparison with the USA, where the half of reported cases is accompanied with the before mentioned lesions. The explanation of the great extent of clinical manifestations spectrum was obtained through indication of monoclonal antibodies (IFA) against 4 borrelia types in blood serum of LB patients: *Borrelia afzelii, B. garinii,* and against two strains of *Borrelia burgdorgeri sensu stricto* isolated in the USA and Czech Republic.

It was found out that the causative factors of 75,5% of LB cases were all three pathogenic for a human types of borrelia of *B.burgdorferi s.l.* complex: in 42,6% of cases there were detected antibodies against *B.garinii,* which cause neuroborreliosis, in 19,8% *B.burgdorferi sensu stricto,* which is connected to locomotor apparatus pathology, and in 27,3% *B.afzelii,* which causes dermal lesions. Every fourth case could be hypothetically caused by other (opportunistically) pathogenic type of borrelia.

3.3.1 Features (spectrum) of neurological lesions

In terms of clinically-epidemiological analysis of laboratory- confirmed cases of LB (1104) neurological symptoms were observed in 236 (21,37%) of patients, among them 55,09% of female and 44,91% of male respectively. The age ranged from 1,5 to 68. It has to be mentioned that the most numerous groups were those of teenagers and young adults from the age group of 11-20 years old (23,31%), and also people of active working age from 31 to 40 years old (16,52%) and from 21 to 30 years old (15,15%).

Central nervous system (204 patients)		Peripheral nervous system (46 patients)	
manifestations	%	manifestations	%
acute encephalitis	17,6	mononeuritis	21,7
meningoencephalitis	9,3	paresthesias (numbness of fingers, feeling cold in extremities)	76,1
meningitis	31,8	hand tremor	2,2
arachnoiditis	0,5	polyneuritis and polyradiculoneuritis	8,69
meningeal symptoms (rigidity neck muscles)	2,9	-	-
convulsions	2,9	-	-
the consequences of the defeat of the cortex cerebral mozka (speech impairment, coordination, sleep, vision, memory, transient loss of consciousness)	9,8	-	-
asthenic-neurotic syndrome (frequent headaches, severe fatigue, headache, nervousness, etc.)	3,4	-	-
epileptic syndrome	0,5	-	-
sluggish paresis of facial muscles	1,47	-	-

Table 4. Neurologic manifestations of Lyme borrelioses patients

Among the manifestations of neuroborreliosis there were observed both lesions of peripheral nervous system (19,49%), which appeared mostly in the acute stage of the disease and those of central nervous system (86,44%), which appeared in acute stage of the disease and in the 2nd stage (dissemination) of LB as well. The lesions of peripheral nervous system in the acute stage were manifested mostly by perceptibility disorders (76,09%) (paresthesia) such as "gooseflesh", "numbness" of fingers, freezing limbs etc, and also by facial, sciatic, lumbar mononeuritis (21,74%), polyneuritis and polyradiculoneuritis (8,69%), and quite rarely by hands tremor (2,17%) (table 4).

The important clinical peculiarity of acute borreliosis in Ukraine are early (occurring in 2-3 week of the disease) transient lesions of central nervous system. The high rates of acute serous encephalitis (17,65%), meningitis (31,86%), meningoencephalitis (9,31%), arachnoiditis (0,49%), were detected mainly in 135 patients from Kherson (41 case), Volyn (53 cases) and Zaporizhia (41) oblasts. Meningitis as an independent form of LB is more often observed in children, while in adults it is combined with spinal and cranial nerves lesions etc. The dominant symptom which prevailed in most cases was a headache of different intensity (14,21%). More often it is a moderate headache, but it can be also frank. Apart from a headache, there are also observed nausea, vomiting (2,45%), edema of a brain (0,98%), convulsions (2,94%), painfulness which accompanies any movements of eye balls (0,49%). In 24,15% of cases the syndrome of general infection was manifested by hyperthermia, asthenia and vertigo. In terms of neurological observation almost all patients have the lack of neck mobility (2,94%). Other meningeal symptoms are observed less often. Cerebrospinal fluid develops lymphocytic pleocytosis, the number of cells–dozens and hundreds in 1 microliter; lymphocytes make 70%-100% of total quantity of cells; quite often, especially in cases of meningoradiculitis, there is an increase in proteins values - sometimes it is above 1-2 millimole/l; the level of glucose can be within norm. In some cases (6,86%) the course of the disease and neurological symptoms (acute initial stage, thermal reaction, rigidity of occiput muscles, extinction of reflexes, inflammation of CSZ etc), LB was very similar to TBE, especially its encephalic-poliomyelitical manifectations, which predetermined preliminary diagnosis TBE, however it wasn't later confirmed in serological tests [Zinchuk, 2007]. Similar indications of LB are observed also in some regions of Russia, however they are rarely observed in patients from any other countries. On the 2 stage of LB the lesions of cerebral cortex were manifested by various encephalic pathologies (9,80%) such as dysphasia, hypotaxia, sleep disturbance, visual and memory impairment, absence. Some patients (3,43%) had some manifestations of asthenically-neurotical syndrome such as frequent headaches, sudden fatigability, migraines, nervousness etc, some patients (1,47%) were observed to have low-intensity paresis of facial muscles, rare cases (0,49%) developed epileptic syndrome. Sixty percent of patients with borreliosic lesions of nervous system developed radicular painfulness followed by peripheral paresis, which are usually manifested in 1,5 months from the beginning of the disease. The indications of progressive vestibular pathology and psychoorganic syndrome were observed relatively rarely. There was observed the development of chronic processes of the disease with slow intensification of symptomatology in 1,27% of patients. The important feature of neuro-borreliosis in Ukraine is absence of migratory erythema in 80,93% of cases, which considerably complicates the diagnostic of the disease. Among patients with lesions of nervous system only 51,27% of cases reported the fact of a tick bite in anamnesis, the rest 48,73% didn't remember anything like that or denied it absolutely. Due to this it can be assumed that there were clings of infected nymphs which are often not noticed. Most patients with borreliosic lesions of nervous system (30%-50%) get sick in the period of June and October after incubative period which lasts from several days to several weeks.

4. Mixed infections

Analysing the current epidemiologic situation with LB one more new peculiarity of great importance has to be mentioned. It must have existed before but for us it has become clear only in recent decades. Here we mean the existence and prevalence in Ukraine of territorial and populational combined foci of transmissible tick-borne infections of viral and bacterial nature – TBE and tick-borne borreliosis. It was first shown in our studies that on the most of the territory of Ukraine TBE and LB are actually epidemiologic 'twins' and differ only in etiological factor. Among main epidemiological characteristics there are the following- the same carrier (*I.ricinus*), which makes the areals of two infection practically concurrent, and reservoirs (*A. flavicollis, Cl. glareolus, A. agrarius, M. arvalis, M. musculus, S. araneus*). The retrospective analysis has shown that most of diseases which were diagnosed previously as TBE (30,78%) and most likely are still being diagnosed as so, are in fact tick-borne borreliosis. In terms of a purposeful serological testing of 227 patients of neurological departments from 7 oblasts with the preliminary diagnosis of TBE and prevailing symptoms of encephalitis, meningitis-encephalitis, viral encephalitis etc, we detected the mixed infection of TBE – LB in 21 (9,3%) patients. Overall in the structure of LB morbidity the cases of mixed with TBE infections made from 5,8% to 7,1% and were detected in 9 oblasts. Analysis of clinical manifestations of mixed infections in 30 patients proved the suppositions as to TBE combined with LB has less complications in its course [Aleksejev, 1996]. Combination of LB with TBE was characterized by acute onset of disease (77,9%) with the development of febrile (52,3%), meningeal (32,8%), focal (5,9%) and asymptomatic forms or with only mild symptoms (9,0%). In the structure of clinical manifestations of LB individual cases there is a predominance of one sign of infection, or a combination thereof, or one of the infections are in latent form. Mutual burdening course of mixed infection TBE-LB was not detected. However, the prevalence of natural foci of LB and TBE with a high incidence of LD in the territory of Ukraine, a large proportion of patients with the transition of the disease in chronic forms of the absence of complete data on the peculiarities of clinical manifestations of disease in the combined infection of Borrelia and TBE virus, the complexity of the objective differential diagnosis and lack of efficacy, require further research in this area.

5. Conclusion

Presented materials so far do not qualify for adequate mapping of the current situation in neuroinfections, ecologically related with ticks in Ukraine. But now the data for individual regions showed that the level of incidence and prevalence, tick-borne infection is obviously a leading position among natural focal zoonoses in Ukraine. Undoubtedly, in the near future with the improvement of laboratory diagnosis number of reported cases of TBE and LB will be increase. Will be expand the spectrum of identified infectious diseases also. So, recently obtained evidence of the existence in Ukraine of natural foci of human granulocytic anaplasmosis (HGA), and identified numerous human cases of mixed infection of LB-HGA, TBE-LB-HGA. It identifies the need to continue clinical and epidemiological studies of tick infections on the territory of Ukraine using standardized criteria for diagnosis (including differential) and the involvement of specialists in various fields.

6. References

Akimov I. & Nebogatkin I. (1997). Some results of the study of ticks in foci of borreliosis in Ukraine. *Bulletin of Zoology*, N° 4, pp. 91-95.

Aleksejev A., Dubinina E.&Vashukova M. (1996). Borrelia as apparent antagonists of tick-borne encephalitis: parasitological and clinical aspects. *Med. Parasitology and Parasitic Diseases*, Vol . 3, N° 3, pp. 3-11.

Baranton G., Postic D., Saint Gisons L., Boerlin P., Piffaretti J., Assous M.&Grimont P.(1992). Delineation of Borrelia burgdorferi sensu stricto, Borrelia garinii spp. Nov., and group VS461 associated with Lyme borreliosis. *Int. J. Syst. Bacteriol.*, Vol. 42, N° 3, pp. 378-383.

Biletska H., Lozinskiy I., Burkalo T., Semenyshyn O., Rogochij E., Markovich V., Sakal' M.&Orel T. (2003). Clinical and epidemiological aspects of mixed infection "tick-borne encephalitis-ixodid tick-borne borrelioses. *Scientific Bulletin of Uzhgorod University. Medical series*, Issue 21, pp. 66-69.

Biletska H., Lozinskiy I.& Semenyshyn O. (2002). Differential diagnosis of mixed-borne infections in Ukraine. *Proceedings of: VI Congress of* infectiologists of Ukraine, September, Odessa, 2002.

Biletska H., Podavalenko A., Semenyshyn O.& Lozinskiy I. (2007). Ecology-epidemiological aspects of spreading the Lyme disease in Ukraine. *Problems of modern medical science and training*, N° 4, pp. 12-14.

Biletska H., Vynograd I., Semenyshyn O., Lozinskiy I., Drul O., Kozlovsky, M, Rogochy E.G.& Sholomey M. (2001). Neurological manifestations of Lyme disease in Ukraine, *Proceedings of: Proc. scientific-practical. Conf. Plenary Session of the Association and infectious disease Ukraine "Neuroinfections. Other infectious diseases"*, Kharkiv, April, 2001.

Canica M.M., Nato F., Merle L., Mazie J. C., Baranton G.& D. Postic. (1993) Monoclonal antibodies for identification of Borrelia afzelii spp. Nov. associated with late cutaneous manifestations of Lyme borreliosis. *Scand. J. Infect. Dis.*, Vol. 25, pp. 441-448.

CDC. Lyme disease - United States, 2003–2005 (2007) *MMWR* 56 (23), pp. 573–576.Retrieved from: http://www.cdc.gov/mmwr/preview/mmwrhtml.

Evstaf'ev I. (2001). Results of a 20-year study of tick-borne encephalitis in Crimea. *Journal of Medical Epidemiology and Immunology*, N° 2, pp. 111-114.

Gratz N. (2005). Vector-borne infectious diseases in Europe, *WHO Regional Office for Europe.* Retrieved from: http://www.euro.who.int/pubrequest.

Kunz Ch. (1992) Die Fruhsommer - Meningoenzephalitis (FSME) in Europa Allgemeinarzt. Vol. 14, N° 7, pp.691-696.

Lozynskiy I (1996). Arboviruses of Forest-steppen Zone and and their importance to the regional infectious diseases. *Dissertation for the degree of the candidate of medical sciences*, 155 pp.

Morochkovski R. (2003) Clinical characteristics of tick-borne encephalitis in Volyn' and optimization of treatment. *Thesis for the degree of the candidate of medical sciences*, 20 pp.

Nebogatkin I.& Semenova N. (1994) Epidemiology and epizootology of Lyme disease in Ukraine. *Ukrainian Scientific-Medical Youth Journal*. N° 1, pp. 61-63.

Naumov, RL & Vasil'ieva I. (2005). Affected populations and the incidence of Borrelia Lyme disease. *Medical Parasitology and Parasitic Diseases*, N° 2, pp. 40-42.

Nijhof A. M., Bodaan C., Postigo M., Nieuwenhuijs H, Opsteegh M, Franssen L, Jebbink. F. & Jongejan F. (2007). Ticks and associated pathogens collected from domestic animals in the Netherlands. *Vector Borne Zoonotic. Dis.*, № 4, pp. 585-595.

Omel'chenko A.A. (1989) Ecology and biological properties of arboviruses selected in south of USSR and their significance in the etiology of seasonal fevers. *Dissertation for the degree of the candidate of medical sciences*, 190 pp.

Randolph S.E.. (2002). The changing incidence of tickborne encephalitis in Europe. *Eurosurveillance Weekly*: June, 2002, Vol. 6, Issue 23

Rudakova S. A., Matusheko E. V., Iakimenko V. V., Tokrevitch N.& Andrejchuk Yu. (2005) A study of possible transovarial and transphase transmission of borreliae by the tick Dermacentor reticulatus (Ixodidae). *Parazitologiia* , Vol. 39, N° 5, pp. 427-432.

Semenyshyn O. (2009). Ecological and epidemiological characteristics of ixodal tick-borne borrelioses in the western Ukrainian region. *Thesis for the degree of the candidate of medical sciences*, 23 pp.

Stanek, G. & Strle F. (2009). Lyme Disease—European Perspective. *Infectious Disease Clinics of North America*, Vol. 22, Issue 2, pp. 327-339.

Stefancikova A., Bhide M., Pet'ko B., Stanko M., Mosansky L., Fricova J., Derdakova M. & Travnicek M (2004). Anti-Borrelia antibodies in rodents: important hosts in ecology of Lyme disease. *Ann. Agric. Environ Med.*, N° 11, pp. 209-213.

Strube C., Montenegro V.M., Epe Ch., Eckelt E.& Schnieder Th. (2010). Establishment of a minor groove binder-probe based quantitative real time PCR to detect Borrelia burgdorferi sensu lato and differentiation of Borrelia spielmanii by ospA-specific conventional PCR. *Parasites & Vectors*, N° 3, pp. 69-76.

Zinchuk A. (2007). Lyme borreliozis detection among patients with neurological disorders. *Practical medicine*, N° 1, pp. 68-72.

Votjakov V., Protas I.&Shdanov V.(1978). *Western Tick-borne Encephalitis*. Medicine, Minsk (Belarus).

Vynograd I.A. (1983). Arboviruses in the Ukrainian SSR and their medical and biological significance. *Dissertation for the degree of the doctor of medical sciences*, 505 pp.

Vynograd I., Biletska H. & Lozynski I. (1996) Tick-borne encephalitis and other arboviruses infections in Ukraine. *Infectious Diseases*, N° 4, pp. 9-13.

Part 3

Japanese Encephalitis

15

Japanese Encephalitis: An Emerging and Spreading Arbovirosis

Shailendra K. Saxena[1], Sneham Tiwari[1], Rakhi Saxena[1], Asha Mathur[2] and Madhavan P.N. Nair[3]

[1]Centre for Cellular and Molecular Biology (CCMB–CSIR), Hyderabad (AP),

[2]Department of General Pathology & Microbiology, Saraswati Medical & Dental College, Lucknow,

[3]Department of Immunology, Institute of NeuroImmune Pharmacology, Herbert Wertheim College of Medicine, Florida International University, Miami, FL,

[1,2]India

[3]USA

1. Introduction

Japanese encephalitis virus (JEV) is a mosquito-borne flavivirus which causes significant epidemics of encephalitis worldwide with 50,000 cases of encephalitis mostly affecting the children below 10 years of age causing 10,000 deaths annually (Saxena 2008, Diagana et al., 2007). It is well distributed all over Asia and posing threat to many other nations (Yamanaka et al., 2010) JEV strong presence can be felt in the south, southeast, and the east regions of Asia (Shimojima et al., 2011). It is transmitted in an enzootic cycle involving water birds, domestic pigs and rice paddy-breeding mosquito's humans and other non-avian vertebrates. Pigs plays role of major amplifying host (Yamanaka et al., 2010). Humans are accidental/dead end hosts of JEV (Schuh et al., 2009) as their immune system cannot sustain high viral titres. Factors underlying the molecular clinical manifestations and pathogenesis of JEV infection are not completely elucidated. JEV consists of five genotypes: GI, GII, GIII, GIV and GV which are distributed worldwide and phylogenetic studies have revealed that GIII is predominant genotype of JEV with 15 strains in Japan and Korea (Schuh et al., 2009). JEV is expanding to the newer horizons as it is evident from the cases reported from the western parts of the globe. In the present scenario there is no specific treatment against JEV strains, few vaccines are available but they cannot treat all the strains of JEV further studies are require for the proper evaluation and their use in treating JEV infections.

2. History

Encephalitis outbreaks have been recorded since early 19th century in countries like Southeast Asia including Japan, Viet Nam, Cambodia, Myanmar, India, Nepal, Malaysia, China, Korea, Taiwan, Thailand and reached to the West including Pakistan and the northeast and southwest of India, also the East (New Guinea), the South (Northern

Australia Archipelago) and it is estimated theoretically to spread further West (Afghanistan). Between 1978 and 1992, 24 imported cases were reported in above regions due to high transmission.

Transmission:	Spread to humans by *Culex* mosquitoes, which pick up the virus from infected pigs.
Symptoms:	One in 200/800 infected people develop clinical signs like high fever and nausea. A quarter of patients with symptoms die; a third of survivors suffer brain damage.
Treatment:	Effective anti-viral drugs have yet to be found. Medicines are given mainly to relieve symptoms.
Prevention:	Vaccination for people at risk, eliminate mosquito breeding grounds, improve drainage, maintain clean piggeries, use insect repellent and mosquito nets

Table 1. Japanese Encephalitis: *at a glance*

Since the 1990s, the transmission of JE virus in humans has extended beyond its original geographical limits as it is evident from the case reports like in 1996, a woman in France suffered from JE after she had visited Thailand, in 1938. JE epidemic reported for first time in restricted seacoast areas of the 'USSR' and it reappeared in 1939. JE was isolated from human in the 'USSR' representing the first genetically characterized strain of JEV from this region, in 1946 major outbreaks of JE were recorded in Korea, in the civilian population in 1949 and among American military personnel in 1950 (Schuh et al., 2009).

Sequencing of JEV strains suggests that JEV is divided into five genotypes (GI–V) (Shimojima et al., 2011), which arose from its ancestor virus in the Indonesia-Malaysia region and evolved into five genotypes: GI, GII, GIII, GIV and GV, out of which GIV and GV are the most divergent which remained confined to the Indonesia-Malaysia region. GI, GII and GIII are the most recent genotypes spread across Asia (Diagana et al., 2007). Phylogenetic characterization in 1930s showed that GIII is predominant genotype of JEV in Japan and Korea since 1935 with 15 strains and GII is present from more than 19 years (Schuh et al., 2009).

GI was first isolated in Cambodia in 1967 and then in China in 1979 while genotype III strains were isolated before the 1970s (Fan et al., 2010). In Vietnam and Japan GIII strains were isolated between 1986 and 1990 and then GI was seen in 1995 and 2002 (Nga et al., 2004) proving that all the strains clustered into two distinct genotypes (III and I) and strains isolated before 1991 belonged to genotype III, whereas those strains isolated after 1994 belonged to genotype I (Ma et al., 2003).

3. New geographical regions covered

JEV Sequencing analysis results exhibiting alarming signal to the new regions as the growing evidences suggests the spreading of different JEV groups to the endemic regions Papua New Guinea and Australia GI includes strains isolated from Northern Thailand,

Cambodia, Korea, China, Japan, Vietnam, Taiwan and Australia between 1967 and the present. GII includes strains isolated from Southern Thailand, Malaysia, Indonesia, Papua New Guinea and Northern Australia between 1970 and 1999, GIII includes strains isolated in temperate regions of Asia from 1935 to the present. GIV includes strains isolated in Indonesia between 1980 and 1981 only, and GV includes a single strain isolated in Singapore in 1952. Sequence analyses of viral genes are further showing that a "genotype shift" from III to I has occurred in Japan since early 1990s, reasons for which remains unclear (Shimojima et al., 2011). Japanese encephalitis (JE) is spreading in the newer areas of northern states of India (Saxena et al., 2006, 2009).

4. Morphology and properties

Flavivirus species, which like the Pestivirus and Hepacivirus, is related to the Flaviviridae family. The Flavivirus species not only includes the JE virus but also dengue, yellow fever and tick-borne encephalitis viruses. JE virus is an enveloped RNA virus with ssRNA as genome. It is spheroidal in shape having cubical symmetry, with size of 40-50 nm. Several non-structural and structural genes are present, where the three structural genes are vitally involved in the capsid formation process and are named as core(C), premembrane (prM) and envelope (E). E is expressed on surface and hence plays an important role in antigenecity.

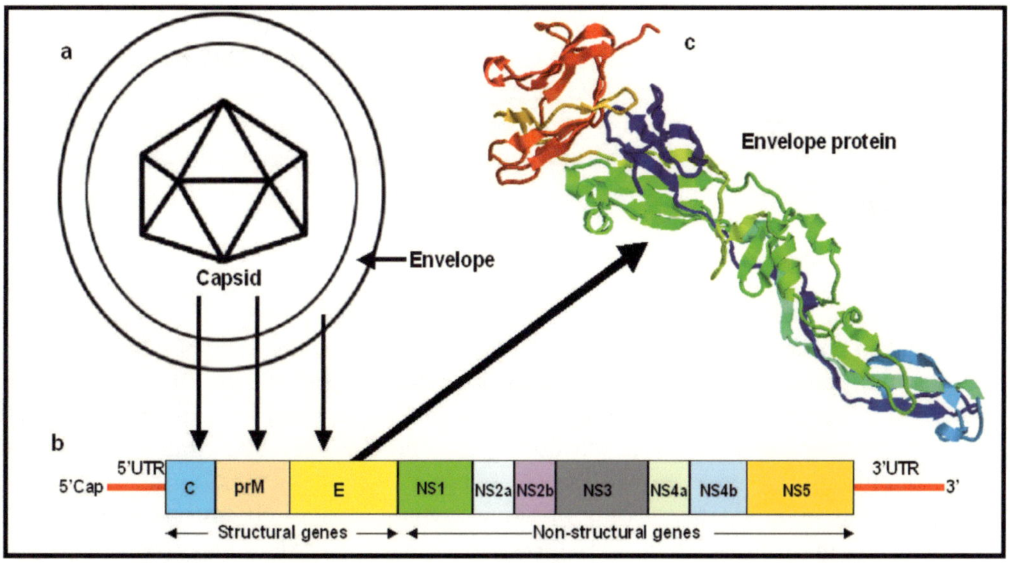

Fig. 1. Japanese encephalitis virus. Japanese encephalitis virus (JEV) structure (A), genomic organization (B), and assimilated structure of the JEV envelope protein (C). JEV genome contains a single open-reading frame (ORF) flanked by 5´ and 3´ UTRs. ORF consists of three structural genes (C, prM and E) and seven nonstructural (NS1 to NS5) genes

5. Genome

JEV isolate from a pool of *Culex tritaeniorhynchus* collected in southern China had genome consisting of 10,965 nucleotides and included a single open reading frame that encodes a

3,432-amino-acid polyprotein (Zhang et al., 2009). The RNA genome is about 11kb in length having positive polar 5'cap but no 3' poly tail. Its genome can be divided into two parts: structural genes (codes for capsid, C; premembrane, prM; and envelope, E) and nonstructural genes (NS1, NS2a, NS2b, NS3, NS4a, NS4b and NS5 are involved in viral replication). NS3 codes for Serine protease and NS5 codes for RNA dependent RNA polymerase, which is cause of mutation, JEV. The functions of other genes are still not understood. Replication of virus happens in cytoplasm and maturation on intracellular membranes (Saxena, 2008).

6. Transmission cycle

JEV was isolated from the brain of an encephalitis patient in Tokyo in 1934, and also from *C. tritaeniorhyncus* mosquitoes in 1938. Studies in Japan, showed pattern of JEV transmission cycle between pigs, mosquitoes, and humans. JE virus is transmitted through a zoonotic cycle between mosquitoes, pigs and water birds. Transmission cycle of JEV was elucidated, where pigs and wild birds played role as amplifying hosts and *Cx. tritaeniorhynchus* as the primary vector species. Pigs are important for pre-epizootic amplification of virus, although sometimes epidemics may rise even in their absence. Humans and horses also are only incidentally infected and are dead-end hosts of the virus due to low level and transient viremia (Misra and Kalita, 2010).

Numerous studies show similar cycles of JEV transmission, although in some cases virus may be detected in mosquitoes prior to amplification in the pigs. Differences in porcine infection rates within countries can also influence human infection, as was evidenced in Sri Lanka, where porcine synchronous seroconversions led to significant transmission to humans (van den et al., 2009) confirmed by enzyme-linked immunosorbent assay (Rajendran et al., 2003).

7. Molecular epidemiology

JEV is classified into 5 genotypes: GI, GII, GIII, GIV, GV. Genotype III (GIII) is widely distributed in Asian countries, including Japan, South Korea, Republic of China, Taiwan, Vietnam, the Philippines, India, Nepal, and Srilanka. By, past decade, JEV GI has been introduced into South Korea, Thailand, and China and has replaced the GIII strains that had been circulating in Japan and Vietnam during the mid-1990s (5). The strains JEV isolated from India till 2007 belonged to GIII (Saxena et al., 2008). JEV emerged in Japan in 1870's, four genotypes of it are recognized presently genotypes I to III are fully sequenced. Complete nucleotide and amino acid sequence of a genotype IV representative, (Indonesian isolate (JKT6468) and it comparison with other fully sequenced genomes has been done. In experimental studies, almost 290 JEV isolates are sequenced showing that all genotypes of JEV circulating in Indonesia- Malaysia region including divergent genotypes GIV and GV which represent the oldest lineages, whereas genotypes GI, GII and GIII circulating in the epidemic and endemic regions are very recent once. Phylogenetic comparisons with other flaviviruses show that it evolved from an African ancestral virus (Solomon *et al.*, 2003). Nucleotide sequencing of C/PrM and E genes, have helped to identify four genotypes of virus. GI includes isolates from northern Thailand, Cambodia, and Korea, GII includes isolates from southern Thailand, Malaysia, Indonesia, and Northern Australia, GIII includes

Japan, China, Taiwan, the Philippines and Asia, and GIV includes isolates from Indonesia. One strain of JEV (Muar strain) is isolated from Singapore in 1952 from a patient, which may represent a fifth genotype. But in some cases this paradigm is violated as in Vietnam epidemic disease occurs in the north and endemic disease occurs in the south.

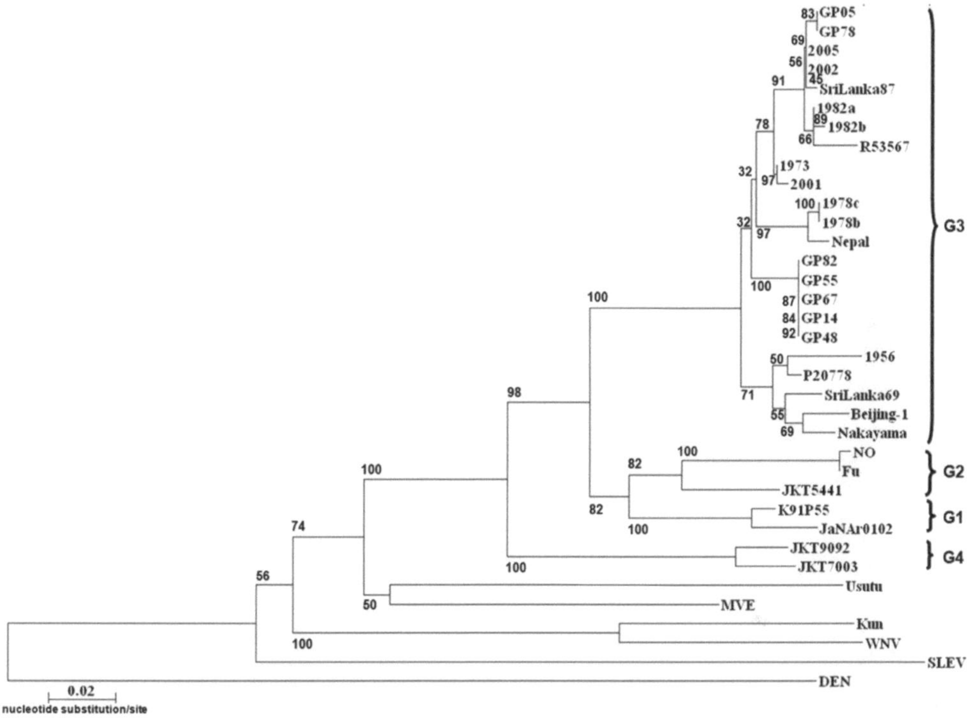

Fig. 2. Sequence phlylogeny of JEV isolates. Sequence phylogeny of Japanese encephalitis virus isolates from the Gorakhpur (India) 2005 epidemic, with reference to other Southeast Asian isolates and flaviviruses based on partial E gene sequence. The tree was generated by neighbor-joining method. Bootstrap values are indicated at the branch points. DEN, WNV, KUN, SLEV and MVE denotes Dengue virus, West Nile virus, Kunjin virus, Saint Louis encephalitis virus and Murray Valley encephalitis virus respectively. (Source: Saxena et al. 2009)

Sequencing and phylogenetic analysis show that JEV strain JKT6468 virus genome is 10,978 nucleotides long and on comparison with 17 sequenced JEV genomes, it was seen that JKT6468 has least similarity, with high nucleotide divergence as compared to GI, GII and G III strains. Analysis has shown that PrM gene has the greatest divergence.

Phylogeny distribution of the JEV strains was based on the E- gene which represents genotypes of the group/groups present in that country. In few instances different genotypes are present within the same country. So the countries are grouped into geographical areas based on geographical proximity, temperature, rainfall, etc which shows dispersed distribution of genotypes (Solomon et al., 2003).

Phylogenetic tree analysis for all JEV strains encircling E, C/PrM, or NS5/3 genes analysis, and GIV, GV comparison with GI, GII, and GIII confirm that the distribution of genotypes have true differences. Other group analysis also shows a significant difference in the geographical distribution of genotypes. All genotypes are present in the Indonesia-Malaysia region, but only the most recently evolved genotypes (I, II, and III) are present in the other geographical regions. C protein and E protein structural analysis shows that JEV isolate from GIV (JKT7003) is found to retain identical sequence to JKT6468. GIII is the most widely distributed genotype and found in India, and it is predicted to eventually reach Australia, and GII might be found in China or Japan (Solomon et al., 2003).

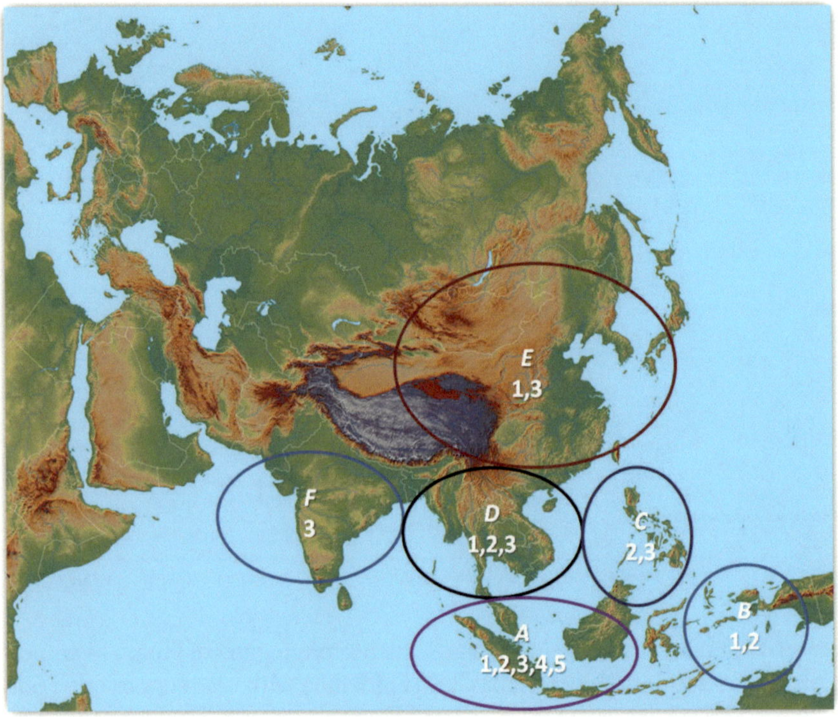

Fig. 3. The geographical distribution and spread of JEV genotypes. Countries are grouped into geographical regions: A, Indonesia (excluding New Guinea) and Malaysia; B, Australia and New Guinea; C, Taiwan and the Philippines; D, Thailand, Cambodia, and Vietnam; E, Japan, Korea, and China; F, India, Sri Lanka, and Nepal. Region A contains all genotypes of JEV, including the oldest. The newer genotypes (I, II, and III) have subsequently spread to other geographical areas. (Source: Solomon et al., 2003)

8. Epidemiology

JEV, transmitted by *Culex spp* mosquitoes, perhaps causes more cases of acute encephalitis than the other arthropod-borne viruses (Richard and John, 2002). JEV is a member of the JEV serological complex, which causes significant morbidity and mortality. The complex consists of eight species and two strains/subtypes including Japanese encephalitis. JEV is the most important member of the JEV group, with an estimated worldwide annual incidence of 45,000 human cases and 10,000 deaths. However, because of insufficient medical facilities and inadequate data collection, JE cases are underreported. Thus, the true annual incidence of encephalitis cases is estimated to be closer to 175,000 (van den et al., 2009). JEV is distributed in temperate and tropical areas of eastern and southern Asia. Its geographic range extends from eastern Asia (China, Japan, Korea, maritime Siberia, Taiwan, the Philippines, and Vietnam), to Southeast Asia and northern Australasia (Cambodia, Indonesia, Laos, Malaysia, Papua New Guinea, Thailand, and the Torres Strait islands of northern Australia), and to southern Asia (Bangladesh, Bhutan, India, Myanmar, Nepal, and Sri Lanka). A single report has also suggested that JEV may occur in Pakistan (Solomon and Winter, 2004). JE is largely a disease of rural areas, especially associated with irrigated rice agriculture. In general, two epidemiological patterns of JEV have been recognized: endemic activity in tropical regions, such as southern Thailand, and epidemic activity in temperate and subtropical regions. In endemic areas, no seasonal pattern exists and sporadic cases of encephalitis occur throughout the year, most often in infants and young children, although cases may peak after the onset of the rainy season. Serological tests have shown that by the time children reach adulthood all have been exposed to JEV and possess neutralizing antibodies. Epidemic activity in temperate and subtropical areas occurs most commonly in summer or early autumn after the rainy season, which may extend from spring to late autumn (van den et al., 2009). Because of its prevalence and mortality JE is a major public health problem in endemic–epidemic regions as due to severe susceptibility of the Children and young adults (Diagana et al., 2007). There is a peak in vector density and virus activity during the north-east monsoon period, October-December (Mani et al., 1991 in endemic zones the percentage of JE antibodies increases with age whereas during an epidemic outbreak both adults and children are equally susceptible (Diagana et al., 2007).

REGION	AREA	SEASON	HOST/VECTOR
Endemic region	Southern India, Southern Vietnam, Southern Thailand, Philippines, Malaysia and Indonesia.	Rainy	Mosquitoes, birds, pigs and human cases are rare.
Intermediary subtropical region	Includes Northern India, Nepal, North and Central Burma, Northern Thailand, Northern Vietnam, Southern China and Bangladesh.	Rainy	Epidemics in contrast, and severe and concentrated among children.
Temperate epidemic region	Northern China, Korea, Taiwan and Southern extremities of Russia. Also Pakistan, Afghanistan, Nile valley, Madagaskar and Oriental Africa.	Summer and Autumn	Postulated explanations are migration of birds, certain irrigation projects, animal smuggling and global warming.

Table 2. JE is primarily found in South East Asian countries. Three epidemiological regions can be distinguished (Diagana et al., 2007)

From past 75 years the focus was on China and Southeast Asia, but now Japanese encephalitis has expanded westward to India and Pakistan, northward to eastern Russia, eastward to the Philippines, and southward to Australia. In the northern region, epidemics occur during the warm summer months, In China, 20 000 symptomatic cases are reported annually. The ratio of symptomatic to symptomless infections is around 1:25 to 1:1000. In areas where Japanese encephalitis is common, it is primarily a paediatric disease; however, more cases are seen in adults in new place of exposure (Richard and John, 2002). Occurrence of JE is more closely related to temperature than to humidity in the atmosphere (Misra and Kalita, 2010). JEV has caused major epidemics as it invaded new areas, often enabled by rice culture and amplification in domesticated swine (Weaver and Reisen, 2010).

9. Geographical distribution

JEV, the most frequent arboviral cause of encephalitis worldwide, has spread throughout most of Asia and as far south as Australia from its putative origin in Indonesia and Malaysia. Here is a brief outlook:

9.1 Japan

Until 1990s, only GIII JE virus was identified in Japan, and then the genotype seemingly shifted to GI. On the basis of molecular epidemiological study in Vietnam, China, and Japan, it was found 8 subgroups of GI JEVs are circulating in East Asia and introduced to Japan through China due to the bird migration and/or infected mosquitoes (Morita, 2009.) JEV infects numerous animal species including humans, horses, pigs, raccoons, wild boars and raccoon dogs recently a study found that it was present in *C. tritaeniorhynchus* feed on small Asian mongooses on Okinawa Island indicating that they are sensitive to JEV (Saito and Nakata et al., 2009). (Ohno et al., 2009). Distribution of JEV has dispersed to new areas due to migratory birds like wild ducks (*Anas poecilorhyncha*) which highlight that there may be circulation of JEV in these captured birds. A sero-epizootiological showed several race horses showing high antibody titer (Sugiura and Shimada, 1999). Serum samples of cattle raised in Saitama and Kagoshima Prefectures also showed antibody titers against JEV (Horimoto et al., 1989).

C. tritaeniorhynchus is major mosquito vector in Japan, but recent surveys show that *C. pipiens* and *Aedes albopictus* as potent competitors too (Konishi, 2005). G1 JEV was also collected from mosquitoes and from swine serum samples collected in Okinawa Island. GI is distributed from northern Thailand to Cambodia and recently expanded to Australia, Vietnam, the Republic of Korea, and Japan (Saito and Taira et al., 2007). Wild boars in the Northern area of the main Okinawa Island in Okinawa Prefecture are infected with JEV which is amplified on pig farms tested for JEV antibody by hemagglutination inhibition assay and IgG enzyme-linked immunosorbent assay (Nidaira et al., 2007).

9.2 Bali/Java

Pigs are effective amplifying hosts for JEV, as antibodies to JEV is present majorly in pigs of bali and java (Yamanaka et al., 2010).

9.3 Thailand

Here the estimated occurrence is more than 40/1000 in hospitalized patients (Diagana et al., 2007) who serve as evidence of acute flavivirus infection. 10% of patients in Bangkok hospitals and 28% patients in southern Thailand were found to have JEV infection (Sonja et al., 2010). JEV genotypes studies in pigs and mosquitoes collected near houses of confirmed human GI JEV cases (Nitatpattana et al., 2008). This surveillance study shows an increase of JEV cases during the rainy-seasons.

9.4 India

Epidemiological investigations incorporating identification of blood meals of vector mosquitoes proved their involvement in the transmission of JEV from the Kuttanadu area, Kerala. *C. tritaeniorhynchus* is highly zoophagic and human feeding and also *Mansonia indiana* and *Ma. uniformis* feed on humans showing significant role played by these mosquitoes in the transmission of JEV (Philip Samuel et al., 2008). JEV activity in endemic areas of Tamil Nadu (southern India) is studied, using ELISA (Tewari et al., 2008). JEV was detected using antigen capture ELISA in dry specimens of the mosquito *C. tritaeniorhynchus* in Karnal (Haryana) (Das et al., 2005). *A. subpictus* serves as a secondary vector in JEV transmission in Cuddalore, Tamil Nadu showing natural transovarial transmission of the virus through *A. subpictus* (Thenmozhi et al., 2006). JE is found endemic in Cuddalore district, TamilNadu (Kabilan et al., 2004). In a serological survey of birds in Kolar District (Karnataka) by hemagglutination-inhibition test it was showed that bird species such as Pond Herons, Little Egrets Grey Partridges and Quails are infected with JEV and play role in the JEV infections (Jamgaonkar et al., 2003) (Rajendran et al., 2003). Three cases of JE were reported for the first time from two villages in Krishnagiri Health Unit district of Tamil Nadu. Sixteen serum samples from patients were sent to the Department of Virology, Calcutta, which is first documentation of concomitant JEV and HIV infection in the eastern India (Neogi et al., 1998).

9.5 Malaysia

JEV is an important encephalitis virus in Malaysia, which was thoroughly studied in Sarawak, Malaysia. JEV is endemic in Sarawak, with cases occurring throughout the year (Wong et al., 2008) a few cases have been reported in tropical Asian countries (Kari et al., 2006). JEV is an important causative agent of viral encephalitis among pediatric admissions in Penang, Malaysia was proved by an IgM capture ELISA (Cardosa et al., 1995). Studies also show encephalitis in Perak, Malaysia with data showing titers of neutralizing antibodies against JEV (Cardosa et al., 1991). JE epidemic occurs sporadically throughout the year and is generally asymptomatic (Sinniah, 1989).

9.6 Philippines

A long-term study in Philippines confirmed acute cases of Japanese encephalitis via IgM-capture ELISA, which detects anti-JEV immunoglobulin M (IgM) in cerebrospinal fluid (CSF) samples (Natividad et al., 2006) (Kari et al., 2006). Mosquitoes were collected from Tagudin, Ilocos Sur Province, Philippines, and found positive for the presence of JEV by the help of microneutralization test (Trosper et al., 1980).

9.7 Korea

Serological survey of JEV infection in goats in Korea provide incidence of positive cases indicating that JEV infection is frequent in goat farms in Korea (Yang et al., 2007).

9.8 Nepal

Regional survey conducted in Nepal for antibody to JEV in pigs, ducks and horses showed positive result for the presence of antibodies against JEV (Pant et al., 2006). Intense transmission of JEV in the area of the British Military Cantonment at Dharan was confirmed by serological studies from the healthy Nepalese from Dharan and animals from the Cantonment farm which indicates rapid transmission of JEV occuring within the Cantonment area. (Henderson, 1983). The first proven outbreak of JE in Kathmandu Valley of Nepal was in 1995 (Zimmerman et al., 1997). Viral studies of serum and cerebro-spinal fluid (CSF) confirm JEV as the causative agent (McCallum, 1991).

9.9 Indonesia

Geographical range of endemic JE is much vast than estimated (Kari et al., 2006), It is no longer rare to tropical Asia, a study was conducted to measure the prevalence with hemagglutination-inhibition (HI) and neutralizing antibodies against JEV in horses of Java, Indonesia indicating a high risk of JEV infection (Widjaja et al., 1995).

9.10 Singapore

Detection of neutralizing antibodies to JEV in a population of wild boars, as well as two human cases of JE in Singapore indicates that JEV may still be actively transmitted in the peripheral part of the Singapore Island (Ting et al., 2004). A study was conducted to determine the presence of prevalence with hemagglutination inhibition (HI) and neutralization antibodies against JEV in wild pigs of an island in Singapore showing positive results for antibodies against JEV (See et al., 2002).

9.11 Cambodia

JEV is an important causative agent of acute encephalitis in Cambodia, this issue still remains unclear, but some survey shows that infection with JEV is the principal cause for it (Srey et al., 2002).

9.12 Taiwan

Sero epidemiological survey of JEV in Taiwan indicated that the JEV vaccination, in conjunction with JEV natural infection, maintains high JEV Neutralizing (NT) antibody level among rural children of Taiwan (Hsu et al., 1997) showing confirmed Japanese encephalitis (JE) cases (Ku et al., 1994).

9.13 Bangkok

Study of JE was conducted in suburban Bangkok and the primary vector species are found to be *C. gelidus* and *C. tritaeniorhynchus*. Human cases occurred from May-July (Gingrich et al., 1987). In a 5 year study, 121 encephalitis patients were admitted to Bangkok Children's Hospital out of which 79 were proved to be JE (Thisyakorn and Nimmannitya, 1985).

9.14 Spain

JEV antigenic complex of *flaviviruses* are recognized as emerging and re-emerging pathogens. Their circulation is recently detected in different mosquito and vertebrate species in several European countries. Serosurvey using a competitive enzyme-linked immunosorbent assay showed seropositivity in Common Coot (*Fulica sp.*), Montagu's Harrier (*Circus sp.*), Black Kite (*Milvus sp.*), Black Vulture, (*Coragyps sp.*), Bonelli's Eagle (*Aquila fasciata*), Spanish Imperial Eagle (*Aquila adalberti*), Egyptian Vulture (*Neophron percnopterus*), and Eurasian Spoonbill (*Platalea leucorodia*) in autumn season. Real-time reverse transcription-polymerase chain reaction indicated that JEV antigenic group circulates in migratory and resident wild bird species (García-Bocanegra et al., 2001).

9.15 Vietnam

JE is an important public health problem in Vietnam (Yen et al., 2010). Many patients are suspected with CNS Infections and children infected with JE virus (JEV), suffered from hemiparesis, meningism including limb paralysis and some of them subsequently became encephalopathic (Solomon T et al., 2008).

9.16 Hawai Island

JEV is emerging arboviruses which is undergoing intercontinental expansion; it is transmitted between mosquito vectors and vertebrate reservoir hosts, including birds. A potential route of JEV introduction from Asia to western North America is via the Hawaiian archipelago also frequent air traffic from both Asia and North America to Hawai increases the chances of flaviviral infection (Nemeth et al., 2010).

9.17 Central China

Studies with four strains of JEV isolated from CSF of aborted fetuses collected in central China through RT-PCR and sequencing, suggested that GIII is the major subtype of JEV, circulating in central China, Fujian, and Heilongjiang (Fan et al., 2010). However, Shanghai isolates belong to GI (Li et al., 2009). GI strain is distributed well in Southeast Asian countries, whereas, genotype III strains in Northern Asia (Fan et al., 2010). Viral encephalitis emerged in Yuncheng city, Shanxi Province was proved to be Japanese encephalitis B (Zhang et al., 2008). Recent JEV isolates from China are divided into two genotypes, genotype 1 and genotype 3; recent JEV isolates from China are grouped into the same clusters within GI and GIII but GIII strains are ancient than GI (Wang et al., 2007).

9.18 Australia

Domestic pigs, act as the amplifying host of JEV (van den Hurk et al., 2008). It appears annually in the Torres Strait in far northern Queensland, Australia, and is proving a threat for invasion in Australian mainland. Sentinel pigs have a tendency to develop detectable viremias to JEV. Since pigs are amplifying hosts for JEV, they are health risk to the public (Ritchie et al., 2007) (van den Hurk et al., 2008). *Culex* mosquitoes in Cape Town (van den Hurk et al., 2006) and Saibai Islands may be responsible for JEV activity (Johansen et al., 2004). Still there are no evidences found to prove JE responsible for enzootic transmission cycles on western Cape York (Johansen et al., 2003). In Western Province of Papua New Guinea, pigs and marsupials were studied indicating marsupials as poor JE virus host (van den Hurk et al., 2003), but they may play a vital role (Mackenzie et al., 2003). Collections from Badu Island community yielded *C. annulirostris* (van den Hurk et al., 2001) and from Croydon, Normanton and Karumba yielded *C. annulirostris skuse* and *C. palpalis* mosquitoes (van den Hurk et al., 2002); (van den Hurk et al., 2003). Mosquitoes from Cape York Peninsula (van den Hurk et al., 2001) and north Queensland appear to have limited transmission on the mainland, nucleotide sequencing indicate that cyclonic winds carried infected mosquitoes from Papua New Guinea to these places (Hanna et al., 1991) and JEV is demonstrating an emergence in the southern part of New Guinea Island (Spicer et al., 1999).

10. Symptoms

Symptomatic JEV infection shows febrile illness, aseptic meningitis or encephalitis which manifests sensorium, seizures and focal neurological deficit and acute flaccid paralysis. A wide variety of movement disorders like Parkinsonian features and dystonia are also seen (Solomon et al., 2004). JE mainly affects thalamus, corpus striatum, brainstem and spinal cord. In some incidences co-infection of JE and cysticercosis occurs because of the involvement of pigs (Misra and Kalita, 2010). JEV is also associated with reproductive failure in swine (Lim et al., 2007) and also causes fever, headache aseptic meningitis,change of consciousness convulsions, vomiting and encephalitis (Yang et al., 2007). Surveys suggest shift clinical manifestation from encephalitis to meningitis (Konishi, 2005). Death is presumed to result from infection, dysfunction and destruction of neurons. Patients for seizures and clinical signs of brainstem herniation are also reported. Findings suggest that seizures and raised ICP may be important causes of death in case of JE (Solomon et al., 2002). The neurologic signs like meningeal signs, hyperreflexia, Babinski's sign, hemiplegia, papilledema and other cranial nerve palsies are also seen. Most children have blood leukocytosis with predominant neutrophils (Poneprasert, 1989; Srivastava et al., 1999).

11. JEV human infections

Infections of humans with JEV produce vast clinical manifestations, ranging from asymptomatic infection like mild febrile illness, acute and lethal meningomyeloencephalitis. Most infections are asymptomatic and cause a nonspecific influenza-like illness. The ratio of symptomatic to asymptomatic cases has occasionally been higher. Sequelae are more frequent in patients having severe and prolonged acute diseases along with coma and focal neurological deficits.

12. Laboratory diagnosis

Laboratory diagnosis of JE is by IgM capture ELISA, which has high sensitivity and specificity. In the absence of specific antiviral therapy, JE is managed by symptomatic and supportive therapies and preventive measures. Encephalitis is an unusual manifestation of human viral infection, whereas many individuals develop systemic viral infections, only a few develop symptomatic infection of the central nervous system (Whitley and Gnann, 2002).

13. Risk

JEV may become epizootic and epidemic if it is introduced unintentionally for commercial use or intentionally for nefarious purposes. Even global warming may also facilitate the distributions of arboviruses, expanding northward into southern Europe, increasing transmission season and capacity of vectors. Greatest health risk of arboviral emergence is due to extensive tropical urbanization and the colonization by highly anthropophilic mosquitoes. Sustained endemic arbovirus transmission, adequate human viremia and vector competence is the minimal requirement to become major human pathogens (Weaver and Reisen, 2010). Recent global warming trends affect vector population dynamics and disease transmission which is measured by hemagglutination-inhibition (HI) antibodies titre tests (Yang et al., 2008). Studies show incidence of dengue virus (DEN) infections in a cohort of Dutch short-term travellers who travelled to endemic areas in Asia, post-travel serological studies were done by DEN immunoglobulin M (IgM) showing that DEN infections are frequent in travellers to endemic areas in Asia (Cobelens et al., 2002).

14. Host immune response

The factors which govern the clinical presentations and outcome of flavivirus infections are not very well understood, but studies are going on at viral virulence determinants and the host immune response. Distribution of the four genotypes across Asia may relate to the different clinical epidemiology. However nucleotide sequence studies of oldest lineages virus, and phylogenetic analyses of all JEV strains, suggest that the origin is best in the Indonesia-Malaysia region (where all genotypes have been found), and there is spread of the more recent genotypes to new geographical areas. Innate immunity, as evidenced by interferon alpha levels, plays an important role in JEV and other flaviviruses. Cellular immunity is less characterized, but CD8+ and CD4+ T cells may play important role (Solomon and Winter, 2004; Tandon et al. 2002). A failure of the humoral immune response may be associated with death from encephalitis caused by JEV.

15. Future risk

There is potential risk of introduction and establishment of JEV in newer areas of the world. JEV is endemic to Asia and when transmitted to humans (accidental host), may lead to JE, mostly in children with a fatality rate up to 30%. The geographical expansion of JEV in Asia shows the ability of arboviruses to rapidly extend their distributions. As for example, studies have shown that California is at risk for JEV introduction because it functions as a hub for international travel and commerce with Asia, indirectly allowing the introduction of mosquitoes infected with JEV. Introduction of JEV in California, might pose challenge to the health sector due to establishment of susceptible mosquito vectors and vertebrate will lead to the flaws in the surveillance of JEV, and cross reactivity of serological test between JEV and other flaviviruses, and may be JE may not be considered as a possible diagnosis, these all will lead to delay and this delay in detection of JEV may pose challenge in eradicating the virus from California so there is need of considerations for future control efforts if JEV emerges in the United States (Nett et al., 2009).

In the last decade had introduction of huge number of encephalitic viruses and the emergence or spread in the Southeast Asian and Western Pacific regions. JEV has spread its wings through the Indonesian archipelago to Papua New Guinea and to the islands of the Torres Strait of northern Australia, and also to Pakistan and new areas in the Indian subcontinent (Mackenzie, 2005). The incidence of JE in recent times is showing an increasing trend. It appears that JE may become one of the major public health problems in India considering the proportion of JEV infections among the encephalitic children (Kabilan et al., 2004).

16. Prevention/vaccination

Vaccination proves to be the best to protect the individual against any disease. In the case of JE, it is essential to immunize the pigs also to interrupt the transmission cycle (Kabilan et al., 2004). Japanese racehorses are vaccinated with inactivated JE vaccine every year which lessens up the JE cases (Konishi et al., 2004). Screening of goats and cattle are also suggested for JE infection risk to the human population (Rajendran et al., 2003). JEV and JEV-induced macrophage-derived factor (MDF) can modulate nitric oxide synthase (NOS) activity in brain and tumor necrosis factor-alpha (TNF-alpha) (Khanna et al., 1991 and Mathur et al 1992; Saxena et al., 2001) NOS activity gets enhanced in JEV or JEV-induced MDF-treated mice (Saxena et al., 2001). The enhanced level of TNF-alpha correlates well with enhanced inducible nitric oxide synthetase (iNOS) activity, thus provide evidence for protective role of iNOS during JEV infection and hence indicate that iNOS may be a key mediator in host innate immune response (Saxena et al., 2000, 2001, 2003). Administration of inactivated mouse-brain derived JEV were reported in Japan and the United States which had some problem (Takahashi et al., 2000). There is continuous need for constant surveillance and monitoring so as to prevent future large outbreaks (Victor et al., 2000). In fact, three doses of mouse-brain vaccine are enough to protect children against the local Taiwan JEV and choice of selection for best strain for a JE vaccine depends on level of Nt Ab [neutralisation antibody] it induces, the molecular epidemiology and antigenic variation. The future vaccine must produce better B- and T-cell memory in the vaccinated populations (Ku et al., 1994) Vaccinia virus (NYVAC) was engineered to express the JEV prM, E, and NS1 genes, the recombinant viruses were tested as vaccine candidates in pigs showing that after immunization, JEV levels detected in the were reduced demonstrating the ability of NYVAC-vectored recombinants to protect pigs from JEV viremia (Konishi et al., 1992). Extracellular HeLa cells produce extracellular subviral particles which were infected with a recombinant vaccinia virus encoding the prM and E gene and were purified. Mice when received a single inoculation of the purified extracellular particles were fully protected against LD50 of JEV (Konishi and Pincus et al., 1992). Although vaccinia recombinants expressing NS1 can provide some protection from lethal JEV infection, recombinants expressing prM and E have higher levels of protective immunity (Konishi et al., 1991). Antipyretics, anticonvulsants, anticerebral edema agents, adequate respiration and nutrition and physical and occupational therapies are needed by patients (Poneprasert, 1989).

17. Acknowledgment

Authors are grateful to Dr Ch. Mohan Rao, Director, Centre for Cellular and Molecular Biology (Council of Scientific and Industrial Research, India), for the encouragement and support for this work. We also thank Mr ML Arvinda Swamy and Ms Kamakshi Dandu for reviewing this manuscript. A NIH Award (R37DA025576) supports S.K.S. and M.P.N.

18. References

Cardosa, M.J., Choo, B.H. and Zuraini, I. (1991). A serological study of Japanese encephalitis virus infections in northern Peninsular Malaysia. *Southeast Asian J Trop Med Public Health* 22(3): 341-346.

Cardosa, M.J., Hooi, T.P. and Kaur, P. (1995). Japanese encephalitis virus is an important cause of encephalitis among children in Penang. *Southeast Asian J Trop Med Public Health* 26(2): 272-275.

Cobelens, F.G., Groen, J., Osterhaus, A.D., Leentvaar-Kuipers, A., Wertheim-van Dillen, P.M. and Kager, P.A. (2002). Incidence and risk factors of probable dengue virus infection among Dutch travellers to Asia. *Trop Med Int Health* 7(4): 331-338.

Das, B.P., Sharma, S.N., Kabilan, L., Lal, S. and Saxena, V.K. (2005). First time detection of Japanese encephalitis virus antigen in dry and unpreserved mosquito Culex tritaeniorhynchus Giles, 1901, from Karnal district of Haryana state of India. *J Commun Dis.* 37(2): 131-133.

Diagana, M., Preux, P.M. and Dumas, M. (2007). Japanese encephalitis revisited. *J Neurol Sci.* 262(1-2): 165-170.

Fan, J.M., Luo, J., Chen, L., Teng, M., Bu, D., Wang, F.Y., Wang, L., Wang, C.Q. and Zhang, G.P. (2010). Genetic analysis of strains of Japanese Encephalitis Virus isolated from swine in central China. *Virus Genes.* 40(3): 357-361.

García-Bocanegra, I., Busquets, N., Napp, S., Alba, A., Zorrilla, I., Villalba, R. and Arenas, A. (2010). Serosurvey of West Nile Virus and Other Flaviviruses of the Japanese Encephalitis Antigenic Complex in Birds from Andalusia, Southern Spain. *Vector Borne Zoonotic Dis.* Dec 13, 2010. [Epub ahead of print].

Gingrich, J.B., Nisalak, A., Latendresse, J.R., Pomsdhit, J., Paisansilp, S., Hoke, C.H.,Chantalakana, C., Satayaphantha, C. and Uechiewcharnkit, K. (1987). A longitudinal study of Japanese encephalitis in suburban Bangkok, Thailand. *Southeast Asian J Trop Med Public Health.* 18(4): 558-566.

Gunakasem, P., Chantrasri, C., Simasathien, P., Chaiyanun, S., Jatanasen, S. and Pariyanonth, A. (1981). Surveillance of Japanese encephalitis cases in Thailand. *Southeast Asian J Trop Med Public Health.* 12(3): 333-337.

Hanna, J.N., Ritchie, S.A., Phillips, D.A., Lee, J.M., Hills, S.L., van den Hurk, A.F., Pyke, A.T., Johansen, C.A. and Mackenzie, J.S. (1999). Japanese encephalitis in north Queensland, Australia, 1998. *Med J Aust.* 170(11): 533-536.

Henderson, A. (1983). Encephalitis in Nepal: the visitation of the goddess of the forest. *J R Army Med Corps* 129(3): 156-162.

Horimoto, M., Sakai, T. and Goto, H. (1989). [Japanese encephalitis virus infection in cattle:a serological survey in Saitama and Kagoshima Prefectures]. *Kansenshogaku Zasshi.* 63(1): 10-14.

Hsu, L.C., Wu, Y.C., Lin, S.R., King, C.C., Ho, M.S., Lu, C.F., Hsu, H.M., Chen, K.T. and Horng, C.B. (1997). [Seroepidemiology of Japanese encephalitis viral infection among 3-6 years old children from mountainous and plains townships located in the northern, central, southern and eastern Taiwan]. *Zhonghua Min Guo Wei Sheng Wu Ji Mian Yi Xue Za Zhi* 30(3): 194-206.

Jamgaonkar, A.V., Yergolkar, P.N., Geevarghese, G., Joshi, G.D., Joshi, M.V. and Mishra, A.C. (2003). Serological evidence for Japanese encephalitis virus and West Nile virus infections in water frequenting and terrestrial wild birds in

Kolar District,Karnataka State, India. A retrospective study. *Acta Virol.* 47(3): 185-188.

Johansen, C.A., Nisbet, D.J., Foley, P.N., Van Den Hurk, A.F., Hall, R.A., Mackenzie, J.S. and Ritchie, S.A. (2004). Flavivirus isolations from mosquitoes collected from Saibai Island in the Torres Strait, Australia, during an incursion of Japanese encephalitis virus. *Med Vet Entomol.* 18(3): 281-287.

Johansen, C.A., Nisbet, D.J., Zborowski, P., van den Hurk, A.F., Ritchie, S.A. and Mackenzie, J.S. (2003). Flavivirus isolations from mosquitoes collected from western Cape York Peninsula, Australia, 1999-2000. *J Am Mosq Control Assoc.* 19(4): 392-396.

Kabilan, L., Rajendran, R., Arunachalam, N., Ramesh, S., Srinivasan, S., Samuel, P.P. and Dash, A.P. (2004). Japanese encephalitis in India: an overview. *Indian J Pediatr.* 71(7): 609-615.

Kabilan, L., Vrati, S., Ramesh, S., Srinivasan, S., Appaiahgari, M.B., Arunachalam, N., Thenmozhi, V., Kumaravel, S.M., Samuel, P.P. and Rajendran, R. (2004). Japanese encephalitis virus (JEV) is an important cause of encephalitis among children in Cuddalore district, Tamil Nadu, India. *J Clin Virol.* 31(2): 153-159.

Kari, K., Liu, W., Gautama, K., Mammen, M.P. Jr., Clemens, J.D., Nisalak, A., Subrata, K., Kim, H.K. and Xu, Z.Y. (2006). A hospital-based surveillance for Japanese encephalitis in Bali,Indonesia. *BMC Med.* 7; 4: 8.

Khanna, N., Agnihotri, M., Mathur, A., and Chaturvedi, U.C. (1991) Neutrophil chemotactic factor produced by Japanese encephalitis virus stimulated macrophages. *Clin Exp Immunol.* 86(2): 299-303.

Konishi, E., Pincus, S., Fonseca, B.A., Shope, R.E., Paoletti, E. and Mason, P.W. (1991). Comparison of protective immunity elicited by recombinant vaccinia viruses that synthesize E or NS1 of Japanese encephalitis virus. *Virology* 185(1): 401-410.

Konishi, E., Pincus, S., Paoletti, E., Laegreid, W.W., Shope, R.E. and Mason, P.W. (1992). A highly attenuated host range-restricted vaccinia virus strain, NYVAC, encoding the prM, E, and NS1 genes of Japanese encephalitis virus prevents JEV viremia in swine. *Virology.* 190(1): 454-458.

Konishi, E., Pincus, S., Paoletti, E., Shope, R.E., Burrage, T. and Mason, P.W. (1992). Mice immunized with a subviral particle containing the Japanese encephalitis virus prM/M and E proteins are protected from lethal JEV infection. *Virology.* 188(2): 714-720.

Konishi, E., Shoda, M. and Kondo, T. (2004). Prevalence of antibody to Japanese encephalitis virus nonstructural 1 protein among racehorses in Japan: indication of natural infection and need for continuous vaccination. *Vaccine.* 22(9-10): 1097-1103.

Konishi, E. (2005). [Clinical and epidemiological aspects of Japanese encephalitis]. *Nippon Rinsho* 63(12): 2138-2142.

Ku, C.C., King, C.C., Lin, C.Y., Hsu, H.C., Chen, L.Y., Yueh, Y.Y. and Chang, G.J. (1994). Homologous and heterologous neutralization antibody responses after immunization with Japanese encephalitis vaccine among Taiwan children. *J Med Virol.* 44(2): 122-131.

Li, Y.T., Zhu, Y.Y. and Jin, B.H. (2009). Epidemiological characteristics of Japanese encephalitis in Shanghai. Zhongguo Yi Miao He Mian Yi. 15(6): 507-10, 561.

Lim, S.I., Kweon, C.H., Tark, D.S., Kim, S.H. and Yang, D.K. (2007). Sero-survey on Aino, Akabane, Chuzan, bovine ephemeral fever and Japanese encephalitis virus of cattle and swine in Korea. *J Vet Sci.* 8(1): 45-49.

Lindenbach, B. D., and Rice, C.M. (2001). Flaviviridae: the viruses and their replication. In D. M. Knipe and P. M. Howley (ed.), *Fields virology*, 4th ed., vol. I: 991-1042.

Ma, S.P., Yoshida, Y., Makino, Y., Tadano, M., Ono, T. and Ogawa, M. (2003). Short report: a major genotype of Japanese encephalitis virus currently circulating in Japan. *Am J Trop Med Hyg.* 69(2): 151-154.

Mackenzie, J.S. (2005). Emerging zoonotic encephalitis viruses: lessons from Southeast Asia and Oceania. *J Neurovirol.* 11(5): 434-440.

Mackenzie, J.S., Johansen, C.A., Ritchie, S.A., van den Hurk, A.F. and Hall, R.A. (2002). Japanese encephalitis as an emerging virus: the emergence and spread of Japanese encephalitis virus in Australasia. *Curr Top Microbiol Immunol.* 267: 49-73.

Mani, T.R., Rao, C.V., Rajendran, R., Devaputra, M., Prasanna, Y., Hanumaiah., Gajanana, A. and Reuben, R. (1991). Surveillance for Japanese encephalitis in villages near Madurai, Tamil Nadu, India. *Trans R Soc Trop Med Hyg* 85(2): 287-291.

Mathur, A., Khanna, N. and Chaturvedi, U.C. (1992). Breakdown of blood-brain barrier by virus-induced cytokine during Japanese encephalitis virus infection. *Int J Exp Pathol.* 73(5): 603-611.

McCallum, J.D. (1991). Japanese encephalitis in southeastern Nepal: clinical aspects in the 1986 epidemic. *J R Army Med Corps.* 137(1): 8-13.

Misra, U.K. and Kalita, J. (2010). Overview: Japanese encephalitis. *Prog Neurobiol.* 91(2): 108-120.

Natividad, F.F., Daroy, M.L., Alonzo, M.T., Matias, R.R., Suarez, L.A. and Inoue, S. (2006). Use of IgM-capture ELISA for confirmation of Japanese encephalitis infections in the Philippines. *Southeast Asian J Trop Med Public Health.* 37(Suppl 3): 136-139.

Nemeth, NM., Bosco-Lauth, AM., Sciulli, RH., Gose, RB., Nagata, MT. and Bowen RA. (2010). Serosurveillance for Japanese encephalitis and West Nile viruses in resident birds in Hawai'i. *J Wildl Dis.* 46(2): 659-664.

Neogi, D.K., Bhattacharya, N., Chakrabarti, T. and Mukherjee, K.K. (1998). Detection of HIV seropositivity during an outbreak of Japanese encephalitis in Manipur. *J Commun Dis.* 30(2): 113-116.

Nerome, R., Tajima, S., Takasaki, T., Yoshida, T., Kotaki, A., Lim, C.K., Ito, M., Sugiyama, A., Yamauchi, A., Yano, T., Kameyama, T., Morishita, I., Kuwayama, M., Ogawa, T., Sahara, K., Ikegaya, A., Kanda, M., Hosoya, Y., Itokazu, K., Onishi, H., Chiya, S., Yoshida, Y., Tabei, Y.,Katsuki, K., Tabata, K., Harada, S. and Kurane, I. (2007). Molecular epidemiological analyses of Japanese encephalitis virus isolates from swine in Japan from 2002 to 2004. *J Gen Virol.* 88(Pt 10): 2762-2768.

Nett, R.J., Campbell, G.L. and Reisen, W.K. (2009). Potential for the emergence of Japanese encephalitis virus in California. *Vector Borne Zoonotic Dis.* 9(5): 511-517.

Nga, P.T., del Carmen Parquet, M., Cuong, V.D., Ma, S.P., Hasebe, F., Inoue, S., Makino, Y., Takagi, M., Nam, V.S. and Morita, K. (2004). Shift in Japanese encephalitis virus (JEV) genotype circulating in northern Vietnam: implications for frequent introductions of JEV from Southeast Asia to East Asia. *J Gen Virol.* 85(Pt 6): 1625-1631.

Nidaira, M., Taira, K., Itokazu, K., Kudaka, J., Nakamura, M., Ohno, A. and Takasaki, T. (2007). Survey of the antibody against japanese encephalitis virus in Ryukyu wild boars (Sus scrofa riukiuanus) in Okinawa, Japan. *Jpn J Infect Dis.* 60(5): 309-311.

Nitatpattana, N., Dubot-Pérès, A., Gouilh, M.A., Souris, M., Barbazan, P., Yoksan, S., deLamballerie, X. and Gonzalez, J.P. (2008). Change in Japanese encephalitis virus distribution, Thailand. *Emerg Infect Dis* (11): 1762-1765.

Olsen, S.J., Supawat, K., Campbell, A.P., Anantapreecha, S., Liamsuwan, S., Tunlayadechanont, S., Visudtibhan, A., Lupthikulthum, S., Dhiravibulya, K., Viriyavejakul, A., Vasiknanonte, P., Rajborirug, K., Watanaveeradej, V., Nabangchang, C., Laven, J., Kosoy, O., Panella, A., Ellis, C., Henchaichon, S., Khetsuriani, N., Powers, A.M., Dowell, S.F. and Fischer, M. (2010). Japanese encephalitis virus remains an important cause of encephalitis in Thailand. *Int J Infect Dis.* 14(10): e888-892.

Pandey, B., Yamamoto, A., Morita, K., Kurosawa, Y., Rai, S., Adhikari, S., Kandel, P. and Kurane, I. (2003). Serodiagnosis of Japanese encephalitis among Nepalese patients by the particle agglutination assay. *Epidemiol Infect.* 131(2): 881-885.

Pant, G.R., Lunt, R.A., Rootes, C.L. and Daniels, P.W. (2006). Serological evidence for Japanese encephalitis and West Nile viruses in domestic animals of Nepal. *Comp Immunol Microbiol Infect Di.s* 29(2-3): 166-175.

Philip Samuel, P., Arunachalam, N., Hiriyan, J. and Tyagi, B.K. (2008). Host feeding pattern of Japanese encephalitis virus vector mosquitoes (Diptera: Culicidae) from Kuttanadu, Kerala, India. *J Med Entomol.* 45(5): 927-932.

Poneprasert, B. (1989). Japanese encephalitis in children in northern Thailand. *Southeast Asian J Trop Med Public Health.* 20(4): 599-603.

Rajendran, R., Thenmozhi, V., Tewari, S.C., Balasubramanian, A., Ayanar, K., Manavalan, R., Gajanana, A., Kabilan, L., Thakare, J.P. and Satyanarayana, K. (2003). Longitudinal studies in South Indian villages on Japanese encephalitis virus infection in mosquitoes and seroconversion in goats. *Trop Med Int Health.* 8(2): 174-181.

Ritchie, S.A., van den Hurk, A.F., Zborowski, P., Kerlin, T.J., Banks, D., Walker, J.A., Lee, J.M., Montgomery, B.L., Smith, G.A., Pyke, A.T. and Smith, I.L. (2007). Operational trials of remote mosquito trap systems for Japanese encephalitis virus surveillance in the Torres Strait, Australia. *Vector Borne Zoonotic Dis* 7(4): 497-506.

Saito, M., Nakata, K., Nishijima, T., Yamashita, K., Saito, A. and Ogura, G. (2009). Proposal for Japanese encephalitis surveillance using captured invasive mongooses under an eradication project on Okinawa Island, Japan. *Vector Borne Zoonotic Dis.* 9(3): 259-266.

Saito, M., Osa, Y. and Asakawa, M. (2009). Antibodies to flaviviruses in wild ducks captured in Hokkaido, Japan: risk assessment of invasive flaviviruses. *Vector Borne Zoonotic Dis.* 9(3): 253-258.

Saxena, S.K. (2008). Japanese encephalitis: perspectives and new developments. *Future Neurol.* 3(5): 515-521.

Saxena, S.K., Mathur, A. and Srivastava, R.C. (2001). Induction of nitric oxide synthase during Japanese encephalitis virus infection: evidence of protective role. *Arch Biochem Biophys.* 391(1): 1-7.

Saxena, S.K., Mathur, A., and Srivastavam R.C. (2003). Inhibition of Japanese encephalitis virus infection by diethyldithiocarbamate is independent of its antioxidant potential. *Antivir Chem Chemother.* 14(2): 91-98.

Saxena, S.K., Mishra, N., Saxena, R., Singh, M., and Mathur, A. (2009). Trend of Japanese encephalitis in North India: evidence from thirty-eight acute encephalitis cases and appraisal of niceties. *J Infect Dev Ctries.* 3(7): 517-530.

Saxena, S.K., Singh, A., and Mathur, A. (2000). Antiviral effect of nitric oxide during Japanese encephalitis virus infection. *Int J Exp Pathol.* 81(2): 165-172.

Saxena, S.K., Singh, M., Pathak, A.K., and Mathur, A. (2006). Reply to 'Encephalitis outbreak finds Indian officials unprepared'. *Nat Med.* 12(3): 269-270.

Schuh, A.J., Li, L., Tesh, R.B., Innis, B.L. and Barrett, A.D. (2010). Genetic characterization of early isolates of Japanese encephalitis virus: genotype II has been circulating since at least 1951. *J Gen Virol.* 91(Pt 1): 95-102.

See, E., Tan, H.C., Wang, D., Ooi, E.E. and Lee, M.A. (2002). Presence of hemagglutination inhibition and neutralization antibodies to Japanese encephalitis virus in wild pigs on an offshore island in Singapore. *Acta Trop.* 81(3): 233-236.

Shimojima, M., Nagao, Y., Shimoda, H., Tamaru, S., Yamanaka, T., Matsumura, T., Kondo, T. and Maeda, K. (2011).Full Genome Sequence and Virulence Analyses of the Recent Equine Isolate of Japanese Encephalitis Virus. *J Vet Med Sci.* Jan 11, 2011 [Epub ahead of print]

Sinniah, M. (1989). A review of Japanese-B virus encephalitis in Malaysia. *Southeast Asian J Trop Med Public Health.* 20(4): 581-585.

Solomon, T. and Winter, P.M. (2004). Neurovirulence and host factors in flavivirus encephalitis--evidence from clinical epidemiology. *Arch Virol Suppl.* (18): 161-670.

Solomon, T., Dung, N.M., Kneen, R., Thao le, T.T., Gainsborough, M., Nisalak, A., Day, N.P.,Kirkham, F.J., Vaughn, D.W., Smith, S. and White, N.J. (2002). Seizures and raised intracranial pressure in Vietnamese patients with Japanese encephalitis. *Brain.* 125(Pt 5): 1084-1093.

Solomon, T., Ni, H., Beasley, D.W., Ekkelenkamp, M., Cardosa, M.J. and Barrett, A.D. (2003). Origin and evolution of Japanese encephalitis virus in southeast Asia. *J Virol.* 77(5): 3091-3098.

Spicer, P.E., Phillips, D., Pike, A., Johansen, C., Melrose, W. and Hall, R.A. (1999). Antibodies to Japanese encephalitis virus in human sera collected from Irian Jaya. Follow-up of a previously reported case of Japanese encephalitis in that region. *Trans R Soc Trop Med Hyg.* 93(5): 511-514.

Srey, V.H., Sadones, H., Ong, S., Mam, M., Yim, C., Sor, S., Grosjean, P., Reynes, J.M.,Grosjean, P. and Reynes, J.M. (2002). Etiology of encephalitis syndrome among hospitalized children and adults in Takeo, Cambodia, 1999-2000. *Am J Trop Med Hyg* 66(2): 200-207.

Srivastava, S., Khanna, N., Saxena, S.K., Singh, A., Mathur, A., and Dhole, T.N. (1999). Degradation of Japanese encephalitis virus by neutrophils. *Int J Exp Pathol.* 80(1): 17-24.

Sugiura, T. and Shimada, K. (1999). Seroepizootiological survey of Japanese encephalitis virus and Getah virus in regional horse race tracks from 1991 to 1997 in Japan. *J Vet Med Sci.* 61(8): 877-881.

Takahashi, H., Pool, V., Tsai, T.F. and Chen, R.T. (2000). Adverse events after Japanese encephalitis vaccination: review of post-marketing surveillance data from Japan and the United States. The VAERS Working Group. *Vaccine.* 18(26):2963-2969.

Tandon, A., Singh, A., Atrishi, E., Saxena, S.K., and Mathur, A. (2002). Alteration in plasma glucose levels in Japanese encephalitis patients. *Int J Exp Pathol.* 83(1): 39-46.

Tewari, S.C., Thenmozhi, V., Arunachalam, N., Philip Samuel, P. and Tyagi, B.K. (2008). Desiccated vector mosquitoes used for the surveillance of Japanese encephalitis virus activity in endemic southern India. *Trop Med Int Health.* 13(2): 286-290.

Thenmozhi, V., Rajendran, R., Ayanar, K., Manavalan, R. and Tyagi, B.K. (2006). Long-term study of Japanese encephalitis virus infection in Anopheles subpictus in Cuddalore district, Tamil Nadu, South India. *Trop Med Int Health.* 11(3): 288-293.

Thisyakorn, U. and Nimmannitya, S. (1985). Japanese encephalitis in Thai children, Bangkok, Thailand. *Southeast Asian J Trop Med Public Health.* 16(1): 93-97.

Ting, S.H., Tan, H.C., Wong, W.K., Ng, M.L., Chan, S.H. and Ooi, E.E. (2004). Seroepidemiology of neutralizing antibodies to Japanese encephalitis virus in Singapore: continued transmission despite abolishment of pig farming? *Acta Trop.* 92(3): 187-191.

Trosper, J.H., Ksiazek, T.G. and Cross, J.H. (1980). Isolation of Japanese encephalitis virus from the Republic of the Philippines. *Trans R Soc Trop Med Hyg.* 74(3): 292-295.

Unni, S.K., Růžek, D., Chhatbar, C., Mishra, R., Johri, M.K. and Singh, S.K. (2011). Japanese encephalitis virus: from genome to infectome. *Microbes Infect.* 13(4): 312-321.

van den Hurk, A.F, Ritchie, S.A, Johansen, C.A, Mackenzie, J.S. and Smith, G.A. (2008). Domestic pigs and Japanese encephalitis virus infection, Australia. *Emerg Infect Dis.* 14(11): 1736-1738.

van den Hurk, A.F., Johansen, C.A., Zborowski, P., Paru, R., Foley, P.N., Beebe, N.W., Mackenzie, J.S. and Ritchie, S.A. (2003). Mosquito host-feeding patterns and implications for Japanese encephalitis virus transmission in northern Australia and Papua New Guinea. *Med Vet Entomol.* 17(4): 403-411.

van den Hurk, A.F., Johansen, C.A., Zborowski, P., Phillips, D.A., Pyke, A.T., Mackenzie, J.S. and Ritchie, S.A .(2001). Flaviviruses isolated from mosquitoes collected during the first recorded outbreak of Japanese encephalitis virus on Cape York Peninsula, Australia. *Am J Trop Med Hyg.* 64(3-4):125-130.

van den Hurk, A.F., Montgomery, B.L., Northill, J.A., Smith, I.L., Zborowski, P., Ritchie, S.A., Mackenzie, J.S. and Smith, G.A. (2006). Short report: the first isolation of Japanese encephalitis virus from mosquitoes collected from mainland Australia. *Am J Trop Med Hyg.* 75(1): 21-25.

van den Hurk, A.F., Nisbet, D.J., Foley, P.N., Ritchie, S.A., Mackenzie, J.S.and Beebe, N.W.(2002). Isolation of arboviruses from mosquitoes (Diptera: Culicidae) collected from the Gulf Plains region of northwest Queensland, Australia. *J Med Entomol.* 39(5):786-792.

van den Hurk, A.F., Nisbet, D.J., Hall, R.A., Kay, B.H., MacKenzie, J.S. and Ritchie, S.A. (2003). Vector competence of Australian mosquitoes (Diptera: Culicidae) for Japanese encephalitis virus. *J Med Entomol.* 40(1): 82-90.

van den Hurk, A.F., Nisbet, D.J., Johansen, C.A., Foley, P.N., Ritchie, S.A. and Mackenzie, J.S. (2001). Japanese encephalitis on Badu Island, Australia: the first isolation of Japanese encephalitis virus from Culex gelidus in the Australasian region and the role of mosquito host-feeding patterns in virus transmission cycles. *Trans R Soc Trop Med Hyg.* 95(6): 595-600.

van den Hurk, A.F., Ritchie, S.A. and Mackenzie, J.S. (2009). Ecology and geographical expansion of Japanese encephalitis virus. *Annu Rev Entomol.* 54: 17-35.

van den Hurk, A.F., Ritchie, S.A., Johansen, C.A., Mackenzie, J.S. and Smith, G.A. (2008). Domestic pigs and Japanese encephalitis virus infection, Australia. *Emerg Infect Dis.* 14(11): 1736-1738.

Victor, T.J., Malathi, M., Ravi, V., Palani, G. and Appavoo, N.C. (2000). First outbreak of Japanese encephalitis in two villages of Dharmapuri district in Tamil Nadu. *Indian J Med Res.* 112: 193-197.

Wang, H.Y., Takasaki, T., Fu, S.H., Sun, X.H., Zhang, H.L., Wang, Z.X., Hao, Z.Y., Zhang, J.K., Tang, Q., Kotaki, A., Tajima, S., Liang, X.F., Yang, W.Z., Kurane, I. and Liang, G.D. (2007). Molecular epidemiological analysis of Japanese encephalitis virus in China. *J Gen Virol.* 88(Pt 3): 885-894.

Weaver, S.C. and Reisen, W.K. (2010). Present and future arboviral threats. *Antiviral Res.* 85(2): 328-345.

Whitley, R.J. and Gnann, J.W. (2002). Viral encephalitis: familiar infections and emerging pathogens. *Lancet.* 359(9305): 507-513. Review.

Widjaja, S., Soekotjo, W., Hartati, S., Jennings, G.B. and Corwin, A.L. (1995). Prevalence of hemagglutination-inhibition and neutralizing antibodies to arboviruses in horses of java. *Southeast Asian J Trop Med Public Health.* 26(1): 109-113.

Wong, S.C., Ooi, M.H., Abdullah, A.R., Wong, S.Y., Krishnan, S., Tio, P.H., Pek, P.C., Lai, B.F.,Mohan, A., Muhi, J., Kiyu, A., Arif, M.T. and Cardosa, M.J. (2008). A decade of Japanese encephalitis surveillance in Sarawak, Malaysia: 1997-2006. *Trop Med Int Health.* 13(1): 52-55.

Yamanaka, A., Mulyatno, K.C., Susilowati, H., Hendrianto, E., Utsumi, T., Amin, M., Lusida, M.I., Soegijanto, S. and Konishi, E. (2010). Prevalence of antibodies to Japanese encephalitis virus among pigs in Bali and East Java, Indonesia, 2008. *Jpn J Infect Dis.* 63(1): 58-60.

Yang, D.K., Kim, B.H., Kweon, C.H., Nah, J.J., Kim, H.J., Lee, K.W., Yang, Y.J. and Mun, K.W. (2008). Serosurveillance for Japanese encephalitis, Akabane, and Aino viruses for Thoroughbred horses in Korea. *J Vet Sci.* 9(4): 381-385.

Yang, D.K., Kweon, C.H., Kim, B.H., Hwang, I.J., Kang, M.I., So, B.J. and Cho, K.O. (2007). The seroprevalence of Japanese encephalitis virus in goats raised in Korea. *J Vet Sci.* 8(2): 197-199.

Yen, NT., Duffy, MR., Hong, NM., Hien, NT., Fischer, M. and Hills, SL. (2010). Surveillance for Japanese encephalitis in Vietnam, 1998-2007. *Am J Trop Med Hyg.* 83(4): 816-819.

Zhang, D.L., Ma, L.B., Fu, S.H., Wang, L.H., Wang, H.Y., Zhang, M., Wei, Z.G., Li, G.G., Cui, X.F., Lei, H.G., Sun, X.H., Lv, X.J., Li, M.H. and Liang, G.D. (2008). [Clinical characteristics and laboratory assay of adult Japanese encephalitis patients in an outbreak in Yuncheng, Shanxi Province, 2006]. *Zhonghua Shi Yan He Lin Chuang Bing Du Xue Za Zhi.* 22(2): 95-97.

Zhang, J.S., Zhao, Q.M., Zhang, P.H., Jia, N. and Cao, W.C. (2009). Genomic sequence of a Japanese encephalitis virus isolate from southern China. *Arch Virol.* 154(7): 1177-1180.

Zimmerman, M.D., Scott, R.M., Vaughn, D.W., Rajbhandari, S., Nisalak, A. and Shrestha, M.P. (1997). Short report: an outbreak of Japanese encephalitis in Kathmandu, Nepal. *Am J Trop Med Hyg.* 57(3): 283-284.

16

Immunobiology of Japanese Encephalitis Virus

Maximilian Larena and Mario Lobigs
Department of Emerging Pathogens and Vaccines, John Curtin School of Medical Research, The Australian National University, Canberra, ACT
Australia

1. Introduction

Japanese encephalitis (JE) is an acute central nervous system inflammatory disease cause by infection with Japanese encephalitis virus (JEV), a small, enveloped, plus-strand RNA virus belonging to the family *Flaviviridae*. It is the leading cause of viral encephalitis in South-East Asia, India and China, where 3 billion people are at risk of contracting the disease (Erlanger *et al.*, 2009). Annually, about 35,000 cases of JE are reported, resulting in about 10,000 deaths and a high incidence of neuropsychiatric deficits among survivors. Treatment of JE patients is supportive and in the absence of availability of antiviral compounds the mainstay of protection against JE is vaccination (Halstead & Thomas, 2011). In the past decades there has been an expansion of the geographic distribution of the virus in Asia and the Asia-Pacific region (van den Hurk *et al.*, 2009) and there is an urgent requirement for improved human and veterinary JE vaccines. An understanding of the immunological responses that lead to recovery from infection with JEV and account for vaccine-mediated protection is important in the design of rational approaches to new treatments and vaccines against the disease, and will be the focus of this review.

1.1 Clinical manifestations

Infection with JEV starts with a bite of an infected *Culex* mosquito, although the possibility of transplacental transmission has been demonstrated in mice, swine and humans (Chaturvedi *et al.*, 1980; Mathur *et al.*, 1981; Morimoto *et al.*, 1972). The infection is largely subclinical with only 1:50 to 1:10,000 human infections resulting in symptomatic disease (Tsai, 2000). The clinical features of infection range from a non-specific febrile illness, aseptic meningitis, poliomyelitis-like syndrome, to a severe meningoencephalomyelitis (Solomon, 2003; Solomon *et al.*, 2000; Solomon *et al.*, 1998). The incubation period is from 5 to 15 days before onset of prodromal symptoms, which include fever, generalized weakness, coryza, diarrhoea, and rigors. Afterwards, patients experience headache, vomiting, decreased sensorium, and convulsion. Then a classic presentation ensues, including dull, flat, mask-like facies with wide unblinking eyes, tremor, generalized hypertonia and cogwheel rigidity. Other signs and symptoms found in a subset of patients include generalized tonic-clonic seizures, focal seizures, upper motor neuron facial nerve palsy, extrapyramidal manifestations, asymmetric paralysis, and mental illness. Occasional extrapyramidal symptoms include non-intention tremors, cogwheel rigidity, head nodding and pill rolling movements, opsoclonus, myoclonus, choreoathetosis, and bizarre facial grimacing and lip smacking (Solomon *et al.*,

2000). The case fatality ratio can be as high as 50-60 % (Tsai, 2000), and one half of the survivors have long-term neurologic or psychiatric sequelae (Solomon, 2003).

1.2 Animal models

JE is also a veterinary disease with occasional fatal outcome in horses, and abortions and abnormal births in pigs (Halstead & Jacobson, 2003). While pigs can act as amplifier host in the transmission cycle of the virus, JEV infection of horses, like that of humans, does not generate sufficient viremia for virus transmission. The clinical course of JE in horses resembles that found in humans (Gould *et al.*, 1964; Lam *et al.*, 2005; Miyake, 1964; Yamanaka *et al.*, 2006). Mice have been most extensively used as a model for studies on the pathogenesis of JEV (Kimura *et al.*, 2010) and show significant similarity to natural human infection. Notably, extraneural infection of adult mice frequently does not result in detectable viremia or virus burden in extraneural tissues, although some animals will develop CNS infection with mostly fatal outcome (Larena *et al.*, 2011). Age, genetic background and route of inoculation are risk factors for severe encephalitis (Grossberg & Scherer, 1966; Larena *et al.*, 2011). The pathologic changes seen in mouse brain infected with JEV are similar to those observed in humans, with perivascular cuffs, cellular infiltrates, and mild vascular damage (German *et al.*, 2006). Interestingly, there is a lack of a dose response in mortality in mice following virus challenge by an extraneural route (Larena *et al.*, 2011). This is thought to reflect, at least in part, induction of more vigorous innate immune responses critical in early control of virus dissemination with increasing amount of virus used for infection (Monath *et al.*, 2003).

To investigate the immunological correlates for recovery and protection from JEV infection, the animal model should resemble the natural infection route and virus dose, and the animals should have a mature immune system and intact blood-brain-barrier. We have shown that in groups of 8- to 12-week-old mice after footpad challenge with 10^3 PFU of JEV (prototype strain Nakayama) ~50% of animals present with clinical signs of infection starting at day 10 post-infection (pi), which included progressive generalized paresis, piloerection and rigidity. Severe neurological impairment demonstrated by ataxia, postural imbalance, and generalized tonic-clonic seizures is evident later in the course of infection, invariably leading to fatality within 24 - 36 h after disease onset (Larena *et al.*, 2011). Histopathological examination at day 10 pi with JEV reveals hallmarks of acute viral encephalitis, including microglial nodules surrounding degenerating neurons, meningeal inflammation, and widespread perivascular leukocytic infiltration. Immunohistochemical staining reveals JEV infected neurons in multiple loci, predominantly localized in the following areas: cerebral cortex, hippocampus, thalamus, brainstem and cerebellum. The initial local site of JEV replication following footpad infection probably involves dendritic cells, given the evidence that they support JEV replication (Aleyas *et al.*, 2009; Cao *et al.*, 2011; Li *et al.*, 2010). Local spread then ensues with peak viremia and splenic viral load, detectable only by real time RT-PCR, peaking at day 2 and day 4, respectively (Larena *et al.*, 2011). Subsequently, virus enters the brain. Putative mechanisms for virus invasion into the CNS include i) hematogenous spread, ii) entry through olfactory neurons, iii) retrograde axonal transport through peripheral nerves, iv) a "Trojan horse" mechanism through infected monocytes and v) transcytosis through the endothelial cells of the blood-brain-barrier. JEV infection of neurons is accompanied by a local inflammatory reaction. This induces the release of chemokines stimulating CCR5-dependent migration of leukocytes into the brain parenchyma (Larena and Lobigs, unpublished). Virus clearance from the CNS is complicated by the irreplaceable nature of neurons and the fact that neuronal damage can be caused directly by virus infection or by infiltrating leukocytes in response to the infection (Griffin, 2011).

2. Innate immunity

2.1 Sensing of the pathogen

Host cells detect distinct conserved molecular signatures (pathogen associated molecular patterns: PAMPs) of invading viruses through germ-line encoded transmembrane or cytosolic pathogen recognition receptors (PRRs) (Bowie & Unterholzner, 2008). This initial sensing and recognition is of paramount importance in viral immunobiology, where activating intracellular signalling cascades ultimately lead to the induction of antiviral, inflammatory and adaptive immune responses. Transmembrane PRRs include C-type lectin receptors (CLRs) and the widely studied toll-like receptors (TLRs), both of which are up-regulated after JEV infection (Gupta & Rao, 2011). CLRs contain carbohydrate recognition domains interacting with mannose, fucose, and glucan carbohydrate structures of pathogens (Geijtenbeek & Gringhuis, 2009). A particular CLR, C-type lectin domain family 5 (CLEC5A), is highly expressed after JEV infection and is associated with a proinflammatory profile (Gupta *et al.*, 2010). Considering the role of CLEC5A in the immunopathology of dengue hemorrhagic fever (Chen et al., 2008), it can be postulated also to have a key role in the pathologic process of JE neuroinflammation.

TLRs are composed of a leucine-rich repeat-containing ectodomain, a transmembrane domain and an intracellular Toll–interleukin 1 receptor (TIR) domain (Kawai & Akira, 2010). The ectodomain mediates recognition of PAMPs, while the intracellular TIR domain mediates downstream signal transduction. TLR signaling, except that via TLR3, requires the TIR-domain adaptor molecule, MyD88, and therefore can be prevented by MyD88 knock-out (Kawai & Akira, 2010). In the absence of MyD88, bone marrow-derived macrophages and dendritic cells infected with JEV have reduced production of inflammatory cytokines interleukin (IL)-6, IL-10, IL-12, and tumour necrosis factor (TNF)-α (Aleyas *et al.*, 2009). This supports a role of TLR signalling through MyD88 in shaping the immune responses to JEV. However, this is not reflected in a markedly altered disease outcome, given that MyD88-/- mice only show a partial impairment in interferon (IFN)-α production and similar susceptibility to JEV in comparison to wild-type mice (Kato *et al.*, 2006), suggesting a redundancy in pathways for recognition of JEV infection.

Cytosolic PRRs are essential for detecting pathogens invading the cytosol. They are classified into nucleotide binding oligomerization domain (NOD)-like and retinoic acid-inducible gene (RIG)-1-like receptors (Wilkins & Gale, 2010). NOD-like receptors, NOD2 and NLRP3, recognize ssRNA and dsRNA, respectively, and have significant antiviral activity through IFN signalling. Both proteins are expected to recognize flaviviral genomic RNA, although their role in JEV infection remains to be investigated. RIG-1-like receptors, also known as RNA helicases, have a conserved DExD/H box helicase domain and a C-terminal regulatory domain among the three recently identified members, RIG-1, melanoma differentiation-associated antigen 5 (MDA-5) and laboratory of genetics and physiology 2 (LGP2) (Wilkins & Gale, 2010). The C-terminal regulatory domain serves as the recognition site for sensing ssRNA and dsRNA. Kato et al (2006) have shown that RIG-1 receptor signaling, but not that via MDA-5, is critical for the antiviral response against JEV: RIG-1-/-, but not MDA-5-/- mice, display impaired type 1 IFN production and increased susceptibility to JEV infection. LGP2 was initially reported as a dominant negative regulator of RIG-1 and MDA-5 signalling (Komuro & Horvath, 2006; Murali *et al.*, 2008); however, Satoh et al (2010) have demonstrated that bone marrow-derived dendritic cells from LGP2-/- mice infected with JEV have an impaired production of IFN-β, indicating that LGP2 functions upstream of RIG-1 and MDA-5 to potentiate viral RNA-induced signalling as a positive regulator.

2.2 Type 1 interferon induction and signalling

Interferons (IFNs) are a group of cytokines first discovered based on their antiviral activity against influenza (Borden *et al.*, 2007). Three families of IFNs, type I, type II and the recently identified type III can be distinguished. Type I IFNs include multiple IFN-α subsets, a single IFN-β, IFN-ω, and the recently discovered IFN-ε (Hardy *et al.*, 2004). All members bind to the same cell surface receptor, and are located in a single gene cluster both in humans and in mice. In addition to their antiviral activity, type I IFNs are key to efficient establishment of the adaptive immune responses (Borden *et al.*, 2007). Type III IFNs (IFN-λ1, -λ2 and -λ3) are new members of the IFN superfamily first discovered in 2003 and shown to be related to type I IFN (Ank *et al.*, 2006). However, they differ by signalling through a receptor complex that is different from that used by type I IFNs. Numerous RNA and DNA viruses induce and are sensitive to IFN-λs, although it remains unclear if type III IFNs are important in the host response against JEV infection. Type II IFN consists of a single cytokine, IFN-γ, and its function in JEV infection is described in Section 2.3.

IFN production after JEV infection was initially documented in mice (Rokutanda, 1969) and later in humans (Burke & Morill, 1987). Early in vitro and in vivo animal studies depicting its significance as an antiviral compound against JEV employed the use of IFN inducers (Ghosh *et al.*, 1990; Taylor *et al.*, 1980) and recombinant IFN-α (Crance et al., 2003). Furthermore, mice deficient in IFN-α receptor infected with JEV show sustained high viremia and fulminant disease (Lee *et al.*, 2004; Lee & Lobigs, 2002; Lobigs *et al.*, 2009), demonstrating that type I IFN is a key tropism determinant of JEV.

IFN gene expression is induced by the binding of PRR-activated transcription factors to their promoters (Borden *et al.*, 2007). They include IFN regulatory factor (IRF) proteins and NF-κB (Honda *et al.*, 2006; Tenoever *et al.*, 2007). In the case of JEV infection, RIG-1-dependent IRF-3 and phosphatidylinositol-3 kinase-dependent NF-κB activation is essential for IFN production (Chang *et al.*, 2006). NF-κB-dependent and NF-κB-independent mechanisms of IFN induction after JEV infection have been suggested by Abraham et al (2010). Binding of IFN to its cognate receptor at the cell surface triggers a signalling cascade, the Janus kinase - signal transducer and activation of transcription (Jak-Stat) pathway, ultimately triggering IFN-stimulated response element and expression of IFN-stimulated genes (ISGs). ISGs serve as mediators of IFN action directed towards initiation of antiviral and immunoregulatory functions (Borden *et al.*, 2007). Antiviral proteins associated with flaviviral infections include double-stranded RNA-activated protein kinase (PKR), the 2′,5′-oligoadenylate synthetases (2′-5′-OAS), ISG15, ISG20, viperin and IFN-induced transmembrane proteins (Brass *et al.*, 2009; Hsiao *et al.*, ; Jiang *et al.*, 2010; Kajaste-Rudnitski *et al.*, 2006; Samuel *et al.*, 2006). Of these, 2′-5′-OAS proteins are the most widely studied and acts through activation of RNase L, a potent endoribonuclease that cleaves viral RNA (Silverman, 2007). The critical role of 2′-5′-OAS in the control of West Nile virus (WNV) infection was first reported in mice (Mashimo *et al.*, 2002; Perelygin *et al.*, 2002) and recently in horses and humans, where distinct OAS1a gene polymorphisms were identified as a risk factor (Lim *et al.*, 2009; Rios *et al.*, 2010). Given the association of OAS with the flavivirus-resistance phenomenon in mice

(Brinton & Perelygin, 2003), this ISG most likely also plays an important role in recovery from JEV infection. ISG-15 is an additional ISG recently documented to be involved in the control of JEV infection (Hsiao *et al.*, 2010).

Considering its antiviral action, the therapeutic potential of recombinant IFN in human cases of JE has been investigated. While an initial study suggested a benefit (Harinasuta *et al.*, 1985), a subsequent randomised double-blind placebo-controlled clinical trial did not (Solomon *et al.*, 2003). The failure to observe a benefit in the larger scale study posed the question of clinical relevance of IFN treatment. It remains to be seen, whether the outcome might differ if higher doses were given, given earlier in the course of infection, or given in combination with other drugs. It is likely that the failure of IFN therapy after an established JEV infection can be attributed to the IFN-antagonistic mechanisms of the virus itself. JEV counteracts the effect of IFN by blocking tyrosine kinase 2 (Tyk2) and Stat activation (Lin *et al.*, 2004). This is mediated by the viral NS5 protein through the activation of protein tyrosine phosphatases (Lin *et al.*, 2006). Additionally, JEV NS4A protein is reported to block IFN action through inhibiting phosphorylation of Stat 1 and Stat 2 (Lin *et al.*, 2008a). Moreover, aside from IFN antagonism at the level of Jak-Stat signalling, JEV is also able to inhibit a downstream antiviral molecule, viperin, by promoting its degradation via a proteasome-dependent mechanism (Chan *et al.*, 2008).

2.3 Cellular factors, chemokines and cytokines

Neutrophil leucocytosis is a unique feature in human cases of JE (Chaturvedi *et al.*, 1979; Singh *et al.*, 2000). A neutrophil chemotactic factor derived from JEV-stimulated macrophages has been reported to induce neutrophilia (Khanna *et al.*, 1991). Additionally, an increased level of the neutrophil chemoattractant, IL-8, found in CSF and serum of JEV infected individuals is significantly associated with neutrophilia and an elevated level of IL-8 in CSF and plasma is linked with adverse clinical outcome (Singh *et al.*, 2000; Winter *et al.*, 2004). This contrasts with a potentially beneficial role of neutrophils in the control of JEV infection by a mechanism involving the degradation of virus via triggering a respiratory burst and the generation of toxic radicals (Srivastava *et al.*, 1999).

Cells of the monocytic lineage and the release of soluble factors thereof have been implicated in JEV pathogenesis. Macrophages predominate the inflammatory cells infiltrating the brain parenchyma of individuals with Japanese encephalitis (Johnson *et al.*, 1985). They are permissive for JEV replication, and provide a putative mechanism for JEV entry into the CNS (Aleyas *et al.*, 2009; Hasegawa *et al.*, 1990; Mathur *et al.*, 1988; Yang *et al.*, 2004). Cathepsin L-mediated processing of the capsid protein appears to play a role in JEV replication in macrophages, since mutant virus resistant to cleavage by the protease has impaired growth in macrophage but not fibroblast or mosquito cell lines (Mori *et al.*, 2007). Microglia are a brain-resident macrophage cell population, which can be infected with JEV for prolonged periods without morphological alteration, suggesting that microglia might serve as a reservoir for viral persistence in the CNS (Thongtan *et al.*, 2010). Local immune responses initiated by microglial cells may provide protection against JEV infection of the CNS. However, microglial activation resulting in elevated levels of proinflammatory cytokines (IL-6, TNF-α, IL-1β) and chemokines (IL-8, RANTES, MCP1) in the CSF and plasma may give rise to irreversible neuronal damage and correlates with an increased mortality rate (Chen *et al.*, 2004; Chen *et al.*, 2010; Ghoshal *et al.*, 2007; Ravi *et al.*, 1997; Saxena *et al.*, 2008; Winter *et al.*, 2004).

Astroyctes were originally classified as a subclass of glial cells with pleiotropic functions for maintainance of CNS homeostasis, and only recently were they shown to be immunocompetent cells (Dong & Benveniste, 2001). JEV infected astrocytes are an important source of chemokines (CCL5 and CXCL10) for migration of leukocytes into the CNS (Bhowmick *et al.*, 2007; Chen *et al.*, 2010).

Lastly, natural killer (NK) and γ/δ T cells form the cytotoxic arm of the innate immune pathways. Both exhibit cellular cytotoxicity by causing apoptotic lysis of virally infected cells, either through a direct cell-cell contact mechanism or, indirectly, by release of soluble cytokines, IFN-γ and TNF-α. An in vitro study has demonstrated the antiviral activity of IFN-γ against JEV (Hasegawa *et al.*, 1990) and we have confirmed a critical role of IFN-γ in recovery from JEV infection using IFN-γ-/- mice, which demonstrate significantly increased mortality relative to wild-type mice (Larena and Lobigs, unpublished). IFN-γ mediates its antiviral effect, at least in part, through induction of nitric oxide (NO) synthase (Karupiah *et al.*, 1993) and an inhibitory effect of NO on JEV growth has been documented (Lin *et al.*, 1997; Saxena *et al.*, 2000). IFN-γ, derived from γ/δ T cells is necessary for the early control of dissemination of WNV, which is closely related to JEV (Wang *et al.*, 2003a). γ/δ T cells may play a protective role at the interface of innate and adaptive immunity, since TCRδ-/- mice display higher susceptibility after secondary challenge with WNV compared to wild-type mice (Wang *et al.*, 2006). It will be interesting to uncover whether γ/δ T cells are also important in experimental models of JEV.

3. Adaptive immunity

Adaptive immunity represents the second wave of immune responses and is characterized by specificity, high potency, and development of memory. For it to become activated, it requires signals from antigen presenting cells of the innate immune system. This can be directly through cell-to-cell communication or, indirectly, by recognition of soluble cytokines. Adaptive immunity is composed of the humoral and cell-mediated immune responses mediated by B and T lymphocytes, respectively. The essential contribution of the adaptive immune responses in recovery from viral infections has been evident from empirical observations in people with defective B cell or T cell development (Fulginiti *et al.*, 1968; Wilfert *et al.*, 1977; Wyatt, 1973).

3.1 B cells

Humoral immunity has paramount protective function in primary JEV infection. The importance of a vigorous, virus-specific, humoral immune response in ameliorating and preventing illness has been documented in human cases of JE (Burke *et al.*, 1987; Libraty *et al.*, 2002; McCallum, 1991) and in animal models by administration of antibody prior or subsequent to infection with JEV (Goncalvez *et al.*, 2008; Gupta *et al.*, 2003; Kimura-Kuroda & Yasui, 1988; Zhang *et al.*, 1989). We have shown that mice genetically defective in B cells and antibody (μMT-/-) develop uncontrolled viremia, viral persistence in peripheral tissues, rapid and widespread viral dissemination into the CNS, and early uniform mortality (Larena *et al.*, 2011). Additionally, transfer of purified JEV-immune B cell fully protects recipient wild-type mice from lethal JEV challenge (Larena *et al.*, 2011).

The early IgM response against JEV is independent of T cell help (Larena *et al.*, 2011), most likely due to the highly ordered and repetitive surface structures of the virion particle

(Spohn & Bachmann, 2008). Neutralizing anti-JEV IgM antibodies are most important in recovery from primary infection. This is supported by the finding that B cell-deficient mice develop detectable virus in both serum and spleen as early as day 4 pi, a time point when neutralizing anti-JEV IgM antibody start to appear in wild-type mice. In addition, CD4+ T cell-deficient mice (MHCII-/-), which have truncated IgM and blunted IgG antibody responses, present with undetectable early viremia, indicating that even suboptimal anti-JEV IgM antibody levels provided a beneficial effect (Larena *et al.*, 2011).

Mechanistically, antibodies elicited against flaviviruses exhibit their action directly by neutralization of infectivity, or indirectly by antibody-dependent cell-mediated cytotoxicity, Fc-γ-receptor-mediated clearance, or complement-mediated cytotoxicity (Pierson *et al.*, 2008). Neutralizing antibodies predominantly target the E protein of the virion, although protective antibodies against prM and NS1 proteins have also been documented (Dewasthaly *et al.*, 2001; Kolaskar & Kulkarni-Kale, 1999; Konishi *et al.*, 1991; Konishi *et al.*, 1992a; Konishi *et al.*, 1992b; Lin *et al.*, 2008b; Lin *et al.*, 1998; Nam *et al.*, 1999; Seif *et al.*, 1995; Wu et al., *2003;* Wu & Lin, *2001;* Xu et al., *2004*). The latter can control JEV infection by their complement-mediated cytolytic potential (Krishna *et al.*, 2009; Lin *et al.*, 2008b; Lin *et al.*, 1998). Antibody neutralizes flavivirus infectivity with high efficiency mainly by interfering with early steps of the viral entry pathway, including attachment, internalisation, and fusion (Butrapet *et al.*, 1998; Crill & Roehrig, 2001; Goncalvez *et al.*, 2008; Nybakken *et al.*, 2005).

3.2 T cells

T cells can be classified phentoypically, on the basis of their antigen receptor usage (α/β vs γ/δ) and their co-receptor expression (CD4 vs. CD8), or functionally (cytotoxic vs helper). Generally, cytotoxic T lymphocytes (CTLs) are predominantly of CD8+ and helper T (Th) cells of CD4+ phenotype. T cells of the γ/δ phenotype recognize non-classical major histocompatibility complex (MHC) antigens and form part of the innate immune response as described earlier. On the other hand, CD8+ and CD4+ α/β T cells recognize MHC-I and MHC-II plus peptide antigen, respectively, and serve as mediators of adaptive immune responses.

3.2.1 CD4+ T cell immune response

Exposure to JEV induces effective CD4+ T cells immunity, characterised by T cell proliferation, production of Th1 and Th2 cytokines, and immunoglobulin class switching (Konishi *et al.*, 1995; Ramakrishna *et al.*, 2003). Putative Th epitopes that elicit virus-specific and flavivirus cross-reactive proliferative responses in immune splenocytes have been mapped in E protein (Kutubuddin *et al.*, 1991). In humans, exposure to live JEV infection or vaccination similarly induces JEV-specific and flavivirus cross-reactive CD4+ T cell responses (Aihara *et al.*, 1998; Konishi *et al.*, 1995). A region of NS3 protein (residues 193 - 324) has been identified as the dominant source of peptide determinants for CD4+ T cells in a healthy JEV-endemic cohort (Kumar *et al.*, 2004a; Kumar *et al.*, 2004c). Patients with severe encephalitis had impaired NS3-specific CD4+ T cell responses, indicating a critical protective role of these immune cells in the pathogenesis of JE (Kumar *et al.*, 2004b).

Multifaceted CD4+ T cells contribute to controlling infection by various mechanisms, including antiviral cytokine production, antibody class switching, direct cytotoxicity, and maintenance CD8+ T cell activity (Zhu *et al.*, 2010). The protective value of JEV-immune CD4+ T cells has been explored in adoptive transfer experiments and genetically deficient mice (Biswas *et al.*, 2009; Larena *et al.*, 2011). The lack of CD4+ T cells in MHCII-/- mice results in a truncated JEV-specific IgM response and significantly blunted immunolgobulin class switching to IgG (Larena *et al.*, 2011). As a consequence, anti-JEV neutralizing activity in MHCII-/- mice increases marginally up to day 8 pi and drops significantly thereafter. This results in an increased viral burden in the CNS late in the course of infection and uniform mortality. Thus, the beneficial effect of JEV-immune CD4+ T cells predominantly involves effective antibody production, thereby preventing virus entry into the CNS.

3.2.2 CD8+ T cell immune response

Early reports demonstrated JEV-specific CD8+ T cell proliferative responses and cytolytic activity in humans and mice after vaccination or exposure to live JEV infection (Konishi *et al.*, 1995; Konishi *et al.*, 1997; Konishi *et al.*, 1998; Murali-Krishna *et al.*, 1995a; Murali-Krishna *et al.*, 1994; 1995b). Peptide determinants recognized by JEV-immune CD8+ cells are starting to be identified: they include a H-2Kd-restricted E protein-derived peptide (CYHASVTDI) (Takada *et al.*, 2000) and a H-2Db-restricted NS4B protein-derived peptide (SAVWNSTTA) (Larena *et al.*, 2011; Trobaugh *et al.*, 2010). The humans CD8+ T cell response against JEV appears to be biased to peptide determinants derived from the NS3 protein (Kumar *et al.*, 2004c; Kumar *et al.*, 2003), as was first reported for the CTL response against the closely related Murray Valley encephalitis virus (MVEV) in mice (Lobigs *et al.*, 1994). This response against determinants in NS3 protein is broadly flavivirus cross-reactive and paradoxically recognises disparate epitopes from JEV and distantly related flaviviruses, but ignores more similar peptides from "self" and other virus families (Regner *et al.*, 2001), suggesting that primary sequence homology is not always the crucial factor in peptide recognition in the cross-reactive cellular immune responses against flaviviruses.

Cytotoxic CD8+ T cells exert their function by lysing virally infected cells directly through Fas-FasL interaction or the perforin-granzymes exocytosis mechanism, and indirectly by release of soluble cytokines, IFN-γ and TNF-α. A dominant protective role of CD8+ T cells was initially reported by Murali-Krishna et al (1996); however, this involved co-injection of a large number of splenocytes with virus into the brain and required co-transfer of CD4+ T cells. In contrast, we have found only a subsidiary role of CD8+ T cells in recovery from JEV infection in a murine model (Larena *et al.*, 2011). Thus, in vivo depletion of CD8+ T cells does not significantly increase susceptibility of mice to virus infection and genetic deficiencies in cytolytic effector pathways of T lymphocytes does not exacerbate the pathogenesis of JEV. However, CD8+ T cells contribute to a significant level to reducing viral load in the CNS of infected Fas-/-, granzymeA/B-/- and CD8+ T cell-depleted mice. Thus, although CD8+ T cells apparently do not provide a significant advantage in terms of survival following JEV infection, they demonstrate a beneficial role in controlling virus growth in the CNS, with the proviso that the latter may occur at the cost of increased immunopathology (Larena *et al.*, 2011).

3.2.3 The contribution of CD8+ T cells to recovery from infection differs between JEV and closely related flaviviruses

Our work and that of others has uncovered a conflicting role of CD8+ T cells in recovery from infection with encephalitic flaviviruses. While essential for virus elimination from the CNS and survival in mouse models of West Nile encephalitis (Shrestha & Diamond, 2004; Shrestha *et al.*, 2006; Wang *et al.*, 2003b; 2004), and a disease-potentiating effect of CTLs was documented in mice infected with MVEV (Licon Luna *et al.*, 2002), the CD8+ T cell response does not markedly affect outcome of infection with JEV (Larena *et al.*, 2011). Notably, mice genetically deficient in the Fas- or perforin-dependent pathways of cytotoxicity show greatly increased susceptibility to virulent lineage I WNV infection (Shrestha & Diamond, 2007), but do not differ from wild-type mice in susceptibility to infection with JEV (Larena et al., 2011) or lineage II WNV strain, Sarafend (Wang *et al.*, 2004), and are more resistant to infection with MVEV (Licon Luna *et al.*, 2002). These findings highlight a difference in pathogenesis between even closely related flaviviruses belonging to the JEV serocomplex (Mullbacher *et al.*, 2004) that most likely involves a difference in the capacity of the cellular immune response to resolve the virus infections in the CNS.

3.2.4 Modulation of MHC-I

MHC-I is expressed on virtually all mammalian cells and the cell surface expression of this class of restriction elements for CTLs is up-regulated as a consequence of infection with JEV and other flaviviruses in a diverse range of cell types from different species (Kesson *et al.*, 2002; Lobigs *et al.*, 2003). Flavivirus-induced up-regulation of MHC-I cell surface expression is, at least in part, IFN-independent (Abraham *et al.*, 2010; Kesson & King, 2001; Mullbacher & Lobigs, 1995), and also includes that of non-classical MHC-I (Abraham *et al.*, 2008). Although the physiological relevance of this phenomenon in virus transmission remains unclear, it has been proposed that the process may contribute to reduced NK cell activity, which is inhibited by engagement with MHC-I by NK cell inhibitory receptors (Hershkovitz *et al.*, 2008; Momburg *et al.*, 2001). It has also been hypothesised that flavivirus-induced up-regulation of MHC-I leads to transient T cell autoimmunity (given the increase in "self" antigen presentation), followed by subsequent suppression of "self"-reactive T cell activity, and that flavivirus infection or live vaccination of humans in the tropics could contribute to the observed lower incidence of overt autoimmunity in the tropics than in temperate climates, where flaviviruses are not endemic (Lobigs *et al.*, 1996).

4. Implications for vaccination against JE

Current vaccines against JE include non-adjuvanted and alum-adjuvanted inactivated vaccines that are licensed internationally, and an attenuated live vaccine predominantly used in China (Beasley *et al.*, 2008; Halstead & Thomas, 2011). There is a clear need for development and licensing of new JE vaccines, which raises the question of immunological correlates for protection against JEV infection that should be targeted by an effective JE vaccine. Our understanding of immune pathways essential for recovery from primary JEV infection emphasises the critical role of neutralising antibody against E protein and the requirement for effective B and CD4+ T cell immune responses, while suggesting a subsidiary contribution of CD8+ T cells to recovery. TLR signalling and type I IFN are also expected to play an important role in induction of effective B cell immunity (Hou *et al.*, 2011; Kasturi *et al.*, 2011; Le Bon *et al.*, 2001). Similar to recovery from primary JEV infection, neutralising antibody against E protein is also key to vaccine-induced protective immunity, with no or only partial protection provided by JEV-immune CD8+ T cell memory (Chen *et al.*, 1999; Konishi *et al.*, 2003; Pan *et al.*, 2001). This evidence highlights that induction of potent and durable memory B cells that produce high-affinity, neutralising antibody against E protein is the prime criterion for efficacy of a vaccine against JEV, in addition to safety and tolerability.

Factor	Outcome after JEV infection
Age	↑ disease severity in younger animals
Route of Infection	intracranial and intranasal = high mortality extraneural = ↓ disease severity
Mouse strain background	impacts on disease outcome
Innate Immunity	
Pathogen Recognition	
Myd88	absence = ↓ production of inflammatory cytokines, no effect on disease severity
RIG-1	absence = ↓ production of type 1 IFN; ↑ disease severity
MDA-5	absence = no effect on production of type 1 IFN; no effect on disease severity
LGP2	absence = ↑ production of type 1 IFN
Interferon Induction and Signalling	
NF-κB	↑ PI3K dependent production of type 1 IFN
IRF-3	↑ RIG-1 dependent production of type 1 IFN
IFN-α	inhibits virus, no effect with treatment of human cases
IFN-α receptor	absence = ↑ disease severity
Jak-stat	inhibited by viral NS4A and NS5 proteins
ISG15	inhibits virus
Viperin	inhibited via proteosome-dependent mechanism
Cellular Factors	
Neutrophils	neutrophilia, intracellular degradation of JEV ↑ release of inflammatory cytokines; ↑ pathology
Macrophage	monocytosis; ↑ migration of monocytes to CNS; ↑ inflammatory cytokines
Microglial Cells	microgliosis; ↑ release of inflammatory cytokines; ↑ pathology
Astrocytes	↑ release of inflammatory cytokines
Other cytokines and chemokines	
IFN-γ	absence = ↑ disease severity
CCR5	absence = ↑ disease severity
Adaptive Immunity	
Effector cells	
B cells	absence = ↑ disease severity
CD4+ T cells	absence = ↑ disease severity
CD8+ Tcells	absence = ↑ CNS viral burden without impact on mortality rate
Cytolytic Pathways	
Perforin	absence = no effect on disease severity
Granzymes A/B	absence = no effect on disease severity
Fas	absence = no effect on disease severity

(↑) increased, (↓) decreased

Table 1. Factors affecting outcome of JEV infection

5. References

Abraham, S., Nagaraj, A. S., Basak, S. & Manjunath, R. (2010). Japanese encephalitis virus utilizes the canonical pathway to activate NF-kappaB but it utilizes the type I interferon pathway to induce major histocompatibility complex class I expression in mouse embryonic fibroblasts. *Journal of Virology* 84, 5485-5493.

Abraham, S., Yaddanapudi, K., Thomas, S., Damodaran, A., Ramireddy, B. & Manjunath, R. (2008). Nonclassical MHC-I and Japanese encephalitis virus infection: induction of H-2Q4, H-2T23 and H-2T10. *Virus Research* 133, 239-249.

Aihara, H., Takasaki, T., Matsutani, T., Suzuki, R. & Kurane, I. (1998). Establishment and characterization of Japanese encephalitis virus-specific, human CD4(+) T-cell clones: flavivirus cross-reactivity, protein recognition, and cytotoxic activity. *Journal of Virology* 72, 8032-8036.

Aleyas, A. G., George, J. A., Han, Y. W., Rahman, M. M., Kim, S. J., Han, S. B., Kim, B. S., Kim, K. & Eo, S. K. (2009). Functional modulation of dendritic cells and macrophages by Japanese encephalitis virus through MyD88 adaptor molecule-dependent and -independent pathways. *Journal of Immunology* 183, 2462-2474.

Ank, N., West, H. & Paludan, S. R. (2006). IFN-lambda: novel antiviral cytokines. J *Interferon Cytokine Research* 26, 373-379.

Beasley, D. W., Lewthwaite, P. & Solomon, T. (2008). Current use and development of vaccines for Japanese encephalitis. *Expert Opinion on Biological Therapy* 8, 95-106.

Bhowmick, S., Duseja, R., Das, S., Appaiahgiri, M. B., Vrati, S. & Basu, A. (2007). Induction of IP-10 (CXCL10) in astrocytes following Japanese encephalitis. *Neuroscience Letters* 414, 45-50.

Biswas, S. M., Ayachit, V. M., Sapkal, G. N., Mahamuni, S. A. & Gore, M. M. (2009). Japanese encephalitis virus produces a CD4+ Th2 response and associated immunoprotection in an adoptive-transfer murine model. *Journal of General Virology* 90, 818-826.

Borden, E. C., Sen, G. C., Uze, G., Silverman, R. H., Ransohoff, R. M., Foster, G. R. & Stark, G. R. (2007). Interferons at age 50: past, current and future impact on biomedicine. *Nature Reviews Drug Discovery* 6, 975-990.

Bowie, A. G. & Unterholzner, L. (2008). Viral evasion and subversion of pattern-recognition receptor signalling. *Nature Reviews Immunology* 8, 911-922.

Brass, A. L., Huang, I. C., Benita, Y., John, S. P., Krishnan, M. N., Feeley, E. M., Ryan, B. J., Weyer, J. L., van der Weyden, L., Fikrig, E., Adams, D. J., Xavier, R. J., Farzan, M. & Elledge, S. J. (2009). The IFITM proteins mediate cellular resistance to influenza A H1N1 virus, West Nile virus, and dengue virus. *Cell* 139, 1243-1254.

Brinton, M. A. & Perelygin, A. A. (2003). Genetic resistance to flaviviruses. *Advances in Virus Research* 60, 43-85.

Burke, D. S. & Morill, J. C. (1987). Levels of interferon in the plasma and cerebrospinal fluid of patients with acute Japanese encephalitis. *Journal of Infectious Diseases* 155, 797-799.

Burke, D. S., Nisalak, A. & Gentry, M. K. (1987). Detection of flavivirus antibodies in human serum by epitope-blocking immunoassay. *Journal of Medical Virology* 23, 165-173.

Butrapet, S., Kimura-Kuroda, J., Zhou, D. S. & Yasui, K. (1998). Neutralizing mechanism of a monoclonal antibody against Japanese encephalitis virus glycoprotein E. *American Journal of Tropical Medicine and Hygiene* 58, 389-398.

Cao, S., Li, Y., Ye, J., Yang, X., Chen, L., Liu, X. & Chen, H. (2011). Japanese encephalitis Virus wild strain infection suppresses dendritic cells maturation and function, and causes the expansion of regulatory T cells. *Virology Journal* 8, 39.

Chan, Y. L., Chang, T. H., Liao, C. L. & Lin, Y. L. (2008). The cellular antiviral protein viperin is attenuated by proteasome-mediated protein degradation in Japanese encephalitis virus-infected cells. *Journal of Virology* 82, 10455-10464.

Chang, T. H., Liao, C. L. & Lin, Y. L. (2006). Flavivirus induces interferon-beta gene expression through a pathway involving RIG-I-dependent IRF-3 and PI3K-dependent NF-kappaB activation. *Microbes and infection* 8, 157-171.

Chaturvedi, U. C., Mathur, A., Chandra, A., Das, S. K., Tandon, H. O. & Singh, U. K. (1980). Transplacental infection with Japanese encephalitis virus. *Journal of Infectious Diseases* 141, 712-715.

Chaturvedi, U. C., Mathur, A., Tandon, P., Natu, S. M., Rajvanshi, S. & Tandon, H. O. (1979). Variable effect on peripheral blood leucocytes during JE virus infection of man. *Clinical and Experimental Immunology* 38, 492-498.

Chen, C. J., Chen, J. H., Chen, S. Y., Liao, S. L. & Raung, S. L. (2004). Upregulation of RANTES gene expression in neuroglia by Japanese encephalitis virus infection. *Journal of Virology* 78, 12107-12119.

Chen, C. J., Ou, Y. C., Lin, S. Y., Raung, S. L., Liao, S. L., Lai, C. Y., Chen, S. Y. & Chen, J. H. (2010). Glial activation involvement in neuronal death by Japanese encephalitis virus infection. *Journal of General Virology* 91, 1028-1037.

Chen, H. W., Pan, C. H., Liau, M. Y., Jou, R., Tsai, C. J., Wu, H. J., Lin, Y. L. & Tao, M. H. (1999). Screening of protective antigens of Japanese encephalitis virus by DNA immunization: a comparative study with conventional viral vaccines. *Journal of Virology* 73, 10137-10145.

Chen, S. T., Lin, Y. L., Huang, M. T., Wu, M. F., Cheng, S. C., Lei, H. Y., Lee, C. K., Chiou, T. W., Wong, C. H. & Hsieh, S. L. (2008). CLEC5A is critical for dengue-virus-induced lethal disease. *Nature* 453, 672-676.

Crance, J. M., Scaramozzino, N., Jouan, A. & Garin, D. (2003). Interferon, ribavirin, 6-azauridine and glycyrrhizin: antiviral compounds active against pathogenic flaviviruses. *Antiviral Research* 58, 73-79.

Crill, W. D. & Roehrig, J. T. (2001). Monoclonal antibodies that bind to domain III of dengue virus E glycoprotein are the most efficient blockers of virus adsorption to Vero cells. *Journal of Virology* 75, 7769-7773.

Dewasthaly, S., Ayachit, V. M., Sarthi, S. A. & Gore, M. M. (2001). Monoclonal antibody raised against envelope glycoprotein peptide neutralizes Japanese encephalitis virus. *Archives of virology* 146, 1427-1435.

Dong, Y. & Benveniste, E. N. (2001). Immune function of astrocytes. *Glia* 36, 180-190.

Erlanger, T. E., Weiss, S., Keiser, J., Utzinger, J. & Wiedenmayer, K. (2009). Past, present, and future of Japanese encephalitis. *Emerging infectious diseases* 15, 1-7.

Fulginiti, V. A., Kempe , C. H., Hathaway, W. E., Pearlman, D. S., Sieber, O. F., Eller, J. J., Joyner, J. J. & Robinson, A. (1968). *Progressive vaccinia in immunologically deficient individuals*, In: Immunologic deficiency diseases in man, vol 4, Bregsma D (ed), pp. 129-144, The National Foundation-March of Dimes, New York.

Geijtenbeek, T. B. & Gringhuis, S. I. (2009). Signalling through C-type lectin receptors: shaping immune responses. *Nature Reviews Immunology* 9, 465-479.

German, A. C., Myint, K. S., Mai, N. T., Pomeroy, I., Phu, N. H., Tzartos, J., Winter, P., Collett, J., Farrar, J., Barrett, A., Kipar, A., Esiri, M. M. & Solomon, T. (2006). A preliminary neuropathological study of Japanese encephalitis in humans and a mouse model. *Transactions of the Royal Society of Tropical Medicine and Hygiene* 100, 1135-1145.

Ghosh, S. N., Goverdhan, M. K., Sathe, P. S., Chelliah, S. C., Naik, S. V., Godbole, P. V. & Banerjee, K. (1990). Protective effect of 6-MFA, a fungal interferon inducer against Japanese encephalitis virus in bonnet macaques. *Indian Journal of Medical Research* 91, 408-413.

Ghoshal, A., Das, S., Ghosh, S., Mishra, M. K., Sharma, V., Koli, P., Sen, E. & Basu, A. (2007). Proinflammatory mediators released by activated microglia induces neuronal death in Japanese encephalitis. *Glia* 55, 483-496.

Goncalvez, A. P., Chien, C. H., Tubthong, K., Gorshkova, I., Roll, C., Donau, O., Schuck, P., Yoksan, S., Wang, S. D., Purcell, R. H. & Lai, C. J. (2008). Humanized monoclonal antibodies derived from chimpanzee Fabs protect against Japanese encephalitis virus in vitro and in vivo. *Journal of Virology* 82, 7009-7021.

Gould, D. J., Byrne, R. J. & Hayes, D. E. (1964). Experimental Infection of Horses with Japanese Encephalitis Virus by Mosquito Bits. *American Journal of Tropical Medicine and Hygiene* 13, 742-746.

Griffin, D. E. (2011). Viral encephalomyelitis. *Public Library of Science Pathogens* 7, e1002004.

Grossberg, S. E. & Scherer, W. F. (1966). The effect of host age, virus dose and route of inoculation on inapparent infection in mice with Japanese encephalitis virus. *Proceedings of the Society for Experimental Biology and Medicine* 123, 118-124.

Gupta, A. K., Lad, V. J. & Koshy, A. A. (2003). Protection of mice against experimental Japanese encephalitis virus infections by neutralizing anti-glycoprotein E monoclonal antibodies. *Acta Virologica* 47, 141-145.

Gupta, N., Lomash, V. & Rao, P. V. (2010). Expression profile of Japanese encephalitis virus induced neuroinflammation and its implication in disease severity. *Journal Clinical Virology* 49, 4-10.

Gupta, N. & Rao, P. L. (2011). Transcriptomic profile of host response in Japanese encephalitis virus infection. *Virology Journal* 8, 92.

Halstead, S. B. & Jacobson, J. (2003). Japanese encephalitis. *Advances in Virus Research* 61, 103-138.

Halstead, S. B. & Thomas, S. J. (2011). New Japanese encephalitis vaccines: alternatives to production in mouse brain. *Expert Review of Vaccines* 10, 355-364.

Hardy, M. P., Owczarek, C. M., Jermiin, L. S., Ejdeback, M. & Hertzog, P. J. (2004). Characterization of the type I interferon locus and identification of novel genes. *Genomics* 84, 331-345.

Harinasuta, C., Nimmanitya, S. & Titsyakorn, U. (1985). The effect of interferon-alpha A on two cases of Japanese encephalitis in Thailand. *Southeast Asian Journal of Tropical Medicine and Public Health* 16, 332-336.

Hasegawa, H., Satake, Y. & Kobayashi, Y. (1990). Effect of cytokines on Japanese encephalitis virus production by human monocytes. *Microbiology and Immunology* 34, 459-466.

Hershkovitz, O., Zilka, A., Bar-Ilan, A., Abutbul, S., Davidson, A., Mazzon, M., Kummerer, B. M., Monsoengo, A., Jacobs, M. & Porgador, A. (2008). Dengue virus replicon expressing the nonstructural proteins suffices to enhance membrane expression of HLA class I and inhibit lysis by human NK cells. *Journal of Virology* 82, 7666-7676.

Honda, K., Takaoka, A. & Taniguchi, T. (2006). Type I interferon [corrected] gene induction by the interferon regulatory factor family of transcription factors. *Immunity* 25, 349-360.

Hou, B., Saudan, P., Ott, G., Wheeler, M. L., Ji, M., Kuzmich, L., Lee, L. M., Coffman, R. L., Bachmann, M. F. & Defranco, A. L. (2011). Selective Utilization of Toll-like Receptor and MyD88 Signaling in B Cells for Enhancement of the Antiviral Germinal Center Response. *Immunity* 34, 375-384.

Hsiao, N. W., Chen, J. W., Yang, T. C., Orloff, G. M., Wu, Y. Y., Lai, C. H., Lan, Y. C. & Lin, C. W. (2010). ISG15 over-expression inhibits replication of the Japanese encephalitis virus in human medulloblastoma cells. *Antiviral Research* 85, 504-511.

Jiang, D., Weidner, J. M., Qing, M., Pan, X. B., Guo, H., Xu, C., Zhang, X., Birk, A., Chang, J., Shi, P. Y., Block, T. M. & Guo, J. T. (2010). Identification of five interferon-induced cellular proteins that inhibit west nile virus and dengue virus infections. *Journal of Virology* 84, 8332-8341.

Johnson, R. T., Burke, D. S., Elwell, M., Leake, C. J., Nisalak, A., Hoke, C. H. & Lorsomrudee, W. (1985). Japanese encephalitis: immunocytochemical studies of viral antigen and inflammatory cells in fatal cases. *Annals of Neurology* 18, 567-573.

Kajaste-Rudnitski, A., Mashimo, T., Frenkiel, M. P., Guenet, J. L., Lucas, M. & Despres, P. (2006). The 2',5'-oligoadenylate synthetase 1b is a potent inhibitor of West Nile virus replication inside infected cells. *Journal of Biological Chemistry* 281, 4624-4637.

Karupiah, G., Xie, Q. W., Buller, R. M., Nathan, C., Duarte, C. & MacMicking, J. D. (1993). Inhibition of viral replication by interferon-gamma-induced nitric oxide synthase. *Science* 261, 1445-1448.

Kasturi, S. P., Skountzou, I., Albrecht, R. A., Koutsonanos, D., Hua, T., Nakaya, H. I., Ravindran, R., Stewart, S., Alam, M., Kwissa, M., Villinger, F., Murthy, N., Steel, J., Jacob, J., Hogan, R. J., Garcia-Sastre, A., Compans, R. & Pulendran, B. (2011). Programming the magnitude and persistence of antibody responses with innate immunity. *Nature* 470, 543-547.

Kato, H., Takeuchi, O., Sato, S., Yoneyama, M., Yamamoto, M., Matsui, K., Uematsu, S., Jung, A., Kawai, T., Ishii, K. J., Yamaguchi, O., Otsu, K., Tsujimura, T., Koh, C. S., Reis e Sousa, C., Matsuura, Y., Fujita, T. & Akira, S. (2006). Differential roles of MDA5 and RIG-I helicases in the recognition of RNA viruses. *Nature* 441, 101-105.

Kawai, T. & Akira, S. (2010). The role of pattern-recognition receptors in innate immunity: update on Toll-like receptors. *Nature Immunology* 11, 373-384.

Kesson, A. M., Cheng, Y. & King, N. J. (2002). Regulation of immune recognition molecules by flavivirus, West Nile. *Viral Immunology* 15, 273-283.

Kesson, A. M. & King, N. J. (2001). Transcriptional regulation of major histocompatibility complex class I by flavivirus West Nile is dependent on NF-kappaB activation. *Journal of Infectious Diseases* 184, 947-954.

Khanna, N., Agnihotri, M., Mathur, A. & Chaturvedi, U. C. (1991). Neutrophil chemotactic factor produced by Japanese encephalitis virus stimulated macrophages. *Clinical and Experimental Immunology* 86, 299-303.

Kimura, T., Sasaki, M., Okumura, M., Kim, E. & Sawa, H. (2010). Flavivirus encephalitis: pathological aspects of mouse and other animal models. *Veterinary Pathology* 47, 806-818.

Kimura-Kuroda, J. & Yasui, K. (1988). Protection of mice against Japanese encephalitis virus by passive administration with monoclonal antibodies. *Journal of Immunology* 141, 3606-3610.

Kolaskar, A. S. & Kulkarni-Kale, U. (1999). Prediction of three-dimensional structure and mapping of conformational epitopes of envelope glycoprotein of Japanese encephalitis virus. *Virology Journal* 261, 31-42.

Komuro, A. & Horvath, C. M. (2006). RNA- and virus-independent inhibition of antiviral signaling by RNA helicase LGP2. *Journal of Virology* 80, 12332-12342.

Konishi, E., Kurane, I., Mason, P. W., Innis, B. L. & Ennis, F. A. (1995). Japanese encephalitis virus-specific proliferative responses of human peripheral blood T lymphocytes. *American Journal of Tropical Medicine and Hygiene* 53, 278-283.

Konishi, E., Kurane, I., Mason, P. W., Shope, R. E. & Ennis, F. A. (1997). Poxvirus-based Japanese encephalitis vaccine candidates induce JE virus-specific CD8+ cytotoxic T lymphocytes in mice. *Virology Journal* 227, 353-360.

Konishi, E., Kurane, I., Mason, P. W., Shope, R. E., Kanesa-Thasan, N., Smucny, J. J., Hoke, C. H., Jr. & Ennis, F. A. (1998). Induction of Japanese encephalitis virus-specific cytotoxic T lymphocytes in humans by poxvirus-based JE vaccine candidates. *Vaccine* 16, 842-849.

Konishi, E., Pincus, S., Fonseca, B. A., Shope, R. E., Paoletti, E. & Mason, P. W. (1991). Comparison of protective immunity elicited by recombinant vaccinia viruses that synthesize E or NS1 of Japanese encephalitis virus. *Virology Journal* 185, 401-410.

Konishi, E., Pincus, S., Paoletti, E., Laegreid, W. W., Shope, R. E. & Mason, P. W. (1992a). A highly attenuated host range-restricted vaccinia virus strain, NYVAC, encoding the prM, E, and NS1 genes of Japanese encephalitis virus prevents JEV viremia in swine. *Virology Journal* 190, 454-458.

Konishi, E., Pincus, S., Paoletti, E., Shope, R. E., Burrage, T. & Mason, P. W. (1992b). Mice immunized with a subviral particle containing the Japanese encephalitis virus prM/M and E proteins are protected from lethal JEV infection. *Virology Journal* 188, 714-720.

Konishi, E., Terazawa, A. & Imoto, J. (2003). Simultaneous immunization with DNA and protein vaccines against Japanese encephalitis or dengue synergistically increases their own abilities to induce neutralizing antibody in mice. *Vaccine* 21, 1826-1832.

Krishna, V. D., Rangappa, M. & Satchidanandam, V. (2009). Virus-specific cytolytic antibodies to nonstructural protein 1 of Japanese encephalitis virus effect reduction of virus output from infected cells. *Journal of Virology* 83, 4766-4777.

Kumar, P., Krishna, V. D., Sulochana, P., Nirmala, G., Haridattatreya, M. & Satchidanandam, V. (2004a). Cell-mediated immune responses in healthy children with a history of subclinical infection with Japanese encephalitis virus: analysis of CD4+ and CD8+ T cell target specificities by intracellular delivery of viral proteins using the human immunodeficiency virus Tat protein transduction domain. *Journal of General Virology* 85, 471-482.

Kumar, P., Sulochana, P., Nirmala, G., Chandrashekar, R., Haridattatreya, M. & Satchidanandam, V. (2004b). Impaired T helper 1 function of nonstructural protein

3-specific T cells in Japanese patients with encephalitis with neurological sequelae. *Journal of Infectious Diseases* 189, 880-891.

Kumar, P., Sulochana, P., Nirmala, G., Haridattatreya, M. & Satchidanandam, V. (2004c). Conserved amino acids 193-324 of non-structural protein 3 are a dominant source of peptide determinants for CD4+ and CD8+ T cells in a healthy Japanese encephalitis virus-endemic cohort. *Journal of General Virology* 85, 1131-1143.

Kumar, P., Uchil, P. D., Sulochana, P., Nirmala, G., Chandrashekar, R., Haridattatreya, M. & Satchidanandam, V. (2003). Screening for T cell-eliciting proteins of Japanese encephalitis virus in a healthy JE-endemic human cohort using recombinant baculovirus-infected insect cell preparations. *Archives of Virology* 148, 1569-1591.

Kutubuddin, M., Kolaskar, A. S., Galande, S., Gore, M. M., Ghosh, S. N. & Banerjee, K. (1991). Recognition of helper T cell epitopes in envelope (E) glycoprotein of Japanese encephalitis, west Nile and Dengue viruses. *Molecular Immunology* 28, 149-154.

Lam, K. H., Ellis, T. M., Williams, D. T., Lunt, R. A., Daniels, P. W., Watkins, K. L. & Riggs, C. M. (2005). Japanese encephalitis in a racing thoroughbred gelding in Hong Kong. *The Veterinary Record* 157, 168-173.

Larena, M., Regner, M., Lee, E. & Lobigs, M. (2011). Pivotal role of antibody and subsidiary contribution of CD8+ T cells to recovery from infection in a murine model of Japanese encephalitis. *Journal of Virology* 85: 5446-55.

Le Bon, A., Schiavoni, G., D'Agostino, G., Gresser, I., Belardelli, F. & Tough, D. F. (2001). Type i interferons potently enhance humoral immunity and can promote isotype switching by stimulating dendritic cells in vivo. *Immunity* 14, 461-470.

Lee, E., Hall, R. A. & Lobigs, M. (2004). Common E protein determinants for attenuation of glycosaminoglycan-binding variants of Japanese encephalitis and West Nile viruses. *Journal of Virology* 78, 8271-8280.

Lee, E. & Lobigs, M. (2002). Mechanism of virulence attenuation of glycosaminoglycan-binding variants of Japanese encephalitis virus and Murray Valley encephalitis virus. *Journal of Virology* 76, 4901-4911.

Li, Y., Ye, J., Yang, X., Xu, M., Chen, L., Mei, L., Zhu, J., Liu, X., Chen, H. & Cao, S. (2010). Infection of mouse bone marrow-derived dendritic cells by live attenuated Japanese encephalitis virus induces cells maturation and triggers T cells activation. *Vaccine* 29, 855-862.

Libraty, D. H., Nisalak, A., Endy, T. P., Suntayakorn, S., Vaughn, D. W. & Innis, B. L. (2002). Clinical and immunological risk factors for severe disease in Japanese encephalitis. *Transactions of the Royal Society of Tropical Medicine and Hygiene* 96, 173-178.

Licon Luna, R. M., Lee, E., Mullbacher, A., Blanden, R. V., Langman, R. & Lobigs, M. (2002). Lack of both Fas ligand and perforin protects from flavivirus-mediated encephalitis in mice. *Journal of Virology* 76, 3202-3211.

Lim, J. K., Lisco, A., McDermott, D. H., Huynh, L., Ward, J. M., Johnson, B., Johnson, H., Pape, J., Foster, G. A., Krysztof, D., Follmann, D., Stramer, S. L., Margolis, L. B. & Murphy, P. M. (2009). Genetic variation in OAS1 is a risk factor for initial infection with West Nile virus in man. *Public Library of Science Pathogens* 5, e1000321.

Lin, C. W., Cheng, C. W., Yang, T. C., Li, S. W., Cheng, M. H., Wan, L., Lin, Y. J., Lai, C. H., Lin, W. Y. & Kao, M. C. (2008a). Interferon antagonist function of Japanese encephalitis virus NS4A and its interaction with DEAD-box RNA helicase DDX42. *Virus Research* 137, 49-55.

Lin, C. W., Liu, K. T., Huang, H. D. & Chen, W. J. (2008b). Protective immunity of E. coli-synthesized NS1 protein of Japanese encephalitis virus. *Biotechnology Letters* 30, 205-214.

Lin, R. J., Chang, B. L., Yu, H. P., Liao, C. L. & Lin, Y. L. (2006). Blocking of interferon-induced Jak-Stat signaling by Japanese encephalitis virus NS5 through a protein tyrosine phosphatase-mediated mechanism. *Journal of Virology* 80, 5908-5918.

Lin, R. J., Liao, C. L., Lin, E. & Lin, Y. L. (2004). Blocking of the alpha interferon-induced Jak-Stat signaling pathway by Japanese encephalitis virus infection. *Journal of Virology* 78, 9285-9294.

Lin, Y. L., Chen, L. K., Liao, C. L., Yeh, C. T., Ma, S. H., Chen, J. L., Huang, Y. L., Chen, S. S. & Chiang, H. Y. (1998). DNA immunization with Japanese encephalitis virus nonstructural protein NS1 elicits protective immunity in mice. *Journal of Virology* 72, 191-200.

Lin, Y. L., Huang, Y. L., Ma, S. H., Yeh, C. T., Chiou, S. Y., Chen, L. K. & Liao, C. L. (1997). Inhibition of Japanese encephalitis virus infection by nitric oxide: antiviral effect of nitric oxide on RNA virus replication. *Journal of Virology* 71, 5227-5235.

Lobigs, M., Arthur, C. E., Mullbacher, A. & Blanden, R. V. (1994). The flavivirus nonstructural protein NS3 is a dominant source of cytotoxic T cell peptide determinants. *Virology Journal* 202, 195-201.

Lobigs, M., Blanden, R. V. & Mullbacher, A. (1996). Flavivirus-induced up-regulation of MHC class I antigens; implications for the induction of CD8+ T-cell-mediated autoimmunity. *Immunological Reviews* 152, 5-19.

Lobigs, M., Larena, M., Alsharifi, M., Lee, E. & Pavy, M. (2009). Live chimeric and inactivated Japanese encephalitis virus vaccines differ in their cross-protective values against Murray Valley encephalitis virus. *Journal of Virology* 83, 2436-2445.

Lobigs, M., Mullbacher, A. & Regner, M. (2003). MHC class I up-regulation by flaviviruses: Immune interaction with unknown advantage to host or pathogen. *Immunology and Cell Biology* 81, 217-223.

Mashimo, T., Lucas, M., Simon-Chazottes, D., Frenkiel, M. P., Montagutelli, X., Ceccaldi, P. E., Deubel, V., Guenet, J. L. & Despres, P. (2002). A nonsense mutation in the gene encoding 2'-5'-oligoadenylate synthetase/L1 isoform is associated with West Nile virus susceptibility in laboratory mice. *Proceedings of the National Academy of Sciences of the United States of America* 99, 11311-11316.

Mathur, A., Arora, K. L. & Chaturvedi, U. C. (1981). Congenital infection of mice with Japanese encephalitis virus. *Infection and Immunity* 34, 26-29.

Mathur, A., Bharadwaj, M., Kulshreshtha, R., Rawat, S., Jain, A. & Chaturvedi, U. C. (1988). Immunopathological study of spleen during Japanese encephalitis virus infection in mice. *British Journal of Experimental Pathology* 69, 423-432.

McCallum, J. D. (1991). Japanese encephalitis in southeastern Nepal: clinical aspects in the 1986 epidemic. Journal of the Royal Army Medical Corps 137, 8-13.

Miyake, M. (1964). The Pathology of Japanese Encephalitis. a Review. *Bulletin of the World Health Organization* 30, 153-160.

Momburg, F., Mullbacher, A. & Lobigs, M. (2001). Modulation of transporter associated with antigen processing (TAP)-mediated peptide import into the endoplasmic reticulum by flavivirus infection. *Journal of Virology* 75, 5663-5671.

Monath, T. P., Guirakhoo, F., Nichols, R., Yoksan, S., Schrader, R., Murphy, C., Blum, P., Woodward, S., McCarthy, K., Mathis, D., Johnson, C. & Bedford, P. (2003). Chimeric live, attenuated vaccine against Japanese encephalitis (ChimeriVax-JE): phase 2 clinical trials for safety and immunogenicity, effect of vaccine dose and schedule, and memory response to challenge with inactivated Japanese encephalitis antigen. *Journal of Infectious Diseases* 188, 1213-1230.

Mori, Y., Yamashita, T., Tanaka, Y., Tsuda, Y., Abe, T., Moriishi, K. & Matsuura, Y. (2007). Processing of capsid protein by cathepsin L plays a crucial role in replication of Japanese encephalitis virus in neural and macrophage cells. *Journal of Virology* 81, 8477-8487.

Morimoto, T., Kurogi, H., Miura, Y., Sugimori, T. & Fujisaki, Y. (1972). Isolation of Japanese encephalitis virus and a hemagglutinating DNA virus from the brain of stillborn piglets. *National Institute of Animal Health Quarterly* 12, 127-136.

Mullbacher, A. & Lobigs, M. (1995). Up-regulation of MHC class I by flavivirus-induced peptide translocation into the endoplasmic reticulum. *Immunity* 3, 207-214.

Mullbacher, A., Regner, M., Wang, Y., Lee, E., Lobigs, M. & Simon, M. (2004). Can we really learn from model pathogens? *Trends in Immunology* 25, 524-528.

Murali, A., Li, X., Ranjith-Kumar, C. T., Bhardwaj, K., Holzenburg, A., Li, P. & Kao, C. C. (2008). Structure and function of LGP2, a DEX(D/H) helicase that regulates the innate immunity response. *Journal of Biological Chemistry* 283, 15825-15833.

Murali-Krishna, K., Ramireddy, B., Ravi, V. & Manjunath, R. (1995a). Recognition of nonstructural protein peptides by cytotoxic T lymphocytes raised against Japanese encephalitis virus. *Microbiology and Immunology* 39, 1021-1024.

Murali-Krishna, K., Ravi, V. & Manjunath, R. (1994). Cytotoxic T lymphocytes raised against Japanese encephalitis virus: effector cell phenotype, target specificity and in vitro virus clearance. *Journal of General Virology* 75, 799-807.

Murali-Krishna, K., Ravi, V. & Manjunath, R. (1995b). Japanese encephalitis virus infection of mouse cell lines: ability to prime mice for generation of virus specific cytotoxic T lymphocytes and differences in CTL recognisable viral determinants. *Archives of Virology* 140, 127-143.

Murali-Krishna, K., Ravi, V. & Manjunath, R. (1996). Protection of adult but not newborn mice against lethal intracerebral challenge with Japanese encephalitis virus by adoptively transferred virus-specific cytotoxic T lymphocytes: requirement for L3T4+ T cells. *Journal of General Virology* 77, 705-714.

Nam, J. H., Wyatt, L. S., Chae, S. L., Cho, H. W., Park, Y. K. & Moss, B. (1999). Protection against lethal Japanese encephalitis virus infection of mice by immunization with the highly attenuated MVA strain of vaccinia virus expressing JEV prM and E genes. *Vaccine* 17, 261-268.

Nybakken, G. E., Oliphant, T., Johnson, S., Burke, S., Diamond, M. S. & Fremont, D. H. (2005). Structural basis of West Nile virus neutralization by a therapeutic antibody. *Nature* 437, 764-769.

Pan, C. H., Chen, H. W., Huang, H. W. & Tao, M. H. (2001). Protective mechanisms induced by a Japanese encephalitis virus DNA vaccine: requirement for antibody but not CD8(+) cytotoxic T-cell responses. *Journal of Virology* 75, 11457-11463.

Perelygin, A. A., Scherbik, S. V., Zhulin, I. B., Stockman, B. M., Li, Y. & Brinton, M. A. (2002). Positional cloning of the murine flavivirus resistance gene. *Proceedings of the National Academy of Sciences of the United States of America* 99, 9322-9327.

Pierson, T. C., Fremont, D. H., Kuhn, R. J. & Diamond, M. S. (2008). Structural insights into the mechanisms of antibody-mediated neutralization of flavivirus infection: implications for vaccine development. *Cell Host & Microbe* 4, 229-238.

Ramakrishna, C., Ravi, V., Desai, A., Subbakrishna, D. K., Shankar, S. K. & Chandramuki, A. (2003). T helper responses to Japanese encephalitis virus infection are dependent on the route of inoculation and the strain of mouse used. *Journal of General Virology* 84, 1559-1567.

Ravi, V., Parida, S., Desai, A., Chandramuki, A., Gourie-Devi, M. & Grau, G. E. (1997). Correlation of tumor necrosis factor levels in the serum and cerebrospinal fluid with clinical outcome in Japanese encephalitis patients. *Journal of Medical Virology* 51, 132-136.

Regner, M., Lobigs, M., Blanden, R. V., Milburn, P. & Mullbacher, A. (2001). Antiviral cytotoxic T cells cross-reactively recognize disparate peptide determinants from related viruses but ignore more similar self- and foreign determinants. *Journal of Immunology* 166, 3820-3828.

Rios, J. J., Fleming, J. G., Bryant, U. K., Carter, C. N., Huber, J. C., Long, M. T., Spencer, T. E. & Adelson, D. L. (2010). OAS1 polymorphisms are associated with susceptibility to West Nile encephalitis in horses. *Public Library of Science One* 5, e10537.

Rokutanda, H. K. (1969). Relationship between viremia and interferon production of Japanese encephalitis virus. *Journal of Immunology* 102, 662-670.

Samuel, M. A., Whitby, K., Keller, B. C., Marri, A., Barchet, W., Williams, B. R., Silverman, R. H., Gale, M., Jr. & Diamond, M. S. (2006). PKR and RNase L contribute to protection against lethal West Nile Virus infection by controlling early viral spread in the periphery and replication in neurons. *Journal of Virology* 80, 7009-7019.

Satoh, T., Kato, H., Kumagai, Y., Yoneyama, M., Sato, S., Matsushita, K., Tsujimura, T., Fujita, T., Akira, S. & Takeuchi, O. (2010). LGP2 is a positive regulator of RIG-I- and MDA5-mediated antiviral responses. *Proceedings of the National Academy of Sciences of the United States of America* 107, 1512-1517.

Saxena, S. K., Singh, A. & Mathur, A. (2000). Antiviral effect of nitric oxide during Japanese encephalitis virus infection. *International Journal of Experimental Pathology* 81, 165-172.

Saxena, V., Mathur, A., Krishnani, N. & Dhole, T. N. (2008). Kinetics of cytokine profile during intraperitoneal inoculation of Japanese encephalitis virus in BALB/c mice model. *Microbes and Infection* 10, 1210-1217.

Seif, S. A., Morita, K., Matsuo, S., Hasebe, F. & Igarashi, A. (1995). Finer mapping of neutralizing epitope(s) on the C-terminal of Japanese encephalitis virus E-protein expressed in recombinant Escherichia coli system. *Vaccine* 13, 1515-1521.

Shrestha, B. & Diamond, M. S. (2004). Role of CD8+ T cells in control of West Nile virus infection. *Journal of Virology* 78, 8312-8321.

Shrestha, B. & Diamond, M. S. (2007). Fas ligand interactions contribute to CD8+ T-cell-mediated control of West Nile virus infection in the central nervous system. *Journal of Virology* 81, 11749-11757.

Shrestha, B., Samuel, M. A. & Diamond, M. S. (2006). CD8+ T cells require perforin to clear West Nile virus from infected neurons. *Journal of Virology* 80, 119-129.

Silverman, R. H. (2007). Viral encounters with 2',5'-oligoadenylate synthetase and RNase L during the interferon antiviral response. *Journal of Virology* 81, 12720-12729.

Singh, A., Kulshreshtha, R. & Mathur, A. (2000). Secretion of the chemokine interleukin-8 during Japanese encephalitis virus infection. *Journal of Medical Microbiology* 49, 607-612.

Solomon, T. (2003). Recent advances in Japanese encephalitis. *Journal of Neurovirology* 9, 274-283.

Solomon, T., Dung, N. M., Kneen, R., Gainsborough, M., Vaughn, D. W. & Khanh, V. T. (2000). Japanese encephalitis. *Journal of Neurology, Neurosurgery, and Psychiatry* 68, 405-415.

Solomon, T., Dung, N. M., Wills, B., Kneen, R., Gainsborough, M., Diet, T. V., Thuy, T. T., Loan, H. T., Khanh, V. C., Vaughn, D. W., White, N. J. & Farrar, J. J. (2003). Interferon alfa-2a in Japanese encephalitis: a randomised double-blind placebo-controlled trial. *Lancet* 361, 821-826.

Solomon, T., Kneen, R., Dung, N. M., Khanh, V. C., Thuy, T. T., Ha, D. Q., Day, N. P., Nisalak, A., Vaughn, D. W. & White, N. J. (1998). Poliomyelitis-like illness due to Japanese encephalitis virus. *Lancet* 351, 1094-1097.

Spohn, G. & Bachmann, M. F. (2008). Exploiting viral properties for the rational design of modern vaccines. *Expert Review of Vaccines* 7, 43-54.

Srivastava, S., Khanna, N., Saxena, S. K., Singh, A., Mathur, A. & Dhole, T. N. (1999). Degradation of Japanese encephalitis virus by neutrophils. *International Journal of Experimental Pathology* 80, 17-24.

Takada, K., Masaki, H., Konishi, E., Takahashi, M. & Kurane, I. (2000). Definition of an epitope on Japanese encephalitis virus (JEV) envelope protein recognized by JEV-specific murine CD8+ cytotoxic T lymphocytes. *Archives of Virology* 145, 523-534.

Taylor, J. L., Schoenherr, C. & Grossberg, S. E. (1980). Protection against Japanese encephalitis virus in mice and hamsters by treatment with carboxymethylacridanone, a potent interferon inducer. *Journal of Infectious Diseases* 142, 394-399.

Tenoever, B. R., Ng, S. L., Chua, M. A., McWhirter, S. M., Garcia-Sastre, A. & Maniatis, T. (2007). Multiple functions of the IKK-related kinase IKKε in interferon-mediated antiviral immunity. *Science* 315, 1274-1278.

Thongtan, T., Cheepsunthorn, P., Chaiworakul, V., Rattanarungsan, C., Wikan, N. & Smith, D. R. (2010). Highly permissive infection of microglial cells by Japanese encephalitis virus: a possible role as a viral reservoir. *Microbes and Infection* 12, 37-45.

Trobaugh, D. W., Yang, L., Ennis, F. A. & Green, S. (2010). Altered effector functions of virus-specific and virus cross-reactive CD8+ T cells in mice immunized with related flaviviruses. *European Journal of Immunology* 40, 1315-1327.

Tsai, T. F. (2000). New initiatives for the control of Japanese encephalitis by vaccination: minutes of a WHO/CVI meeting, Bangkok, Thailand, 13-15 October 1998. *Vaccine* 18 Suppl 2, 1-25.

van den Hurk, A. F., Ritchie, S. A. & Mackenzie, J. S. (2009). Ecology and geographical expansion of Japanese encephalitis virus. *Annual review of Entomology* 54, 17-35.

Wang, T., Gao, Y., Scully, E., Davis, C. T., Anderson, J. F., Welte, T., Ledizet, M., Koski, R., Madri, J. A., Barrett, A., Yin, Z., Craft, J. & Fikrig, E. (2006). Gamma delta T cells facilitate adaptive immunity against West Nile virus infection in mice. *Journal of Immunology* 177, 1825-1832.

Wang, T., Scully, E., Yin, Z., Kim, J. H., Wang, S., Yan, J., Mamula, M., Anderson, J. F., Craft, J. & Fikrig, E. (2003a). IFN-gamma-producing gamma delta T cells help control murine West Nile virus infection. *Journal of Immunology* 171, 2524-2531.

Wang, Y., Lobigs, M., Lee, E. & Mullbacher, A. (2003b). CD8+ T cells mediate recovery and immunopathology in West Nile virus encephalitis. *Journal of Virology* 77, 13323-13334.

Wang, Y., Lobigs, M., Lee, E. & Mullbacher, A. (2004). Exocytosis and Fas mediated cytolytic mechanisms exert protection from West Nile virus induced encephalitis in mice. *Immunology and Cell Biology* 82, 170-173.

Wilfert, C. M., Buckley, R. H., Mohanakumar, T., Griffith, J. F., Katz, S. L., Whisnant, J. K., Eggleston, P. A., Moore, M., Treadwell, E., Oxman, M. N. & Rosen, F. S. (1977). Persistent and fatal central-nervous-system ECHOvirus infections in patients with agammaglobulinemia. *New England Journal of Medicine* 296, 1485-1489.

Wilkins, C. & Gale, M., Jr. (2010). Recognition of viruses by cytoplasmic sensors. Current Opinion in Immunology 22, 41-47.

Winter, P. M., Dung, N. M., Loan, H. T., Kneen, R., Wills, B., Thu le, T., House, D., White, N. J., Farrar, J. J., Hart, C. A. & Solomon, T. (2004). Proinflammatory cytokines and chemokines in humans with Japanese encephalitis. *Journal of Infectious Diseases* 190, 1618-1626.

Wu, K. P., Wu, C. W., Tsao, Y. P., Kuo, T. W., Lou, Y. C., Lin, C. W., Wu, S. C. & Cheng, J. W. (2003). Structural basis of a flavivirus recognized by its neutralizing antibody: solution structure of the domain III of the Japanese encephalitis virus envelope protein. *Journal of Biological Chemistry* 278, 46007-46013.

Wu, S. C. & Lin, C. W. (2001). Neutralizing peptide ligands selected from phage-displayed libraries mimic the conformational epitope on domain III of the Japanese encephalitis virus envelope protein. *Virus Research* 76, 59-69.

Wyatt, H. V. (1973). Poliomyelitis in hypogammaglobulinemics. *Journal of Infectious Diseases* 128, 802-806.

Xu, G., Xu, X., Li, Z., He, Q., Wu, B., Sun, S. & Chen, H. (2004). Construction of recombinant pseudorabies virus expressing NS1 protein of Japanese encephalitis (SA14-14-2) virus and its safety and immunogenicity. *Vaccine* 22, 1846-1853.

Yamanaka, T., Tsujimura, K., Kondo, T., Yasuda, W., Okada, A., Noda, K., Okumura, T. & Matsumura, T. (2006). Isolation and genetic analysis of Japanese encephalitis virus from a diseased horse in Japan. *Journal of Veterinary Medical Science* 68, 293-295.

Yang, K. D., Yeh, W. T., Chen, R. F., Chuon, H. L., Tsai, H. P., Yao, C. W. & Shaio, M. F. (2004). A model to study neurotropism and persistency of Japanese encephalitis virus infection in human neuroblastoma cells and leukocytes. *Journal of General Virology* 85, 635-642.

Zhang, M. J., Wang, M. J., Jiang, S. Z. & Ma, W. Y. (1989). Passive protection of mice, goats, and monkeys against Japanese encephalitis with monoclonal antibodies. *Journal of Medical Virology* 29, 133-138.

Zhu, J., Yamane, H. & Paul, W. E. (2010). Differentiation of effector CD4 T cell populations. *Annual Review of Immunology* 28, 445-489.

17

Japanese Encephalitis Virus: Innate and Adaptive Immunity

Sojan Abraham*, Shwetank,
Gaurav Kumar and Ramanathapuram Manjunath
Department of Biochemistry, Indian Institute of Science, Bangalore, India

1. Introduction

Japanese encephalitis virus (JEV) is a flavivirus that is one of the major causes of encephalitis in Eastern and Southern Asia with recent observations marking its spread to newer geographical regions. Flaviviruses, in general consitutute a global health threat since many of them are endemic in large parts of the Americas, Africa and Australia in addition to Asia and suitable vaccines are unavailable for many of them. JEV causes serious inflammation of the brain, which may lead to permanent brain damage, and has a high mortality rate. More than three billion people live in JE endemic areas and JEV is estimated to cause 45,000 human cases of disease and 10000 deaths per year (Solomon and Winter, 2004; van den Hurk et al., 2009).

The occurrence of encephalitic epidemics in humans due to this virus have been recognized from 1870s in Japan where it was termed Japanese B encephalitis to distinguish it from type A encephalitis caused by sleeping sickness. The first prototype Nakayama strain was isolated and established in 1935 from the brain of a fatal case from Tokyo, Japan. This was closely followed by virus isolation from *Culex tritaeniorrhynchus* in 1936 confirming earlier suspicions that mosquitoes served as the transmission vector (Solomon et al., 2000).

JEV transmission occurs through a zoonotic cycle involving mosquitoes as an important intermediate maintenance and replicative vector. Vertebrates, chiefly pigs and ardeid birds act as amplifying hosts. Only those animals that develop high viraemias are significant in this natural enzootic cycle. Humans are infected only coincidently when bitten by an infected mosquito and are dead end hosts. Human to human transmission is yet to be documented, possibly due to the presence of transient viraemia. The absence of high serum viraemia prevents the virus from being picked up during mosquito bites. Pigs play a major role in the transmission cycle with respect to human infection since they are often bred close to humans whereas herons, egrets and other ardeid birds are important for maintenance and overwintering of this virus. Among the other vertebrates, horses also develop central nervous system (CNS) infections and are considered as dead end hosts. Rodents are relatively refractory to infections while amphibians, reptiles and bats can also be infected (Mackenzie et al., 2004). JEV does not cause encephalitis in pigs and birds although it is

* Present Address: Department of Biomedical Sciences, Center of excellence for infectious diseases, Paul. L. Foster School of Medicine, Texas Tech University Health Sciences Center, El Paso, TX, USA

known to result in abortions in pigs (D.S. Burke and Leake, 1988). Thus the incidence of JEV induced disease correlates with rising mosquito densities and increased human contact with amplifying vertebrate hosts. As a result, activities such as deforestation and irrigation that are associated with farming as well as increases in temperatures and precipitation that occurs during monsoons favor JEV infection and propagation. Not surprisingly, seasonal JEV epidemics are associated in the tropics with the beginning of the monsoon season (Umenai et al., 1985). The increased rainfall during the monsoon season has been shown to be followed by an increase in mosquito breeding leading to seroconversion in farm animals and later human encephalitis (Mani et al., 1991) in Southern India as well as in other northern areas of Vietnam, Thailand and Korea, Japan and China (Erlanger et al., 2009; Hoke et al., 1988).
Under laboratory conditions *Culex* species *Cx. tritaeniorrhynchus, Cx. geldius, Cx. pseudovishnui and Cx. fuscocephala* have found to be very efficient vectors for JEV transmission (Solomon, 2006; Solomon, 2004). However, JEV has also been isolated from other species of mosquitoes as well. JEV has been isolated from ten different species of *Culex*, four different species of *Anopheles* and three different species of *Mansonia* mosquitoes (Reuben and Gajanana, 1977). Among various *Culex* species, *Cx. tritaeniorrhychus* has been found to be a very efficient vector for JEV replication and transmission. It breeds predominantly in paddy fields and is the primary vector for transmission of JEV throughout Southeast Asia (Takahashi, 1976).

2. Epidemiology

A major epidemic involving encephalitis was observed in Japan in 1924 with over 6000 cases and 3797 deaths which was followed by another large outbreak in 1935 and then, annual outbreaks from 1946 to 1952. Subsequently, outbreaks were reported in China in 1940 and in Korea in 1949 and in other Asian countries which include Thailand, Vietnam, Burma, Bangladesh, Indonesia, Malaysia, the Philippines, Sri Lanka, India, and Taiwan where epidemics have been reported since 1950s. JE was reported from Russia in 1938 while a large epidemic was reported in North Vietnam and North Thailand in the 1960s (Endy and Nisalak, 2002).
JE is now being described from newer geographical areas and was reported from Australian Torres straits island as well as the mainland in 1995 and 1998 (Mackenzie et al., 2002; Hanna et al., 1999). The factors contributing to this geographical spread could be multifold including several environmental and ecological factors as well as the ability of humans to travel and birds to migrate. The former was exemplified by the isolation of another flavivirus, WNV from New York in 1999 (Lanciotti et al., 1999).
In India, JEV was first diagnosed in 1955 in Vellore, North Arcot district of Tamil Nadu (Kabilan et al., 2004). Major outbreaks were reported in West Bengal in 1973 with 700 cases and 300 deaths. This was followed by another epidemic in 1976 in the same region. Other outbreaks have been reported in several other states of India which include Bihar, Andhra Pradesh, Assam, Manipur, Uttar Pradesh, Karnataka, Madhya Pradesh, Maharashtra and Haryana (Kabilan et al., 2004).
Broadly three epidemiological regions have been associated with JE (Rodhain, 1996):

1. Temperate epidemic region: In temperate regions such as Northern China, Korea, Japan, Taiwan and Southern Russia, the extreme low temperatures of the winters do not allow mosquito transmission. However, in the summer and autumn months, the thaw and increase in temperatures allows mosquito transmission, possibly leading to large epidemics.

2. Endemic region: In southern regions of India, Southern Vietnam, Thailand, the Phillipines, Malayasia and Indonesia, JEV is endemic due to the constant presence of mosquitoes and the bird-mosquito-pig cycle gains predominance.
3. Intermediate subtropical region: In Northern India, Burma, Northern Thailand, Northern Vietnam and Southern China and Bangladesh, JEV transmission occurs continuously at low levels. However, it increases soon after the monsoon and rainy season. Unexposed children are mostly affected in such regions since the adults in the region would have been exposed at some time to the virus.

JEV causes disease mostly in new born children and young adults. Most infections in adults are asymptomatic, at most having flu-like symptoms and rarely cause disease. However, immunologically naïve adults are susceptible to the disease and they could be affected when epidemics occur for the first time in their geographical area. The estimated ratio of symptomatic to asymptomatic infection varies from 1 in 25 to 1 in 1000 (Solomon and Winter, 2004). The incidence of symptomatic JE infection is influenced by several factors including previous exposure to flaviviruses, age-related differences, different immunological and genetic factors as well as efficiency of available surveillance procedures. The occurrence of high levels of neutralizing antibodies in children aged above 14 years, possibly due to natural exposure and subclinical infections decreases the susceptibility of these older age groups.

3. Clinical features

JEV normally infects children below 15 years and man to man transmission of JEV is not detected. The incubation period after the infected mosquito bite is not exactly known, but varies from 1-6 days normally. The onset of illness can be abrupt, acute, subacute or gradual. Progression of disease can be divided into three stages: (i) the prodromal stage preceding CNS features (ii) an encephalitis stage marked by CNS symptoms and (iii) the late stage noticeable by recovery or persistence of signs of CNS injury (Misra and Kalita, 2010; Huy et al., 1994; Kumar et al., 1993). Definitive clinical diagnosis is not possible in prodromal stage, but is characterized by high grade fever, with or without rigors, headache, general malaise, nausea and vomiting. The prodromal stage usually lasts 1-6 days. It can be as short as less than 24 hr or as long as 14 days. The initial symptoms in children are usually nausea, vomiting and abdominal pains that are associated with acute abdominal syndromes. The encephalitic stage is characterized by altered sensorium, convulsions, neck stiffness, muscular rigidity and abnormal movements, speech impairment, mask-like face, tremors in finger, eyes, eyelids and tongue. The late stage is characterized by the persistent signs of CNS injury such as mental impairment, increased deep tendon reflexes, paresis either of the upper or lower motor neuron type, epilepsy, abnormal movements and behavioral abnormalities. Case fatality rates for JEV range from 0-30% (Burke et al., 1985). Children who survive take several weeks to regain the neurological functions. However, only one third of the affected children recover the normal neurological functions. 30% of survivors have persistent motor deficits like weakness of upper and lower motor neurons. 20% of the patients suffer from severe cognitive and language impairment and some patients show further convulsions. Some patients are observed to exhibit mild sequelae such as learning disabilities and behavioral problems (Kumar et al., 1993). Chronic progressive encephalitis and relapse, caused by persistence of virus in the CNS has been reported in a small number of patients (Pradhan et al., 2001; Ravi et al., 1993). The details involving the clinical presentation of JE have been reviewed (Misra and Kalita, 2010).

4. Structural and genome organization

4.1 RNA genome

JEV is a RNA virus belonging to the *Flavivirus* genus of the family *Flaviviridae.* The *Flaviviridae* is a large family of viruses responsible for causing severe disease and mortality in humans and animals. The family consists of three genera: *Flavivirus, Pestivirus* and *Hepacivirus.* Among the three, *Flavivirus* is the largest genus and includes several viruses including dengue virus (DNV), Japanese encephalitis virus (JEV), tick-borne encephalitis virus (TBEV), West Nile virus (WNV) and yellow fever virus (YFV). Most members of the *Flavivirus* genus are arthropod-borne or arboviruses, which indicates the requirement of a blood sucking arthropod to complete their life cycle. Few of the members have no known vector. The genus contains over 70 viruses, of which approximately 40 are mosquito borne, 16 are tick borne and 18 have no known vector (Heinz et al., 2000). Flaviviruses are serologically related and are classified based on cross-neutralization assays using polyclonal sera into 12 sero-complexes (D.S Burke and Monath, 2001; Gubler, 2002). The important ones are the dengue serological group, Japanese encephalitis serological group and yellow fever virus group. JEV belongs to the JE serocomplex which also includes St. Louis encephalitis virus (SLE), West Nile Virus (WNV), Kunjin virus (KUNV), Murray Valley encephalitis virus (MVEV), Cacipacore virus (CPCV), Kautango virus (LOUV), Alfuy virus (ALFV), Usutu virus (USUV) and Yaounde virus (YAOV). JEV has been grouped into 5 genotypes (I -V) based on the phylogenetic analysis of PrM and E encoding genes and different genotypes are found in different climatic regions (Heinz et al., 2000; Nitatpattana et al., 2008; Solomon, 2006).

The complete nucleotide sequence of JEV was reported in 1990 (McMinn, 1997) and shows that it consists of a single stranded, positive-polarity 11kb long RNA. The 3′ end of the genome lacks a poly-A-tail and a type 1 cap (m7GpppAmp) is found at the 5′ end. Flaviviral genome RNAs are also characterized by their high purine content and low CG and UA doublet frequencies (Rice et al., 1985). Untranslated regions (UTR) that contain highly conserved sequences and secondary structures are located at the 5′ and 3′ end of the JEV genome and are 95 and 585 nucleotides long respectively (Sumiyoshi et al., 1987). Host cell and viral proteins are involved in the conversion of the positive sense RNA into a negative sense RNA through a double stranded replicative form (dsRF) after the first round of translation. The negative sense RNA acts as a template for the synthesis of progeny positive sense RNAs that is packaged with viral proteins and assembled into infectious virus particles. Approximately 10-100 fold excess plus strands exist relative to negative strands at any given time within an infected cell. Several cellular and viral proteins such as EF-1α (Davis et al., 2007), TIA-1 (Li et al., 2002) and YB-1 (Paranjape and Harris, 2007) have been reported to bind the UTRs and regulate flaviviral translation and replication. In the case of JEV, FBP1 represses JEV protein expression by interacting with the 3′ and 5′ UTRs (Chien et al., 2011) and La autoantigen facilitates replication by interacting with the 3′ UTR. The role of various host cell factors in flaviviral infection and replication has been reviewed in detail elsewhere (Pastorino et al., 2010).

The RNA genome of JEV contains a single long open reading frame that codes for a polyprotein which is cleaved by host and viral encoded proteases to form three structural and seven non-structural proteins (Fig 1). The N-terminal end of the polyprotein encodes the three structural proteins called capsid (C), a glycosylated membrane protein precursor (prM) and an envelope protein (E). The prM is cleaved to precursor (pr) and membrane protein (M) during JEV maturation. These structural proteins are followed by seven non-structural (NS) proteins (NS1-NS2A-NS2B-NS3-NS4A-NS4B-NS5) (Chambers et al., 1990). The structural proteins finally become components of the mature infectious viral particle while the non-structural proteins take part in the process of polyprotein processing, viral RNA synthesis and virus morphogenesis within the infected cell. Signal sequences direct the polyprotein precursor into the host endoplasmic reticulum (ER) with NS1 and the exogenous domains of prM and E facing the lumen while C, NS3 and NS5 are cytoplasmic. The mature viral proteins are formed by post and cotranslational cleavage of the polyprotein by NS3 in the cytoplasm and ER resident host proteases. Both the processes of polyprotein processing and RNA replication are thought to occur in distinct but adjacent compartments composed of convoluted membranes and vesicle packets containing dsRNA (Salonen et al., 2005; Welsch et al., 2009). The process of virus assembly occurs in the lumen of the rough endoplasmic reticulum (RER) while the final maturation of virus particles occurs in the trans-golgi network and involves the cleavage of prM to M by furin-like protease. This is a step that causes conformational rearrangements of the E protein and is essential for converting fusion incompetent, non-infectious virus particles to mature infectious virions (Yu et al., 2008). These mature viruses exit the host cell as packages of virions.

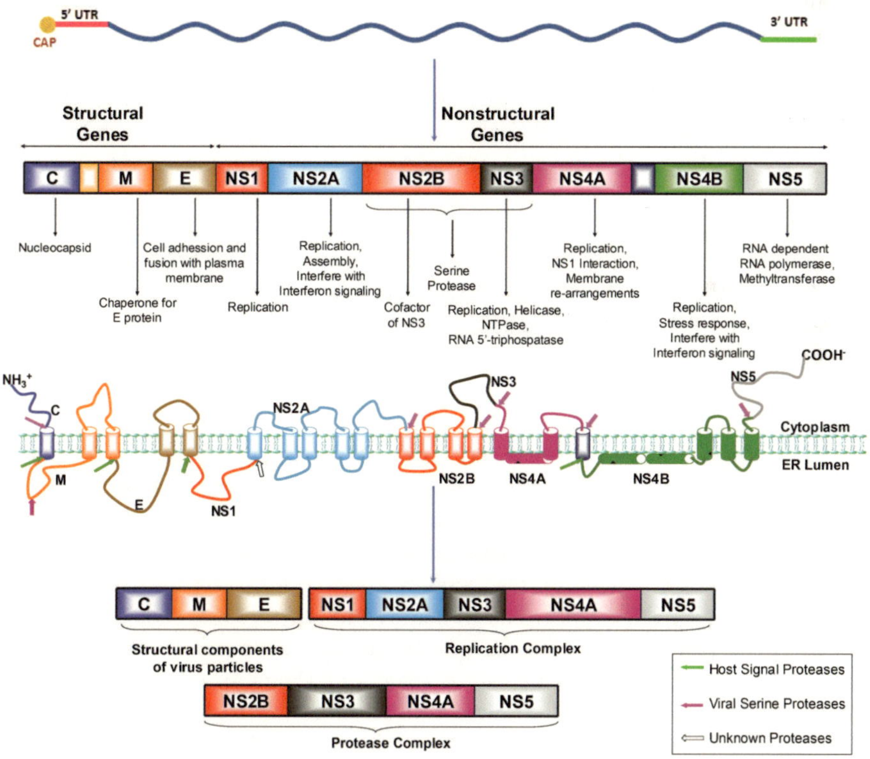

Fig. 1. Schematic diagram of Japanese encephalitis virus genome and polyprotein organization. 11 kb ssRNA JEV genome can be divided into four regions - 5'Cap and 5'UTR, Structural Protein coding gene regions, Nonstructural Protein coding gene regions and 3'UTR. It codes for ~ 380 kDa polyprotein which is further processed by several host and viral proteases to give rise to individual proteins. These individual proteins can assemble together to give rise to structural complexes made up of capsid (C), matrix (M) and envelope (E) proteins. The nonstructural proteins take part in virus replication and assembly within infected cells but do not form part of the mature virus particle that is released (adapted from Assenberg et al., J. Virol (2009) 83: 12895-12906

The RNA genome is packed into a particle by the viral capsid protein (C) in a host-derived lipid bilayer containing the viral envelope protein (E) that participates in receptor binding, membrane fusion and viral assembly. The virus gains access to local fibroblasts when it is deposited at a local site during the mosquito bite where it replicates leading to transient serum viraemia. Both hsp70 (Das et al., 2009b) and integrin molecules (Chu and Ng, 2004) have been shown to act as viral receptors for JEV and WNV respectively. Subsequent viral entry occurs by receptor mediated endocytosis (Lee et al., 2008) involving clathrin coated vesicles (Nawa et al., 2003). Low endosomal pH induces a structural reorganization of the E protein and mediates the fusion of the viral and host cell membranes resulting in the release of the viral nucleocapsid into the cytoplasm (Rey et al., 1995). Infectious virus is released 12 hrs post infection (p.i.) as studied in infected cell lines but viral RNA synthesis can be observed as early as 3 hrs after infection and host macromolecular synthesis is not significantly inhibited by the virus at these times. Although a wide variety of host cells including arthropod cells support virus infection, monocytes, macrophages and dendritic cells are believed to be the main cells that support the spread of this virus into the visceral organs and thence into the CNS in vertebrates. Maximum virus titres vary considerably from cell type to cell type. Although the virus infections in arthropod cells are generally noncytopathic, they are cytocidal in vertebrate cells (Chambers et al., 1990). The period of transient viraemia is followed by the viral invasion of the CNS either through hematogenous spread or by the breakage of the blood-brain barrier and entry through endothelial cells in the cerebrum (Liu et al., 2008). CNS infection is associated with perivascular cuffing that is rich in B cells and the infected parenchyma is invaded by inflammatory macrophages that enter to phagocytose infected and dying cells. Parenchymal damage associated with JEV infection is mainly due to the inflammatory reactions triggered by such invading leukocytes as well as the direct virus- induced cellular apoptotic processes that occur within the CNS.

4.2 Viral proteins

4.2.1 The Capsid and matrix protein

The C protein is highly basic in nature and forms the nucleocapsid along with the genomic RNA. The C protein is a small (12-14 kDa) highly positively charged protein that contains a C-terminal hydrophobic region that is preceded by a hydrophilic region and a central hydrophobic region. It is known to have both N-terminal and C-terminal modifications (Chambers et al., 1990). Cathepsin L mediated processing of this protein has been shown to play an important role in JEV replication in neural and macrophage cells (Mori et al., 2007). Monoclonal antibodies that have been made to the Dengue 4 virus C protein have been shown to localize in the nucleus of the infected cell (Tadano et al., 1989) and nuclear localization of C has been shown to enhance JEV replication in infected cells (Mori et al., 2005). The prM (~26 kDa) is a glycoprotein precursor to the M structural protein and possesses several N-linked glycosylation sites that are conserved in the JE serogroup while the N terminal 'pr' segment contains six conserved cysteine residues, all of which form disulfide bridges (Chambers et al., 1990). A single N-linked glycosylation site has been identified on prM that is essential for the release of JE virus particles from infected cells as well as its ability to cause pathogenesis (Kim et al., 2008). A valine to alanine change at aa76 has been associated with escape from antibody neutralization in MVE (McMinn et al., 1995). Anti-prM antibodies were shown to have low virus-neutralizing activity (Takegami et al., 1982) but its biological significance has not been elucidated. The role of C protein in eliciting B cell responses is yet unclear.

4.2.2 The envelope protein

The envelope (E) protein (~ 53 kDa) is the major virion surface protein with 180 copies existing as head to tail dimers on the virus surface as shown for Dengue viruses (Kuhn et al., 2002). It contains about 500 amino acids and two potential glycosylation sites and mediates viral attachment and fusion to cell membranes of receptor-bearing cells. These properties of E protein are responsible for its glycosylation as well as generating virus neutralizing, haemagglutination inhibiting and fusion blocking antibodies. A feature that distinguishes this structure from that of many others is that the orientation of the E-head to tail homodimers is parallel rather than perpendicular to the membrane as would be expected of a viral glycoprotein spike (Heinz and Allison, 2000). The formation of the E protein homodimer found in the mature virus particle takes place just before the release of the mature virus particle and is associated with the cleavage of the closely associated prM protein to M by a furin-like protease (Yu et al., 2008). While the immunogenicity of the flaviviral E protein has led to the generation of many monoclonal antibodies that were used to understand virus structure, they have also been used to evaluate antigenic drift of related viruses, analysis of the replication cycle as well as in virus detection and diagnostic tools (Roehrig, 2003).

The crystal structure of E protein of JEV has been deduced from knowledge based homology modeling approach using 2Å crystal structure of the E protein of TBEV (Rey et al., 1995) as template (Kolaskar and Kulkarni-Kale, 1999) as well as recombinant subviral particles (RSPs). The RSPs were found to be icosahedral with 30 dimers arranged in a T=1 lattice. Lateral dimer-dimer interactions appear to involve contacts between a loop in domain II on one side and a groove in domains I and III on the other side. The crystal structure of E protein of the Dengue virus type 2 S1 strain has also been found to be nearly identical to that of TBEV protein (Modis et al., 2003). In addition, all of the 12 cysteines present in TBEV and the six disulfide bonds assigned to them are absolutely conserved. Three distinct domains (I, II, III) were elucidated in the E protein and this structure has been assumed for all flavivirus E proteins. These domains directly correspond to the antigenic domains C, A and B respectively, which had been previously defined using monoclonal antibodies to examine the antigenic structure of the TBEV envelope protein. Based on the E protein model of Kolaskar and Kulkarni (1999), domain I contains 128 amino acid residues from 1-51,137-196 and 293-311. The second domain (II) consists of 171 amino acid residues from 52-136 and 197-292 and the IIIrd domain is a contiguous stretch of 100 amino acid residues from 310-411. Domain III contains an IgC immunoglobulin-like domain (Lin and Wu, 2003), that is a unique feature not found in other viral envelopes and an integrin binding motif RGD at aa387-389. This integrin binding motif has been suggested to be involved in viral attachment to the target cell (Mandl et al., 2000; Rey et al., 1995) while amino acids 98-110 of domain II has been suggested to form a barrel shaped fusion peptide that is responsible for initiating the fusion of the virus to endosomal target membranes (Allison et al., 2001; Rey et al., 1995). A unique transmembrane hairpin present in the E protein is needed for this membrane fusion event (Fritz et al., 2011). Recently, a broadly flavivirus cross-neutralizing epitope has been characterized within this fusion loop (Deng et al., 2011). Thus, many of the JEV neutralizing epitopes/regions have been found in these two domains with predominance in Domain III (Table 1). Peptides from this region have also been useful for serological diagnosis (Chavez et al., 2010). However, the binding site of a strongly neutralizing monoclonal antibody (mAb) against JEV (Kimura-Kuroda and Yasui, 1983) was shown to be at the junction area of the Domain I and II and being distant from the virus-target cell attachment site (Morita et al., 2001). Several neutralizing antibodies have been shown to bind the C-terminal E region aa280-414 (Mason et al., 1987). Fragment (aa205-456) that was obtained by CNBr cleavage of the purified E protein has also been shown to induce neutralizing antibodies (Srivastava et al., 1990). Overall, six neutralization regions have been identified based on escape variant analysis of different flaviviruses including JEV. These are region 1, aa66-72 and 112; region 2, aa123-128; region 3, aa155 and 158; region 4, aa171, 181 and 293, region 5, aa52, 136 and 270 -279; region 6, aa307-311, 333 and 384-385. These regions are found on the outer, upper or lateral surfaces of the E-glycoprotein. Many of these regions of the E protein that are associated with neutralizing epitopes have been used in various immunization approaches to develop vaccines and have been detailed later in the chapter.

Envelope Domain	Amino Acid Number	Property of neutralization epitope/region	Reference
I, III	303-396	Binds several anti-JEV neutralizing antibodies	(Mason et al., 1989)
II, III III	205-456 375-457	Fragments obtained by CNBr cleavage Induces neutralizing antibodies in mice	(Srivastava et al., 1990)
III	319-500	Protein A fusion protein eluted from electrophoretic gels induces neutralizing antibodies and protection in mice	(Srivastava et al., 1991)
II III	270 333	Monoclonal antibody neutralization escape variant	(Cecilia and Gould, 1991)
III III	373-500 373-399	Protein A or GST fusion peptide induces neutralizing antibodies	(Seif, Morita, and Igarashi, 1996; Seif et al., 1995)
II II II II	52 126 136 275	Monoclonal antibody neutralization escape variant	(Morita et al., 2001)
I	149-163	Monoclonal antibody raised to synthetic peptide E149-163 neutralizes JEV	(Dewasthaly et al., 2001)
I II III	307-309 327-333 386-390	Phage-display libraries used to select neutralizing peptide ligands	(Wu et al., 2004)
I, III	292-500	Purified E292-500 induces neutralizing antibodies and protects in mice	(Chia et al., 2001)
III	373-399	E373-399 expressed as a fusion protein with JGM virus like particles induce neutralizing antibodies and protection in mice	(Saini and Vrati, 2003)

Table 1. Some Neutralization Epitopes/Regions in the E protein of JEV

4.2.3 The NS1 protein

NS1 is a secreted glycoprotein that is highly conserved across flaviviruses and has been hypothesized to aid in immune evasion. Flaviviral NS1 has been shown to inhibit complement activation both in solution and on cell surfaces (Chung et al., 2006a) due to its ability to bind and recruit the complement regulatory protein factor H. The protein is highly immunogenic and some studies report the protective nature of anti-NS1 antibodies both by immunization and passive transfer (Chung et al., 2006b; Schlesinger et al., 1986). The NS1 protein is not incorporated into the mature virion and has been found in the serum of infected individuals and animals (Alcon et al., 2002) but its high immunogenicity, serotype-specific nature of the antibodies and the identification of a conserved B cell epitope on NS1 of JEV suggests that NS1 is a virus-specific serological antigen (Wang et al., 2009). Monoclonal antibodies have been used to define antigenic domains at the N and C- termini of JEV NS1. Antibody-based assays using anti-NS1 antibodies have also been designed to differentiate between JEV and WNV infections (Kitai et al., 2011).

Multiple forms of NS1 are present in flavivirus infected cells and a protein containing NS1 and a portion of NS2A (NS1′) is found within cells and extracellular fluid of JEV infected cells. The membrane associated forms are hypothesized to form during its dimerization and are detected after 30 minutes of viral protein synthesis (Chambers et al., 1990). It has been shown to be a GPI anchored protein (Jacobs et al., 2000; Winkler et al., 1989) and the GPI anchor is believed to be added to the C-terminus by an ER resident enzyme.

The JE serocomplex NS1 contains 12 conserved cysteines that form disulfide bonds and three N-linked glycosylation sites. Two of these sites are conserved in all mosquito-borne flaviviruses and correspondingly, at least two N-linked oligosaccharide chains are present in the cell-associated and extracellular NS1 and NS1′ in JEV infected cells. Mutations in these N-linked glycosylation sites led to significant defects in RNA replication indicating its important role in virus replication (Chambers et al., 1990).

NS1 (48 kDa) induces a strong antibody response due to its presence both on the surface as well as in secretory form, apart from being present intracellularly in virus induced vesicle packets (Fan and Mason, 1990) and extracellular nonvirion forms. This ability of NS1 to induce a strong antibody response prompted its evaluation for protective efficacy in mice models immunized with either recombinant vaccinia virus (VACV) expressing the NS1 gene or recombinant DNA based immunizations (Lin et al., 1998; Konishi et al., 1991). These results indicate that immunizations with NS1 can provide only low protection from JEV infection, as compared to that elicited by the E protein alone. The secreted form has been named as the soluble complement fixing (SCF) antigen due to its ability to fix complement (Brandt et al., 1970). A recent study has shown that the *E. coli* expressed NS1 protein induces protective humoral immune response in mice during JEV infection (Lin et al., 2008b). A synthetic NS1 peptide has been shown to reconstitute lysis of uninfected syngeneic targets by anti-JEV specific CTL (Murali-Krishna et al., 1996) and anti NS1 antibodies have been shown to reduce virus production from infected cells (Krishna et al., 2009).

4.2.4 The NS2A & NS2B protein

The NS2 protein has two relatively hydrophobic components - NS2A (~25 kDa) and NS2B (~16 kDa) with short hydrophilic segments. NS2A forms part of the replication complex, inhibits IFN production (Liu et al., 2006a) and is also involved in the biogenesis of Kunjin virus-induced membranes that take part in virus assembly (Leung et al., 2008). It has also been shown to bind to the 3′ UTR of viral RNA (Mackenzie et al., 1998). Little information is available regarding NS2A from JEV, but studies with YFV and KUNV suggests that this membrane spanning protein is generated when NS1-2A is cleaved by an ER resident protease at the N-terminal end while its C-terminus is generated by virus encoded NS3 serine protease in the cytoplasm (Falgout and Markoff, 1995). Mutants that block the latter cleavage as well as immunogold localization studies suggest an important role for NS2A in virus replication. Mutations at Lys190 of NS2A and other suppressor mutations in NS3 suggest that NS2A interacts with NS3 in infectious particle production. Similarly, the NS2B protein also complexes with NS3 and is a required cofactor for NS3 serine protease activity as well as its proper folding. NS2B has also been suggested to modulate membrane permeability during JEV infection. Very little information is available regarding their antigenic structure but other studies suggest that NS2A and NS2B may take part in viral RNA assembly (Leung et al., 2008; Lindenbach and Rice, 2003; Kummerer and Rice, 2002).

4.2.5 The NS3 protein

The NS3 protein is the second largest viral protein (70 kDa) and is a multifunctional membrane-associated protein with protease, helicase and RNA triphosphatase activities. The serine protease is required for polyprotein processing (Pastorino et al., 2010; Assenberg et al., 2009) while the helicase/NTPase activity is needed for unwinding the double stranded replicative form of RNA and the RNA triphosphatase activity is needed for capping nascent viral RNA (Bollati et al., 2009). Much of the available information about NS3 has been derived from crystallographic studies of the MVEV protein that is a member of the JEV serogroup. Recent structural data reveal that this single protein has two segregated domains connected by a linker domain (residues 169-181). The relative orientation of these domains differs between different flaviviruses and the helicase and protease activities are independent of each other (Assenberg et al., 2009).

Residues 1 to 169 mediate the trypsin-like serine protease activity and contain the characteristic catalytic triad (Asp-His-Ser) as well as a highly specific substrate recognition sequence that is conserved in all flaviviruses (Chambers et al., 1990). The presence of an aberrant fold makes its structure different from the canonical trypsin structure and makes it dependent on a noncovalent association with a 47 amino acid hydrophilic stretch of NS2B for its proteolytic activity. NS3 cleaves at the C-terminal side of highly conserved dibasic residues located between NS2A/NS2B, NS2B/NS3, NS3/NS4A, NS4B/NS5.

Residues 170 to 619 mediate the activities of RNA strand separation and (poly)nucleotide hydrolysis. The structure of this region has been solved for JEV (Yamashita et al., 2008) and other flaviviruses (Luo et al., 2008; Wu et al., 2005). These studies show that NS3 is a member of the DEAH/D family of helicase superfamily (SF2) containing the Walker A and B motifs that are responsible for NTP and Mg^{2+} binding. It's abilities to separate nascent from template RNA strands and to unwind RNA secondary structure in the 3′ untranslated region is presumed to assist RNA replication. The RNA 5′ triphosphatase activity is thought to facilitate viral RNA capping by removing the terminal γ-phosphate. In addition to its interaction with NS2B which is a cofactor required for its proteolytic activity, NS3 has also been shown to interact with NS5 as a result of which its helicase/NTPase activity is stimulated. The NS3 protein of JEV has also been shown to interact with Src resulting in NS3 tyrosine phosphorylation although the significance of this phosphorylation is still unclear (Raung et al., 2007). Thus, its multifunctional activities have made NS3 an attractive target for antiviral strategies.

4.2.6 The NS4A & NS4B protein

Flaviviruses mediate late cytoplasmic membrane rearrangements that occur after the virus latency period in order to facilitate efficient RNA replication (Westaway et al., 1997). Such rearrangements that involve microtubules and microtubule-associated proteins may facilitate efficient JEV replication by enabling intracellular trafficking of viral components. A certain threshold of viral RNA replication was found to be required for the formation of these structures indicating that cellular membrane biogenesis was closely linked to viral RNA replication and protein synthesis. Three types of membrane structures are induced called convoluted membranes (CM), paracrystalline arrays (PC) and vesicle packets. The CMs are derived from the RER while the vesicle packets are derived from the trans-golgi region of infected host cells. Antibody staining for virus and host-specific proteins reveals that each of these structures perform specific functions during viral replication. Although not shown for JEV, studies with KUNV and WNV suggest that flaviviral NS4A protein mediates these cytoplasmic membrane rearrangements. The cleavage of the NS4A-4B polyprotein intermediate by the NS3-2B protease serves as the signal for the induction of cellular membrane biogenesis and allows NS4A targeting to the golgi complex where viral replication occurs. The exact nature of NS4A cleavage fragments that are involved in these processes as well as the role of NS4A and NS4B in viral replication is still unclear (Roosendaal et al., 2006). Information about posttranslational modifications despite the presence of a conserved, potential N-linked glycosylation site in the C-terminal portion of NS4B is also not clear (Chambers et al., 1990). However, it has recently been demonstrated that the peptidyl-prolyl isomerase (PPIase) function of cyclophilin B (CypB) is essential for JEV replication and that CypB interacts with NS4A in JEV infected cells (Kambara et al., 2011). Also, NS4A has been shown to function as an IFN antagonist (Lin et al., 2008a).

4.2.7 The NS5 protein

NS5 is the largest (105 kDa) and most highly conserved flaviviral protein that has been crystallized and characterized clearly. Like NS3, NS5 is also a multifunctional protein and contains two distinct enzymatic activities of S-adenosyl methyltransferase and RNA-dependent RNA polymerase (RdRp) (Davidson, 2009; Kim et al., 2007) that are separated by an interdomain region. The former resides in the N-terminal domain and is probably involved in performing sequential N7 and 2′ O methylations after the terminal γ phosphate is removed by NS3 during the capping process. The RdRp activity that resides in the C terminal domain of NS5 is majorly responsible for *de novo* initiation of viral RNA synthesis. NS5 can be phosphorylated by a serine/threonine kinase and this phosphorylated form has been shown to localize to the nucleus presumably via the nuclear localization signals that are found in its NS3-interacting interdomain region. In addition to its interaction with the C terminal domain of NS3 as mentioned above, NS5 may also be involved in interactions with several other nonstructural proteins that may be required for its association with other replicase components (Khromykh et al., 1996) and to facilitate virus replication, maturation and assembly. It has also been shown that NS5 has a phosphatase activity which reverses Stat-1 phosphorylation and inhibits IFN responses (Lin et al., 2006).

5. Immune responses to JEV

Both innate and adaptive immune responses are activated in response to JEV infection and have been shown to reduce serum viraemia and viral loads in infected tissues. These immunological responses – both humoral and cellular are the subject of active investigation. Humoral responses play a central role in protection against JEV. However, cell mediated immune responses contributing to this end are not fully understood. In fact, both clinical and experimental data clearly show that IgM and IgG humoral immune responses act in conjunction with cellular immune responses to prevent virus dissemination and persistence as well as resolution of CNS infection. Ironically, the same protective immune responses can also become pathological and cause immune-mediated damage to the host.

5.1 Humoral immune response to JEV

The presence of IgM in the cerebrospinal fluid (CSF) of patients within 5-7 days appears to be a positive prognostic indicator in patients infected with JEV for the first time. Raised IgM levels are present seven days after infection with JEV in the sera and CSF of most symptomatic patients (Solomon et al., 2000). However, raised IgM levels are observed only in the serum but not in the CSF of asymptomatic patients. Maximal levels of serum IgM occur from about day 9 onwards after the onset of clinical disease. Isolation of virus has been possible only in patients who lack the primary IgM response and is usually associated with fatal outcome. Hence diagnostic tests are based on the capture of anti-JEV IgM from patient sera (Shrivastva et al., 2008; Ravi et al., 2006). This primary IgM response leads to class switching and production of IgG by 30 days after infection only in patients who survive. Neutralizing antibodies lead to inhibition of virus replication and virus spread in the initial stages while in encephalitic patients, antibody mediated inhibition of virus replication leads to the inhibition of the cytopathic effects of the virus and hence less tissue damage.

Protection from JEV challenge has been shown to be mainly antibody dependant and virus neutralizing antibodies alone are sufficient for conferring protection. Passive immunization of neutralizing monoclonal antibodies raised against E protein protects mice from lethal challenge with JEV (Zhang et al., 1989; Kimura-Kuroda and Yasui, 1988). Sub-viral particles consisting of prM in addition to E proteins were highly effective in generating a protective immune response in mice against JEV (Konishi et al., 1992b; Mason et al., 1991). The critical role of antibodies in protection against JEV has also been shown using mice lacking immunoglobulins (Pan et al., 2001) as mentioned later in the chapter. It has been shown that humanized monoclonal antibodies derived from chimpanzees protect mice from lethal JEV challenge. These protective antibodies were against different domains of E protein and exhibited high neutralizing activities against a broad spectrum of JEV genotype strains (Goncalvez et al., 2008).

Antibody responses have been observed against many nonstructural proteins but none except anti-NS1 antibodies were protective in nature. However, even these could provide only low protection from JEV infection. A recent study has shown that the *E. coli* expressed NS1 protein induces protective humoral immune response in mice during JEV infection (Lin et al., 2008b). The low level of protective immunity of NS1 was previously proposed to rely on the NS1-specific antibody-dependent complement-mediated cytolysis of the JEV-infected cells (Lin et al., 1998). However, anti NS1 antibodies can directly effect reduction in virus titres from infected cells (Krishna et al., 2009). Immunization of mice with recombinant vaccinia viruses that express various JEV gene products such as E, prM, M and NS1 have also been reported to confer protection against lethal JEV challenge in mice (Konishi et al., 1992a; Mason et al., 1991; Yasuda et al., 1990).

Enhanced neurovirulence of JEV has also been reported in mouse models by passive transfer of virus-specific antibodies. Such enhanced neurovirulence is thought to be mediated by antibody dependent enhancement (ADE) of virus infection due to the internalization of antibody-virus complexes into cells via Fcγ or complement receptors (Gould and Buckley, 1989). The role of non-neutralizing antibodies in increasing infection via antibody dependent enhancement (ADE) is still unclear although this has been thought to contribute to the immunopathological activity of anti-flaviviral humoral responses. ADE has been observed with DNV (Kliks et al., 1989), YFV (Gould and Buckley, 1989) and other flaviviruses.

It has also been shown that oral immunization of mice with live JEV generates a brisk and protective immune response. It was also observed that more robust IgG1 antibody response against JEV occurs following oral infections compared to intraperitoneal (i.p) or subcutaneous (s.c) infections in C57BL/6 and Swiss albino mice (Ramakrishna et al., 2003). However, oral immunization of mice with JEV envelope protein that was expressed in *E. coli* also led to the generation of low neutralizing titre antibodies that were not protective. This result was ascribed to the lack of glycosylation and lack of correct folding in the *E. coli* expressed protein.

Despite the presence of comprehensive data that point out the important role of antibodies in protection, differences in the role of humoral responses in different flaviviruses are evident in studies that utilize mice lacking B cell function. In the case of WNV, mice lacking B cells are more susceptible to the disease while such mice show no change in disease severity in the case of dengue virus (Diamond et al., 2003).

5.2 Cell mediated immune response to JEV

The activation of T cell immunity during JEV infection is an area of intense scrutiny but its role is less clear. In early studies, thymus-deprived mice showed an impaired anti-JEV antibody response indicating the importance of T cell responses in generating B cell immunity to JEV infection (Mori et al., 1970). Similarly, the suppression of T cell function in spider monkeys that are normally resistant to JEV-induced disease resulted in their susceptibility (Nathanson and Cole, 1970). Life long cell mediated immunity could be conferred by passive transfer of immune spleen T cells in mice (Jia and Huang, 1983). The role of T cells in JEV infection was indicated in infection studies involving T cell deficient (nu/nu) nude mice, wherein it was observed that T cells were required for recovery (Lad et al., 1993) and protection after i.p. challenge with JEV (Miura et al., 1990). Adoptive transfer studies had shown that adult but not newborn mice were protected from JEV infection when JEV primed purified T cells were given intracerebral (i.c.) along with 10 x LD_{50} JEV. It was also shown that $CD4^+$ and $CD8^+$ T cells were necessary in protection from JEV and depletion of either population abrogated the protective ability of transferred effectors (Murali-Krishna et al., 1996). However, other reports have not supported a role for T cells in protection from JEV infection (Pan et al., 2001). In their study, neither enriched JEV primed T cells nor B cells were able to protect mice from JEV infection. Further, in their JEV challenge experiments in immunoglobulin (Ig), $CD4^+$ or $CD8^+$ T knockout mice immunized with envelope DNA vaccine, it was observed that protection was abrogated only in Ig and $CD4^+$ knockout mice but not in $CD8^+$ knockout mice suggesting that only $CD4^+$ but not $CD8^+$ T cells were required for protection. Nonetheless, $CD8^+$ T cell activation may contribute to disease pathogenesis in the case of other flaviviruses. It has been shown that mice lacking perforin and Fas/FasL expression were protected from MVEV-induced disease (Licon Luna et al., 2002). Similarly a immunopathological role for $CD8^+$ T cells has been reported for dengue virus (An et al., 2004).

JEV specific T cell responses were observed in peripheral blood mononuclear cells (PBMCs) collected from vaccinees who had received a purified formalin inactivated JEV vaccine as well as JEV patients (Konishi et al., 1995). Both $CD4^+$ and $CD8^+$ T cell subsets directed against structural proteins were observed in PBMCs isolated from vaccinees that are directed against structural proteins. In contrast, PBMCs from JEV patients showed $CD4^+$ and $CD8^+$ responses to nonstructural or C proteins.

Nonstructural proteins play a major role in the initiation of T cell responses and among the non-structural proteins, NS3 is the major target of JEV-specific cell mediated immune responses, whereas NS5 is the weakest. In another study, cytolytic $CD4^+$ T cell clones have been generated from PBMCs of individuals immunized with inactivated JEV vaccine (Aihara et al., 1998). These $CD4^+$ CTLs recognized the envelope protein and were flavivirus cross reactive in nature. The significance of such $CD4^+$ T cells in an *in vivo* context is not clear. NS3 protein (region aa193-324) is a dominant source of epitopes for both $CD4^+$ and $CD8^+$ T cells in PBMCs isolated from children belonging to a JE endemic region of India. NS3 stimulated IFN-γ production by both the $CD4^+$ and $CD8^+$ T cells indicates that a Th1 immune response to the NS3 protein may be a critical determinant of immune control during JEV infection (Kumar et al., 2004a; Kumar et al., 2004b). Recombinant JEV domain III has also been shown to elicit a Th1 type of response in Balb/c mice (Verma et al., 2009).

JEV infection using the mouse model has been reported to result in differential secretion of cytokines in the brain, spleen and sera that depended on the route of inoculation. This differential secretion could influence the overall balance between Th1 and Th2 predominance after infection and thus determine its outcome. The expression of IL-4 and IL-10 increased immediately after intracerebral (i.c.) challenge with virus and decreased later as virus load increased with concomitant increases in the expression of TNFα and IFN-γ. The levels of IL-4 and TNFα but not IL-10 and IFN-γ increased in the serum of these challenged animals (Saxena et al., 2008a). However, intraperitoneal challenge resulted in an increase in the expression of all these cytokines in the spleen (Saxena et al., 2008b). Thus, while TNFα and IFN-γ could be involved in rapid virus clearance from the periphery, they could exacerbate inflammation within the CNS.

Recent reports suggest that different flaviviruses are able to infect dendritic cells (DCs) both *in vitro* and *in vivo* and alter their phenotype and function (Cao et al., 2011). JEV is able to infect macrophages as well as dendritic cells derived from the bone marrow and spleen but it appears to have dual action on these two different antigen presenting cells of the immune system. Macrophages and DCs are antigen presenting cells that produce several cytokines such as TNFα and IL-6 upon virus infection or activation (Zhang et al., 2001). DC maturation is associated with increased antigen presentation, increased synthesis and secretion of proinflammatory cytokines such as TNFα, IL-12 and IL-6, upregulation of costimulatory molecules such as CD80, CD86 and CD40 and alteration of chemokine receptors (Kawai and Akira, 2006). They are also the principal cells that express toll-like receptor (TLR) molecules for pathogen recognition and therefore, important for innate immune responses. JEV infection of macrophages resulted in increased synthesis of cytokines and costimulatory markers but JEV infection of DCs *in vitro* led to suppressed activation, enhanced CCL2 (MCP-1) release and more prominently secretion of IL-10, a cytokine that suppresses T cell response (Pestka et al., 2004). All these mediators namely TNFα, IL-10, CCL2 and type I IFNs are crucial modulators of viral infections and have the ability to alter the polarization of Th1 and Th2 cells. Endogenous IL-10 has also been shown to decrease during JEV infection (Swarup et al., 2007a) using immuno-histochemical approaches. However, the observation that infected DCs activated Foxp3+ regulatory T (Treg) cells suggests that JEV may have the ability to suppress ongoing immune responses although this ability may not be sufficient to suppress the virus-triggered inflammatory response. Taken together with the observation that the highly efficient vaccine strain SA14-14-2 of JEV stimulated DC function and suppressed Foxp3+ Treg cells suggests an important role for dendritic cells in the JEV mediated disease process (Li et al., 2011). JEV infection has also been found to result in the

depletion of splenic $CD8\alpha^+CD11c^+$ DCs as well as suppression of MHC-I mediated antigen presentation leading to suppression of $CD8^+$ T cells (Aleyas et al., 2010).
DCs play a critical role in antigen presentation and alterations in DC function will lead to altered adaptive immune responses. However, DCs are also capable of initiating innate immune responses against viruses through TLRs that are expressed on the cell surface or intracellularly. TLRs use the pan adaptor MyD88 molecule to transduce downstream TLR signaling events. The cytokine profile induced in JEV infected DCs from wild type mice was considerably reduced in DCs that were obtained from TLR2 and TLR3 deficient mice. JEV-induced functional impairment of DCs finally led to altered $CD4^+$ and $CD8^+$ T cell function. It is hence significant that this was mediated through MyD88 dependent and independent signalling pathways implicating the involvement of TLRs in JEV pathogenesis (Aleyas et al., 2009). TLR3 plays a role in WNV entry into the CNS and has been shown to play an important immunopathological role in the WNV induced CNS disease. TLR3 deficient mice show an impaired microglial TNFα response and hence decreased primary neuronal damage and absence of encephalitis (Wang et al., 2004). All these observations suggest that JEV can modulate both adaptive and innate immunity.

6. Pathogenesis

Altered cytokine secretion profiles and the balance between proinflammatory and anti-inflammatory cytokines determine the outcome of disease processes. Immunoprotective responses to JEV infection lead to the secretion of proinflammatory cytokines in the initial phases but overproduction of these cytokines shift the balance and cause neuronal injury. JEV infection in humans is associated with elevated levels of proinflammatory mediators such as IFNα, TNFα, MIF, IL-8, IL-6, (CCL5) RANTES, Cox-2, IL-1β and (CCL2) MCP-1 (Ghoshal et al., 2007; Burke and Morill, 1987) in the CSF and/or serum. Increasing levels of such cytokines in the serum and CSF of JEV patients have been correlated with higher mortality rates (Ravi et al., 1997).
Activation of CNS cells such as microglia and astrocytes is a major histological feature of JEV infection both in animals and humans infected with JEV, MVE and WNV. JEV is a neurotropic virus and infects relatively immature neurons (Kimura-Kuroda et al., 1993), astrocytes and microglial cells which might serve as a reservoir for the virus (Thongtan et al., 2010). Several studies report the interaction of JEV with microglia and astrocytes leading to production of chemokines, inflammatory mediators and neuronal degeneration. The chemokines, CCL5 and CCL2 that are produced from JEV infected cells (Das et al., 2009a; Chen et al., 2004) result in the extravasation of activated T cells and macrophages into the brain and leads to the stimulation of microglial cells within the CNS. IL-6, MCP-1 and RANTES promote leukocyte infiltration into the brain while IP10 production by infected astrocytes leads to infiltration of NK cells and monocytes (Bhowmick et al., 2007).
Neuronal degeneration as a consequence of JEV infection may be brought about directly or indirectly. Direct effects of JEV within neurons are due to virus replication leading to cytopathicity and cell death while indirect effects are due to the action of inflammatory mediators that are produced as a result of virus infection (Ghosh and Basu, 2009). Cytotoxic effects can be the result of oxidative stress caused by the overproduction of reactive oxygen species (ROS), free radical derivatives of molecular oxygen and hydrogen peroxide. JEV has been shown to activate the ROS mediated pathway (Lin et al., 2004b) and JEV infection of primary neurons/glia, mixed glia, microglia and astrocytes results in the stimulation of

RANTES production (Chen et al., 2004). TNFα and IL-1 released during the inflammatory processes occurring in the JEV infected CNS play an important role in the induction of RANTES gene expression. These responses along with other proinflammatory cytokines increase upon JEV infection of cells within the CNS and lead to uncontrolled microglial activation and neuronal cell death. Although activated astroglial cells have the ability to neutralize the toxic effects of free radicals, they may be unable to deal with the uncontrolled inflammatory effects of JEV infection (Ghosh and Basu, 2009). In addition to the triggering of an inflammatory cascade, JEV has been shown to inhibit the proliferation of neural progenitor stem cells and thus block the replenishment of damaged neural cells which could be one of the reasons for the sequelae that are observed in surviving JEV patients. Nitric oxide (NO) is also another antiviral factor secreted from the infiltrating leukocytes and blocks virus replication (Lin et al., 1997) but the high levels of NO produced cause oxidative bystander damage leading to further neuronal damage. NO plays an important role in other flaviviral infections as well and has been reviewed elsewhere (King et al., 2007).

Programmed cell death (PCD) or apoptosis is a prominent consequence of flaviviral replication within infected cells and the ensuing release of inflammatory mediators such as TNFα (Ghosh and Basu, 2009). JEV infection triggers perturbation of ER homeostasis and the unfolded protein response, thus accelerating ER stress-induced apoptosis (Liao et al., 1997). Apoptosis can also be mediated by the virus induced release of ROS which is an antiviral defense response. JEV infection has been shown to cause apoptosis of neuroblastoma cells and activates caspase 8 and 9 in a FADD-independent and mitochondrion-dependent manner (Tsao et al., 2008). JEV non structural protein NS3 along with NS2B expression enhances apoptosis via caspase-3 activation as well as decreased mitochondrial membrane potential in human medulloblastoma cells (Yang et al., 2009).

Many of the observations made above have been supported by the results obtained recently from genomic expression profiling. Whole genomic expression profiling by cDNA microarray of JEV infected mouse brain cerebral cortex (Gupta and Rao, 2011) revealed the activation of several genes participating in immune response, inflammatory response, cell adhesion, defense response, proteolysis, endocytosis and chemokine signaling. Several other genes involved with the cell cycle, endocytosis, leukotriene metabolism, signal transduction, transcription, cell adhesion and apoptosis were downregulated during the course of disease. Significantly, genes encoding caspases 1 and 5 characteristic of the inflammasome complex were upregulated supporting the occurrence of inflammation during JEV infection. Although the exact manner in which the plethora of upregulated genes play a role in JEV mediated disease is still to be worked out, it is significant that many lectin receptors, TLR 2 and 3, OAS family, guanylate nucleotide binding proteins and TRIM family of proteins are among those that are altered. In general, these results corroborate the expression profiles that have been reported for WNV (Koh and Ng, 2005; Venter et al., 2005).

7. Interferons, MHC and NF-κB mediated regulation

IFNs play a major role in viral infections and the importance of type-I and type-II IFN in controlling viral infection was clearly demonstrated in mice which are unresponsive to either IFN-α/β or IFN-γ (Muller et al., 1994). Type-I IFN mediated immune response is the main innate immune mechanism of the host against viral infection. IFNs are one of the best characterized components of the immune system. They act in paracrine fashion to induce gene expression through the engagement of cell surface IFN receptors and by activating the

Jak-Stat signaling pathway. The coordinated activities of multiple cellular transcription factors such as IRFs, NF-κB, and c-Jun/ATF-2 are responsible for the induction of type-1 IFNs during viral infection (Doly et al., 1998; Wathelet et al., 1998). During JEV infection, both NF-κB and interferon regulatory factor-3 (IRF3) mediated signaling events are involved in the induction of IFN-β (Chang et al., 2006). WNV infection has been shown to induce IFN-β and several IFN-stimulated genes (ISG) late in the infection of cultured cells due to the delayed activation of IRF-3 (Fredericksen et al., 2004). High levels of IFN-α have been detected in patients with dengue fever or dengue hemorrhagic fever (Kurane et al., 1993). IFN-α activity was also detected in the plasma and cerebrospinal fluid specimens from patients infected with JEV (Winter et al., 2004; Burke and Morill, 1987). Type-I IFNs are produced by most cell types soon after viral infection whereas, IFN-γ is produced by a restricted set of cells of the immune system such as NK cells, $CD4^+$ T helper 1 (Th1) cells and CTLs. Although IFN-γ may play a protective role, it has been shown that lethality was less severe in WNV infected IFN-γ knockout mice suggesting that IFN-γ may be a contributory factor in the establishment of immunopathology (King et al., 2007).

Pretreatment of cell cultures with IFN-α and IFN-β inhibits the replication of flaviviruses including JEV, YFV and WNV (Ajariyakhajorn et al., 2005; Samuel and Diamond, 2005; Scherbik et al., 2007) However, the use of IFN-α in clinical trials for the treatment of JEV infection has not been successful (Solomon et al., 2003). This may be because many flaviviruses such as JEV, WNV and KUNV have developed different strategies to overcome the antiviral activities of type-I IFNs (Liu et al., 2005; Munoz-Jordan et al., 2005; Guo et al., 2005; Lin et al., 2004a; Munoz-Jordan et al., 2003). NS2A of WNV prevents the translocation of Stat1 and Stat2 into the nucleus by preventing their phosphorylation (Liu et al., 2006a). JEV is known to escape from the action of IFNs by preventing both Tyk2 tyrosine phosphorylation as well as Stat activation, thereby blocking the IFN stimulated Jak-Stat signaling (Lin et al., 2004a). This inhibition of Tyk2 tyrosine phosphorylation and Stat activation is mediated by the nonstructural protein NS5 of JEV (Lin et al., 2006). It has recently been shown that JEV encoded NS4A is able to block the phosphorylation of Stat1 and Stat2 but not Tyk2 activation in response to IFN-α/β (Lin et al., 2008a). In addition to IFNs, ISGs 49, 54 and 56 as well as the double stranded RNA activated protein kinase (PKR) and 2′,5′-oligoadenylate synthetase may play important roles in flavivirus infections (King et al., 2007).

NF-κB induced transcriptional activation plays an important role in the production of type-I IFNs during viral infection and the consequent initiation of antiviral immune responses. Many viruses have evolved different strategies either to disrupt or activate NF-κB signaling and modulate host immune response with the help of viral proteins. The NF-κB activation by viruses such as HIV-1, HTLV-1, HHV8, EBV and Influenza virus serves different functions such as to promote viral replication, to prevent virus-induced apoptosis as well as to modulate cellular apoptosis and growth (Hiscott et al., 2006; Hiscott et al., 2001). It has been shown that both JEV and WNV infections induce NF-κB activation (Kesson and King, 2001; Liao et al., 2001).

There are 2 different pathways of NF-κB activation, the classical or canonical pathway and the alternate or noncanonical pathway. The NF-κB factor is a dimer composed of different Rel proteins and is retained in the cytoplasm of a resting cell by three inhibitor proteins, IκBα, IκBβ and IκBε. In the canonical pathway, stimulus-responsive phosphorylation of the IκBs by IκB kinase (IKK) complex leads to their degradation to allow for nuclear translocation of the NF-κB dimers. The IKK complex is composed of two catalytic subunits, IKK1 (IKKα), and IKK2 (IKKβ) and the regulatory subunit IKK3 (NEMO). IKK1 kinase is dispensable for the canonical pathway of NF-κB activation (Scheidereit, 2006). However, the noncanonical pathway critically depends on IKK1 activity for NF-κB signaling. Hence mutant mouse embryonic fibroblasts lacking in any one of these kinases or the Rel counterparts have been used to dissect the roles of the canonical and noncanonical pathways (Basak and Hoffmann, 2008). Both the classical and the alternate NF-κB signaling pathways play important but distinct roles in the functioning of the immune system. The classical pathway is largely responsible for the regulation of inflammation as well as the control of proliferation and apoptosis of lymphoid cells during the immune response. In contrast, the alternate pathway is associated with the development of lymphoid organs that ensure the mounting of an effective immune response. JEV infection also activates NF-κB in glial cells and primary mouse brain astrocytes (Abraham et al., 2008; Liao et al., 2001). Using $IKK1^{-/-}$, $IKK2^{-/-}$, $IKK3^{-/-}$ and $IKK1^{-/-}IKK2^{-/-}$ double mutant as well as $RelA^{-/-}cRel^{-/-}p50^{-/-}$ triple mutant mouse embryonic fibroblasts infected with JEV, it has been shown that JEV activates the classical pathway of NF-κB activation in a IKK2- and IKK3- but not IKK1-dependent manner that involved RelA and p50 complexes. NF-κB dependent and independent mechanisms also critically determined type I IFN induction in JEV infected MEFs (Abraham et al., 2010).

In addition to its involvement in immune responses, apoptosis and the cell cycle (Bonizzi and Karin, 2004), NF-κB has been shown to play a major role in flavivirus-mediated induction of MHC-I (Cheng et al., 2004). Both NF-κB dependent and independent mechanisms regulate WNV-induced MHC-I expression on infected cells. MHC molecules play an important role in host responses to viral infection and the consequences of virus infection on the expression of MHC molecules are varied. Many viruses such as HIV, MCMV, HCMV, AdV and EBV are known to decrease the expression of MHC molecules upon infection (Lilley and Ploegh, 2005). On the other hand, WNV induces the cell surface expression of both MHC-I and MHC-II molecules (Kesson et al., 2002) and the induced MHC-II was functionally intact in mouse brain astrocytes since it was associated with better recognition by a class II MHC reactive T cell line (Liu et al., 1989). In contrast to WNV, JEV infection of primary mouse brain astrocytes induces MHC-I but is unable to induce MHC-II. JEV-induced MHC-I expression was also associated with induced transcription of molecules involved in antigen processing and presentation such as *Tap1, Tap2, Tapasin, Lmp2, Lmp*7 and *Lmp10* (Abraham and Manjunath, 2006). The absence of MHC-II induction during JEV infection could be important because it may lead to the initiation of an immune response which is different from other flaviviral infections that induce the expression of MHC-II molecules. Again, in contrast to WNV, the use of knockout MEFs showed that JEV-mediated induction of classical MHC-I molecules remained unaffected in NF-κB defective cells but was completely dependent on type I IFNs (Abraham et al., 2010).

In contrast to classical MHC molecules, the nonclassical MHC molecules do not belong to a single group of structurally and functionally homologous proteins and normally have lower cell surface expression. They play an important role in bridging adaptive and innate immune responses. Nonclassical MHC-I family members include gene products from HLA-E, F, G and H in humans and H2-Q, H2-T and H2-M regions in mice (Shawar et al., 1994). JEV infection of primary mouse brain astrocytes induced the expression of nonclassical MHC-I or class Ib molecules in addition to the induction of classical MHC-I molecules (Abraham and Manjunath, 2006). Given the distinct regulations of the classical and nonclassical MHC-I molecules, it was of interest to evaluate the role of the NF-κB pathway in nonclassical MHC-I gene expression.

We analyzed the role of NF-κB mediated signaling in the induction of nonclassical MHC-I molecules during JEV infection. WT, IKK1-/-, IKK2-/- and IKK3-/- MEFs were harvested at different time intervals p.i. and expression of nonclassical MHC-I molecules was analyzed by semi quantitative RT-PCR analysis. As shown in Figure 2A, JEV infection induced the transcription of Qa-1, T10 and Qb1 in IKK1-/-, IKK2-/- and IKK3-/- MEFs. To further validate this observation that the induction of nonclassical MHC-I molecules during JEV infection occurs independent of NF-κB activation, IKK1-/-IKK2-/- double mutant MEFs were harvested at different time intervals p.i. and expression of nonclassical MHC-I molecules was analyzed by semiquantitative RT-PCR. As shown in Figure 2B, JEV infection induced the transcription of Qa-1 and Qb1 in IKK1-/-IKK2-/- MEFs confirming our results that JEV-induced expression of Qa-1 and Qb1 occurs independent of NF-κB activation. The role of type-I IFNs in the induction of nonclassical MHC-I molecules during JEV infection was then determined. IFNAR-/- and IFNGR-/- MEFs were harvested at different time intervals p.i. and the expression of Qa-1, Qb1 and T10 was analyzed by RT-PCR analysis as above. As shown in Figure 2B, our RT-PCR results demonstrated that JEV-induced expression of nonclassical MHC-I molecules, Qa-1 and Qb1 was completely abrogated in IFNAR-/- MEFs but not in IFNGR-/- MEFs. In contrast, the expression of T10 was not altered in IFNAR-/- and IFNGR-/- MEFs. Thus, our results clearly show that JEV-induced expression of Qb1 and Qa-1 was dependent on type-I IFN mediated signaling. In contrast, the induction of T-10 was independent of type-I IFN mediated signaling.

The functional role of the induced nonclassical molecule T10 in the activation of γδ T cells was further analyzed. JEV infected cells were added to a cloned γδ T cell clone called G8 that responds by secretion of IL-2 upon specific recognition of the T10 molecule on the surface of cells. The G8 clone was kindly provided by Dr Chien, Stanford university school of medicine, USA. As shown in Fig 2C, exposure of G8 to JEV infected H-6 cells resulted in IL-2 secretion suggesting that the induced T10 on H6 could be functional. However, the relevance of this observation in the larger *in vivo* context is still unclear.

The involvement of γδ T cells has been shown in the case of WNV but no information is available with JEV. Mice deficient in TCRδ (TCRδ-/-) were found to be more susceptible to WNV infection and exhibited higher viral titres in blood and lymph organs (Wang et al., 2003). A higher IFN-γ production and enhanced perforin expression in splenic T cells in WT mice as compared to TCRδ-/- mice was proposed to be responsible for higher survival of WT mice in WNV infection. In a recent report, it has been shown that WNV is capable of infecting γδ T-cells which leads to maturation of dendritic cells by production of IFN-γ, TNF-α and IL-6, thus facilitating adaptive immune responses as well (Fang et al., 2010).

The avidity of T cell-target interactions and the threshold for T cell activation is the result of both specific (MHC-I associated) as well as nonspecific interactions due to adhesion molecules such as ICAM-1 (Lebedeva et al., 2005). Hence, virus-induced alterations in ICAM-1 and/or VCAM-1 expression can lead to alterations not only in T cell activation but also in the leukocyte subsets attaching to the infected cells and consequently altering host cell-virus interactions. In addition to inhibition of IFN signaling, flaviviruses have been shown to modulate the expression of MHC and adhesion molecules such as VCAM and ICAM on the cell surface. Using endothelial cells, it has also been shown that flaviviruses such as WNV increases the cell surface expression of adhesion molecules such as ICAM-1, VCAM-1 as well as E-selectin. These changes were mediated by WNV in a NF-κB dependent but IFN and TNF independent manner (Shen et al., 1997).

We have reported that the cell surface expression of adhesion molecules ICAM-1 and VCAM-1 was significantly induced on primary astrocyte cultures but not hepatoma cells, L929 and 3T3 fibroblasts. Hence we observed that the JEV induced the cell surface expression of adhesion molecules does not occur uniformly on all cell types (Abraham et al., 2008). Since NF-κB transcriptionally controls the expression of ICAM-1 and VCAM-1, we further analyzed the role of NF-κB in the induction of adhesion molecules by JEV. Only VCAM-1 but not ICAM-1 was induced by JEV on mouse embryonic fibroblasts (MEFs) and knockout MEFs are the cell types that are generally utilized for analyzing the role of this transcriptional factor in gene induction studies. Hence WT (wild type), IKK1$^{-/-}$, IKK2$^{-/-}$ and IKK3$^{-/-}$ MEFs were harvested at different time intervals p.i. and expression of VCAM-1 was analyzed by flow cytometry. As shown in Figure 3, JEV infection induced the cell surface expression of VCAM-1 in IKK1$^{-/-}$MEFs but not in IKK2$^{-/-}$ and IKK3$^{-/-}$ MEFs. The basal level of expression of VCAM-1 was high in IKK2$^{-/-}$ and IKK3$^{-/-}$ MEFs. We also analyzed the status of VCAM-1 in IKK1$^{-/-}$IKK2$^{-/-}$ double knockout and RelA$^{-/-}$cRel$^{-/-}$p50$^{-/-}$triple knockout MEFs upon JEV infection by flow cytometry. As shown in Figure 3, JEV-induced expression of VCAM-1 was completely abrogated in both mutants. The basal level of expression of VCAM-1 was high in IKK1$^{-/-}$IKK2$^{-/-}$ MEFs whereas, it was low in RelA$^{-/-}$cRel$^{-/-}$p50$^{-/-}$ MEFs. This lack of induction of VCAM-1 in RelA$^{-/-}$cRel$^{-/-}$p50$^{-/-}$ MEFs indicates that the canonical pathway of NF-κB mediated signaling events are involved in the induction of VCAM-1 during JEV infection.

To determine whether JEV infection induces the expression of VCAM-1 molecules on MEFs deficient in IFN signaling, WT, IFNAR$^{-/-}$ and IFNGR$^{-/-}$ MEFs were harvested at different time intervals p.i. and the expression of VCAM-1 was analyzed by flow cytometry. As shown in the Figure 3, there was no induction of VCAM-1 on both IFNAR$^{-/-}$ and IFNGR$^{-/-}$ MEFs during JEV infection. All these results indicated that both NF-κB and type-I IFNs play a major role in the induction of VCAM-1 during JEV infection.

It has been reported that the induction of VCAM-1 molecules in response to TNF-α treatment is mediated by the coordinated activity of NF-κB and IRF-1 (Neish et al., 1995). It has also been reported that the Concanavalin A (Con A) induced expression of VCAM-1 is reduced in IRF-1$^{-/-}$ hepatic cells as compared to that of WT cells (Jaruga et al., 2004). These results point to the importance of IRF-1 in the induction of VCAM-1 molecules. However, to our surprise there was no increase of VCAM-1 on JEV infected IFNAR$^{-/-}$ MEFs but it has also been reported that IL-6 mediated induction of IRF-1 was reduced in IFNAR$^{-/-}$ MEFs as compared to that of WT MEFs (Mitani et al., 2001). Hence, we believe that the defective activity of IRF-1 in IFNAR$^{-/-}$ MEFs may be responsible for the lack of induction of VCAM-1 on IFNAR$^{-/-}$ MEFs upon JEV infection. This brings forth the possibility that even during JEV infection, the coordinated activity of both NF-κB and IRF-1 might be responsible for the induction of VCAM-1. At the same time there is one report which shows that IRF-1 is not activated upon JEV infection of human A549 cells (Chang et al., 2006) but the effects of JEV infection could be different on human cells. The mechanism of induction of ICAM-1 during JEV infection could not be characterized using knockout MEFs because ICAM-1 was induced only in astrocytes but not in MEFs.

8. Vaccines and viral inhibitors

Given the importance of flavivirus mediated encephalitis worldwide, it is not surprising that considerable efforts are underway to develop several antiviral strategies against these viruses. These efforts include the development of antiviral drugs that inhibit not only the virus and its interactions with the host but also the development of vaccines that are aimed at strengthening antiviral immune responses as well as mosquito vector control measures to stop the spread of virus.The current vaccines that are under study are the inactivated mouse brain derived vaccine, the inactivated cell culture vaccines, the live attenuated vaccine, and the chimeric yellow fever/JE virus vaccine.

The BIKEN (JE-VAX) vaccine is derived from formalin inactivated JEV infected mouse brain and a crude inactivated version was tested in Japan as early as 1930s. The currently available version was in use from 1966. Mouse brain derived inactivated JE vaccines are based on genotype-III strains Nakayama or Beijing-1. It is prepared by clarification of Nakayama or Beijing JEV infected mouse brain suspensions by low speed centrifugation, followed by formalin inactivation, ultrafiltration, ammonium sulphate precipitation, ultracentrifugation through a 40% sucrose density gradient and dialysis (Takaku et al., 1968; Oya, 1988). This vaccine has been found to induce both JE specific and flavivirus cross reactive HLA restricted $CD4^+$ cytotoxic T cells directed against the envelope protein of the virus (Aihara et al., 1998). Vaccinated individuals exposed to infection with JEV have both memory B- and T-cell and CTL responses to the envelope protein (Aihara et al., 1998; Konishi et al., 1995). Adverse reactions have also been observed in field trials with this vaccine. These include injection site reactions (erthema, swelling, tenderness) in approximately 20% volunteers and systemic side effects (fever, headache, malaise, rashes, chills, dizziness, myaglia, nausea, vomiting and abdominal pain) in 5-10% of volunteers (Andersen and Ronne, 1991; Ruff et al., 1991; Poland et al., 1990; Hoke et al., 1988). This vaccine finds limited use in developing countries because of its high cost and has been discontinued from 2005 (Tauber et al., 2007).

Effective formalin Inactivated cell culture derived vaccine was first produced and used in China since 1960s. This was prepared from JEV infected primary hamster kidney (PHK) cells (Tsai et al., 1999). The inactivated Beijing-3 virus produced from PHK cells is the P-3 vaccine. Concerns about the presence of animal proteins in this vaccine led to development of cell culture vaccine from Vero cells infected with SA14-14-2 strain of JEV that has been adapted to PDK-8 (primary dog kidney cells). Its protective efficacy was tested in mice and phase I clinical trials (Srivastava et al., 2001). Similarly, another vaccine was derived from Vero cells infected with the Beijing strain of JEV. Phase I clinical trial of this Vero cell culture derived vaccine in 269 adult males identified a low rate of mild adverse events and greater or equivalent seroconversion rates compared to mouse brain derived vaccine (Kuzuhara et al., 2003; Sugawara et al., 2002). A vero cell-derived inactivated JE vaccine containing the purified, inactivated JEV strain SA14-14-2 with aluminum hydroxide as adjuvant has passed the Phase III randomized controlled trial (Tauber et al., 2007). A new inactivated vaccine licensed in US, Europe and Australia is also prepared from SA14-14-2 grown in Vero cells and is called IC-51 (IXIARO).

Another important vaccine is the live attenuated SA14-14-2 vaccine, which is derived via extensive passage series in primary hamster kidney cells, followed by UV irradiation, plaque purification and passage in hamsters and suckling mice (Ni et al., 1994; Aihara et al., 1991). SA14-14-2 was licensed in china in 1988 and provides 80-96% protection after a single dose and further studies in China have shown 97.5% efficacy after 2 doses 1 year apart (Tandan et al., 2007; Hennessy et al., 1996; Xin et al., 1988). Seroconversion of 99-100% and neutralizing antibody titres of 1:50 to 1:150 has been observed in field trials with this vaccine in China and South Korea (Tsai, 2000; Sohn et al., 1999; Tsai et al., 1999). Very few side effects were observed. It is now being used in Indian, Nepal and Sri Lanka.

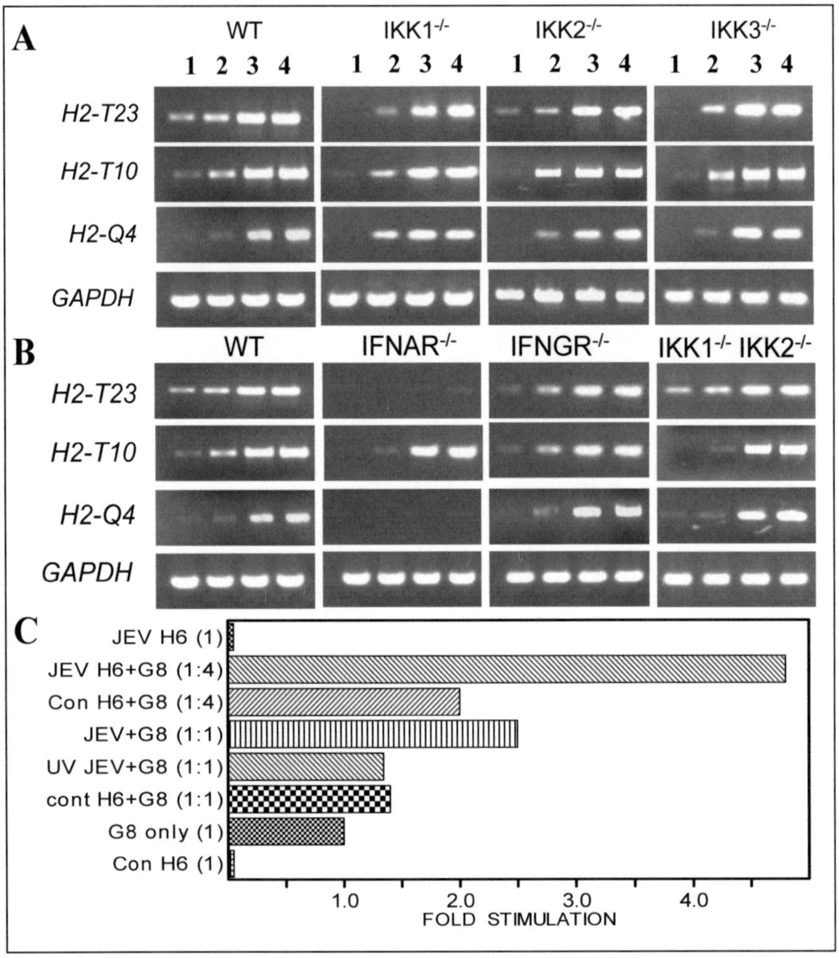

Fig. 2. JEV infection and expression of nonclassical MHC-I molecules in wild type (WT) and mutant MEFs. Panel A represents the semi quantitative RT-PCR analysis carried out for 35 cycles with uninfected and JEV infected WT, IKK1-/-, IKK2-/- and IKK3-/- MEFs. Panel B represents the semi quantitative RT-PCR analysis carried out for 35 cycles with uninfected and JEV infected WT, IFNAR-/-, IFNGR-/- and IKK1-/-IKK2-/- double mutant MEFs. Lane 1 represents the result obtained from cells that were mock infected for 36 hr while lanes 2-4 represent results obtained from cells infected for 12, 24 and 36 hr. Protocols, procedures and gene specific primers used are published elsewhere (Abraham *et al.*, 2010). Panel C represents IL-2 secretion from G8, γδ T cell clone upon activation with JEV infected H6 hepatoma cells. G8 cells were cultured for 24 hr alone (G8 only) or with H6 cells (Cont H6+G8), JEV infected H6 (JEV H6+G8) and H6 infected with UV inactivated JEV (UV JEV H6+G8). Uninfected H6 (Con H6) and infected H6 cultures were also cultured separately and the cell culture supernatants collected after 24 hr of stimulation were evaluated for IL-2 secretion by ELISA (BD biosciences). Values in parenthesis represent the ratios of G8:H6 cells used when 10^3 H6 cells were used for all cultures. Data from one of two different experiments are represented as fold stimulation relative to the IL-2 secretion from G8 cultured alone for 24 hr. The G8 clone was obtained as a kind gift from Dr. YH Chien, Stanford University School of Medicine, California, USA (Crowley *et al.*, 1997)

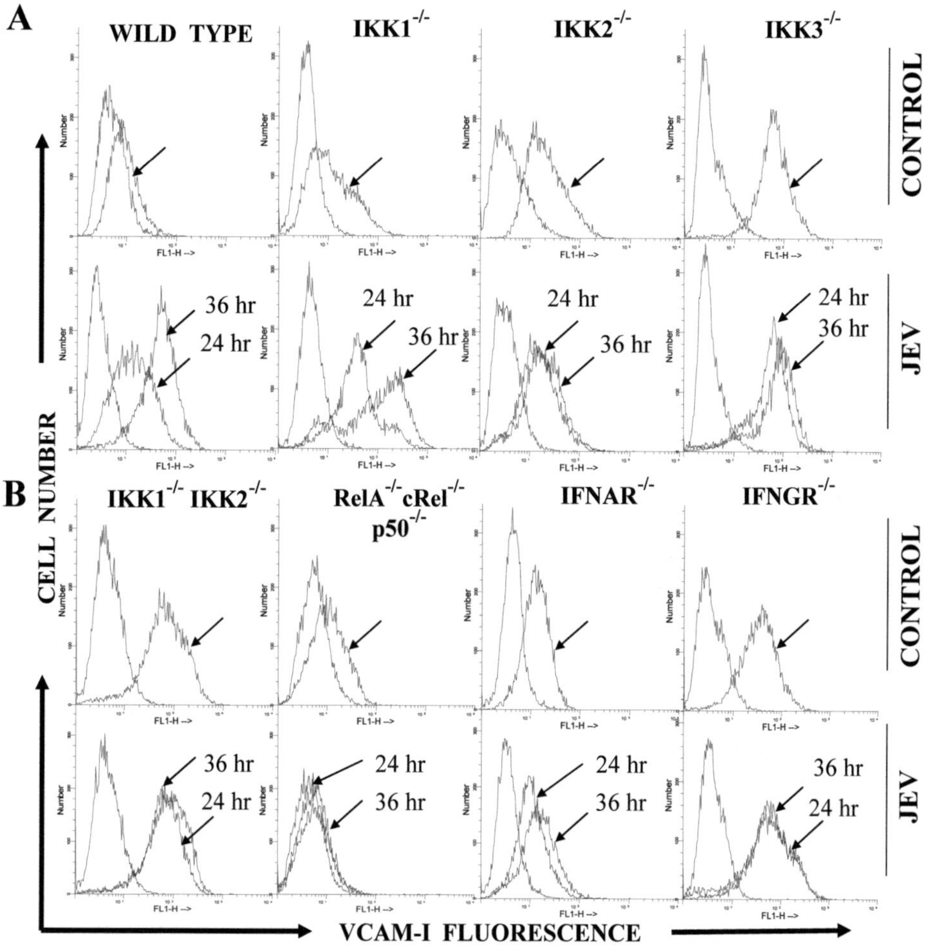

Fig. 3. JEV infection and expression of VCAM-1 on Wild type and knockout mouse embryo fibroblasts (MEFs) defective in NF-κB and interferon signaling. Wild type and knockout MEFs were infected with JEV for 24 and 36 hr and the cell surface expression of VCAM-1 was analyzed by flow cytometry. Panel A: As indicated, the upper panel (CONTROL) represents uninfected cells while the lower panel (JEV) represents infected WT, IKK1-/-, IKK2-/- and IKK3-/- cells. Panel B: As indicated, the upper panel (CONTROL) represents uninfected cells while the lower panel (JEV) represents infected IKK1-/-IKK2-/- double mutant, RelA-/-cRel-/-p50-/- triple mutant, IFNAR-/- and IFNGR-/- cells. Unmarked histograms represent staining with FITC conjugated secondary antibody alone in both panels while arrow-marked histograms in the upper panel indicate staining with unlabeled primary antibody (clone 429; anti CD 106) followed by FITC conjugated secondary antibody. They represent basal VCAM-1 expression in uninfected cells. In the lower panel, the arrows represent 24 and 36 hr post infection. Protocols, procedures and nomenclature followed are published elsewhere (Abraham *et al.*, 2010)

A chimeric yellow fever/JE virus vaccine was constructed by Chambers *et al.* (1999) by substitution of prM and E genes from the highly attenuated YFV strain (strain YF17D) with that of JEV. Studies in mice and monkey models have shown that this chimeric vaccine was highly immunogenic and protects the animals against lethal JEV i.c. challenge (Monath et al., 2000; Guirakhoo et al., 1999; Monath et al., 1999). Phase I and II clinical trials of the vaccine have been carried out and it was found to be well tolerated and induced neutralizing antibodies in 100% of naïve and yellow fever virus immune participants. In both trials it was found that a single dose of the chimeric vaccine was sufficient to elicit high titre of neutralizing antibodies (Monath et al., 2003; Monath et al., 2002). Although this vaccine was developed using genotype III virus, it stimulates protective antibodies against other genotypes as well (Beasley et al., 2004).

In addition to the development of the vaccines mentioned above, numerous studies have utilized the importance of protective epitopes in the E and NS1 protein as the basis for development of subunit vaccines to JEV. These attempts show varying degrees of protection in mouse models and use three different approaches using 1) direct protein immunization, 2) recombinant pox viruses and 3) recombinant DNA. These are discussed below:

Direct protein immunizations

These studies have evaluated different mouse model systems to evaluate the protection offered after immunization with JEV antigens in the form of recombinant subviral particles produced from cell lines, synthetic and CNBr cleaved fragments of E protein or different JEV antigens isolated from different expression systems either in the crude or purified forms.

It is known that non-infectious extracellular particles (EP) containing the M and E proteins without the nucleocapsid are secreted from BHK and Vero cells infected with a JEV prM-E-NS1-NS2A gene recombinant vaccinia virus (Mason et al., 1991). These EPs have been thought to be a promising candidate for a second generation JE subunit vaccine. Mice immunized with EPs produced from HeLa cells infected with recombinant vaccinia viruses expressing prM and E genes of JEV showed good neutralizing antibody titres and 100% protection (Konishi et al., 1992b) as well as long lasting virus specific memory T cells in mice (Konishi et al., 1997b). Similar success in affording protection was achieved with EPs from cell lines stably transformed with plasmid DNA encoding prM and E genes of JEV (Kojima et al., 2003; Hunt et al., 2001).

The C-terminal region (aa280-414) of the E protein binds several neutralizing antibodies. Hence this region or its fragments have been used in approaches that utilized their isolation from several expression systems. A protein fragment containing the C-terminal aa319-500 of the E protein was expressed along with the N-terminal 65 amino acid residues of NS1 in *E. coli* as a fusion protein with protein A. Mice immunized with this fragment produced significant protection and good neutralizing antibody titres (Srivastava et al., 1991). Mice immunized with the C-terminal region (aa280-414) of the E protein that was overexpressed in *E. coli* alone failed to generate significant protection and neutralizing antibodies. Hence, it is possible that that the N-terminal 65 amino acids of NS1 protein could have played some role in protection against viral challenge. A 27 amino acid (aa372-399) stretch within this C-terminal E fragment expressed in *E. coli,* either as a fusion protein with protein A or GST produces neutralizing antibodies (Seif et al., 1996). Immunization of mice with the same 27 amino acid peptide expressed as fusion protein with Johnson Grass Mosaic (JGM) virus-like particles also produced neutralizing antibody titres and protection was observed upon i.c. challenge with JEV (Saini and Vrati, 2003).

Expression of JEV proteins using a different expression system such as the baculovirus system has also produced moderate protection. Significant neutralizing antibody titres and moderate protection have been shown in mice immunized with recombinant baculovirus-infected spodoptera cells expressing either E protein or a polyprotein including prM, E, NS1, NS2A, NS2B and N-terminal 28 amino acids residues of NS3 (McCown et al., 1990).

Expression of different fragments of the envelope protein reported to bind neutralizing antibodies on the surface of *Saccharomyces cerevisiae* also led to the generation of anti-JEV antibodies. However, they were not protective in mice suggesting the importance of conformational determinants for protection (Upadhyaya and Manjunath, 2009). Immunization of mice with a crude extract of *Saccharomyces cerevisiae* expressing the E protein produced only low titre neutralizing antibodies (Fujita et al., 1987).

Recombinant Pox virus based immunizations

Recombinant vaccinia viruses can also be used to generate protective immunity to JEV. Neutralizing antibodies and significant levels of protection were generated by immunizing mice with recombinant vaccinia viruses expressing prM and E genes (Yasuda et al., 1990) as well as vaccinia viruses expressing prM-E-NS1-NS2A genes of JEV. Subsequent studies introduced prM and E genes into highly attenuated strains of vaccinia viruses such as NYVAC, ALVAC and MVA (Konishi et al., 1997a; Konishi et al., 1992a; Nam et al., 1999). These approaches in mice were then followed by testing the efficacy of recombinant vaccinia virus system in humans. Highly attenuated strains of vaccinia viruses NYVAC/ALVAC expressing prM and E genes of JEV (called as NYVAC-JE and ALVAC-JE) were well tolerated in volunteers but were more reactogenic as compared to volunteers immunized with licensed form of inactivated JEV vaccine. Studies revealed that NYVAC-JE induced neutralizing antibody responses only in vaccinia non-immunised recipients, vaccinia immunized volunteers failed to develop protective antibodies. NYVAC-JE was more effective in inducing antibody responses as compared to ALVAC-JE (Kanesa-thasan et al., 2000).

Recombinant DNA based immunizations

DNA vaccines have been successful against several viral infections. Immunization using recombinant DNA constructs expressing prM-E or NS1 alone and the efficient protection obtained in mice was first reported in 1998 (Lewis and Babiuk, 1999; Lin et al., 1998). A parallel report (Konishi et al., 1998) using mice immunized with DNA constructs expressing prM-E genes of JEV showed only low levels of neutralizing antibodies but 100% protection was observed upon lethal challenge of mice with JEV. $CD8^+$ CTL response to E protein was also induced following immunization with recombinant DNA constructs. Plasmid encoding NS1 gene alone was able to afford good protection as compared to previous studies (Konishi et al., 1992a; McCown et al., 1990). The protective efficacy of several genes of JEV (C, E, NS1, NS3 and NS5) by DNA based immunization have been evaluated in mice (Chen et al., 1999). In this study only the E gene construct afforded significant protection either by i.m. immunization or by gene gun immunization but they also did not detect neutralizing antibodies before challenge in these mice. Thus, it appears that mechanism of protection induced by recombinant DNA immunization is different as compared to other immunization systems. Neutralizing antibodies were observed to be weak or absent in another DNA based vaccine attempt (Ashok and Rangarajan, 2002). The efficacy of various routes (i.d., i.v, i.m., i.p.) of immunization with plasmid DNA encoding prM and E was tested when delivered along with colloidal gold. They found that i.v. and i.d. routes generated a stronger anti-E response as compared to other routes of immunization (Zhao et al., 2003).

The studies discussed above demonstrate the potential and efficacy of various vaccines employed to generate protective immunity to JEV. Various other antiflaviviral agents that have been studied are listed in Table 2.

Sl no	Antiviral Agent	Target	System used	Reference
1	Rana catesbeiana ribonuclease (RC-RNase)	enhances apoptosis in JEV-infected cells	BHK21 cells	(Lee et al., 2011)
2	Mycophenolic acid	immunosuppressant	Mouse *In vivo*	(Sebastian et al., 2011)
3	Peptide-conjugated phosphorodiamidate morpholino oligomers (PPMOs)	JEV 3' cyclization sequence (3'CSI)	Vero (epithelial), Neuro2A (neuronal), J774E cells (macrophage)	(Anantpadma et al., 2010)
4	Octaguanidinium dendrimer-conjugated Morpholino	3′ and 5′ UTRs	Mouse, *in vivo*	(Nazmi et al., 2010)
5	Cell-penetrating peptide (CPP)-PNA conjugates	cis-acting signals at the 5'-untranslated region (UTR), 3'-UTR, and genome cyclization motifs	BHK-21 cells	(Yoo et al., 2009)
6	Pentoxifylline	virus assembly and/or release	Cell line and mouse *in vivo* mouse	(Sebastian et al., 2009)
7	Aloe-emodin (compounds from Chinese herbal medicine)	upregulates expression of IFN-stimulated genes such as dsRNA-activated protein kinase and 2',5'-oligoisoadenylate synthase	Human HL-CZ promonocyte cells and TE-671 medulloblastoma cells	(Lin et al., 2008c)
8	Bovine lactoferrin	binding to cell surface expressed heparan sulfate	CHO cells	(Chien et al., 2008)
9	Arctigenin (a plant lignin)	antiviral, neuroprotective, anti-inflammatory, antioxidative effects	Mouse *In vivo*	(Swarup et al., 2008)
10	Minocycline	anti-inflammatory and antiapoptotic drug	Mouse *In vivo*	(Mishra and Basu, 2008)
11	N-methylisatin-beta-Thiosemicarbazone (MIBT) derivative (SCH 16)	inhibit JEV replication	BHK-21 and PS cells	(Sebastian et al., 2008)
12	Rosmarinic acid	antiviral and anti-inflammatory effects	Mouse *In vivo*	(Swarup et al., 2007b)
13	N-nonyl-deoxynojirimycin (NN-DNJ), an alkyl iminosugar derivative	inhibits ER α-glucosidases I and II	BHK-21 cells	(Wu et al., 2002)

Sl no	Antiviral Agent	Target	System used	Reference
14	Bafilomycin A1	vacuolar-type proton (V-H+) pump inhibitor	Vero cells	(Andoh et al., 1998)
15	siRNA	NS5	BHK-21 cells	(Qi et al., 2008)
16	siRNA	NS1	Vero cells	(Liu et al., 2006b)
17	siRNA	cd loop-coding sequence in domain II of the viral Envelope protein	BHK-21, vero, Neuro2A cells	(Kumar et al., 2006)
18	DNAZyme	3'-NCR	J774E murine macrophage & mouse *in vivo*	(Appaiahgari and Vrati, 2007)

Table 2. Antiviral agents for JEV

9. Conclusions

Flaviviruses have developed several strategies to counter the antiviral responses that are activated in the host. It is now apparent that they can inhibit both adaptive and innate immune responses such as antigen presentation, inhibition of complement factors and interferon. However, some of these strategies that may have evolved to enhance virus survival such as activation of transcriptional factors result in the activation of inflammatory host responses as well. This results in damage to the CNS, a tissue where replenishment and renewal of damage tissue is more difficult. Virus-induction of MHC molecules is also a host response that leads to antiviral mechanisms in the long run such as activation of CTL. It is believed that all these responses are aimed at inhibition of NK cells that may kill virus infected cells immediately after infection. However, the activation of nonclassical MHC molecules by JEV could be considered as a viral strategy to the inhibit NK cells since several nonclassical MHC molecules bind to NK receptors leading to their inhibition. The presence of inflammatory responses *in vivo* highlights its importance in influencing the differences that may occur during *ex vivo* and *in vitro* studies when compared to *in vivo* studies. Hence apart from the development of new approaches to eradicate the disease, a basic understanding of the nature by which this virus alters the balance between protective and immunopathological mechanisms triggered within the infected host is also important.

10. Acknowledgements

Experimental work done was supported by a grant from CSIR and the DBT, Government of India. Cytometry operations were performed by Omana Joy and M. Vamsi. Wild type and mutant MEFs were obtained from Inder Verma (Salk Institute of Biological Sciences, La Jolla), CA, Marc Schmidt Supprian (Harvard Medical School, Boston, MA) and Alexander Hoffmann (University of California, San Diego, CA) and Otto Haller (University of Frieburg, Germany) as acknowledged in Abraham et al., 2010.

11. References

Abraham, S. and Manjunath, R. (2006) Induction of classical and nonclassical MHC-I on mouse brain astrocytes by Japanese encephalitis virus. Virus Res 119(2), 216-20.

Abraham, S., Nagaraj, A.S., Basak, S. and Manjunath, R. (2010) Japanese encephalitis virus utilizes the canonical pathway to activate NF-kappaB but it utilizes the type I interferon pathway to induce major histocompatibility complex class I expression in mouse embryonic fibroblasts. J Virol 84(11), 5485-93.

Abraham, S., Yaddanapudi, K., Thomas, S., Damodaran, A., Ramireddy, B. and Manjunath, R. (2008) Nonclassical MHC-I and Japanese encephalitis virus infection: induction of H-2Q4, H-2T23 and H-2T10. Virus Res 133(2), 239-49.

Aihara, H., Takasaki, T., Matsutani, T., Suzuki, R. and Kurane, I. (1998) Establishment and characterization of Japanese encephalitis virus-specific, human CD4(+) T-cell clones: flavivirus cross-reactivity, protein recognition, and cytotoxic activity. J Virol 72(10), 8032-6.

Aihara, S., Rao, C.M., Yu, Y.X., Lee, T., Watanabe, K., Komiya, T., Sumiyoshi, H., Hashimoto, H. and Nomoto, A. (1991) Identification of mutations that occurred on the genome of Japanese encephalitis virus during the attenuation process. Virus Genes 5(2), 95-109.

Ajariyakhajorn, C., Mammen, M.P., Jr., Endy, T.P., Gettayacamin, M., Nisalak, A., Nimmannitya, S. and Libraty, D.H. (2005) Randomized, placebo-controlled trial of nonpegylated and pegylated forms of recombinant human alpha interferon 2a for suppression of dengue virus viremia in rhesus monkeys. Antimicrob Agents Chemother 49(11), 4508-14.

Alcon, S., Talarmin, A., Debruyne, M., Falconar, A., Deubel, V. and Flamand, M. (2002) Enzyme-linked immunosorbent assay specific to Dengue virus type 1 nonstructural protein NS1 reveals circulation of the antigen in the blood during the acute phase of disease in patients experiencing primary or secondary infections. J Clin Microbiol 40(2), 376-81.

Aleyas, A.G., George, J.A., Han, Y.W., Rahman, M.M., Kim, S.J., Han, S.B., Kim, B.S., Kim, K. and Eo, S.K. (2009) Functional modulation of dendritic cells and macrophages by Japanese encephalitis virus through MyD88 adaptor molecule-dependent and -independent pathways. J Immunol 183(4), 2462-74.

Aleyas, A.G., Han, Y.W., George, J.A., Kim, B., Kim, K., Lee, C.K. and Eo, S.K. (2010) Multifront assault on antigen presentation by Japanese encephalitis virus subverts CD8+ T cell responses. J Immunol 185(3), 1429-41.

Allison, S.L., Schalich, J., Stiasny, K., Mandl, C.W. and Heinz, F.X. (2001) Mutational evidence for an internal fusion peptide in flavivirus envelope protein E. J Virol 75(9), 4268-75.

An, J., Zhou, D.S., Zhang, J.L., Morida, H., Wang, J.L. and Yasui, K. (2004) Dengue-specific CD8+ T cells have both protective and pathogenic roles in dengue virus infection. Immunol Lett 95(2), 167-74.

Anantpadma, M., Stein, D.A. and Vrati, S. (2010) Inhibition of Japanese encephalitis virus replication in cultured cells and mice by a peptide-conjugated morpholino oligomer. J Antimicrob Chemother 65(5), 953-61.

Andersen, M.M. and Ronne, T. (1991) Side-effects with Japanese encephalitis vaccine. Lancet 337(8748), 1044.

Andoh, T., Kawamata, H., Umatake, M., Terasawa, K., Takegami, T. and Ochiai, H. (1998) Effect of bafilomycin A1 on the growth of Japanese encephalitis virus in Vero cells. J Neurovirol 4(6), 627-31.

Appaiahgari, M.B. and Vrati, S. (2007) DNAzyme-mediated inhibition of Japanese encephalitis virus replication in mouse brain. Mol Ther 15(9), 1593-9.

Ashok, M.S. and Rangarajan, P.N. (2002) Protective efficacy of a plasmid DNA encoding Japanese encephalitis virus envelope protein fused to tissue plasminogen activator signal sequences: studies in a murine intracerebral virus challenge model. Vaccine 20(11-12), 1563-70.

Assenberg, R., Mastrangelo, E., Walter, T.S., Verma, A., Milani, M., Owens, R.J., Stuart, D.I., Grimes, J.M. and Mancini, E.J. (2009) Crystal structure of a novel conformational state of the flavivirus NS3 protein: implications for polyprotein processing and viral replication. J Virol 83(24), 12895-906.

Basak, S. and Hoffmann, A. (2008) Crosstalk via the NF-kappaB signaling system. Cytokine Growth Factor Rev 19(3-4), 187-97.

Beasley, D.W., Li, L., Suderman, M.T., Guirakhoo, F., Trent, D.W., Monath, T.P., Shope, R.E. and Barrett, A.D. (2004) Protection against Japanese encephalitis virus strains representing four genotypes by passive transfer of sera raised against ChimeriVax-JE experimental vaccine. Vaccine 22(27-28), 3722-6.

Bhowmick, S., Duseja, R., Das, S., Appaiahgiri, M.B., Vrati, S. and Basu, A. (2007) Induction of IP-10 (CXCL10) in astrocytes following Japanese encephalitis. Neurosci Lett 414(1), 45-50.

Bollati, M., Milani, M., Mastrangelo, E., Ricagno, S., Tedeschi, G., Nonnis, S., Decroly, E., Selisko, B., de Lamballerie, X., Coutard, B., Canard, B. and Bolognesi, M. (2009) Recognition of RNA cap in the Wesselsbron virus NS5 methyltransferase domain: implications for RNA-capping mechanisms in Flavivirus. J Mol Biol 385(1), 140-52.

Bonizzi, G. and Karin, M. (2004) The two NF-kappaB activation pathways and their role in innate and adaptive immunity. Trends Immunol 25(6), 280-8.

Brandt, W.E., Chiewslip, D., Harris, D.L. and Russell, P.K. (1970) Partial purification and characterization of a dengue virus soluble complement-fixing antigen. J Immunol 105(6), 1565-8.

Burke, D.S., Lorsomrudee, W., Leake, C.J., Hoke, C.H., Nisalak, A., Chongswasdi, V. and Laorakpongse, T. (1985) Fatal outcome in Japanese encephalitis. Am J Trop Med Hyg 34(6), 1203-10.

Burke, D.S. and Morill, J.C. (1987) Levels of interferon in the plasma and cerebrospinal fluid of patients with acute Japanese encephalitis. J Infect Dis 155(4), 797-9.

Cao, S., Li, Y., Ye, J., Yang, X., Chen, L., Liu, X. and Chen, H. (2011) Japanese encephalitis Virus wild strain infection suppresses dendritic cells maturation and function, and causes the expansion of regulatory T cells. Virol J 8, 39.

Cecilia, D. and Gould, E.A. (1991) Nucleotide changes responsible for loss of neuroinvasiveness in Japanese encephalitis virus neutralization-resistant mutants. Virology 181(1), 70-7.

Chambers, T.J., Hahn, C.S., Galler, R. and Rice, C.M. (1990) Flavivirus genome organization, expression, and replication. Annu Rev Microbiol 44, 649-88.

Chambers, T.J., Nestorowicz, A., Mason, P.W. and Rice, C.M. (1999) Yellow fever/Japanese encephalitis chimeric viruses: construction and biological properties. J Virol 73(4), 3095-101.

Chang, T.H., Liao, C.L. and Lin, Y.L. (2006) Flavivirus induces interferon-beta gene expression through a pathway involving RIG-I-dependent IRF-3 and PI3K-dependent NF-kappaB activation. Microbes Infect 8(1), 157-71.

Chavez, J.H., Silva, J.R., Amarilla, A.A. and Moraes Figueiredo, L.T. (2010) Domain III peptides from flavivirus envelope protein are useful antigens for serologic diagnosis and targets for immunization. Biologicals 38(6), 613-8.

Chen, C.J., Chen, J.H., Chen, S.Y., Liao, S.L. and Raung, S.L. (2004) Upregulation of RANTES gene expression in neuroglia by Japanese encephalitis virus infection. J Virol 78(22), 12107-19.

Chen, H.W., Pan, C.H., Liau, M.Y., Jou, R., Tsai, C.J., Wu, H.J., Lin, Y.L. and Tao, M.H. (1999) Screening of protective antigens of Japanese encephalitis virus by DNA immunization: a comparative study with conventional viral vaccines. J Virol 73(12), 10137-45.

Cheng, Y., King, N.J. and Kesson, A.M. (2004) Major histocompatibility complex class I (MHC-I) induction by West Nile virus: involvement of 2 signaling pathways in MHC-I up-regulation. J Infect Dis 189(4), 658-68.

Chia, S.C., Leung, P.S., Liao, C.P., Huang, J.H. and Lee, S.T. (2001) Fragment of Japanese encephalitis virus envelope protein produced in Escherichia coli protects mice from virus challenge. Microb Pathog 31(1), 9-19.

Chien, H.L., Liao, C.L. and Lin, Y.L. (2011) FUSE binding protein 1 interacts with untranslated regions of Japanese encephalitis virus RNA and negatively regulates viral replication. J Virol 85(10), 4698-706.

Chien, Y.J., Chen, W.J., Hsu, W.L. and Chiou, S.S. (2008) Bovine lactoferrin inhibits Japanese encephalitis virus by binding to heparan sulfate and receptor for low density lipoprotein. Virology 379(1), 143-51.

Chu, J.J. and Ng, M.L. (2004) Infectious entry of West Nile virus occurs through a clathrin-mediated endocytic pathway. J Virol 78(19), 10543-55.

Chung, K.M., Liszewski, M.K., Nybakken, G., Davis, A.E., Townsend, R.R., Fremont, D.H., Atkinson, J.P. and Diamond, M.S. (2006a) West Nile virus nonstructural protein NS1 inhibits complement activation by binding the regulatory protein factor H. Proc Natl Acad Sci U S A 103(50), 19111-6.

Chung, K.M., Nybakken, G.E., Thompson, B.S., Engle, M.J., Marri, A., Fremont, D.H. and Diamond, M.S. (2006b) Antibodies against West Nile Virus nonstructural protein NS1 prevent lethal infection through Fc gamma receptor-dependent and -independent mechanisms. J Virol 80(3), 1340-51.

Crowley, M.P., Reich, Z., Mavaddat, N., Altman, J.D. and Chien, Y. (1997) The recognition of the nonclassical major histocompatibility complex (MHC) class I molecule, T10, by the gammadelta T cell, G8. J Exp Med 185(7), 1223-30.

D.S Burke and Monath, T.P. (2001) Flaviviruses. In: D.M. Knipe and P.M. Howley (Eds), Fields Virology fourth ed., pp. 1043–1125. Vol. I. Lippincott Williams and Wilkins, Philadelphia.

D.S. Burke and Leake, C.J. (1988) Japanese encephalitis. In: T.P. Monath (Ed), The Arboviruses: Epidemiology and Ecology, pp. 63-92. Vol. III. CRC Press, Boca Raton, FL.

Das, S., Ghosh, D. and Basu, A. (2009a) Japanese encephalitis virus induce immuno-competency in neural stem/progenitor cells. PLoS One 4(12), e8134.

Das, S., Laxminarayana, S.V., Chandra, N., Ravi, V. and Desai, A. (2009b) Heat shock protein 70 on Neuro2a cells is a putative receptor for Japanese encephalitis virus. Virology 385(1), 47-57.

Davidson, A.D. (2009) Chapter 2. New insights into flavivirus nonstructural protein 5. Adv Virus Res 74, 41-101.

Davis, W.G., Blackwell, J.L., Shi, P.Y. and Brinton, M.A. (2007) Interaction between the cellular protein eEF1A and the 3'-terminal stem-loop of West Nile virus genomic RNA facilitates viral minus-strand RNA synthesis. J Virol 81(18), 10172-87.

Deng, Y.Q., Dai, J.X., Ji, G.H., Jiang, T., Wang, H.J., Yang, H.O., Tan, W.L., Liu, R., Yu, M., Ge, B.X., Zhu, Q.Y., Qin, E.D., Guo, Y.J. and Qin, C.F. (2011) A broadly flavivirus cross-neutralizing monoclonal antibody that recognizes a novel epitope within the fusion loop of E protein. PLoS One 6(1), e16059.

Dewasthaly, S., Ayachit, V.M., Sarthi, S.A. and Gore, M.M. (2001) Monoclonal antibody raised against envelope glycoprotein peptide neutralizes Japanese encephalitis virus. Arch Virol 146(7), 1427-35.

Diamond, M.S., Shrestha, B., Marri, A., Mahan, D. and Engle, M. (2003) B cells and antibody play critical roles in the immediate defense of disseminated infection by West Nile encephalitis virus. J Virol 77(4), 2578-86.

Doly, J., Civas, A., Navarro, S. and Uze, G. (1998) Type I interferons: expression and signalization. Cell Mol Life Sci 54(10), 1109-21.

Endy, T.P. and Nisalak, A. (2002) Japanese encephalitis virus: ecology and epidemiology. Curr Top Microbiol Immunol 267, 11-48.

Erlanger, T.E., Weiss, S., Keiser, J., Utzinger, J. and Wiedenmayer, K. (2009) Past, present, and future of Japanese encephalitis. Emerg Infect Dis 15(1), 1-7.

Falgout, B. and Markoff, L. (1995) Evidence that flavivirus NS1-NS2A cleavage is mediated by a membrane-bound host protease in the endoplasmic reticulum. J Virol 69(11), 7232-43.

Fan, W.F. and Mason, P.W. (1990) Membrane association and secretion of the Japanese encephalitis virus NS1 protein from cells expressing NS1 cDNA. Virology 177(2), 470-6.

Fang, H., Welte, T., Zheng, X., Chang, G.J., Holbrook, M.R., Soong, L. and Wang, T. (2010) gammadelta T cells promote the maturation of dendritic cells during West Nile virus infection. FEMS Immunol Med Microbiol 59(1), 71-80.

Fredericksen, B.L., Smith, M., Katze, M.G., Shi, P.Y. and Gale, M., Jr. (2004) The host response to West Nile Virus infection limits viral spread through the activation of the interferon regulatory factor 3 pathway. J Virol 78(14), 7737-47.

Fritz, R., Blazevic, J., Taucher, C., Pangerl, K., Heinz, F.X. and Stiasny, K. (2011) The unique transmembrane hairpin of the flavivirus fusion protein E is essential for membrane fusion. J Virol 85(9), 4377-85.

Fujita, H., Sumiyoshi, H., Mori, C., Manabe, S., Takagi, M., Yoshida, I., Morita, K., Fuke, I., Fukai, K. and Igarashi, A. (1987) Studies in the development of Japanese encephalitis vaccine: expression of virus envelope glycoprotein V3 (E) gene in yeast. Bull World Health Organ 65(3), 303-8.

Ghosh, D. and Basu, A. (2009) Japanese encephalitis-a pathological and clinical perspective. PLoS Negl Trop Dis 3(9), e437.

Ghoshal, A., Das, S., Ghosh, S., Mishra, M.K., Sharma, V., Koli, P., Sen, E. and Basu, A. (2007) Proinflammatory mediators released by activated microglia induces neuronal death in Japanese encephalitis. Glia 55(5), 483-96.

Goncalvez, A.P., Chien, C.H., Tubthong, K., Gorshkova, I., Roll, C., Donau, O., Schuck, P., Yoksan, S., Wang, S.D., Purcell, R.H. and Lai, C.J. (2008) Humanized monoclonal antibodies derived from chimpanzee Fabs protect against Japanese encephalitis virus in vitro and in vivo. J Virol 82(14), 7009-21.

Gould, E.A. and Buckley, A. (1989) Antibody-dependent enhancement of yellow fever and Japanese encephalitis virus neurovirulence. J Gen Virol 70 (Pt 6), 1605-8.

Gubler, D.J. (2002) The global emergence/resurgence of arboviral diseases as public health problems. Arch Med Res 33(4), 330-42.

Guirakhoo, F., Zhang, Z.X., Chambers, T.J., Delagrave, S., Arroyo, J., Barrett, A.D. and Monath, T.P. (1999) Immunogenicity, genetic stability, and protective efficacy of a recombinant, chimeric yellow fever-Japanese encephalitis virus (ChimeriVax-JE) as a live, attenuated vaccine candidate against Japanese encephalitis. Virology 257(2), 363-72.

Guo, J.T., Hayashi, J. and Seeger, C. (2005) West Nile virus inhibits the signal transduction pathway of alpha interferon. J Virol 79(3), 1343-50.

Gupta, N. and Rao, P.L. (2011) Transcriptomic profile of host response in Japanese encephalitis virus infection. Virol J 8, 92.

Hanna, J.N., Ritchie, S.A., Phillips, D.A., Lee, J.M., Hills, S.L., van den Hurk, A.F., Pyke, A.T., Johansen, C.A. and Mackenzie, J.S. (1999) Japanese encephalitis in north Queensland, Australia, 1998. Med J Aust 170(11), 533-6.

Heinz, F.X. and Allison, S.L. (2000) Structures and mechanisms in flavivirus fusion. Adv Virus Res 55, 231-69.

Heinz, F.X., Collet, M.S., H., P.R., Gould, E.A., Howard, C.R., Houghton, M., M., M.R.J., Rice, C.M. and J., T.H. (2000) Family *Flaviviridae*. In: M.H.V. Regenmortel, C.M. Fauquet, D.H.L. Bishop, E. Carstens, M.K. Estes, S. Lemon, J. Maniloff, M. M. A, D. McGeoch, C.R. Pringle and R.B. Wickner (Eds), Virus Taxonomy: 7th International Committie for the Taxanomy of Viruses, pp. 859-878. Academic Press, San Diego.

Hennessy, S., Liu, Z., Tsai, T.F., Strom, B.L., Wan, C.M., Liu, H.L., Wu, T.X., Yu, H.J., Liu, Q.M., Karabatsos, N., Bilker, W.B. and Halstead, S.B. (1996) Effectiveness of live-attenuated Japanese encephalitis vaccine (SA14-14-2): a case-control study. Lancet 347(9015), 1583-6.

Hiscott, J., Kwon, H. and Genin, P. (2001) Hostile takeovers: viral appropriation of the NF-kappaB pathway. J Clin Invest 107(2), 143-51.

Hiscott, J., Nguyen, T.L., Arguello, M., Nakhaei, P. and Paz, S. (2006) Manipulation of the nuclear factor-kappaB pathway and the innate immune response by viruses. Oncogene 25(51), 6844-67.

Hoke, C.H., Nisalak, A., Sangawhipa, N., Jatanasen, S., Laorakapongse, T., Innis, B.L., Kotchasenee, S., Gingrich, J.B., Latendresse, J., Fukai, K. and et al. (1988) Protection against Japanese encephalitis by inactivated vaccines. N Engl J Med 319(10), 608-14.

Hunt, A.R., Cropp, C.B. and Chang, G.J. (2001) A recombinant particulate antigen of Japanese encephalitis virus produced in stably-transformed cells is an effective noninfectious antigen and subunit immunogen. J Virol Methods 97(1-2), 133-49.

Huy, B.V., Tu, H.C., Luan, T.V. and Lindqvist, R. (1994) Early mental and neurological sequelae after Japanese B encephalitis. Southeast Asian J Trop Med Public Health 25(3), 549-53.

Jacobs, M.G., Robinson, P.J., Bletchly, C., Mackenzie, J.M. and Young, P.R. (2000) Dengue virus nonstructural protein 1 is expressed in a glycosyl-phosphatidylinositol-linked form that is capable of signal transduction. FASEB J 14(11), 1603-10.

Jaruga, B., Hong, F., Kim, W.H. and Gao, B. (2004) IFN-gamma/STAT1 acts as a proinflammatory signal in T cell-mediated hepatitis via induction of multiple chemokines and adhesion molecules: a critical role of IRF-1. Am J Physiol Gastrointest Liver Physiol 287(5), G1044-52.

Jia, F.L. and Huang, Z.X. (1983) [Cell-mediated immunity in mice infected with Japanese encephalitis virus. II. Passive transfer of immune spleen T cells for life protection in infected mice]. Zhongguo Yi Xue Ke Xue Yuan Xue Bao 5(1), 68-9.

Kabilan, L., Rajendran, R., Arunachalam, N., Ramesh, S., Srinivasan, S., Samuel, P.P. and Dash, A.P. (2004) Japanese encephalitis in India: an overview. Indian J Pediatr 71(7), 609-15.

Kambara, H., Tani, H., Mori, Y., Abe, T., Katoh, H., Fukuhara, T., Taguwa, S., Moriishi, K. and Matsuura, Y. (2011) Involvement of cyclophilin B in the replication of Japanese encephalitis virus. Virology 412(1), 211-9.

Kanesa-thasan, N., Smucny, J.J., Hoke, C.H., Marks, D.H., Konishi, E., Kurane, I., Tang, D.B., Vaughn, D.W., Mason, P.W. and Shope, R.E. (2000) Safety and immunogenicity of NYVAC-JEV and ALVAC-JEV attenuated recombinant Japanese encephalitis virus--poxvirus vaccines in vaccinia-nonimmune and vaccinia-immune humans. Vaccine 19(4-5), 483-91.

Kawai, T. and Akira, S. (2006) Innate immune recognition of viral infection. Nat Immunol 7(2), 131-7.

Kesson, A.M., Cheng, Y. and King, N.J. (2002) Regulation of immune recognition molecules by flavivirus, West Nile. Viral Immunol 15(2), 273-83.

Kesson, A.M. and King, N.J. (2001) Transcriptional regulation of major histocompatibility complex class I by flavivirus West Nile is dependent on NF-kappaB activation. J Infect Dis 184(8), 947-54.

Khromykh, A.A., Harvey, T.J., Abedinia, M. and Westaway, E.G. (1996) Expression and purification of the seven nonstructural proteins of the flavivirus Kunjin in the E. coli and the baculovirus expression systems. J Virol Methods 61(1-2), 47-58.

Kim, J.M., Yun, S.I., Song, B.H., Hahn, Y.S., Lee, C.H., Oh, H.W. and Lee, Y.M. (2008) A single N-linked glycosylation site in the Japanese encephalitis virus prM protein is critical for cell type-specific prM protein biogenesis, virus particle release, and pathogenicity in mice. J Virol 82(16), 7846-62.

Kim, Y.G., Yoo, J.S., Kim, J.H., Kim, C.M. and Oh, J.W. (2007) Biochemical characterization of a recombinant Japanese encephalitis virus RNA-dependent RNA polymerase. BMC Mol Biol 8, 59.

Kimura-Kuroda, J., Ichikawa, M., Ogata, A., Nagashima, K. and Yasui, K. (1993) Specific tropism of Japanese encephalitis virus for developing neurons in primary rat brain culture. Arch Virol 130(3-4), 477-84.

Kimura-Kuroda, J. and Yasui, K. (1983) Topographical analysis of antigenic determinants on envelope glycoprotein V3 (E) of Japanese encephalitis virus, using monoclonal antibodies. J Virol 45(1), 124-32.

Kimura-Kuroda, J. and Yasui, K. (1988) Protection of mice against Japanese encephalitis virus by passive administration with monoclonal antibodies. J Immunol 141(10), 3606-10.

King, N.J., Getts, D.R., Getts, M.T., Rana, S., Shrestha, B. and Kesson, A.M. (2007) Immunopathology of flavivirus infections. Immunol Cell Biol 85(1), 33-42.

Kitai, Y., Kondo, T. and Konishi, E. (2011) Non-structural protein 1 (NS1) antibody-based assays to differentiate West Nile (WN) virus from Japanese encephalitis virus infections in horses: effects of WN virus NS1 antibodies induced by inactivated WN vaccine. J Virol Methods 171(1), 123-8.

Kliks, S.C., Nisalak, A., Brandt, W.E., Wahl, L. and Burke, D.S. (1989) Antibody-dependent enhancement of dengue virus growth in human monocytes as a risk factor for dengue hemorrhagic fever. Am J Trop Med Hyg 40(4), 444-51.

Koh, W.L. and Ng, M.L. (2005) Molecular mechanisms of West Nile virus pathogenesis in brain cell. Emerg Infect Dis 11(4), 629-32.

Kojima, A., Yasuda, A., Asanuma, H., Ishikawa, T., Takamizawa, A., Yasui, K. and Kurata, T. (2003) Stable high-producer cell clone expressing virus-like particles of the Japanese encephalitis virus e protein for a second-generation subunit vaccine. J Virol 77(16), 8745-55.

Kolaskar, A.S. and Kulkarni-Kale, U. (1999) Prediction of three-dimensional structure and mapping of conformational epitopes of envelope glycoprotein of Japanese encephalitis virus. Virology 261(1), 31-42.

Konishi, E., Kurane, I., Mason, P.W., Innis, B.L. and Ennis, F.A. (1995) Japanese encephalitis virus-specific proliferative responses of human peripheral blood T lymphocytes. Am J Trop Med Hyg 53(3), 278-83.

Konishi, E., Kurane, I., Mason, P.W., Shope, R.E. and Ennis, F.A. (1997a) Poxvirus-based Japanese encephalitis vaccine candidates induce JE virus-specific CD8+ cytotoxic T lymphocytes in mice. Virology 227(2), 353-60.

Konishi, E., Pincus, S., Fonseca, B.A., Shope, R.E., Paoletti, E. and Mason, P.W. (1991) Comparison of protective immunity elicited by recombinant vaccinia viruses that synthesize E or NS1 of Japanese encephalitis virus. Virology 185(1), 401-10.

Konishi, E., Pincus, S., Paoletti, E., Laegreid, W.W., Shope, R.E. and Mason, P.W. (1992a) A highly attenuated host range-restricted vaccinia virus strain, NYVAC, encoding the prM, E, and NS1 genes of Japanese encephalitis virus prevents JEV viremia in swine. Virology 190(1), 454-8.

Konishi, E., Pincus, S., Paoletti, E., Shope, R.E., Burrage, T. and Mason, P.W. (1992b) Mice immunized with a subviral particle containing the Japanese encephalitis virus prM/M and E proteins are protected from lethal JEV infection. Virology 188(2), 714-20.

Konishi, E., Win, K.S., Kurane, I., Mason, P.W., Shope, R.E. and Ennis, F.A. (1997b) Particulate vaccine candidate for Japanese encephalitis induces long-lasting virus-specific memory T lymphocytes in mice. Vaccine 15(3), 281-6.

Konishi, E., Yamaoka, M., Khin Sane, W., Kurane, I. and Mason, P.W. (1998) Induction of protective immunity against Japanese encephalitis in mice by immunization with a plasmid encoding Japanese encephalitis virus premembrane and envelope genes. J Virol 72(6), 4925-30.

Krishna, V.D., Rangappa, M. and Satchidanandam, V. (2009) Virus-specific cytolytic antibodies to nonstructural protein 1 of Japanese encephalitis virus effect reduction of virus output from infected cells. J Virol 83(10), 4766-77.

Kuhn, R.J., Zhang, W., Rossmann, M.G., Pletnev, S.V., Corver, J., Lenches, E., Jones, C.T., Mukhopadhyay, S., Chipman, P.R., Strauss, E.G., Baker, T.S. and Strauss, J.H. (2002) Structure of dengue virus: implications for flavivirus organization, maturation, and fusion. Cell 108(5), 717-25.

Kumar, P., Lee, S.K., Shankar, P. and Manjunath, N. (2006) A single siRNA suppresses fatal encephalitis induced by two different flaviviruses. PLoS Med 3(4), e96.

Kumar, P., Sulochana, P., Nirmala, G., Chandrashekar, R., Haridattatreya, M. and Satchidanandam, V. (2004a) Impaired T helper 1 function of nonstructural protein 3-specific T cells in Japanese patients with encephalitis with neurological sequelae. J Infect Dis 189(5), 880-91.

Kumar, P., Sulochana, P., Nirmala, G., Haridattatreya, M. and Satchidanandam, V. (2004b) Conserved amino acids 193-324 of non-structural protein 3 are a dominant source of peptide determinants for CD4+ and CD8+ T cells in a healthy Japanese encephalitis virus-endemic cohort. J Gen Virol 85(Pt 5), 1131-43.

Kumar, R., Mathur, A., Singh, K.B., Sitholey, P., Prasad, M., Shukla, R., Agarwal, S.P. and Arockiasamy, J. (1993) Clinical sequelae of Japanese encephalitis in children. Indian J Med Res 97, 9-13.

Kummerer, B.M. and Rice, C.M. (2002) Mutations in the yellow fever virus nonstructural protein NS2A selectively block production of infectious particles. J Virol 76(10), 4773-84.

Kurane, I., Innis, B.L., Nimmannitya, S., Nisalak, A., Meager, A. and Ennis, F.A. (1993) High levels of interferon alpha in the sera of children with dengue virus infection. Am J Trop Med Hyg 48(2), 222-9.

Kuzuhara, S., Nakamura, H., Hayashida, K., Obata, J., Abe, M., Sonoda, K., Nishiyama, K., Sugawara, K., Takeda, K., Honda, T., Matsui, H., Shigaki, T., Kino, Y., Mizokami, H., Tanaka, M., Mizuno, K. and Ueda, K. (2003) Non-clinical and phase I clinical trials of a Vero cell-derived inactivated Japanese encephalitis vaccine. Vaccine 21(31), 4519-26.

Lad, V.J., Gupta, A.K., Goverdhan, M.K., Ayachit, V.L., Rodrigues, J.J. and Hungund, L.V. (1993) Susceptibility of BL6 nude (congenitally athymic) mice to Japanese encephalitis virus by the peripheral route. Acta Virol 37(4), 232-40.

Lanciotti, R.S., Roehrig, J.T., Deubel, V., Smith, J., Parker, M., Steele, K., Crise, B., Volpe, K.E., Crabtree, M.B., Scherret, J.H., Hall, R.A., MacKenzie, J.S., Cropp, C.B., Panigrahy, B., Ostlund, E., Schmitt, B., Malkinson, M., Banet, C., Weissman, J., Komar, N., Savage, H.M., Stone, W., McNamara, T. and Gubler, D.J. (1999) Origin of the West Nile virus responsible for an outbreak of encephalitis in the northeastern United States. Science 286(5448), 2333-7.

Lebedeva, T., Dustin, M.L. and Sykulev, Y. (2005) ICAM-1 co-stimulates target cells to facilitate antigen presentation. Curr Opin Immunol 17(3), 251-8.

Lee, C.J., Lin, H.R., Liao, C.L. and Lin, Y.L. (2008) Cholesterol effectively blocks entry of flavivirus. J Virol 82(13), 6470-80.

Lee, Y.H., Wei, C.W., Wang, J.J. and Chiou, C.T. (2011) Rana catesbeiana ribonuclease inhibits Japanese encephalitis virus (JEV) replication and enhances apoptosis of JEV-infected BHK-21 cells. Antiviral Res 89(3), 193-8.

Leung, J.Y., Pijlman, G.P., Kondratieva, N., Hyde, J., Mackenzie, J.M. and Khromykh, A.A. (2008) Role of nonstructural protein NS2A in flavivirus assembly. J Virol 82(10), 4731-41.

Lewis, P.J. and Babiuk, L.A. (1999) DNA vaccines: a review. Adv Virus Res 54, 129-88.

Li, W., Li, Y., Kedersha, N., Anderson, P., Emara, M., Swiderek, K.M., Moreno, G.T. and Brinton, M.A. (2002) Cell proteins TIA-1 and TIAR interact with the 3' stem-loop of the West Nile virus complementary minus-strand RNA and facilitate virus replication. J Virol 76(23), 11989-2000.

Li, Y., Ye, J., Yang, X., Xu, M., Chen, L., Mei, L., Zhu, J., Liu, X., Chen, H. and Cao, S. (2011) Infection of mouse bone marrow-derived dendritic cells by live attenuated Japanese encephalitis virus induces cells maturation and triggers T cells activation. Vaccine 29(4), 855-62.

Liao, C.L., Lin, Y.L., Wang, J.J., Huang, Y.L., Yeh, C.T., Ma, S.H. and Chen, L.K. (1997) Effect of enforced expression of human bcl-2 on Japanese encephalitis virus-induced apoptosis in cultured cells. J Virol 71(8), 5963-71.

Liao, C.L., Lin, Y.L., Wu, B.C., Tsao, C.H., Wang, M.C., Liu, C.I., Huang, Y.L., Chen, J.H., Wang, J.P. and Chen, L.K. (2001) Salicylates inhibit flavivirus replication independently of blocking nuclear factor kappa B activation. J Virol 75(17), 7828-39.

Licon Luna, R.M., Lee, E., Mullbacher, A., Blanden, R.V., Langman, R. and Lobigs, M. (2002) Lack of both Fas ligand and perforin protects from flavivirus-mediated encephalitis in mice. J Virol 76(7), 3202-11.

Lilley, B.N. and Ploegh, H.L. (2005) Viral modulation of antigen presentation: manipulation of cellular targets in the ER and beyond. Immunol Rev 207, 126-44.

Lin, C.W., Cheng, C.W., Yang, T.C., Li, S.W., Cheng, M.H., Wan, L., Lin, Y.J., Lai, C.H., Lin, W.Y. and Kao, M.C. (2008a) Interferon antagonist function of Japanese encephalitis virus NS4A and its interaction with DEAD-box RNA helicase DDX42. Virus Res 137(1), 49-55.

Lin, C.W., Liu, K.T., Huang, H.D. and Chen, W.J. (2008b) Protective immunity of E. coli-synthesized NS1 protein of Japanese encephalitis virus. Biotechnol Lett 30(2), 205-14.

Lin, C.W., Wu, C.F., Hsiao, N.W., Chang, C.Y., Li, S.W., Wan, L., Lin, Y.J. and Lin, W.Y. (2008c) Aloe-emodin is an interferon-inducing agent with antiviral activity against Japanese encephalitis virus and enterovirus 71. Int J Antimicrob Agents 32(4), 355-9.

Lin, C.W. and Wu, S.C. (2003) A functional epitope determinant on domain III of the Japanese encephalitis virus envelope protein interacted with neutralizing-antibody combining sites. J Virol 77(4), 2600-6.

Lin, R.J., Chang, B.L., Yu, H.P., Liao, C.L. and Lin, Y.L. (2006) Blocking of interferon-induced Jak-Stat signaling by Japanese encephalitis virus NS5 through a protein tyrosine phosphatase-mediated mechanism. J Virol 80(12), 5908-18.

Lin, R.J., Liao, C.L., Lin, E. and Lin, Y.L. (2004a) Blocking of the alpha interferon-induced Jak-Stat signaling pathway by Japanese encephalitis virus infection. J Virol 78(17), 9285-94.

Lin, R.J., Liao, C.L. and Lin, Y.L. (2004b) Replication-incompetent virions of Japanese encephalitis virus trigger neuronal cell death by oxidative stress in a culture system. J Gen Virol 85(Pt 2), 521-33.

Lin, Y.L., Chen, L.K., Liao, C.L., Yeh, C.T., Ma, S.H., Chen, J.L., Huang, Y.L., Chen, S.S. and Chiang, H.Y. (1998) DNA immunization with Japanese encephalitis virus nonstructural protein NS1 elicits protective immunity in mice. J Virol 72(1), 191-200.

Lin, Y.L., Huang, Y.L., Ma, S.H., Yeh, C.T., Chiou, S.Y., Chen, L.K. and Liao, C.L. (1997) Inhibition of Japanese encephalitis virus infection by nitric oxide: antiviral effect of nitric oxide on RNA virus replication. J Virol 71(7), 5227-35.

Lindenbach, B.D. and Rice, C.M. (2003) Molecular biology of flaviviruses. Adv Virus Res 59, 23-61.

Liu, T.H., Liang, L.C., Wang, C.C., Liu, H.C. and Chen, W.J. (2008) The blood-brain barrier in the cerebrum is the initial site for the Japanese encephalitis virus entering the central nervous system. J Neurovirol 14(6), 514-21.

Liu, W.J., Wang, X.J., Clark, D.C., Lobigs, M., Hall, R.A. and Khromykh, A.A. (2006a) A single amino acid substitution in the West Nile virus nonstructural protein NS2A disables its ability to inhibit alpha/beta interferon induction and attenuates virus virulence in mice. J Virol 80(5), 2396-404.

Liu, W.J., Wang, X.J., Mokhonov, V.V., Shi, P.Y., Randall, R. and Khromykh, A.A. (2005) Inhibition of interferon signaling by the New York 99 strain and Kunjin subtype of West Nile virus involves blockage of STAT1 and STAT2 activation by nonstructural proteins. J Virol 79(3), 1934-42.

Liu, X., Cao, S., Zhou, R., Xu, G., Xiao, S., Yang, Y., Sun, M., Li, Y. and Chen, H. (2006b) Inhibition of Japanese encephalitis virus NS1 protein expression in cell by small interfering RNAs. Virus Genes 33(1), 69-75.

Liu, Y., King, N., Kesson, A., Blanden, R.V. and Mullbacher, A. (1989) Flavivirus infection up-regulates the expression of class I and class II major histocompatibility antigens on and enhances T cell recognition of astrocytes in vitro. J Neuroimmunol 21(2-3), 157-68.

Luo, D., Xu, T., Hunke, C., Gruber, G., Vasudevan, S.G. and Lescar, J. (2008) Crystal structure of the NS3 protease-helicase from dengue virus. J Virol 82(1), 173-83.

Mackenzie, J.M., Khromykh, A.A., Jones, M.K. and Westaway, E.G. (1998) Subcellular localization and some biochemical properties of the flavivirus Kunjin nonstructural proteins NS2A and NS4A. Virology 245(2), 203-15.

Mackenzie, J.S., Gubler, D.J. and Petersen, L.R. (2004) Emerging flaviviruses: the spread and resurgence of Japanese encephalitis, West Nile and dengue viruses. Nat Med 10(12 Suppl), S98-109.

Mackenzie, J.S., Johansen, C.A., Ritchie, S.A., van den Hurk, A.F. and Hall, R.A. (2002) Japanese encephalitis as an emerging virus: the emergence and spread of Japanese encephalitis virus in Australasia. Curr Top Microbiol Immunol 267, 49-73.

Mandl, C.W., Allison, S.L., Holzmann, H., Meixner, T. and Heinz, F.X. (2000) Attenuation of tick-borne encephalitis virus by structure-based site-specific mutagenesis of a putative flavivirus receptor binding site. J Virol 74(20), 9601-9.

Mani, T.R., Rao, C.V., Rajendran, R., Devaputra, M., Prasanna, Y., Hanumaiah, Gajanana, A. and Reuben, R. (1991) Surveillance for Japanese encephalitis in villages near Madurai, Tamil Nadu, India. Trans R Soc Trop Med Hyg 85(2), 287-91.

Mason, P.W. (1989) Maturation of Japanese encephalitis virus glycoproteins produced by infected mammalian and mosquito cells. Virology 169(2), 354-64.

Mason, P.W., McAda, P.C., Dalrymple, J.M., Fournier, M.J. and Mason, T.L. (1987) Expression of Japanese encephalitis virus antigens in Escherichia coli. Virology 158(2), 361-72.

Mason, P.W., Pincus, S., Fournier, M.J., Mason, T.L., Shope, R.E. and Paoletti, E. (1991) Japanese encephalitis virus-vaccinia recombinants produce particulate forms of the structural membrane proteins and induce high levels of protection against lethal JEV infection. Virology 180(1), 294-305.

McCown, J., Cochran, M., Putnak, R., Feighny, R., Burrous, J., Henchal, E. and Hoke, C. (1990) Protection of mice against lethal Japanese encephalitis with a recombinant baculovirus vaccine. Am J Trop Med Hyg 42(5), 491-9.

McMinn, P.C. (1997) The molecular basis of virulence of the encephalitogenic flaviviruses. J Gen Virol 78 (Pt 11), 2711-22.

McMinn, P.C., Marshall, I.D. and Dalgarno, L. (1995) Neurovirulence and neuroinvasiveness of Murray Valley encephalitis virus mutants selected by passage in a monkey kidney cell line. J Gen Virol 76 (Pt 4), 865-72.

Mishra, M.K. and Basu, A. (2008) Minocycline neuroprotects, reduces microglial activation, inhibits caspase 3 induction, and viral replication following Japanese encephalitis. J Neurochem 105(5), 1582-95.

Misra, U.K. and Kalita, J. (2010) Overview: Japanese encephalitis. Prog Neurobiol 91(2), 108-20.

Mitani, Y., Takaoka, A., Kim, S.H., Kato, Y., Yokochi, T., Tanaka, N. and Taniguchi, T. (2001) Cross talk of the interferon-alpha/beta signalling complex with gp130 for effective interleukin-6 signalling. Genes Cells 6(7), 631-40.

Miura, K., Onodera, T., Nishida, A., Goto, N. and Fujisaki, Y. (1990) A single gene controls resistance to Japanese encephalitis virus in mice. Arch Virol 112(3-4), 261-70.

Modis, Y., Ogata, S., Clements, D. and Harrison, S.C. (2003) A ligand-binding pocket in the dengue virus envelope glycoprotein. Proc Natl Acad Sci U S A 100(12), 6986-91.

Monath, T.P., Guirakhoo, F., Nichols, R., Yoksan, S., Schrader, R., Murphy, C., Blum, P., Woodward, S., McCarthy, K., Mathis, D., Johnson, C. and Bedford, P. (2003) Chimeric live, attenuated vaccine against Japanese encephalitis (ChimeriVax-JE): phase 2 clinical trials for safety and immunogenicity, effect of vaccine dose and schedule, and memory response to challenge with inactivated Japanese encephalitis antigen. J Infect Dis 188(8), 1213-30.

Monath, T.P., Levenbook, I., Soike, K., Zhang, Z.X., Ratterree, M., Draper, K., Barrett, A.D., Nichols, R., Weltzin, R., Arroyo, J. and Guirakhoo, F. (2000) Chimeric yellow fever virus 17D-Japanese encephalitis virus vaccine: dose-response effectiveness and extended safety testing in rhesus monkeys. J Virol 74(4), 1742-51.

Monath, T.P., McCarthy, K., Bedford, P., Johnson, C.T., Nichols, R., Yoksan, S., Marchesani, R., Knauber, M., Wells, K.H., Arroyo, J. and Guirakhoo, F. (2002) Clinical proof of principle for ChimeriVax: recombinant live, attenuated vaccines against flavivirus infections. Vaccine 20(7-8), 1004-18.

Monath, T.P., Soike, K., Levenbook, I., Zhang, Z.X., Arroyo, J., Delagrave, S., Myers, G., Barrett, A.D., Shope, R.E., Ratterree, M., Chambers, T.J. and Guirakhoo, F. (1999) Recombinant, chimaeric live, attenuated vaccine (ChimeriVax) incorporating the envelope genes of Japanese encephalitis (SA14-14-2) virus and the capsid and nonstructural genes of yellow fever (17D) virus is safe, immunogenic and protective in non-human primates. Vaccine 17(15-16), 1869-82.

Mori, R., Kimoto, K. and Takeya, K. (1970) The role of the thymus in antibody production and in resistance to Japanese encephalitis virus infection. Arch Gesamte Virusforsch 29(1), 32-8.

Mori, Y., Okabayashi, T., Yamashita, T., Zhao, Z., Wakita, T., Yasui, K., Hasebe, F., Tadano, M., Konishi, E., Moriishi, K. and Matsuura, Y. (2005) Nuclear localization of Japanese encephalitis virus core protein enhances viral replication. J Virol 79(6), 3448-58.

Mori, Y., Yamashita, T., Tanaka, Y., Tsuda, Y., Abe, T., Moriishi, K. and Matsuura, Y. (2007) Processing of capsid protein by cathepsin L plays a crucial role in replication of Japanese encephalitis virus in neural and macrophage cells. J Virol 81(16), 8477-87.

Morita, K., Tadano, M., Nakaji, S., Kosai, K., Mathenge, E.G., Pandey, B.D., Hasebe, F., Inoue, S. and Igarashi, A. (2001) Locus of a virus neutralization epitope on the Japanese encephalitis virus envelope protein determined by use of long PCR-based region-specific random mutagenesis. Virology 287(2), 417-26.

Muller, U., Steinhoff, U., Reis, L.F., Hemmi, S., Pavlovic, J., Zinkernagel, R.M. and Aguet, M. (1994) Functional role of type I and type II interferons in antiviral defense. Science 264(5167), 1918-21.

Munoz-Jordan, J.L., Laurent-Rolle, M., Ashour, J., Martinez-Sobrido, L., Ashok, M., Lipkin, W.I. and Garcia-Sastre, A. (2005) Inhibition of alpha/beta interferon signaling by the NS4B protein of flaviviruses. J Virol 79(13), 8004-13.

Munoz-Jordan, J.L., Sanchez-Burgos, G.G., Laurent-Rolle, M. and Garcia-Sastre, A. (2003) Inhibition of interferon signaling by dengue virus. Proc Natl Acad Sci U S A 100(24), 14333-8.

Murali-Krishna, K., Ravi, V. and Manjunath, R. (1996) Protection of adult but not newborn mice against lethal intracerebral challenge with Japanese encephalitis virus by adoptively transferred virus-specific cytotoxic T lymphocytes: requirement for L3T4+ T cells. J Gen Virol 77 (Pt 4), 705-14.

Nam, J.H., Wyatt, L.S., Chae, S.L., Cho, H.W., Park, Y.K. and Moss, B. (1999) Protection against lethal Japanese encephalitis virus infection of mice by immunization with the highly attenuated MVA strain of vaccinia virus expressing JEV prM and E genes. Vaccine 17(3), 261-8.

Nathanson, N. and Cole, G.A. (1970) Fatal Japanese encephalitis virus infection in immunosuppresed spider monkeys. Clin Exp Immunol 6(1), 161-6.

Nawa, M., Takasaki, T., Yamada, K., Kurane, I. and Akatsuka, T. (2003) Interference in Japanese encephalitis virus infection of Vero cells by a cationic amphiphilic drug, chlorpromazine. J Gen Virol 84(Pt 7), 1737-41.

Nazmi, A., Dutta, K. and Basu, A. (2010) Antiviral and neuroprotective role of octaguanidinium dendrimer-conjugated morpholino oligomers in Japanese encephalitis. PLoS Negl Trop Dis 4(11), e892.

Neish, A.S., Read, M.A., Thanos, D., Pine, R., Maniatis, T. and Collins, T. (1995) Endothelial interferon regulatory factor 1 cooperates with NF-kappa B as a transcriptional activator of vascular cell adhesion molecule 1. Mol Cell Biol 15(5), 2558-69.

Ni, H., Burns, N.J., Chang, G.J., Zhang, M.J., Wills, M.R., Trent, D.W., Sanders, P.G. and Barrett, A.D. (1994) Comparison of nucleotide and deduced amino acid sequence of the 5' non-coding region and structural protein genes of the wild-type Japanese encephalitis virus strain SA14 and its attenuated vaccine derivatives. J Gen Virol 75 (Pt 6), 1505-10.

Nitatpattana, N., Dubot-Peres, A., Gouilh, M.A., Souris, M., Barbazan, P., Yoksan, S., de Lamballerie, X. and Gonzalez, J.P. (2008) Change in Japanese encephalitis virus distribution, Thailand. Emerg Infect Dis 14(11), 1762-5.

Oya, A. (1988) Japanese encephalitis vaccine. Acta Paediatr Jpn 30(2), 175-84.

Pan, C.H., Chen, H.W., Huang, H.W. and Tao, M.H. (2001) Protective mechanisms induced by a Japanese encephalitis virus DNA vaccine: requirement for antibody but not CD8(+) cytotoxic T-cell responses. J Virol 75(23), 11457-63.

Paranjape, S.M. and Harris, E. (2007) Y box-binding protein-1 binds to the dengue virus 3'-untranslated region and mediates antiviral effects. J Biol Chem 282(42), 30497-508.

Pastorino, B., Nougairede, A., Wurtz, N., Gould, E. and de Lamballerie, X. (2010) Role of host cell factors in flavivirus infection: Implications for pathogenesis and development of antiviral drugs. Antiviral Res 87(3), 281-94.

Pestka, S., Krause, C.D., Sarkar, D., Walter, M.R., Shi, Y. and Fisher, P.B. (2004) Interleukin-10 and related cytokines and receptors. Annu Rev Immunol 22, 929-79.

Poland, J.D., Cropp, C.B., Craven, R.B. and Monath, T.P. (1990) Evaluation of the potency and safety of inactivated Japanese encephalitis vaccine in US inhabitants. J Infect Dis 161(5), 878-82.

Pradhan, S., Gupta, R.K., Singh, M.B. and Mathur, A. (2001) Biphasic illness pattern due to early relapse in Japanese-B virus encephalitis. J Neurol Sci 183(1), 13-8.

Qi, W.B., Hua, R.H., Yan, L.P., Tong, G.Z., Zhang, G.H., Ren, T., Wu, D.L. and Liao, M. (2008) Effective inhibition of Japanese encephalitis virus replication by small interfering RNAs targeting the NS5 gene. Virus Res 132(1-2), 145-51.

Ramakrishna, C., Ravi, V., Desai, A., Subbakrishna, D.K., Shankar, S.K. and Chandramuki, A. (2003) T helper responses to Japanese encephalitis virus infection are dependent on the route of inoculation and the strain of mouse used. J Gen Virol 84(Pt 6), 1559-67.

Raung, S.L., Chen, S.Y., Liao, S.L., Chen, J.H. and Chen, C.J. (2007) Japanese encephalitis virus infection stimulates Src tyrosine kinase in neuron/glia. Neurosci Lett 419(3), 263-8.

Ravi, V., Desai, A., Balaji, M., Apte, M.P., Lakshman, L., Subbakrishna, D.K., Sridharan, G., Dhole, T.N. and Ravikumar, B.V. (2006) Development and evaluation of a rapid IgM capture ELISA (JEV-Chex) for the diagnosis of Japanese encephalitis. J Clin Virol 35(4), 429-34.

Ravi, V., Desai, A.S., Shenoy, P.K., Satishchandra, P., Chandramuki, A. and Gourie-Devi, M. (1993) Persistence of Japanese encephalitis virus in the human nervous system. J Med Virol 40(4), 326-9.

Ravi, V., Parida, S., Desai, A., Chandramuki, A., Gourie-Devi, M. and Grau, G.E. (1997) Correlation of tumor necrosis factor levels in the serum and cerebrospinal fluid with clinical outcome in Japanese encephalitis patients. J Med Virol 51(2), 132-6.

Reuben, R. and Gajanana, A. (1997) Japanese encephalitis in India. Indian J Pediatr 64(2), 243-51.

Rey, F.A., Heinz, F.X., Mandl, C., Kunz, C. and Harrison, S.C. (1995) The envelope glycoprotein from tick-borne encephalitis virus at 2 A resolution. Nature 375(6529), 291-8.

Rice, C.M., Lenches, E.M., Eddy, S.R., Shin, S.J., Sheets, R.L. and Strauss, J.H. (1985) Nucleotide sequence of yellow fever virus: implications for flavivirus gene expression and evolution. Science 229(4715), 726-33.

Rodhain, F. (1996) [Recent data on the epidemiology of Japanese encephalitis]. Bull Acad Natl Med 180(6), 1325-37; discussion 1338-40.

Roehrig, J.T. (2003) Antigenic structure of flavivirus proteins. Adv Virus Res 59, 141-75.

Roosendaal, J., Westaway, E.G., Khromykh, A. and Mackenzie, J.M. (2006) Regulated cleavages at the West Nile virus NS4A-2K-NS4B junctions play a major role in rearranging cytoplasmic membranes and Golgi trafficking of the NS4A protein. J Virol 80(9), 4623-32.

Ruff, T.A., Eisen, D., Fuller, A. and Kass, R. (1991) Adverse reactions to Japanese encephalitis vaccine. Lancet 338(8771), 881-2.

Saini, M. and Vrati, S. (2003) A Japanese encephalitis virus peptide present on Johnson grass mosaic virus-like particles induces virus-neutralizing antibodies and protects mice against lethal challenge. J Virol 77(6), 3487-94.

Salonen, A., Ahola, T. and Kaariainen, L. (2005) Viral RNA replication in association with cellular membranes. Curr Top Microbiol Immunol 285, 139-73.

Samuel, M.A. and Diamond, M.S. (2005) Alpha/beta interferon protects against lethal West Nile virus infection by restricting cellular tropism and enhancing neuronal survival. J Virol 79(21), 13350-61.

Saxena, V., Mathur, A., Krishnani, N. and Dhole, T.N. (2008a) An insufficient anti-inflammatory cytokine response in mouse brain is associated with increased tissue pathology and viral load during Japanese encephalitis virus infection. Arch Virol 153(2), 283-92.

Saxena, V., Mathur, A., Krishnani, N. and Dhole, T.N. (2008b) Kinetics of cytokine profile during intraperitoneal inoculation of Japanese encephalitis virus in BALB/c mice model. Microbes Infect 10(10-11), 1210-7.

Scheidereit, C. (2006) IkappaB kinase complexes: gateways to NF-kappaB activation and transcription. Oncogene 25(51), 6685-705.

Scherbik, S.V., Stockman, B.M. and Brinton, M.A. (2007) Differential expression of interferon (IFN) regulatory factors and IFN-stimulated genes at early times after West Nile virus infection of mouse embryo fibroblasts. J Virol 81(21), 12005-18.

Schlesinger, J.J., Brandriss, M.W., Cropp, C.B. and Monath, T.P. (1986) Protection against yellow fever in monkeys by immunization with yellow fever virus nonstructural protein NS1. J Virol 60(3), 1153-5.

Sebastian, L., Desai, A., Madhusudana, S.N. and Ravi, V. (2009) Pentoxifylline inhibits replication of Japanese encephalitis virus: a comparative study with ribavirin. Int J Antimicrob Agents 33(2), 168-73.

Sebastian, L., Desai, A., Shampur, M.N., Perumal, Y., Sriram, D. and Vasanthapuram, R. (2008) N-methylisatin-beta-thiosemicarbazone derivative (SCH 16) is an inhibitor of Japanese encephalitis virus infection in vitro and in vivo. Virol J 5, 64.

Sebastian, L., Madhusudana, S.N., Ravi, V. and Desai, A. (2011) Mycophenolic acid inhibits replication of Japanese encephalitis virus. Chemotherapy 57(1), 56-61.

Seif, S.A., Morita, K. and Igarashi, A. (1996) A 27 amino acid coding region of JE virus E protein expressed in E. coli as fusion protein with glutathione-S-transferase elicit neutralizing antibody in mice. Virus Res 43(1), 91-6.

Seif, S.A., Morita, K., Matsuo, S., Hasebe, F. and Igarashi, A. (1995) Finer mapping of neutralizing epitope(s) on the C-terminal of Japanese encephalitis virus E-protein expressed in recombinant Escherichia coli system. Vaccine 13(16), 1515-21.

Shawar, S.M., Vyas, J.M., Rodgers, J.R. and Rich, R.R. (1994) Antigen presentation by major histocompatibility complex class I-B molecules. Annu Rev Immunol 12, 839-80.

Shen, J., SS, T.T., Schrieber, L. and King, N.J. (1997) Early E-selectin, VCAM-1, ICAM-1, and late major histocompatibility complex antigen induction on human endothelial cells by flavivirus and comodulation of adhesion molecule expression by immune cytokines. J Virol 71(12), 9323-32.

Shrivastva, A., Tripathi, N.K., Parida, M., Dash, P.K., Jana, A.M. and Lakshmana Rao, P.V. (2008) Comparison of a dipstick enzyme-linked immunosorbent assay with commercial assays for detection of Japanese encephalitis virus-specific IgM antibodies. J Postgrad Med 54(3), 181-5.

Sohn, Y.M., Park, M.S., Rho, H.O., Chandler, L.J., Shope, R.E. and Tsai, T.F. (1999) Primary and booster immune responses to SA14-14-2 Japanese encephalitis vaccine in Korean infants. Vaccine 17(18), 2259-64.

Solomon, T. (2004) Flavivirus encephalitis. N Engl J Med 351(4), 370-8.

Solomon, T. (2006) Control of Japanese encephalitis--within our grasp? N Engl J Med 355(9), 869-71.

Solomon, T., Dung, N.M., Kneen, R., Gainsborough, M., Vaughn, D.W. and Khanh, V.T. (2000) Japanese encephalitis. J Neurol Neurosurg Psychiatry 68(4), 405-15.

Solomon, T., Dung, N.M., Wills, B., Kneen, R., Gainsborough, M., Diet, T.V., Thuy, T.T., Loan, H.T., Khanh, V.C., Vaughn, D.W., White, N.J. and Farrar, J.J. (2003) Interferon alfa-2a in Japanese encephalitis: a randomised double-blind placebo-controlled trial. Lancet 361(9360), 821-6.

Solomon, T. and Winter, P.M. (2004) Neurovirulence and host factors in flavivirus encephalitis--evidence from clinical epidemiology. Arch Virol Suppl(18), 161-70.

Srivastava, A.K., Morita, K. and Igarashi, A. (1990) Immunogenicity of peptides cleaved by cyanogen bromide from Japanese encephalitis virus envelope glycoprotein E. Acta Virol 34(3), 228-38.

Srivastava, A.K., Morita, K., Matsuo, S., Tanaka, M. and Igarashi, A. (1991) Japanese encephalitis virus fusion protein with protein A expressed in Escherichia coli confers protective immunity in mice. Microbiol Immunol 35(10), 863-70.

Srivastava, A.K., Putnak, J.R., Lee, S.H., Hong, S.P., Moon, S.B., Barvir, D.A., Zhao, B., Olson, R.A., Kim, S.O., Yoo, W.D., Towle, A.C., Vaughn, D.W., Innis, B.L. and Eckels, K.H. (2001) A purified inactivated Japanese encephalitis virus vaccine made in Vero cells. Vaccine 19(31), 4557-65.

Sugawara, K., Nishiyama, K., Ishikawa, Y., Abe, M., Sonoda, K., Komatsu, K., Horikawa, Y., Takeda, K., Honda, T., Kuzuhara, S., Kino, Y., Mizokami, H., Mizuno, K., Oka, T. and Honda, K. (2002) Development of Vero cell-derived inactivated Japanese encephalitis vaccine. Biologicals 30(4), 303-14.

Sumiyoshi, H., Mori, C., Fuke, I., Morita, K., Kuhara, S., Kondou, J., Kikuchi, Y., Nagamatu, H. and Igarashi, A. (1987) Complete nucleotide sequence of the Japanese encephalitis virus genome RNA. Virology 161(2), 497-510.

Swarup, V., Ghosh, J., Duseja, R., Ghosh, S. and Basu, A. (2007a) Japanese encephalitis virus infection decrease endogenous IL-10 production: correlation with microglial activation and neuronal death. Neurosci Lett 420(2), 144-9.

Swarup, V., Ghosh, J., Ghosh, S., Saxena, A. and Basu, A. (2007b) Antiviral and anti-inflammatory effects of rosmarinic acid in an experimental murine model of Japanese encephalitis. Antimicrob Agents Chemother 51(9), 3367-70.

Swarup, V., Ghosh, J., Mishra, M.K. and Basu, A. (2008) Novel strategy for treatment of Japanese encephalitis using arctigenin, a plant lignan. J Antimicrob Chemother 61(3), 679-88.

Tadano, M., Makino, Y., Fukunaga, T., Okuno, Y. and Fukai, K. (1989) Detection of dengue 4 virus core protein in the nucleus. I. A monoclonal antibody to dengue 4 virus reacts with the antigen in the nucleus and cytoplasm. J Gen Virol 70 (Pt 6), 1409-15.

Takahashi, M. (1976) The effects of environmental and physiological conditions of Culex tritaeniorhynchus on the pattern of transmission of Japanese encephalitis virus. J Med Entomol 13(3), 275-84.

Takaku, K., Yamashita, T. and Osanai, T. (1968) Japanese encephalitis purified vaccine. Biken J. 11, 25-39

Takegami, T., Miyamoto, H., Nakamura, H. and Yasui, K. (1982) Biological activities of the structural proteins of Japanese encephalitis virus. Acta Virol 26(5), 312-20.

Tandan, J.B., Ohrr, H., Sohn, Y.M., Yoksan, S., Ji, M., Nam, C.M. and Halstead, S.B. (2007) Single dose of SA 14-14-2 vaccine provides long-term protection against Japanese encephalitis: a case-control study in Nepalese children 5 years after immunization. Vaccine 25(27), 5041-5.

Tauber, E., Kollaritsch, H., Korinek, M., Rendi-Wagner, P., Jilma, B., Firbas, C., Schranz, S., Jong, E., Klingler, A., Dewasthaly, S. and Klade, C.S. (2007) Safety and immunogenicity of a Vero-cell-derived, inactivated Japanese encephalitis vaccine: a non-inferiority, phase III, randomised controlled trial. Lancet 370(9602), 1847-53.

Thongtan, T., Cheepsunthorn, P., Chaiworakul, V., Rattanarungsan, C., Wikan, N. and Smith, D.R. (2010) Highly permissive infection of microglial cells by Japanese encephalitis virus: a possible role as a viral reservoir. Microbes Infect 12(1), 37-45.

Tsai, T.F. (2000) New initiatives for the control of Japanese encephalitis by vaccination: minutes of a WHO/CVI meeting, Bangkok, Thailand, 13-15 October 1998. Vaccine 18 Suppl 2, 1-25.

Tsai, T.F., GJ, C. and YX, Y. (1999) Japanese encephalitis vaccines, 672-710 pp. WB Saunders and Company, Philadelphia.

Tsao, C.H., Su, H.L., Lin, Y.L., Yu, H.P., Kuo, S.M., Shen, C.I., Chen, C.W. and Liao, C.L. (2008) Japanese encephalitis virus infection activates caspase-8 and -9 in a FADD-independent and mitochondrion-dependent manner. J Gen Virol 89(Pt 8), 1930-41.

Umenai, T., Krzysko, R., Bektimirov, T.A. and Assaad, F.A. (1985) Japanese encephalitis: current worldwide status. Bull World Health Organ 63(4), 625-31.

Upadhyaya, B. and Manjunath, R. (2009) Baker's yeast expressing the Japanese encephalitis virus envelope protein on its cell surface: induction of an antigen-specific but non-neutralizing antibody response. Yeast 26(7), 383-97.

van den Hurk, A.F., Ritchie, S.A. and Mackenzie, J.S. (2009) Ecology and geographical expansion of Japanese encephalitis virus. Annu Rev Entomol 54, 17-35.

Venter, M., Myers, T.G., Wilson, M.A., Kindt, T.J., Paweska, J.T., Burt, F.J., Leman, P.A. and Swanepoel, R. (2005) Gene expression in mice infected with West Nile virus strains of different neurovirulence. Virology 342(1), 119-40.

Verma, S.K., Gupta, N., Pattnaik, P., Babu, J.P., Rao, P.V. and Kumar, S. (2009) Antibodies against refolded recombinant envelope protein (domain III) of Japanese encephalitis virus inhibit the JEV infection to Porcine Stable Kidney cells. Protein Pept Lett 16(11), 1334-41.

Wang, B., Hua, R.H., Tian, Z.J., Chen, N.S., Zhao, F.R., Liu, T.Q., Wang, Y.F. and Tong, G.Z. (2009) Identification of a virus-specific and conserved B-cell epitope on NS1 protein of Japanese encephalitis virus. Virus Res 141(1), 90-5.

Wang, T., Scully, E., Yin, Z., Kim, J.H., Wang, S., Yan, J., Mamula, M., Anderson, J.F., Craft, J. and Fikrig, E. (2003) IFN-gamma-producing gamma delta T cells help control murine West Nile virus infection. J Immunol 171(5), 2524-31.

Wang, Y., Lobigs, M., Lee, E. and Mullbacher, A. (2004) Exocytosis and Fas mediated cytolytic mechanisms exert protection from West Nile virus induced encephalitis in mice. Immunol Cell Biol 82(2), 170-3.

Wathelet, M.G., Lin, C.H., Parekh, B.S., Ronco, L.V., Howley, P.M. and Maniatis, T. (1998) Virus infection induces the assembly of coordinately activated transcription factors on the IFN-beta enhancer in vivo. Mol Cell 1(4), 507-18.

Welsch, S., Miller, S., Romero-Brey, I., Merz, A., Bleck, C.K., Walther, P., Fuller, S.D., Antony, C., Krijnse-Locker, J. and Bartenschlager, R. (2009) Composition and three-dimensional architecture of the dengue virus replication and assembly sites. Cell Host Microbe 5(4), 365-75.

Westaway, E.G., Khromykh, A.A., Kenney, M.T., Mackenzie, J.M. and Jones, M.K. (1997) Proteins C and NS4B of the flavivirus Kunjin translocate independently into the nucleus. Virology 234(1), 31-41.

Winkler, G., Maxwell, S.E., Ruemmler, C. and Stollar, V. (1989) Newly synthesized dengue-2 virus nonstructural protein NS1 is a soluble protein but becomes partially hydrophobic and membrane-associated after dimerization. Virology 171(1), 302-5.

Winter, P.M., Dung, N.M., Loan, H.T., Kneen, R., Wills, B., Thu le, T., House, D., White, N.J., Farrar, J.J., Hart, C.A. and Solomon, T. (2004) Proinflammatory cytokines and chemokines in humans with Japanese encephalitis. J Infect Dis 190(9), 1618-26.

Wu, H.H., Chen, C.T., Lin, Y.L. and Lee, S.T. (2004) Sub-fragments of the envelope gene are highly protective against the Japanese encephalitis virus lethal infection in DNA priming--protein boosting immunization strategies. Vaccine 22(5-6), 793-800.

Wu, J., Bera, A.K., Kuhn, R.J. and Smith, J.L. (2005) Structure of the Flavivirus helicase: implications for catalytic activity, protein interactions, and proteolytic processing. J Virol 79(16), 10268-77.

Wu, S.F., Lee, C.J., Liao, C.L., Dwek, R.A., Zitzmann, N. and Lin, Y.L. (2002) Antiviral effects of an iminosugar derivative on flavivirus infections. J Virol 76(8), 3596-604.

Xin, Y.Y., Ming, Z.G., Peng, G.Y., Jian, A. and Min, L.H. (1988) Safety of a live-attenuated Japanese encephalitis virus vaccine (SA14-14-2) for children. Am J Trop Med Hyg 39(2), 214-17.

Yamashita, T., Unno, H., Mori, Y., Tani, H., Moriishi, K., Takamizawa, A., Agoh, M., Tsukihara, T. and Matsuura, Y. (2008) Crystal structure of the catalytic domain of Japanese encephalitis virus NS3 helicase/nucleoside triphosphatase at a resolution of 1.8 A. Virology 373(2), 426-36.

Yang, T.C., Shiu, S.L., Chuang, P.H., Lin, Y.J., Wan, L., Lan, Y.C. and Lin, C.W. (2009) Japanese encephalitis virus NS2B-NS3 protease induces caspase 3 activation and mitochondria-mediated apoptosis in human medulloblastoma cells. Virus Res 143(1), 77-85.

Yasuda, A., Kimura-Kuroda, J., Ogimoto, M., Miyamoto, M., Sata, T., Sato, T., Takamura, C., Kurata, T., Kojima, A. and Yasui, K. (1990) Induction of protective immunity in animals vaccinated with recombinant vaccinia viruses that express PreM and E glycoproteins of Japanese encephalitis virus. J Virol 64(6), 2788-95.

Yoo, J.S., Kim, C.M., Kim, J.H., Kim, J.Y. and Oh, J.W. (2009) Inhibition of Japanese encephalitis virus replication by peptide nucleic acids targeting cis-acting elements on the plus- and minus-strands of viral RNA. Antiviral Res 82(3), 122-33.

Yu, I.M., Zhang, W., Holdaway, H.A., Li, L., Kostyuchenko, V.A., Chipman, P.R., Kuhn, R.J., Rossmann, M.G. and Chen, J. (2008) Structure of the immature dengue virus at low pH primes proteolytic maturation. Science 319(5871), 1834-7.

Zhang, M.J., Wang, M.J., Jiang, S.Z. and Ma, W.Y. (1989) Passive protection of mice, goats, and monkeys against Japanese encephalitis with monoclonal antibodies. J Med Virol 29(2), 133-8.

Zhang, Y., Chirmule, N., Gao, G.P., Qian, R., Croyle, M., Joshi, B., Tazelaar, J. and Wilson, J.M. (2001) Acute cytokine response to systemic adenoviral vectors in mice is mediated by dendritic cells and macrophages. Mol Ther 3(5 Pt 1), 697-707.

Zhao, Z., Wakita, T. and Yasui, K. (2003) Inoculation of plasmids encoding Japanese encephalitis virus PrM-E proteins with colloidal gold elicits a protective immune response in BALB/c mice. J Virol 77(7), 4248-60.

18

Genetic Evolution of Japanese Encephalitis Virus

Ching-Kai Chuang and Wei-June Chen
Department of Public Health and Parasitology, Chang Gung University
Taiwan

1. Introduction

Japanese encephalitis (JE) is widely distributed in most areas of Asia, particularly in eastern, southern, and southeastern Asia (Rosen 1986). It expanded to the Torres Strait of northern Australia in 1999, and has now become widespread in Australia (Mackenzie, 1999; Mackenzie et al., 2004). Mass vaccinations were implemented in a number of Asian countries such as Japan, Korea, China, Taiwan, Thailand, and India, leading to declines in the incidences of JE (Wu et al., 1999; Monath, 2002; Erlanger et al., 2009). Generally, swine serve as an amplifying host in the transmission cycle of the JE virus (JEV) (fig. 1), giving it an important role in the maintenance of the JEV in nature (Nidaira et al., 2009). Due to changes in the socioeconomic status, households that breed swine have sharply decreased in Japan and many other countries (Yoshida et al., 2005). Despite, an estimated 3 billion persons living in countries with endemic JE, it causes about 30,000~50,000 cases per year (Solomom, 2004; van den Hurk et al., 2008); among these, there are estimated to be 10,000~15,000 human deaths yearly worldwide (Erlanger et al., 2009). The potential for the emergence of frontiers of JEV is now a new concern (Nett et al., 2009; van den Hurk et al., 2009).

The etiological agent of JE is one of about 70 members of the genus *Flavivirus* that belongs to the family Flaviviridae (Monath & Heinz, 1996). JEV frequently causes encephalitic diseases through bites by rice-field breeding *Culex* mosquitoes (van den Hurk et al., 2009; Unni et al., 2011), especially *Culex tritaeneorhynchus* which is a species that breeds in paddy fields (Lindenbach & Rice, 2001). This suggests that most species of JE vectors are rural mosquitoes. In association with seasonal fluctuations in mosquito population densities, JE cases mostly appear during the summer, particularly May to October in most endemic areas (Rosen, 1986). In spite of this, other mosquitoes classified in different genera including *Armigeres, Aedes, Anopheles,* and *Mansonia* have also been documented to be a potential vector (Chen et al., 2000; Deng et al., 2009; Weng et al., 1999).

The JE virion is about ca. 50 nm in diameter (Westaway et al., 1985); its genome contains linear, single-stranded positive-sense RNA (~11 kb in length) (Chambers et al., 1990). The genomic RNA of the JEV comprises a 5' untranslated region (UTR), a longer 3' UTR, and an intervening single open reading frame (ORF) (Chambers et al., 1990) that encodes 3 structural proteins in the order of the capsid (C), membrane (prM/M), and envelope (E), followed by 7 non-structural proteins (NS1~NS5) (Chambers et al., 1990; Sumiyoshi et al., 1987). The functions of some viral proteins are now clearer. Among these, protein E is the major component of the viral envelope which binds to host cell surface receptors (Ren et al., 2007) and is also involved in membrane fusion between the virion and host late endosomes (Stiasny & Heinz, 2006). NS3 is an enzyme with both serine protease and NTPase/helicase activities (Assenberg et al., 2009), while NS5 was confirmed to be a RNA-dependent RNA polymerase as well as a methyltransferase (Lescar & Canard, 2009; Zhou et al., 2007).

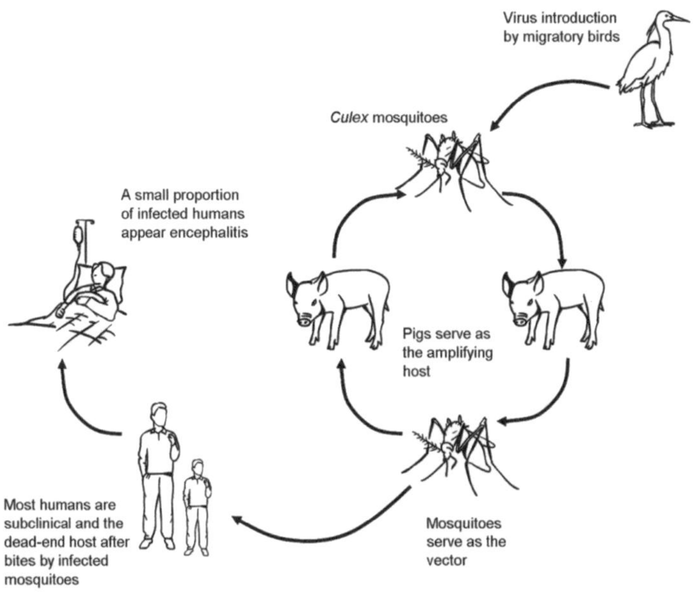

Fig. 1. Transmission cycle of Japanese encephalitis virus in nature. A proportion of infected humans exhibit encephalitis and are a dead-end host after being bitten by infected mosquitoes

In general, the JEV replicates inefficiently and thus causes delayed low-titer viremia in hosts (Shope & Sather, 1979). The central nervous system (CNS) is the principal target of infection by the JEV (Ravi et al., 1994). However, the virus is usually cleared from the CNS by an immune response before the development of encephalitis (McMinn et al., 1996). This thus leads to a relatively high number of subclinical infections in humans or those who rapidly recover from clinical symptoms, defined as a dead-end host (Mathur et al., 1987, Ravi et al., 1994). It is estimated that about 1 in 25~1000 humans with infections, depending on the endemicity, exposure to mosquitoes, preexisting antibodies to flaviviruses, and viral strain differences (Mackenzie et al., 2004; Solomon and Vaughn, 2002), will exhibit clinical symptoms (Konishi & Suzuki, 2002). Despite this, the case fatality rate of JE can be as high as 25%~30% (Burke & Leake, 1988); 15%~50% of the survivors may end up with sequelae of neurologic impairment and/or mental retardation (Monath, 2002).

2. The route through which JEV enters the CNS

The JEV tends to infect the CNS in dead-end hosts, *i.e.*, humans (Johnson et al., 1985; Johnson, 1987). However, it is not clear how the virus gains entry into the CNS from the peripheral circulation (Myint et al., 2007). Theoretically, after the bite of an infected mosquito, the JEV is amplified in dermal tissues and then lymph nodes via migration of dendritic (Langerhans) cells before invading the CNS (Johnson et al., 2000; Solomon et al., 2000). A variety of flaviviruses were speculated to enter the CNS via the olfactory pathway (Monath et al., 1996), across cerebral capillary endothelial cells (Liou and Hsu, 1998), or virion budding on the parenchymal side after replication in endothelial cells (McMinn et al., 1996). Nevertheless, features including the diffuse infection throughout the brain and no viral antigens in the choroid plexus or ependyma indicate that viruses probably enter the CNS via a hematogenous route (Kimura-Kuroda et al., 1992), especially with a status of severe viremia (Yamada et al., 2004).

In both animals and humans, the blood-brain barrier (BBB) generally prevents viral invasion of the CNS (Ballabh et al., 2004), unless it has been disrupted, resulting in increased permeability and inflammatory cell infiltration (Muller et al., 2005). The BBB integrity was observed to evidently be weakened in the primary phase of JEV infection, showing modified distribution of occludin, a tight-junction (TJ) component protein of the BBB (Liu et al., 2008). Increased permeability of the BBB actually allows peripheral blood monocytes (PBMCs) to migrate from the peripheral blood into brain tissues (Stephens *et al.*, 2003; Diamond & Klein, 2004). Normally, lymphocytes constantly enter the CNS in small numbers (Hickey et al., 1991), but their presence in the CNS may increase in response to viral infections (Griffin et al., 1992).

PBMCs isolated from inoculated mice were detected to be infected by the JEV (Chuang et al., 2003; Liu et al., 2009). Leukocytes move across endothelial cells of capillaries at sites where TJs appear to be dissociated (Liu et al., 2008), suggesting that the JEV enters brain tissues via penetration of infected PBMCs. Uniquely, this pathway of penetration may begin at the cerebrum, not in the cerebellum (Liu et al., 2008). Destruction of the BBB can be caused by apoptosis of astrocytes and/or neurons (Suri & Banerjee, 1995; Tseng et al., 2011). Viral replication in peripheral tissues may also trigger a Toll-like receptor inflammatory response that alters the BBB (Wang et al., 2004). The stimulus capable of causing changes in BBB permeability can also be derived from the effects of the chemokine, monocyte chemoattractant protein (MCP)-1 (Stamatovic et al., 2005; Yamada et al., 2004).

3. Pathogenesis of the JEV

The JEV infects a variety of brain tissues with a characteristic pattern of mixed intensity of hypodense lesions in the thalamus, basal ganglia, and midbrain (Kalita & Misra, 2000, 2002). Most JE patients present typical clinical symptoms including headaches, vomiting, an altered mental state, as well as dystonia, rigidity, and a characteristic mask-like facies (Chuang et al., 2002). Clinically, movement disorders are frequently seen in patients who survive the acute phase of JE (Misra & Kalita, 1997), implying that sensorimotor neuropathy eventually occurs. It is now known that encphealitis associated with flaviviral infections may cause Guillain-Barré-like syndrome, showing a demyelinating feature in sensorimotor tissues of the brain (Sejvar et al., 2005). This suggests that demyelination is an important step causing disruption of motor coordination during JEV infection.

The JEV has repeatedly been demonstrated to infect neurons in brains of experimental animals and humans (Johnson et al., 1985; Yamada et al., 2004) and is usually not cleared from tissues by elicited antibodies (Desai et al., 1995). Generally, encephalitic flaviviruses induce apoptosis in infected neurons and subsequently cause fatal outcomes to the host (Liu et al., 2008; Nargi-Aizenman & Griffin, 2001; Samuel et al., 2007; Xia et al, 2001). This possibly occurs by way of reactive oxygen specie-mediated induction of matrix metalloproteinase-9 expression and subsequent activation of nuclear factor-κB (Tung et al., 2010). Neuronal death, which is widely seen in JEV-infected mouse brains, is probably important for induction of axonal injury and demyelination (Meyer et al., 2001; Tsunoda et al., 2003). Demyelination is a common feature in brains infected with encephalitic viruses (Stohlman & Hinton, 2001); this is the process by which axons lose myelin that normally serves as an insulator, resulting in loss of balance and coordination, although it may vary among patients (Sarma, 2010). In fact, demyelination is rather common in mouse brains infected with the JEV; this is supposed to be triggered by T cell-mediated autoimmunity against the myelin basic protein (MBP), a component of myelin (Grigoriadis & Hadjigeorgiou, 2006; Tseng et al., 2011). In other words, the JEV, which normally causes inflammation and neuronal degeneration in the CNS, eventually induces the proliferation of specific T cells which mediate autoimmunity to destroy components of axon-surrounding myelin such as MBP (Tseng et al., 2011).

4. Origin and genetic diversity of the JEV

The first JE epidemic in history was reported in Japan in 1871 (van den Hurk et al., 2009); however, the causal virus was not isolated until 1935 (Rosen, 1986). There are 2 epidemiological patterns of JE: one restrictedly occurs in tropical zones including South India, Indonesia, Malaysia, Singapore, and southern Thailand with no seasonal preference, and the other mainly occurs in northern parts of tropical zones, such as China, Taiwan, Japan, Korea, Nepal, and northern parts of Myanmar, India, and Viet Nam (Umenai et al., 1985). The JEV in temperate areas is supposedly re-introduced by migratory birds or bats and/or is wind-borne (Rosen, 1986; Solomon et al., 2003).

Phylogenic studies revealed that the JEV possesses genetic diversity among strains, through which the origin, evolution, and spread of the virus were theoretically determined (Gould, 2002; Gould et al., 2004). It seems that the JEV originated from an ancestral virus in the Indonesia-Malaysia region, and subsequently evolved there into the different genotypes before they spread across Asia (Solomon et al., 2003). It was estimated that the ancestor common to all genotypes of JEV arose within the last 300 years (Uchil & Satchidanandam, 2001).

Major alterations in the genome of resulting viral variants frequently occur in the envelope (E) protein (Deubel et al., 1993; Trent et al., 1983, 1987). Based on the nucleotide sequences of the C/PrM and E genes, 5 genotypes (I~V) of the JEV were identified (fig. 2); these probably originated from the ancestral virus and evolved into the different genotypes (Solomon et al., 2003). Geographically, genotype I includes isolates from Korea, India, Cambodia, Laos, and northern Thailand (Fan et al., 2010; Fulmali et al., 2011; Wang et al., 2007, 2010;); genotype II includes isolates from Malaysia, Sarawak, Indonesia, southern Thailand, and northern Australia (Pyke et al., 2001); genotype III includes isolates widely distributed in Asian countries with temperate climates, including Japan, Taiwan, China, India, Sri Lanka, Nepal, Viet Nam, and the Philippines (Chen et al., 1990; Mackenzie et al., 2004; Wang et al., 2007); and genotype IV includes isolates from Indonesia (Chen et al., 1992). The last one identified was genotype V, which includes isolates with a restricted distribution in India (Solomon et al., 2003; Uchil & Satchidanandam, 2001). Based on the composition of nucleotides and amino acids, strains belonging to genotype II are the most similar to genotype I (9.1%~10.7% difference), followed by genotype III (10.2%~11.7% difference), and genotype IV (16.2%~16.6% difference) (Schuh et al., 2011). The phylogenetic tree presented here shows that genotype V is the most distant from genotype I. This newly identified genotype was suggested to have originated from Malaysia (Solomon et al., 2003). Nevertheless, it must be noted that the genetic similarity does not necessarily match their epidemiological distributions (Schuh et al., 2011).

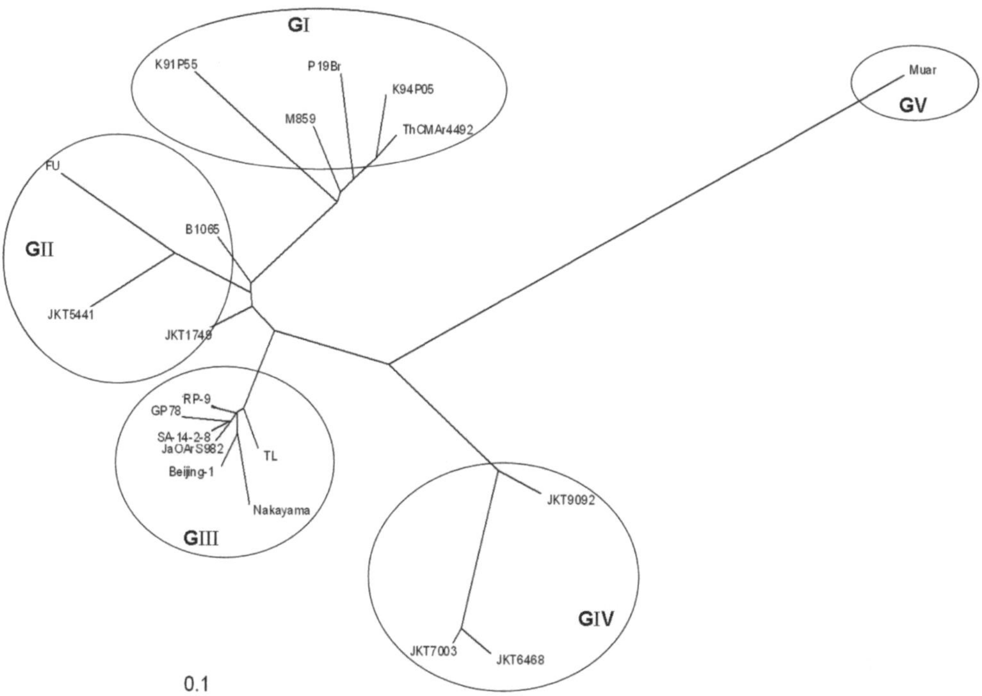

Fig. 2. Unrooted phylogenetic analysis of 17 homologs of protein E of the Japanese encephalitis virus showing that this protein can be divided into 5 clades or genotypes. Genotype I: K91P55 (U34928), M859 (U70410), P19Br (U70416), K94P05 (AF045551), and ThCMAr4492 (D45362); genotype II: B1065 (U70388), FU (AF217620), JKT5441 (U70406), and JKT1749 (U70405); genotype III: RP-9 (AF014161), GP78 (AF075723), SA-14-2-8 (U15763), JaOArS982 (M18370), Beijing-1 (L48961), Nakayama (EF571853), and TL (AF098737); genotype IV: JKT7003 (U70408), JKT6468 (AY184212), and JKT9092 (U70409); and genotype V: Muar (HM596272). The analysis used the Neighbor-joining method within the PHYLIP 3.6 software package with 500 bootstraps (Felsenstein, 2005) after sequence alignment with the Clustal W package (Thompson et al., 1994)

In fact, intra-genotypic groupings can occur (Ali & Igarashi, 1997; Wang et al., 2007), among which genotypes IV and V are the most divergent genotypes and are thought to represent the oldest lineages (Misra & Kalita, 2010). Genotype III can further be divided into 3 clusters among strains isolated in Taiwan (Huang et al., 2010). It is interesting that genotype III was the major one in Japan before 1991, while most isolates after 1995 were identified as belonging to genotype I (Ma et al., 2003; Morita, 2009). A similar phenomenon or even genotype replacement was also seen in many other countries in Asia (Huang et al., 2010; Morita, 2009; Nitatpathana et al., 2008). This suggests that the flow or a shift of genotypes between endemic regions is possible (fig. 3). Eventually, genotype I, which is genetically close to those from Malaysia, was found to have been introduced and co-circulated with and/or ultimately replaced the existing genotype III in many Asian countries (Fulmali et al., 2011; Huang et al., 2010; Ma et al., 2003; Nga et al., 2004; Pyke et al., 2001; Wang et al., 2007; Yoshida et al., 2005; Yun et al., 2010). Putatively, the introduced genotype I originated from Southeast Asia (Nabeshima et al., 2009; Nga et al., 2004); which has been an important region for emerging pathogens (Solomon et al., 2003). Wind-blown infected mosquitoes flying with air currents during the typhoon season supposedly played a role in the geographic expansion (Ritchie & Rochester, 2001).

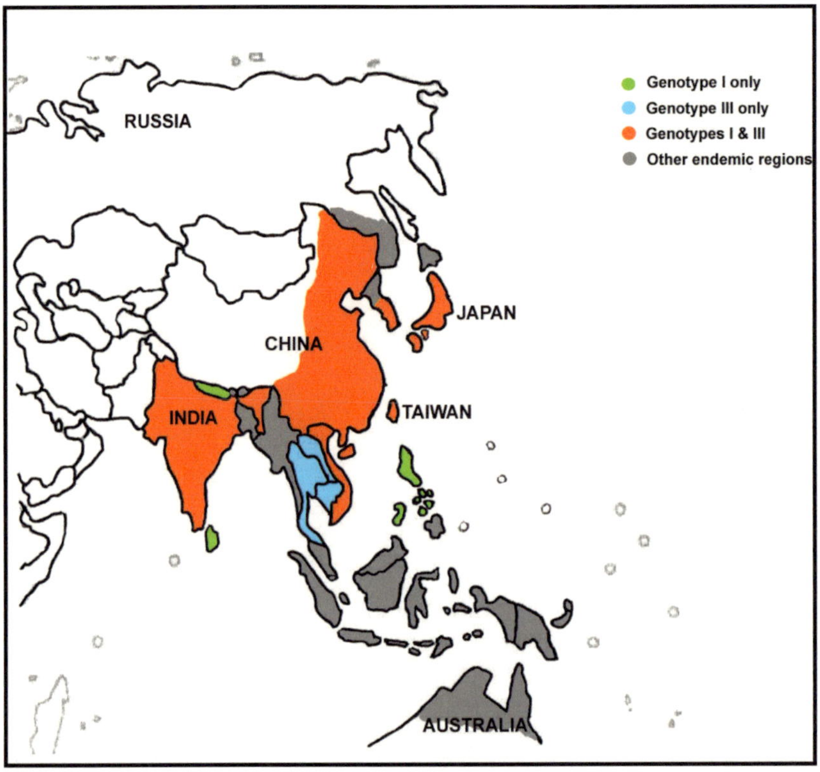

Fig. 3. Japanese encephalitis virus (JEV) is widely distributed in most Asian countries (gray). Among the 5 genotypes of JEV, genotype III (blue) has been predominant in most northeast Asian countries such as Taiwan, China, Japan, Korea, Viet Nam, Thailand, and even India. Genotype I (green) was putatively introduced by wind-blown infected mosquitoes, for example, during the typhoon season. Nowadays, the mixed occurrence of both genotypes (orange) has become common in such regions

5. Mutations and evolution of the JEV in nature

RNA genomes of flaviviruses evolve rather rapidly compared to DNA-based organisms. Generally, RNA viruses evolve rapidly, with approximately 6 orders of magnitude higher rates of nucleotide substitutions compared to DNA viruses (Jenkins et al., 2002). It seems that horizontal gene transfer of the virus between host cells increases its genetic diversity.

Therefore, it is important to see how genetic diversity occurs, either by investigating the molecular epidemiology or evolution of flaviviruses. Unlike re-assortments of RNA segments that frequently occur in the influenza virus (Khiabanian et al., 2009), flaviviruses readily change nucleotides in their genomes due to a lack of proof-reading and mismatch repair abilities (Holland, 1996). This error-prone nature of RNA synthesis triggers mutations which are an important source of RNA virus diversity. They, in turn, form a variety of genetically related variants known as "quasispecies" and are responsible for the pathogenesis and tissue distribution of viruses (Holmes, 2004).

Natural mutations with lower virulence were isolated from field-caught mosquitoes (Chiou & Chen, 2001), leading to circulation in a human population with a low incidence of the disease (Chen et al., 2000). Among most viruses, mutations serve as the major source of genetic change; which in turn creates strains that may be either lethal or advantageous. The E protein is known to be the major component on the surface of flaviviral virions (Adams et al., 1995; Rey et al., 1995), and generally plays a role in interactions with molecule(s) or receptor(s) on cell membranes when the virus infects host cells (Martinez-Barragan & del Angel, 2001; Ramos-Castaneda et al., 1997; Rothwell et al., 1996). Passage of flaviviruses in cultured cells was demonstrated to induce genetic changes in the E protein (Marchette et al., 1990), causing phenotypic alterations, *e.g.*, viral virulence (Cao et al., 1995; Hasegawa et al., 1992).

As mentioned, phenotypic changes may be caused by mutations in the E protein (fig. 4), which include antigenicity, pathogenicity, virulence, persistence, or interactions with host cells (Cecilia & Gould, 1991; Chiou et al., 2007; Chung et al., 1996; Hasegawa et al., 1994; Lee & Lobigs, 2002; Mangada & Takegami, 1999; Ni & Barrett, 1996; Nitayaphan et al., 1990; Wu et al., 1998). It was reported that a single mutation at E-123 (Ser→Arg) in the JEV significantly increases the virulence in mice, indicating that this nucleotide may be responsible for the pathogenicity of the JEV (Tajima et al., 2010). In Neuro-2a cells, a higher-virulent variant (CJN-S1) of the JEV with a mutation at E-138 (Glu→Lys) was isolated from human brain tissues in a relatively short time of passage. The same mutation was also reported to evidently affect multiple steps of the life cycle of the JEV (Zhao et al., 2005), including reduced neurotropism and attenuated virulence (Chen et al., 1996; Ni & Barrett, 1998). The specific step of such an effect is its ability to attach and penetrate (Liu et al., 2004), leading to lower virulence in host cells (Chiou & Chen, 2007). In the meantime, mutations at E-306 (Glu→Lys) (T1P1-S1) and E-389 (Asp→Asn) (CC27-S6) were also observed to possess a higher affinity for heparin sulfate and to form small plaques (Chiou et al., 2005). Apparently, the E protein is not the only site of the viral genome related to phenotype determination of the JEV. A single N-linked glycosylation site in the prM protein of the JEV was documented to be critical for the pathogenicity of the virus in mice (Kim et al., 2008).

Factors affecting the genetic diversity of the JEV may be complex and remain to be worked out. In a study of E/NS1 protein of another flavivirus (dengue), the genetic composition changed with passages of cultured cells (Chen et al., 2003). In fact, 1 (E-53) and 2 amino acids (NS1-178 and NS1-181) had mutated after 30 passages in Vero cells, while no changes were observed in viruses serially passaged in C6/36 cells (Chen et al., 2003). This reflects a feature by which mutations occur more slowly in arboviruses, either alphaviruses or flaviviruses, than in other RNA viruses (Weaver et al., 1992). Perhaps, antioxidant defenses that protect mosquito cells from apoptosis in response to the virus may play an important role in reducing the occurrence of viral mutations (Chen et al., 2011).

Heparan sulfate, a glycosaminoglycan (GAG), on the surface of all adherent cells is known to modulate the actions of a number of extracellular ligands (Bernfield et al., 1999). Clusters consisting of E protein residues 49, 138, 306, or 389/390 on the surface of JE virions may define molecular determinants for GAG binding and concomitant virulence attenuation in human adenocarcinoma (SW13) cells (Lee et al., 2004). Additionally, the JEV strain with the mutation of Glu-306-Lys in the E protein was found to increase its binding ability with highly sulfated forms of GAGs in Neuro-2a cells (Chiou et al., 2005). This implies that GAGs, particularly highly sulfated forms (Su et al., 2001), in host cells can be important as a tool to screen viral strains (Chiou et al., 2005).

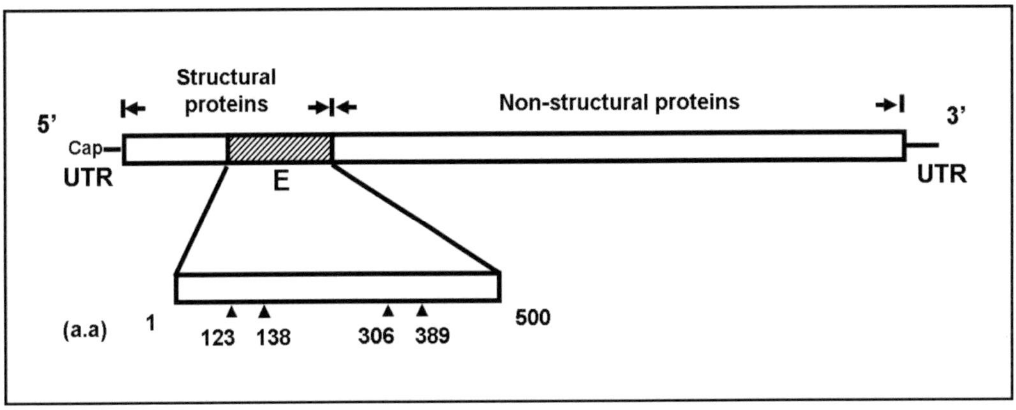

Fig. 4. Phenotypic changes through mutations in the E protein may determine viral characteristics, such as the antigenicity, pathogenicity, virulence, persistence, and interactions with host cells. Several amino acids, including E123, E138, E306, and E389, were demonstrated to be important in the ability of the Japanese encephalitis virus to interact with a host

Viral evolution generally occurs as a result of genetic variations and selection of variants from large viral populations, producing a new genetic makeup which can pass from generation to the next. Due to the differential fates of flaviviruses in vertebrate and mosquito cells (Chen et al., 2003), patterns of genetic evolution may differ between viruses replicating in these 2 types of host cells. Experimental evidence showed that slower mutations of arboviruses, either alphaviruses or flaviviruses, may occur in mosquito cells by applying the brake on the evolution of these viruses (Vasilakis et al., 2009). The evolution of viruses depends on the mutation-selection balance. It was hypothesized that the JEV changes its genetic composition under certain circumstances in vertebrate cells. In contrast, either positive or negative selection can occur in mosquito cells, selecting fitter variants.

6. RNA recombination in the JEV

As mentioned, RNA viruses evolve rapidly compared to DNA viruses, with approximately 6 orders of magnitude higher rates of nucleotide substitutions (Jenkins et al., 2002). In addition, genetic exchanges via re-assortment of RNA segments are known to occur in segmented RNA-containing viruses such as the influenza virus (Khiabanian et al., 2009), rotavirus (Gentsch et al., 2005), bluetongue virus (Carpi et al., 2010), and so forth. RNA recombinations are now believed to be one mechanism exploited by many viruses, which serve as a strategy for evolution (Worobey & Holmes, 1999). This was found in the poliovirus (Ledinko, 1963), flaviviruses (Cristina & Colina, 2006; Twiddy & Holmes, 2003), and others (Rohayem et al., 2005). Most notably, western equine encephalitis virus, a member of the genus *Alphavirus*, is thought to have originated from a recombination between an eastern equine encephalitis-like virus and a Sindbis-like virus, giving rise to a completely new virus (Hahn et al., 1988). Similarly, the Singapore S275/90 strain of dengue 1 virus very likely arose from a recombination between a Djibouti/Cambodia lineage ancestor and an Abidjan lineage ancestor (Tolou et al., 2001).

Genetic diversity derived from spontaneous mutations and the introduction of new strains through migratory birds increase the possibility of RNA recombination in the JEV (Rosen, 1986). Accumulating data from phylogenetic analyses indicate that the recombinant forms of the JEV may have appeared in Korea and Thailand (Twiddy & Holmes, 2003). It is now believed that 2 putative recombinants isolated from Korea (K82P01 and K91P55) appear to have parental strains originating in Japan and Korea, while one from Thailand (Thailand 82) has parental strains originating in Thailand and China (Twiddy & Holmes, 2003).

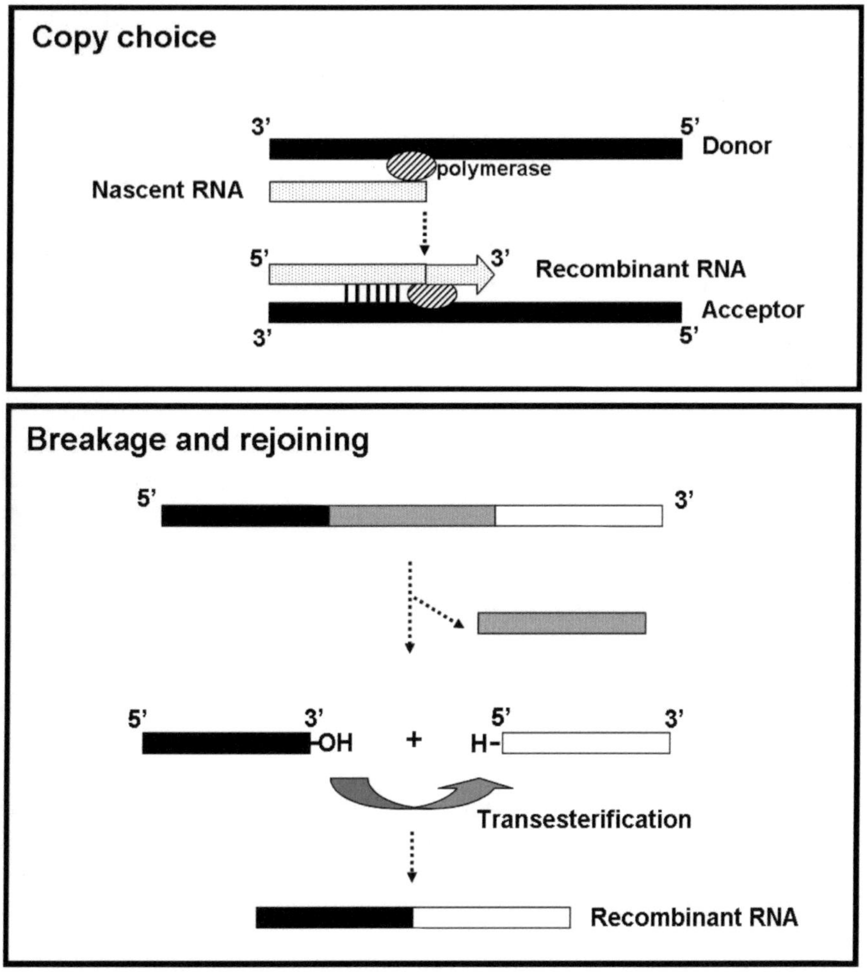

Fig. 5. Two possible mechanisms were proposed for the occurrence of RNA recombination: (i) the copy choice mechanism and (ii) breakage and rejoining (Lai, 1992)

In general, recombination follows 2 possible mechanisms (fig. 5): (1) a copy choice mechanism and (2) breakage and rejoining (Lai, 1992). The breaking and rejoining pathway is commonly seen with DNA but usually not with RNA recombinations (Jarvis & Kirkegaard, 1991, 1992). In contrast, a copy choice mechanism for RNA recombination was demonstrated to occur in the poliovirus; in which templates are switched by viral RNA-dependent RNA polymerase (RdRp) switches during negative-strand synthesis (Kirkegaard & Baltimore, 1986). This may also be the mechanism of RNA recombination in other RNA viruses such as coronaviruses and plant viruses (Makino et al., 1986; Sztuba-Solunsk et al., 2011).

There are 3 types of RNA recombinations (fig. 6), including precisely homologous, imprecisely (aberrantly) homologous, and non-homologous, which are known to occur in RNA viruses (Alejska et al., 2001). Of these, the precisely homologous recombination through a template-switching (copy-choice) mechanism is probably the most common type (Wierzchoslawski & Bujarski, 2006). We recently provided experimental evidence showing that genetically different JEV strains can simultaneously infect a single BHK-21 or C6/36 cell, resulting in the occurrence of genetic exchange or RNA recombination. It probably follows the copy choice mechanism with the precisely homologous recombination type (Chuang & Chen, 2009).

Secondary structures are probably essential for the occurrence of RNA (Hsue et al., 2000; Wierzchoslawski & Bujarski, 2006). It is particularly important that the structure of the acceptor RNA affects the occurrence of RNA recombinations in the case of HIV (Abdeladim et al., 2003). The stability of the secondary structure eventually promotes the frequency of template-switching RNA recombinations (Nagy & Jozef, 1997; White & Morris, 1995). In the JEV, changes in specific secondary structures eventually affect the frequency of RNA recombinations (Chuang & Chen, 2009).

Recently, AU-rich sequences were mentioned as being more efficient at promoting recombination, compared to GC-rich sequences, in single-stranded, positive-sense genomic RNA (Shapka & Nagy, 2004). However, AU-rich sequences do not really exist, and the AU content was $< 50\%$ in the region favoring crossovers in Japanese encephalitis according our recent study (Chuang & Chen, 2009). Perhaps the nucleotide composition of the sequence is not crucial in determining RNA recombinations of the JEV. Because neither deletions nor insertions of nucleotides were shown to occur in the crossover region, the precisely homologous recombination is believed to be the predominant, if not the only, type of RNA recombination between JEVs. This is consistent with the inference from previous observations that AU-rich sequences usually decrease the accuracy of crossovers, leading to imprecisely or aberrantly homologous recombinations of viral RNA (Nagy & Bujarski, 1996).

Rates of recombination in many single-stranded RNA viruses appear to be low (Chare et al., 2006; Worobey & Holmes, 1999), and RNA recombination is thought to have played some roles in the co-evolution of viruses with genetic conflicts (Turner & Chao, 1998) and the development of strains with increased virulence and transmission potential (Holmes et al., 1999). Moreover, RNA recombination was found more frequently in BHK-21 than C6/36 cells, indicating that mammalian cells are more crucial in determining RNA recombinations (Schneider & Roossinch, 2001). This causes higher rates of genetic variants in mammalian cells, and only those with fitness are selected, which possibly also operates in mosquito cells.

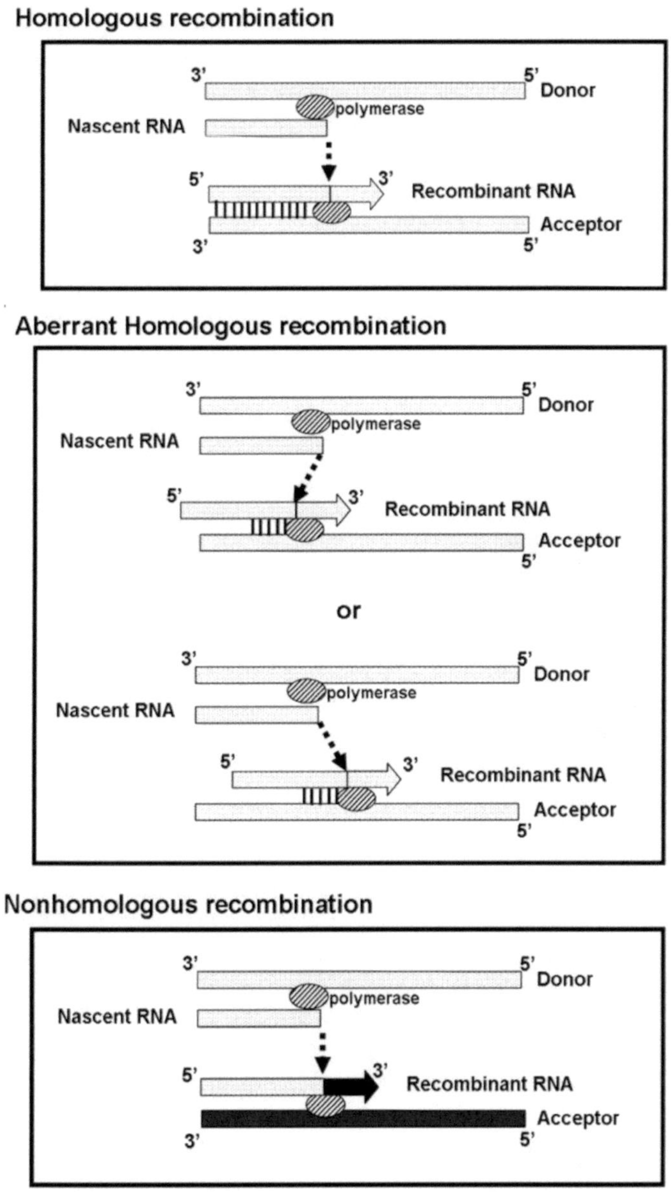

Fig. 6. Putatively, there are 3 types of RNA recombinations: (i) homologous (precisely), (ii) aberrantly (imprecise) homologous, and (iii) non-homologous (Alejska et al., 2001)

7. Conclusions and perspectives

Because of underlying mutation and genetic recombinations, the JEV probably evolves in a very similar way to that which governs other organisms. Nowadays, new mass-sequencing techniques are more popular and have revealed a greater diversity of flaviviruses than ever thought (Kuno et al., 1998). Due to the small size and probably the fragility, virus evolution cannot possibly be investigated from so-called fossil viruses, if there are any. However, genetic diversity in nature provides information, facilitating an understanding of the existence of viral evolution. Maintenance of genetic diversity can theoretically reduce the rapid loss of fitness due to Muller's ratchet during passage of the virus from 1 host to another. Evolutionary, this is beneficial for a virus that has shifted to a new environmental niche or selective regimen, serving as a factor helping a virus escape from accumulated deleterious effects in a virus population.

Most flaviviruses comprise multiple genotypes or strains which potentially determine the virulence and epidemiology of the diseases. Mutation(s) of the viral genome followed by selection in host cells are the commonest way to form a new viral strain, the phenotypes of which may be more virulent or attenuated. Understanding changes in genomic RNA can help better elucidate evolving viruses as well as their clinical significance. Accumulating evidence suggests that RNA recombination is also one mechanism creating diversity of viruses, producing more unpredictable results during their evolution. A special concern is the possibility of genetic exchange between different populations of the virus (Tolou et al., 2001). As a result, it is particularly worthwhile noting whether or not live-attenuated vaccine strains experience crossing-over with wild viruses during the synthesis of new RNA (Becher et al., 2001; Holmes et al., 1999).

8. Acknowledgment

This work was financial supported by National Science Council of Taiwan (NSC99-2320-B-182-012-MY3) and partially by Chang Gung Memorial Hospital (CMRPD190161). The authors would like to thank Mr. Wei-Ting Chen for figure sketching.

9. References

Abdeladim, M.; Lucette, P.; Torsten, U.; Michel, V.; Henri, B. & Matteo, N. (2003). Evidence for a mechanism of recombination during reverse transcription dependent on the structure of the acceptor RNA. *Journal of Biological Chemistry*, 278, pp. 15973-15982.

Adams, S. C.; Broom, A. K.; Sammels, L. M.; Hartnett, A. C.; Howard, M. J.; Coelen, R. J.; Mackenzie, J. S. & Hall, R. A. (1995). Glycosylation and antigenic variation among Kunjin virus isolates. *Virology*, 206, pp. 49-56.

Alejska, M.; Kurzyñska-Kokorniak, A.; Broda, M.; Kierzek, R. & Figlerowicz, M. (2001) How RNA viruses exchange their genetic material. *Acta Biochimic. Polonica*, 48, pp. 391-407.

Ali, A. & Igarashi, A. (1997). Antigenic and genetic variations among Japanese encephalitis virus strains belonging to genotype 1. *Microbiology and Immunology*, 41, pp. 241-52.

Assenberg, R.; Mastrangelo, E.; Walter, T. S.; Verma, A.; Milani, M.; Owens, R. J.; Stuart, D. I.; Grimes, J. M. & Mancini, E. J. (2009). Crystal structure of a novel conformational state of the flavivirus NS3 protein: implications for polyprotein processing and viral replication. *Journal of Virology*, 83, pp. 12895-12906.

Ballabh, P.; Braun, A. & Nedergaard, M. (2004). The blood-brain barrier: an overview: structure, regulation, and clinical implications. *Neurobiology of Disease*, 16, pp. 1-13.

Becher, P.; Orlich, M. & Thiel, H. J. (2001). RNA recombination between persisting pestivirus and a vaccine strain: generation of cytopathogenic virus and induction of lethal disease. *Journal of Virology*, 75, pp. 6256-6264.

Bernfield, M.; Götte, M.; Park, P. W.; Reizes, O.; Fitzgerald, M. L.; Lincecum, J. & Zako, M. (1999). Functions of cell surface heparan sulfate proteoglycans. *Annual Review of Biochemistry,* 68, pp. 729-777.

Burke, D.S. & Leake, C. J. (1988). Japanese encephalitis, In: *The Arboviruses: Epidemiology and Ecology,* T. P. Monath, (Ed.), 63-92, CRC, Boca Raton, Florida, USA.

Cao, J. X.; Ni, H.; Wills, M. R.; Campbell, G. A.; Sil, B. K.; Ryman, K. D.; Kitchen, I. & Barrett, A. D. (1995). Passage of Japanese encephalitis virus in HeLa cells results in attentuation of virulence in mice. *Journal of General Virology,* 76, pp. 2757-2764.

Carpi, G.; Holmes, E. C. & Kitchen, A. (2010). The evolutionary dynamics of bluetongue Virus. *Journal of Molecular Evolution,* 70, pp. 583-592.

Cecilia, D. & Gould, E. A. (1991). Nucleotide changes responsible for loss of neuroinvasiveness in Japanese encephalitis virus neutralization-resistant mutants. *Virology,* 181, pp. 70-77.

Chambers, T. J.; Hahn, C. S.; Galler, R. & Rice, C. M. (1990). Flavivirus genome organization, expression, and replication. *Annual Review of Microbiology,* 44, pp. 649-688.

Chare, E. R. & Holmes, E. C. (2006). A phylogenetic survey of recombination frequency in plant RNA viruses. *Archive of Virology,* 151, pp. 933-946.

Chen, L. K.; Lin, Y. L.; Liao, C. L.; Lin, C. G.; Huang, Y. L.; Yeh, C. T.; Lai, S. C.; Jan, J. T. & Chin, C. (1996). Generation and characterization of orang-tropism mutants of Japanese encephalitis *in vivo* and *in vitro. Virology,* 223, pp. 79-88.

Chen, T. H.; Tang, P.; Yang, C. F.; Kao, L. H.; Lo, Y. P.; Chuang, C. K.; Shih, Y. T. & Chen, W. J. (2011). Antioxidant defense is one of the mechanisms by which mosquito cells survive dengue 2 viral infection. *Virology,* 410, pp. 410-417.

Chen, W. J.; Wu, H. R. & Chiou, S. S. (2003). E/NS1 modifications of dengue 2 virus after serial passages in mammalian and/or mosquito cells. *Intervirology,* 46, pp. 289-295.

Chen, W. J.; Dong, C. F.; Chiou, L. Y. & Chuang, W. L. (2000). Potential role of *Armigeres subalbatus* (Diptera: Culicidae) in the transmission of Japanese encephalitis virus in the absence of rice culture on Liu-Chiu Islet, Taiwan. *Journal of Medical Entomology,* 37, pp. 108-113.

Chen, W. R.; Rico-Hesse, R. & Tesh, R. B. (1992). A new Genotype of Japanese Encephalitis Virus from Indonesia. *American Journal of Tropical Medicine and Hygiene,* 47, pp. 61-69.

Chen, W. R.; Tesh, R. B. & Rico-Hesse, R. (1990). Genetic variation of Japanese encephalitis virus in nature. *Journal of General Virology,* 71, pp. 2915-2922.

Chiou, S. S. & Chen, W. J. (2001). Mutations in the NS3 gene and 3′-NCR of Japanese encephalitis virus isolated from an unconventional ecosystem and implications for natural attenuation of the virus. *Virology,* 289, pp. 129-136.

Chiou, S. S. & Chen, W. J. (2007). Phenotypic changes in the Japanese encephalitis virus after one passage in Neuro-2a cells: Generation of attenuated strains of the virus. *Vaccine,* 26, pp. 15-23.

Chiou, S. S.; Liu, H.; Chuang, C. K.; Lin, C. C. & Chen, W. J. (2005). Fitness of Japanese encephalitis virus to Neuro-2a cells is determined by interactions of viral envelope protein with highly sulfated glycosaminoglycans on the cell surface. *Journal of Medical Virology,* 76, 2005, 583-592.

Chiou, S. S.; Tsai, K. H.; Huang, C. G.; Liao, Y. K. & Chen, W. J. (2007). High antibody prevalence in an unconventional ecosystem is related to circulation of a low-virulent strain of Japanese encephalitis virus. *Vaccine*, 25, pp. 1437-1443.

Chuang, C. K. & Chen, W. J. (2009). Experimental evidence that RNA recombination occurs in the Japanese encephalitis virus. *Virology*, 394, pp. 186-197.

Chuang, C. K.; Chiou, S. S.; Liang, L. C. & Chen, W. J. (2003). Detection of Japanese encephalitis virus inside peripheral blood mononuclear cells of mouse using *in situ* RT-PCR. *American Journal of Tropical Medicine and Hygiene*, 69, pp. 648-651.

Chuang, Y. M.; Kwan, S. Y.; Lirng, J. F.; Tiu, C. M. & Pan, P. J. (2002). Radiological and manometric diagnosis of cricopharyngeal dysphagia in a Japanese encephalitis survivor. *European Journal of Neurology*, 9, pp. 407−411.

Chung, Y. J.; Nam, J. H.; Ban, S. L. & Cho, H. W. (1996). Antigenic and genetic analysis of Japanese encephalitis viruses isolated from Korea. *American Journal of Tropical Medicine and Hygiene*, 55, pp. 91-97.

Cristina, J. & Colina, R. (2006). Evidence of structural genomic region recombination in hepatitis C virus. *Virology Journal*, 3, pp. 53.

Deng, S.; Zhang, H. & Li, J. (2009). Distribution characteristics of mosquitoes and their natural infection with Japanese encephalitis virus in Yunnan province. *Chinese Journal of Vector Biology and Control*, 20, pp. 344-348.

Desai, A.; Shankar, S. K.; Chandramuki, A. & Gourie-Devi, M. (1995). Japanese encephalitis virus antigen in the human brain and its topographic distribution. *Acta* Neuropathologica, (Berl.) 89, pp. 368-73.

Deubel, V.; Nogueira, M.; Drouet, M. T.; Zeller, H.; Reynes, J. M. & Do, Q. H. (1993). Direct sequencing of genomic cDNA fragments amplified by the polymerase chain reaction for molecular epidemiology of dengue 2 viruses. *Archive of Virology*, 129, pp. 197-210.

Diamond, S. M., & Klein, R. S. (2004). West Nile virus: crossing the blood-brain barrier. *Nature Medicine*, 10, pp. 1294-1295.

Erlanger, T. E.; Weiss, S.; Keiser, J.; Utzinger, J. & Wiedenmayer, K. (2009). Past, present, and future of Japanese encephalitis. *Emerging Infectious Diseases*, 15, pp. 1-7.

Fan, J. M.; Luo, J.; Chen, L.; Teng, M.; Bu, D.; Wang, F. Y.; Wang, L.; Wang, C. Q. & Zhang, G. P. (2010). Genetic analysis of strains of Japanese encephalitis virus isolated from swine in central China. *Virus Gene*, 40, pp. 357–361.

Felsenstein, J. (2005). PHYLIP (Phylogeny Inference Package) version 3.6: Department of Genome Science, University of Washington, Seattle, USA.

Fulmali, P. V.; Sapkal, G. N.; Athawale, S.; Gore, M. M.; Mishra, A. C. & Bondre, V. P. (2011). Introduction of Japanese encephalitis virus genotype I, India. *Emerging Infectious Diseases*, 17, pp. 319-321.

Gentsch, J. R.; Laird, A. R.; Bielfelt, B.; Griffin, D. D.; Banyaim, K.; Ramachandran, M.; Jain, V.; Cunliffe, N. A.; Nakagomi, O.; Kirkwood, C. D.; Fischer, T. K.; Parashar, U. D.; Bresee, J. S.; Jiang, B. & Glass, R. I. (2005). Serotype diversity and reassortment between human and animal rotavirus strains: implications for rotavirus vaccine programs. *Journal of Infectious Diseases*, 192 (Suppl 1), pp. S146-S159.

Gould, E. A. (2002). Evolution of Japanese encephalitis serocomplex viruses. *Curr. Top. Microbiology and Immunology*, 267, pp. 391-404.

Gould, E. A.; Moss, S. R. & Turner, S. L. (2004). Evolution and dispersal of encephalitic flavivruses. *Archive of Virology, (Suppl.)* 18, pp. 65-84.

Griffin, D. E.; Levine, B.; Tyor, W. R. & Irani, D. N. (1992). The immune response in viral encephalitis. *Seminars in Immunology,* 4, pp. 111-119.

Grigoriadis, N. & Hadjigeorgiou, G. M. (2006). Virus-mediated autoimmunity in multiple sclerosis. *Journal of Autoimmune Diseases,* 3, pp. 1.

Hahn, C.S.; Lustig, S.; Strauss, E. G. & Strauss, J. H. (1988). Western equine encephalitis virus is a recombinant virus. *Proceedings of the National Academy of Sciences,* 85, pp. 5997-6001.

Hasegawa, H.; Yoshida, M.; Fujita, S. & Kobayashi, Y. (1994). Comparison of structural proteins among antigenically different Japanese encephalitis virus strains. *Vaccine,* 12, pp. 841-844.

Hasegawa, H.; Yoshida, M.; Shiosaka, T.; Fujita, S. & Kobayashi, Y. (1992). Mutations in the envelope protein of Japanese encephalitis virus affect entry into cultured cells and virulence in mice. *Virology,* 191, pp. 158-165.

Hickey, W. F.; Hsu, B. L. & Kimura, H. (1991). T-lymphocyte entry into the central nervous system. *Journal of Neuroscience Research,* 28, pp. 254-260.

Holland, J. J. (1996). Evolving virus plaques. *Proceedings of the National Academy of Sciences,* 93, pp. 545-546.

Holland, J.; Spindler, K.; Horodyski, F.; Grabau, E.; Nichol, S. & VandePol, S. (1982). Rapid evolution of RNA genomes. *Science,* 215, pp. 1577-1585.

Holmes, E. C. (2004). The phylogeography of human viruses. *Molecular Ecology,* 13, pp. 745-756.

Holmes, E. C.; Worobey, M., & Rambaut, A. (1999). Phylogenetic evidence for recombination in dengue virus. *Molecular Biology and Evolution,* 16, pp. 405-409.

Hsue, B.; Hartshorne, T. & Masters, P. S. (2000). Characterization of an essential RNA secondary structure in the 3' untranslated region of the murine coronavirus genome. *Journal of Virology,* 74, pp. 6911-6921.

Huang, J. H.; Lin, T. H.; Teng, H. J.; Su, C. L.; Tsai, K. H.; Lu, L. C.; Lin, C.; Yang, C. F.; Chang, S. F.; Liao, T. L.; Yu, S. K.; Cheng, C. H.; Chang, M. C.; Hu, H, C. & Shu, P. Y. (2010). Molecular epidemiology of Japanese encephalitis virus, Taiwan. *Emerging Infectious Diseases,* 16, pp. 876-878.

Jarvis, T. C. & Kirkegaard, K. (1991). The polymerase in its labyrinth: mechanisms and implications of RNA recombination. *Trends in Genetics,* 7, pp. 186-191.

Jarvis, T. C. & Kirkegaard, K. (1992). Poliovirus RNA recombination: mechanistic studies in the absence of selection. *EMBO Journal,* 11, pp. 3135-3145.

Jenkins, G. M.; Rambaut, A.; Pybus, O. G. & Holmes, E. C. (2002). Rates of molecular evolution in RNA viruses: a quantitative phylogenetic analysis. *Journal of Moleculaar Evolution,* 54, pp. 152-161.

Johnson, L. J.; Halliday, G. M. & King, N. J. (2000). Langerhans cells migrate to local lymph nodes following cutaneous infection with an arbovirus. *Journal of Investigative Dermatology* 114, pp. 560-568.

Johnson, R. T. (1987).The pathogenesis of acute viral encephalitis and postinfectious encephalomyelitis. *Journal of Infectious Diseases,* 155, pp. 359-364.

Johnson, R. T.; Burke, D. S.; Elwell, M.; Leake, C. J.; Nisalak, A.; Hoke, C. H. & Lorsomrudee, W. (1985). Japanese encephalitis: Immunocytochemical studies of viral antigen and inflammatory cells in fatal cases. *Annals of Neurology,* 18, pp. 567-573.

Kalita, J. & Misra, U. K. (2000). Comparison of CT and MRI findings in the diagnosis of Japanese encephalitis. *Journal of Neurological Science,* 174, pp. 3-8.

Kalita, J. & Misra, U. K. (2000). Neurophysiological changes in Japanese encephalitis. *Neurology India,* 50, pp. 262-266.

Khiabanian, H.; Trifonov, V. & Rabadan, R. (2009). Reassortment patterns in swine influenza viruses. *PLoS ONE,* 4, pp. e7366.

Kim, J. M.;Yun, S. I.; Song, B. H.; Hahn, Y. S.; Lee, C. H.; Oh, H. W. & Lee, Y. M. (2008). A single N-linked glycosylation site in the Japanese encephalitis virus prM protein is critical for cell type-specific prM protein biogenesis, virus particle release, and pathogenicity in mice. *Journal of Virology,* 82, pp. 7846-7862.

Kimura-Kuroda, J.; Ichikawa, M.; Ogata, A.; Nagashima, K.; Yasui, K. (1992). Specific tropism of Japanese encephalitis virus for developing neurons in primary rat brain culture. *Archive of Virology,* 130, pp. 477-484.

Kirkegaard, K. & Baltimore, D. (1986). The mechanism of RNA recombination in poliovirus. *Cell,* 47, pp. 433-443.

Konishi, E. & Suzuki, T. (2002). Ratios of subclinical to clinical Japanese encephalitis (JE) virus infections in vaccinated populations: evaluation of an inactivated JE vaccine by comparing the ratios with those in unvaccinated populations. *Vaccine,* 21, pp. 98-107.

Kuno, G.; Chang, G. J.; Tsuchiya, K. R.; Karabatsos, N. & Cropp, C. B. (1998). Phylogeny of the genus *Flavivirus*. *Journal of Virology,* 72, pp. 73-83.

Lai, M. M. (1992). RNA recombination in animal and plant viruses. *Micribiology and Molecular Biology Review,* 56, pp. 61-79.

Ledinko, N. (1963).Genetic recombination with poliovirus type 1: studies of crosses between a normal horse serum-resistant mutant and several guanidine-resistant mutants of the same strain. *Virology,* 20, pp. 107-119.

Lee, E. & Lobigs, M. (2002). Mechanism of virulence attenuation of glycosaminoglycans-binding variants of Japanese encephalitis virus and Murray Valley encephalitis Virus. *Journal of Virology,* 76, pp. 4901-4911.

Lee, E.; Hall, R. A. & Lobigs, M. (2004). Common E protein determinants for attenuation of glycosaminoglycan-binding variants of Japanese encephalitis and West Nile viruses. *Journal of Virology,* 78, pp. 8271-8280.

Lescar, J. & Canard, B. (2009). RNA-dependent RNA polymerases from flaviviruses and Picornaviridae. *Current Opinion in Structural Biology,* 19, pp. 759-767.

Lindenbach, B. D. & Rice, C. M. (2001). Flaviviridae: the viruses and their replication, In: *Fields Virology, vol. 1. 4th ed,* D. M. Knipe & P. M. Howley, (Eds.), 991-1041. Lippincott Williams & Wilkins Publishers, Philadelphia, PA, USA.

Liou, M. L. & Hsu, C. Y. (1998). Japanese encephalitis virus is transported across the cerebral blood vessels by endocytosis in mouse brain. *Cell and Tissue Research,* 293, pp. 389-394.

Liu, H.; Chiou, S. S. & Chen, W. J. (2004). Differential binding efficiency between the envelope protein of Japanese encephalitis virus variants with heparan sulfate on the cell surface. *Journal of Medical Virology,* 72, pp. 618-624.

Liu, T. H.; Liang, L. C.; Wang, C. C.; Liu, H. C. & Chen, W. J. (2008). The blood-brain barrier in the cerebrum is the initial site for the Japanese encephalitis virus entering the central nervous system. *Journal of Neurovirology,* 14, pp. 514-521.

Liu, Y.; Chuang, C. K. & Chen, W. J. (2009). *In situ* reverse-transcription loop-mediated isothermal amplification (in situ RT-LAMP) for detection of Japanese encephalitis viral RNA in host cells. *Journal of Clinical Virology,* 46, pp. 49-54.

Ma, S. P.; Yoshida, Y.; Makino, Y.; Tadano, M.; Ono, T. & Ogawa, M. (2003). A major genotype of Japanese encephalitis virus currently circulating in Japan. *American Journal of Tropical Medicine and Hygiene,* 69, pp. 151-154.

Mackenzie, J. S. (1999). Emerging viral diseases: an Australian perspective. *Emerging Infectious Diseases,* 5, pp.1-8.

Mackenzie, J. S.; Gubler, D. J. & Petersen, L. R. (2004). Emerging flaviviruses: the spread and resurgence of Japanese encephalitis, West Nile and dengue viruses. *Nature Medicine,* 10, pp. S98-S109.

Mackenzie, J. S.; Williams, D. T. & Smith, D. W. (2007). Japanese encephalitis virus: the geographic distribution, incidence, and spread of a virus with a propensity to emerge in new areas. In: *Emerging viruses in human populations,* E. Tabor, (Ed.), 201-268, Elsevier, Amsterdam, Netherlands.

Mangada, M. N. M. & Takegami, T. (1999). Molecular characterization of the Japanese encephalitis virus representative immunotype strain JaGAr 01. *Virus Research,* 59, pp. 101-112.

Marchette, N. J.; Dubois, D. R.; Larsen, L. K.; Summers, P. L.; Kraiselburd, E. G.; Gubler, D. J. & Eckels, K. H. (1990). Preparation of an attenuated dengue 4 (341750 Carib) virus vaccine. I. Pre-clinical studies. *American Journal of Tropical Medicine and Hygiene,* 43, pp. 212-218.

Martinez-Barragan, J. J. & del Angel, R. M. (2001). Identification of putative coreceptor on Vero cells that participates in dengue 4 virus infection. *Journal of Virology,* 75, pp. 7818-7827.

Mathur, A.; Kulshreshtha, R. & Chaturvedi, U. C. (1987). Induction of secondary immune response by reactivated Japanese encephalitis virus in latently infected mice. *Immunology,* 60, pp. 481-484.

McMinn, P. C.; Dalgarno, L. & Weir, R. C. (1996). A comparison of the spread of Murray Valley viruses of high or low neuroinvasiveness in the tissues of Swiss mice after peripheral inoculation. *Virology,* 220, pp. 414-423.

Meyer, R.; Weissert, R.; Diem, R.; Storch, M. K.; Graaf, K. L.; Kramer, B. & Bähr, M. (2001). Acute neuronal apoptosis in a rat model of multiple sclerosis. *The Journal of Neuroscience,* 21, pp. 6214-6220.

Misra. U. K. & Kalita, J. (1997). Movement disorders in Japanese encephalitis. *Journal of Neurology,* 244, pp. 299–303.

Misra. U. K. & Kalita, J. (2010). Overview: Japanese encephalitis. *Progress in Neurobiology,* 91, pp. 108-120.

Monath, T. P. (2002). Japanese encephalitis vaccines: current vaccines and future prospects. *Current Topics in Microbiology and Immunology,* 267, pp. 105-138.

Monath, T. P., and F. X. Heinz. (1996). Flaviviruses, In: *Fields Virology,* 3rd ed., B. N. Fields, D. M. Knipe, P. M. Howley, R. M. Chanock, J. P. Melnick, T. P. Monath, B.

Roizman, & S. E. Strauss, (Eds.), 961-1034, Lippincott-Raven Publishers, Philadelphia, USA.

Morita, K. (2009). Molecular epidemiology of Japanese encephalitis in East Asia. *Vaccine,* 27, pp. 7131-7132.

Muller, D. M.; Pender, M. P. & Greer, J. M. (2005). Blood-brain barrier disruption and lesion localization in experimental autoimmune encephalomyelitis with predominant cerebella and brainstem involvement. *Journal of Neuroimmunology,* 160, pp. 162-169.

Myint, K. S. A.; Gibbons, R. V.; Perng, G. C. & Solomon, T. (2007). Unraveling the neuropathogenesis of Japanese encephalitis. *Transactions of the Royal Society of Tropical Medicine and Hygiene,* 101, pp. 955-956.

Nabeshima, T.; Loan, H. T. K.; Sumiyoshi, M.; Haruda, Y.; Nga, P. H.; Huong, V. T.; Parquet, M. C.; Hasebe, F. & Morita, K. (2009). Evidence of frequent introduction of Japanese encephalitis virus from south-east Asia and continental east Asia to Japan. *Journal of General Virology,* 90, pp. 827-832.

Nagy, P. D. & Bujarski, J. J. (1996). Homologous RNA recombination in brome mosaic virus: AU-rich sequences decrease the accuracy of crossovers. *Journal of Virology,* 70, pp. 415-426.

Nagy, P. D. & Jozef, J. B. (1997). Engineering of homologous recombination hotspots with AU-rich sequences in Brome mosaic virus. *Journal of Virology,* 71, pp. 3799-3810.

Nargi-Aizenman, J. L. & Griffin, D. E. (2001). Sindbis virus-induced neuronal death is both necrotic and apoptotic and is ameliorated by N-methyl-D-aspartate receptor antagonists. *Journal of Virology,* 75, pp. 7114-7121.

Nett, R. J.; Campbell, G. L. & Reisen, W. K. (2009). Potential for the emergence of Japanese encephalitis virus in California. *Vector Borne and Zoonotic Diseases,* 9, pp. 511-517.

Nga, P. T.; del Carmen Parquet, M.; Cuong, V. D.; Ma, S. P.; Hasebe, F.; Inoue, S.; Mikino, Y.; Takagi, M.; Nam, V. S. & Morita, K. (2004). Shift in Japanese encephalitis virus (JEV) genotype circulating in northern Vietnam: implications for frequent introductions of JEV from Southeast Asia to East Asia. *Journal of General Virology,* 85, pp. 1625-1631.

Ni, H. & Barrett, A. D. T. (1998). Attenuation of Japanese encephalitis virus by selection of its mouse brain membrane receptor preparation escape variants. *Virology,* 241, pp. 30-36.

Ni, H. & Barrett, A. D. T. (1996).Molecular differences between wild-type Japanese encephalitis virus strains of high and low mouse neuroinvasiveness. *Journal of General Virology,* 77, pp. 1449-1455.

Nidaira, M.; Taira, K.; Okano. S.; Shinzato, T.; Morikawa, T.; Tokumine. M.; Asato, Y.; Tada, Y.; Miyagi, K.; Matsuda, S.; Itokazu, K.; Kydaka, J.; Nakamura, M. & Tamanaha, K. (2009). Survey of Japanese encephalitis in pigs on Miyako, Ishigaki, Kume, and Yonaguri islands in Okinawa, Japan. *Japanese Journal of Infectious Diseases,* 62, pp. 220-224.

Nitatpattana, N.; Dubot-Pérès, A.; Gouilh, M. A.; Souris, M.; Barbazan, P.; Yoksan, S.; de Lamballerie, X. & Gonzalez, J. P. (2008). Change in Japanese encephalitis virus distribution, Thailand. *Emerging Infectious Diseases,* 14, pp. 1762-1765.

Nitayaphan, S.; Grant, J. A. & Chang, G. J. (1990). Nucleotide sequence of the virulent SA-14 strain of Japanese encephalitis virus and its attenuated vaccine derivative, SA14-14-2. *Virology,* 177, pp. 541-552.

Pyke, A. T.; Williams, D. T.; Nisbet, D. J.; van den Hurk, A. F.; Taylor, C. T.; Johansen, C. A.; Macdonald, J.; Hall, R. A.; Simmons, R. J.; Mason, R. J.; Lee, J. M.; Ritchie, S. A.; Smith, G. A. & Mackenzie, J. S. (2001). The appearance of a second genotype of Japanese encephalitis virus in the Australasian region. *American Journal of Tropical Medicine and Hygiene,* 65, pp. 747-753.

Ramos-Castaneda, J.; Imbert, J. L.; Barron, B. L. & Ramos, C. (1997). A 65-kDa trypsin-sensible membrane cell protein as a possible receptor for dengue virus in cultured neuroblastoma cells. *Journal of Neurovirology,* 3, pp. 435-440.

Ravi, V.; Taly, A. B.; Shankar, S. K.; Shenoy, P. K.; Desai, A.; Nagaraja, D.; Gourie-Devi, M. & Chandramuki, A. (1994). Association of Japanese encephalitis virus infection with Guillain–Barré syndrome in endemic area of South India. *Acta Neurologica Scandinavica,* 90, pp. 67-72.

Ren, J.; Ding, T.; Zhang, W.; Song, J. & Ma, W. (2007). Does Japanese encephalitis virus share the same cellular receptor with other mosquito-borne flaviviruses on the C6/36 mosquito cells? *Virology Journal,* 4, pp. 83.

Rey, F. A.; Heinz, F. X.; Mandl, C.; Kunz, C. & Harrison, S. C. (1995). The envelope glycoprotein from tick-borne encephalitis virus at 2 Å resolution. *Nature,* 375, pp. 291-298.

Ritchie, S. A. & Rochester, W. (2001).Wind-blown mosquitoes and introduction of Japanese encephalitis into Australia. *Emerging Infectious Diseases,* 7, pp. 900-903.

Rohayem, J.; Münch, J. & Rethwilm, A. (2005). Evidence of recombination in the norovirus capsid gene. *Journal of Virology,* 79, pp. 4977-4990.

Rosen, L. (1986). The natural history of Japanese encephalitis virus. *Annual Review of Microbiology,* 40, pp. 395-414.

Rothwell, S. W.; Putnak, R. & LaRussa, V. E. (1996). Dengue-2 virus infection of human bone marrow characterization of Dengue-2 antigen-positive stromal cells. *American Journal of Tropical Medicine and Hygiene,* 54, pp. 503-510.

Samuel, M. A.; Morrey, J. D. & Diamond, M. S. (2007). Caspase 3-dependent cell death of neurons contributes to the pathogenesis of West Nile virus encephalitis. *Journal of Virology,* 81, pp. 2614-2623.

Sarma, J. D. (2010). A mechanism of virus-induced demyelination. *Interdisciplinary perspectives on infectious diseases,* Article ID 109239.

Schneider, W. L. & Roossinck, M. J. (2001). Genetic diversity in RNA virus quasispecies is controlled by host-virus interactions. *Journal of Virology* 75, pp. 6566-6571.

Schuh, A. J.; Tesh, R. B. & Barrett, A. D. T. (2011). Genetic characterization of Japanese encephalitis virus genotype II strains isolated from 1951 to 1978. *Journal of General Virology,* 92, pp. 516-527.

Sejvar, J. J.; Bode, A. V.; Marfin, A. A.; Campbell, G. L.; Ewing, D.; Mazowiecki, M.; Pavot, P. V.; Schmitt, J.; Pape, J.; Biggerstaff, B. J. & Petersen, L. R. (2005). West Nile virus-associated flaccid paralysis. *Emerging Infectious Diseases,* 11, pp. 1021-1027.

Shapka, N. & Nagy, P. D. (2004). The AU-Rich RNA recombination hot spot sequence of Brome mosaic virus is functional in tombusviruses: implications for the mechanism of RNA recombination. *Journal of Virology,* 78, pp. 2288-2300.

Shope, R. E. & Sather, G. E. (1979). Arboviruses, In: *Diagnostic procedures for viral, rickettsial, and chlamydial infections, 5th ed.,* E. H. Lennette & N. J. Schmidt , (Ed.), 767-814. American Public Health Association, Inc., Washington, D.C., USA.

Solomon, T. & Vaughn, D. W. (2002). Pathogenesis and clinical features of Japanese encephalitis and West Nile virus infections. *Current Topics in Microbiology and Immunology*, 267, pp. 171−194.

Solomon, T. (2004). Flavivirus encephalitis. *New England Journal of Medicine*, 351, pp. 370-378.

Solomon, T.; Dung, N. M.; Kneen, R.; Gainsborough, M.; Vaughn, D. W.; Khanh, V. T. (2000). Japanese encephalitis. *Journal of Neurology, Neurosurgery & Psychiatry*, 68, pp. 405-415.

Solomon, T.; Ni, H.; Beasley, D. W. C.; Ekkelenkamp, M.; Cardosa, M. J. & Barrett A. D. T. (2003). Origin and evolution of Japanese encephalitis virus in Southeast Asia. *Journal of Virology*, 77, pp. 3091-3098.

Stamatovic, S. M.; Shakui, P.; Keep, R. F.; Moore, B. B.; Kunkel, S. L.; Van Rooijen, N. & Andjelkovic, A. V. (2005). Monocyte chemoattractant protein-1 regulation of blood-brain barrier permeability. *Journal of Cerebral Blood Flow & Metabolism*, 25, pp. 593–606.

Stephens, E. B.; Singh, D. K.; Kohler, M. E.; Jackson, M.; Pacyniak, E. & Berman, N. E. J. (2003). The primary phase of infection by pathogenic simian-human immunodeficiency virus results in disruption of the blood-brain barriers. *AIDS Research and Human Retroviruses*, 19, pp. 837−846.

Stiasny, K. & Heinz, F. X. (2006). Flavivirus membrane fusion. *Journal of General Virology*, 87, pp. 2755–2766.

Stohlman, S. A. & Hinton, D. R. (2001). Viral induced demyelination. *Brain Pathology*, 11, pp. 92-106.

Su, C. M.; Liao, C. L.; Lee, Y. L.; Lin, Y.-L. (2001). Highly sulfated forms of heparin sulfate are involved in Japanese encephalitis virus infection. *Virology*, 286, pp. 206-215.

Sumiyoshi, H.; Mori, C.; Fuke, I.; Morita, K.; Kuhara, S.; Kondou, J.; Kikuchi, Y.; Nagamatu, H. & Igarashi, A. (1987). Complete nucleotide of the Japanese encephalitis virus genome RNA. *Virology*, 161, pp. 479-510.

Suri, N. K. & Banerjee, K. (1995). Growth and cytopathic effect of Japanese encephalitis in astrocyte-enriched cell cultures from neonatal mouse brains. *Acta Virologica*, 39, pp. 143-148.

Sztuba-Solinska, J.; Urbanowicz, A.; Figlerowicz, M. & Bujarski, J. J. (2011). RNA-RNA recombination in plant virus replication and evolution. *Annual Review of Phytopathology*, 49, (in press)

Tajima, S.; Nerome, R.; Nukui, Y.; Kato, F.; Takasaki, T. & Kurane, I. (2010). A single mutation in the Japanese encephalitis virus E protein (S123R) increases its growth rate in mouse neuroblastoma cells and its pathogenicity in mice. *Virology*, 396, pp. 298-304.

Thompson, J. D.; Hinggins, D. G. & Gibson, T. J. (1994). CLUSTAL W: improving the sensitivity of progressive multiple sequence alignment through sequence weighting, position specific gap penalties and weight matrix choice. *Nucleic Acid Research*, 22, pp. 4673-4680.

Tolou, H. J. G.; Couissinier-Paris, P.; Durand, J. P.; Mercier, V.; de Pina, J. J.; de Micco, P.; Billoir, F.; Charrel, R. N. & de Lamballerie, X. (2001). Evidence for recombination in natural populations of dengue virus type 1 based on the analysis of complete genome sequences. *Journal of General Virology*, 82, pp. 1283-1290.

Trent, D. W.; Grant, J. A.; Rosen, L. & Monath, T. P. (1983). Genetic variation among dengue 2 viruses of different geographic origin. *Virology*, 128, pp. 271-284.

Trent, D. W.; Kinney, R. M.; Johnson, B. J.; Vorndam, A.V.; Grant, J. A.; Deubel, V.; Rice, C.M. & Hahn, C. (1987). Partial nucleotide sequence of St. Louis encephalitis virus RNA: structural proteins, NS1, NS2a, and NS2b. *Virology*, 156, pp. 293-304.

Tseng, Y. F.; Wang, C. C.; Liao, S. K.; Chuang, C. K. & Chen, W. J. (2011). Autoimmunity-related demyelination in infection by Japanese encephalitis virus. Journal: *Journal of Biomedical Science*, 18, pp. 20.

Tsunoda, I.; Kuang, L. Q.; Libbey, J. E. & Fujinami, R. S. (2003). Axonal injury heralds virus-induced demyelination. *The American Journal of Pathology*, 162, pp. 1259-1269.

Tung, W. H.; Tsai, H. W.; Lee, I. T.; Hsieh, H. L.; Chen, W. J.; Chen, Y. L. & Yang, C. M. (2010). Japanese encephalitis virus induces matrix metalloproteinase-9 expression via the ROS/MAPKs-dependent NF-κB signaling pathway in rat brain astrocytes. *British Journal of Pharmacology*, 161, pp. 1566-1583.

Turner, P. E. & Chao, L. (1998). Sex and evolution of intrahost competition in RNA virus φ6. *Genetics*, 150, pp. 523-532.

Twiddy, S. S. & Holmes, E. C. (2003). The extent of homologous recombination in members of the genus Flavivirus. *Journal of General Virology*, 84, pp. 429-440.

Uchil, P. D. & Satchidanandam, V. (2001). Phylogenetic analysis of Japanese encephalitis virus: envelope gene based analysis reveals a fifth genotype, geographic clustering, and multiple introductions of the virus into the Indian subcontinent. *American Journal of Tropical Medicine and Hygiene*, 65, pp. 242-251.

Umenai, T.; Krzysko, R.; Bektimirov, T. A. & Assaad, F. A. (1985). Japanese encephalitis: current worldwide status. *Bulletin of World Health Organization*, 63, 625-631.

Unni, S. K.; Růžek, D.; Chhatbar, C.; Mishra, R.; Johri, M. K.; Singh, S. K. (2011). Japanese encephalitis virus: From genome to infectome. *Microbes and Infection*, 13, pp. 312-321.

van den Hurk, A. F.; Ritchie, S. A. & Mackenzie, J. S. (2009). Ecology and geographical expansion of Japanese encephalitis virus. *Annual Review of Entomology*, 54, pp. 17-35.

van den Hurk, A. F.; Ritchie, S. A.; Johansen, C. A.; Mackenzie, J. S. & Smith, G. A. (2008). Domestic pigs and Japanese encephalitis virus infection, Australia. *Emerging Infectious Diseases*, 14, pp. 1173-1178.

Vasilakis, N; Deardorff, E. R.; Kenney, J. L.; Rossi, S. L. & Hanley, K.A. (2009) Mosquitoes put the brake on arbovirus evolution: experimental evolution reveals slower mutation accumulation in mosquito than vertebrate cells. *PLoS Pathogens*, 5, pp. e1000467.

Wang, H.; Takasaki, T.; Fu, S, Sun, X.; Zhang, H.; Wang, Z.; Hao, Z.; Zhang, J.; Tang, Q.; Kotaki, A.; Tajima, S.; Liang, X.; Yang, W.; Kurane, I. & Liang, G. (2007). Molecular epidemiological analysis of Japanese encephalitis virus in China. *Journal of General Virology*, 88, pp. 885-894.

Wang, L.; Fu, S.; Zhang, H.; Ye, X.; Yu, D.; Deng, Z.; Yuan, J.; Zhai, Y.; Li, M.; Lv, Z.; Chen, W.; Jiang, H.; Gao, X.; Cao, Y.; Wang, H.; Tang, Q. & Liang, G. (2010). Identification and isolation of Genotype-I Japanese encephalitis virus from encephalitis patients. *Virology Journal*, 7, pp. 345.

Wang, T.; Town, T.; Alexopoulou, L.; Anderson, J. F.; Fikrig, E. & Flavell, R. A. (2004). Toll-like receptor 3 mediates West Nile virus entry into the brain causing lethal encephalitis. *Nature Medicine,* 10, pp. 1366–1373.

Weaver, S. C.; Rico-Hesse, R. & Scott, T. W. (1992). Genetic diversity and slow rates of evolution in New World alphaviruses. *Current Topics in Micriobiology and Immunology,* 176, pp. 99-117.

Weng, M. H.; Lien, J. C.; Wang, Y. M,.; Lin, C. C.; Lin, H. C. & Chin, C. (1999). Isolation of Japanese encephalitis virus from mosquitoes collected in Northern Taiwan between 1995 and 1996. *Journal of Microbiology, Immunology, and Infection,* 32, pp. 9-13.

Westaway, E. G.; Brinton, M. A.; Gaidamovich, S, Y.; Horzinek, M. C.; Igarashi, A.; Kääriäinen, L.; Lvov, D. K.; Porterfield, J. S.; Russell, P. K. & Trent, D. W. (1985). Flaviviridae. *Intervirology,* 24, pp. 183-192.

White, K. A. & Morris, T. J. (1995). RNA determinants of junction site selection in RNA virus recombinants and defective interfering RNAs. *RNA,* 1, pp. 1029-1040.

Whitley, R. J. & Gnann, J. W. (2002). Viral encephalitis: familiar infections and emerging pathogens. *Lancet,* 359, pp. 507–513.

Wierzchoslawski, R. & Bujarski, J. (2006). Efficient *in vitro* system of homologous recombination in Brome mosaic bromovirus. *Journal of Virology,* 80, pp. 6182-6187.

Worobey, M. & Holmes, E. C. (1999). Evolutionary aspects of recombination in RNA viruses. *Journal of General Virology,* 80, pp. 2535-2543.

Wu, S. C.; Lian, W. C.; Hsu, L. C.; Wu, Y. C. & Liau. M. Y. (1998). Antigenic characterization of nine wild-type Taiwanese isolates of Japanese encephalitis virus as compared with two vaccine strains. *Virus Research,* 55, pp. 83-91.

Wu, Y. C.; Huang, Y. S.; Chien, L. J.; Lin, T. L.; Yueh, Y. Y.; Tseng, W. L.; Chang,K. J. & Wang, G. R. (1999). The epidemiology of Japanese encephalitis on Taiwan during 1966-1997. *American Journal of Tropical Medicine and Hygiene,* 61, pp. 78-84.

Xia, S. Y.; Guzman, Ha.; Zhang, H.; Travassos, da Rosa. A. P. A. & Tesh, R. B. (2001). West Nile virus infection in the golden hamster (*Mesocricetus auratus)*: a model for West Nile encephalitis. *Emerging Infectious Diseases,* 7, pp. 714–722.

Yamada, M.; Nakamura, K.; Yoshii, M. & Kaku, Y. (2004). Nonsuppurative encephalitis in piglets after experimental inoculation of Japanese encephalitis flavivirus isolated from pigs. *Veterinary Pathology,* 41, pp. 62–67.

Yoshida, Y.; Tabei, Y.; Hasegawa, M.; Nagashima, M. & Morozumi, S. (2005). Genotypic analysis of Japanese encephalitis virus strains isolated from swine in Tokyo, Japan. *Japanese Journal of Infectious Diseases,* 58, pp. 259-261.

Yun, S. M.; Cho, J. E.; Ju, Y. R.; Kim. S. Y.; Ryou, J.; Han, M. G.; Choi, W. Y. & Jeong, Y. E. (2010). Molecular epidemiology of Japanese encephalitis virus circulating in South Korea, 1983-2005. *Virology Journal,* 7, pp. 127.

Zhao, Z.; Date, T.; Li, Y.; Kato, T.; Miyamoto, M.; Yasui, K. & Wakita, T. (2005). Characterization of the E-138 (Glu/Lys) mutation in Japanese encephalitis virus by using a stable, full-length, infectious cDNA clone. *Journal of General Virology,* 86, pp. 2209-2220.

Zhou, Y.; Ray, D.; Zhao, Y.; Dong, H.; Ren, S.; Li, Z.; Guo, Y.; Bernard, K. A.; Shi, P. Y. & Li, H. (2007). Structure and function of flavivirus NS5 methyltransferase. *Journal of Virology,* 81, pp. 3891-3903.

When Japanese Encephalitis Virus Invaded Eastern Hemisphere – The History of the Spread of Virus Genotypes

Guillaume Le Flohic[1] and Jean-Paul Gonzalez[1,2]
[1]*Centre International de Recherches Médicales de Franceville,*
[2]*Ministère Français des Affaires Etrangères & Européennes*
[1]*Gabon*
[2]*France*

1. Introduction

1.1 Japanese Encephalitis expansion

Japanese Encephalitis (JE) was first clinically identified in 1871 in Japan and known as "summer encephalitis". In 1924, during an outbreak of encephalitis, important studies were carried out at the Tokyo Research Institute of Infectious Disease (Mackenzie et al., 2007). Subsequently, a virus was isolated of a brain of a patient deceased of Japanese summer encephalitis and named "Japanese encephalitis type B" (JEB) in order to distinguish it, by that time, from another intensively circulating pandemic encephalitis, the "von Economo encephalitis", initially named "Encephalitis Lethargica" (von Economo, 1931), and named afterward "type A encephalitis". Then, in 1933, the virus responsible of JEB was reisolated and ultimately characterized in 1934, when it was experimentally inoculated into monkey brain and successfully reproduced the disease (Rosen, 1986; Showa in Seiichi & Teizo, 2002[1]; Hayashi, *in* Asim A. Jani, 2009[2]).

From Japan, until the late 1990s, Japanese encephalitis virus (JEV) was known to actively circulate in South East Asia, extending its eastern range towards Korea, Chinese mainland, Taiwan and Philippines, and then further West towards India and Pakistan. Major epidemics occurred in the 1960s and JE appeared endemic within the Indochinese Peninsula including Cambodia, Laos, Thailand and Vietnam, and further on to Malaysia, Burma, Singapore (rare cases), Brunei (Erlanger et al., 2009). Then, within the following four decades, JE occupied subsequently most of the Asian continent from Pakistan to Sri Lanka on the east of its range (Igarashi et al., 1994; Solomon et al., 2000; Nga et al., 2004; van den Hurk et al., 2009) and then Bangladesh, Nepal (Terai region). Furthermore, in the mean time, JEV emerged among unaffected area of Asia as in Papua New Guinea, Far East Russia (maritime Siberia), and subsequently crossed the Torres Strait toward Northern Australia where it was isolated and emerged for the first time within the Australian continent (Hanna

---

[1] Seiichi Iwao, Teizo Iyanaga, *Dictionnaire historique du Japon, Volume I*, Maisonneuve & Larose, 2002 (ISBN 9782706815751) p. 441
[2] http://emedicine.medscape.com/article/233802-diagnosis

et al., 1999). Limited outbreaks were also reported from the two Western Pacific Islands of Guam and Saipan, respectively in 1947-48 and 1990, but the enzootic cycle might be not sustainable and the virus was therefore very probably introduced there (Richards et al., 2010; Fisher et al., 2010).

1.2 Japanese Encephalitis epidemiology

In nature, JEV is essentially transmitted by *Culex* mosquito species to wild and domestic birds and pig herds. In the transmission cycle, humans are accidental and dead-end hosts. The most prevalent vector for human infection is *Culex tritaeniorhynchus* which breeds in pools of stagnant water such as rice fields (Keiser et al., 2005; Richards et al., 2010). However, about fifteen other mosquito species belonging to genus *Anopheles, Aedes, Armigeres, Mansonia* and *Culex* and other species of true flies are recognized to carry the virus, but all of them are not equally competent to transmit the virus to new hosts (Mackenzie et al., 2007). Moreover, pigs are attractive hosts that are generally asymptomatic and are important virus amplifiers. As a consequence, human living close industrial or familial piggeries are at higher risk of transmission (Nitatpattana et al., 2011).

1.3 Japanese Encephalitis syndrome

In terms of human morbidity and mortality, JE is one of the most important and widespread causes of arboviral encephalitis worldwide, with an estimated 35,000 to 50,000 cases and 10,000 deaths annually in Asia (Tsai, 2000). It is estimated that three billion people are at risk of infection. Human infections are generally asymptomatic (1 in 1000 cases), while 25% of symptomatic infections will present brain inflammatory signs and, among them, a quarter may result in permanent neurological and psychiatric sequel with a 25% mortality rate (Vaughn & Hoke, 1992; Solomon & Vaughn, 2002).

1.4 Japanese Encephalitis Virus

JEV is a *Flavivirus* of the *Flaviviridae* family and a member of the Japanese encephalitis eponym serogroup, including ten antigenically related virus species as: Alfuy, Koutango, Kokobera, Kunjin, Murray Valley encephalitis, Japanese encephalitis, Stratford, Usutu, West Nile and St. Louis encephalitis viruses. JEV consists of a lipo-glicoprotein envelope surrounding a nucleocapsid of a single-stranded positive-sense RNA of 11-Kb nucleotide. A single open reading frame is flanked by two 5′ and 3′ untranslated regions (UTRs), and carry genes coding for structural proteins including a capsid (C), a membrane (cleavage product of a pre-membrane protein PrM), an envelope (E), and seven nonstructural (NS) proteins (Sumiyoshi et al., 1987). Based on nucleotide sequencing of C/PrM and E genes, four virus genotypes have been distinguished (Chen et al., 1990; Chen et al., 1992): genotype I (GI), genotype II (GII) and genotype III (GIII) are distributed all over the geographical area of Asia, and genotype IV (GIV) includes isolates from Eastern Indonesia (Solomon et al., 2003). In addition, a JEV strain named Muar, isolated once in Singapore from a patient who originated from Malaysia, may represents a fifth genotype (GV) (Hasegawa et al., 1994; Uchil & Satchidanandam, 2001). Although this fifth genotype remained uncertain, it has been recently argued that it would be the most genetically different from the other JEV four genotypes (GI to GIV) (Mohammed et al., 2011). Furthermore, this fifth genotype is believed to be the oldest of the JEV lineage which would have originated from an ancestral virus in the mid 1500s in the Indonesia-Malaysia region. As suggested by Solomon et al. (2003), the

JEV is supposed to have evolved in other genotypes from the most divergent and probably oldest genotypes (GIV and GV), that have only be found in Indonesia-Malaysia region, and that JEV has spread from this region across Asia.

Although it was classically accepted that genotypes I and III occurred mostly in epidemic regions (temperate region of Asia), while GII and GIV were associated with endemic disease (tropical region), and ultimately postulated that differences in strain virulence could explain the clinical epidemiology (Chen et al., 1990; Chen et al., 1992; Williams et al., 2000), limited experimental assay on mice were not conclusive (Solomon et al., 2003). Moreover, several more recent observations tend to discard this hypothesis and suggest that genotypes could be found indifferently within former epidemic or endemic area. Thus, two JEV strains belonging to GI were isolated in the Australasian region (Pyke et al., 2001) and strains of the genotype II have been shown to use to circulate in Korea before 1970's (Schuh et al., 2010, 2011).

1.5 Japanese Encephalitis vaccine

Currently, three JEV vaccines are in use (Guirakhoo et al., 1999 ; Chang et al., 2000): (i) a formalin-inactivated, mouse brain-derived vaccine, based on the wild-type Nakayama or Beijing-1 strains, has been used internationally since the 1960s; (ii) a cell culture-derived inactivated vaccine; (iii) a cell culture-derived live attenuated vaccine, in China only. All vaccine types were developed from GIII JEV strains. Vaccine campaigns dramatically reduced the burden of the disease particularly in Japan, Korea, Taiwan, Sri Lanka, Thailand and Vietnam.

2. Materials and methods

2.1 Data collection

Among 563 wild strains investigated, 512 Japanese encephalitis virus strains could be fully characteristics from the available literature, GenBank Nucleotide database (www.ncbi.nlm.nih.gov/nuccore/), and possibly from Virus Sequence Database (http://kcdc.labkm.net/vsd/) and the database from Journal of General Virology (vir.sgmjournals.org/content/vol90/issue4/images/data/827/.../TableS1.xls). The literature review was achieved by using both generalist web search engines such as Google and Google Scholar, and scientific web search engines such as PubMed, Springerlink, ScienceDirect and Web of Science. It aimed at identifying an exhaustive panel of different JEV strains, and also at gathering a maximum of information on them as for date of sample collection and/ or virus isolation, site of collection, country, host, genotypes, sequence used for genotyping, GenBank accession number, and original reference when available. Keywords used for searching were: Japanese encephalitis virus; genotypes; genome; strains; phylogeny; molecular; epidemiology. Several different combinations and different suffixes were used; for instance, we used genom(e) as well as genom(ic). Then, articles were selected depending on their degree of relevance for the study, which were initially evaluated through the examination of the abstract. Then, to be selected, each article needed to meet the following criteria:

- Study of wild strain of Japanese encephalitis virus and
- Availability of the main features of the strain(s) including circumstances of viral isolation (i.e.: country, host, year of isolation and/or collection), and virological and molecular characteristics (i.e.: genes of interest, sequences).

The year of sample collection was a key data for the temporal analysis of virus genotypes dispersion and a particular attention was required to identify the year (and the site) of sampling collection, the year of virus isolation, and the year of publication.
However, for the selection, no particular attention was paid to the year of publication of articles. Nevertheless, since molecular techniques used for genetic, phylogenetic and epidemiologic studies are quite recent, the most recent articles from mid 90's to 2011 were deeply reviewed. These articles were especially interesting because they integrate isolates that were previously characterized, to increase the relevance of their analysis. Language accepted was English. When available, abstract in English of studies published in other languages were integrated to our review when they provided isolate name, of which characteristics were presented in GenBank database.
All available sequences of interest for genotyping were crossrefered with the corresponding one of GenBank, allowing checking for accuracy of the data presented in those articles, and consequently imprecision or even mistakes were identified and corrected.
The number of times that each strain was cited was recorded, also JEV strain descriptions were carefully compared as many studies often used the same strains and, in some instances, with different name.
On the one hand, this analysis aimed at enriching the total amount of specific data for each strain. On the other hand, it was used to identify erroneous data introduced by authors during the process of data collection from the original sources.

2.2 Identification of homogeneous regions

Countries were grouped together into distinct regions depending on biological, physical, anthropogenic and geographic factors. First, geopolitics criteria were used to associate several neighbouring states such as India and Sri Lanka. Secondly, since the epidemiology of JEV is strongly dependant on agroclimatic features (Solomon et al., 2000; Bi et al., 2003; Keiser et al., 2005), land use and climatic conditions were taken into account. In the context of climate change and rapid expansion of human activities, many studies have been conducted for the last two decades and have provided a large amount of updated information on these topics. On the one hand, regions that are characterized by the same vegetation and the same climatic conditions were defined as homogenous ecoregions (Olson et al., 2001). On the other hand, land use, and in particular irrigated and paddy fields areas, was considered, given the strong relationship existing between rice field density and mosquito populations, especially *Cx. tritaeniorhynchus* (Richards et al., 2010), and given the role of flooded rice system on JE outbreaks (Akiba et al., 2001; Keiser et al., 2005). Regarding both ecoregions and land use, we determined regions, which were also consistent with those proposed by Solomon et al. (2003). Moreover, since China is a very large country consisting in multiple different biomes ranging over the territory, for which the classification has been subject to several studies (Ni, 2001), it was divided in four parts, two of them being then integrated into already defined regions, one of them constituting one single region. The last area, including the Tibet, Xinjiang and Qinghai Provinces, was considered irrelevant for our study because JE is absent and no strain was collected there[3]. Grouping of Chinese provinces was achieved following precipitation variation, land use and ecoregions.

[3] Fischer et al., 2010 In: Travelers' Health - Yellow Book, Chapter 2: Japanese Encephalitis; available at wwwnc.cdc.gov/travel/yellowbook/2010/chapter-2/japanese-encephalitis.aspx

3. Results

3.1 Statistics on data collected

45 relevant articles from 1984 to 2011 were used for the data retrieval, of which most of the first author affiliation was Japanese, Chinese, Indian, Australian, South Korean and US American (Fig. 1).

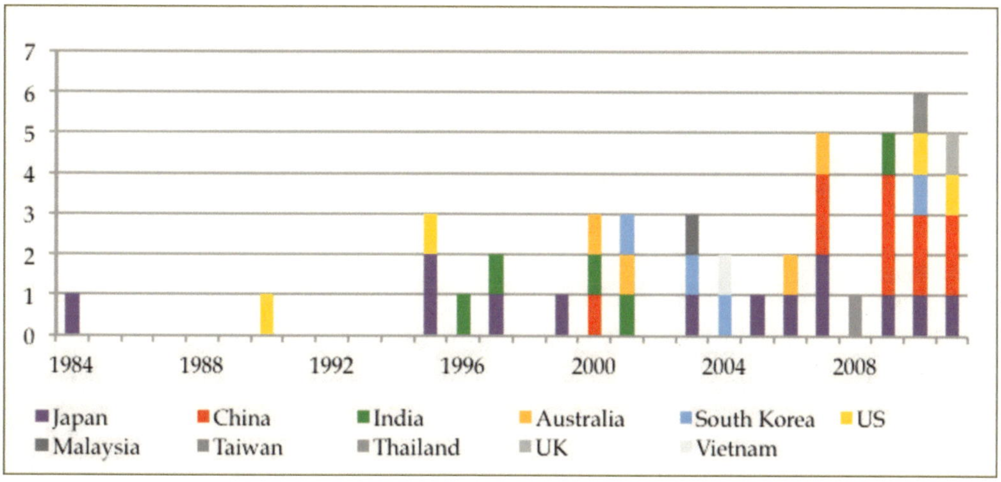

Fig. 1. Temporal distribution of the 45 selected articles and the country of their first author affiliations

A total amount of 2113 strains were integrated to these articles, among which 591 were strictly different wild strains. Vaccine strains were all excluded. Number of appearance of strains among studies ranged from 1 to 44, Beijing-1 being the strains the most cited. On the 591 strains available, 530 (89.7%) were referenced in the GenBank Nucleotide database.

In parallel, 886 sequences of 686 different strains were extracted from the GenBank Nucleotide database. Therefore, thanks to the cross-reference between all resources available, 564 distinct strains were investigated. Among them, the year of collection of 537 (95.2%), the country of collection of 562 (99.6%) and genotype of 526 (93.3%) strains were available. Complete information on 1/ the year of collection, 2/ the location of collection and 3/ genotypes was achieved on 500 (88.7%) strains. As we considered 20 years-time period, the amount of strains reached 511 (90.9%). Furthermore, while parts of countries or whole countries were integrated to larger region (see below 3.2 Region identification), three Chinese JEV strains that failed at being localized in an administrative division were unuseful. Eventually, 508 (90.1%) wild strains were integrated to our study on the spatiotemporal evolution of JEV genotypes in Asia.

Strains were collected from 1935 to 2009 in 16 countries of South Asia (India, Nepal and Sri Lanka), East Asia (China, Japan, South Korea, Russia, Taiwan, the Philippines, and Vietnam), of Southeast Asia (Cambodia, Thailand, Indonesia and Malaysia) and Northern Australasia (Papua New Guinea, the Torres Strait islands of northern Australia and northern Australia mainland) (Fig. 2). Number of strains collected in each country ranges from 1 to 158 (Japan). With Japan, China and Taiwan were the countries where larger amount of strains was collected, respectively accounting for 28.1%, 24.4% and 16.4% of the 562 strains for which location was available.

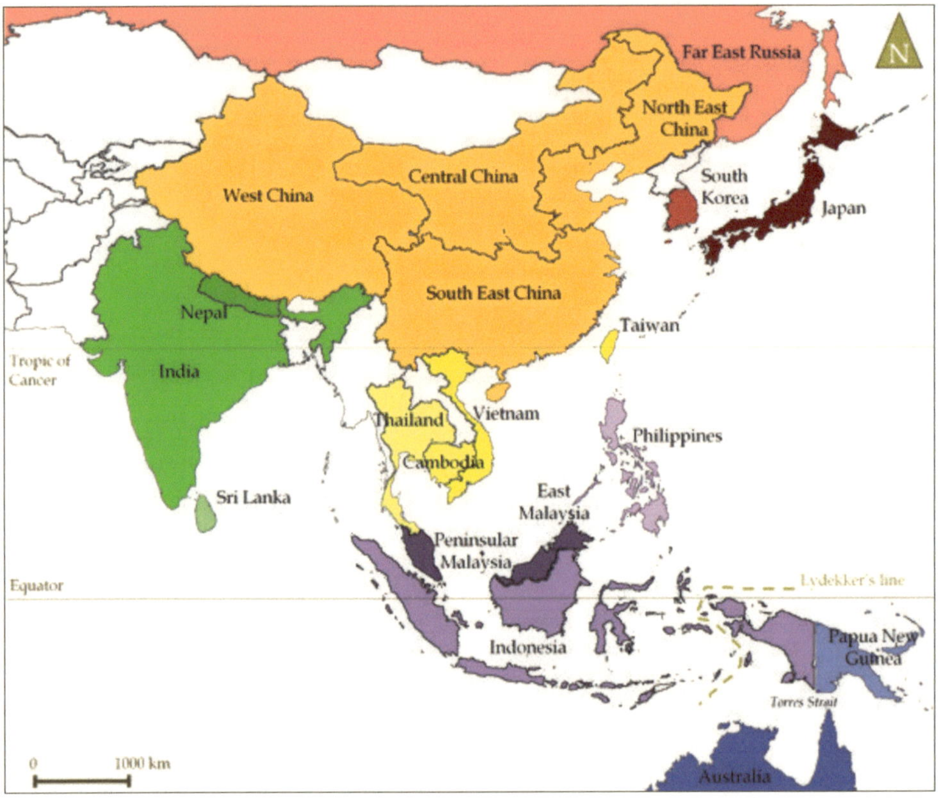

Fig. 2. Map of Asia: the 16 countries from which 562 JEV strains were collected between 1935 and 2009. Each shade of colour corresponds to one of the seventeen countries

3.2 Region identification

Regarding biotic, abiotic and anthropogenic features, we classified the 16 countries into six different regions (Fig. 3). First, the biogeoraphic realms separated the countries in three areas: Paleoarctic, Indo-Malay and Australasia realms (Olson et al., 2001). The Paleoarctic realm comprised Russia, Japan, Korea and northern part of China and was considered as the first region.

Within the Indo-Malay realm, Indian peninsula was separated from the Indochinese peninsula following a geographic east-west separation. On the east, the Indian peninsula included India, Nepal and Sri Lanka, plus Bangladesh, Buthan and Pakistan, and represented the second region. Further west, the Indochinese peninsula comprising Thailand, Cambodia and Vietnam plus Laos and Burma, and South China and Taiwan, were considered as the third region characterized by tropical climate and large cover of rice fields (Xiao et al., 2006). Then, peninsular Malaysia, east Malaysia and Indonesia constituted, with the Philippines, the fourth region. However, since Indonesia is a very fragmented country composed by very numerous islands stretching over 4,500 km from east to west and over 1,500 km from north to south, we considered the Lydekker's line to separate Australasia and the Oriental realm. Indeed, the Lydekker's line snaking through the Indonesian islands represents one of the ecological boundaries between the Sunda Shelf and the Sahul Shelf, which illustrates a great difference of biodiversity between ecosystems under similar climatic conditions (Cox, 2001; van den Bergh et al., 2001). Consequently, on the opposite side of the Lydekker's line, northern Australian mainland, Torres Strait Islands, Papua New Guinea were associated with the West Indonesian provinces of the Western New Guinea region, and therefore constituted the fifth region.

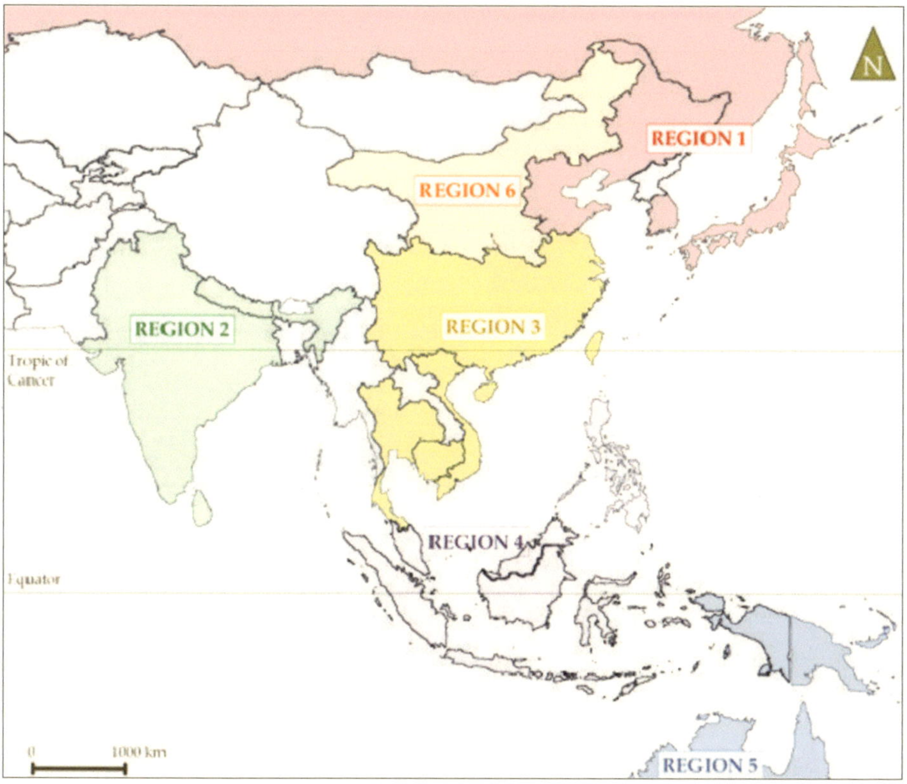

Fig. 3. Map of Asia: the six regions.
Region 1 in red; Region 2 in green; Region 3 in yellow; Region 4 in purple; Region 5 in blue, Region 6 in orange

China: as presented above, we defined an area on the south of the country as belonging to the same region than Vietnam, Thailand and Cambodia. This region was part of the Indo-Malay realm (Olson et al., 2001) and was mostly characterized by high precipitation and a tropical climate with high rice crop production (Frolking et al. 2002; Xiao et al., 2005). South China included the 14 (51.2%) following provinces (or other administrative divisions): Anhui, Fujian, Guangdong, Guangxi, Guizhou, Hainan, Hunan, Hubei, Jiangsu, Jiangxi, Shanghai, Sichuan, Yunnan and Zhejiang. Further north, 6 provinces (22.2%) (Gansu, Henan, Inner Mongolia, Ningxia, Shanxi and Shaanxi) represented the sixth and last region and were characterized by lower rice crop production in temperate climate and higher altitude of Central China. Finally, the last 7 (26.0%) northern provinces of the country (Beijing, Hebei, Heilongjiang, Jilin, Liaoning, Shandong and Tianjin) were associated with Far East Russia, Japan and Korea peninsula, all under temperate environment (Olson et al., 2001). Altogether, these six regions were used to describe the temporal evolution of the JE genotypes (Fig. 3).

3.3 Historic of the JEV genotypes in Asia

Over the 80 years of survey, from 1930's to 2000's, JEV have been actively circulating in Asia (Fig. 4). Historically, JEV was first identified in 1935 in Japan (Table 1).

Regions	Countries	Genotypes					Number of strains
		I	II	III	IV	V	
Reg. 1	Japan	1991	1959	1935			158
Reg. 1	Far East Russia			1943			1
Reg. 1	South Korea	1991		1946			37
Reg. 1	North East China	2002		1949			15
Reg. 2	India			1956			23
Reg. 2	Sri Lanka			1969			3
Reg. 2	Nepal			1985			3
Reg. 3	South East China	1979		1954			100
Reg. 3	Taiwan	2008		1958			92
Reg. 3	Vietnam	2001		1962			18
Reg. 3	Thailand	1979	1983	1964			40
Reg. 3	Cambodia	1967					2
Reg. 3	Hong Kong		2000				1
Reg. 4	Malaysia	1994	1968	1965		1952	18
Reg. 4	Indonesia		1978	1979	1980		15
Reg. 4	Philippines			1984			1
Reg. 5	Australia	2000	1995				10
Reg. 5	Papua New Guinea		1997				3
Reg. 6	Central China	2004		1954			18

Table 1. Year of collection of the first strain of each genotype in the 6 regions and 19 areas of Asia

Then the virus was detected in Far East Russia, South Korea and China (1940's), then in Malaysia, India and Taiwan (1950's), then Vietnam, Thailand, Cambodia and Sri Lanka (1960's), Indonesia (1970's), Philippines, Nepal (1980's), Australia, Papua New Guinea (1990's) and finally in Hong Kong in early 2000's. Thus, after the first isolation of the virus in 1930's, a large amount of strains was isolated during the following decades. Their genotype was usually defined through the comparison of sequences between representatives of each genotype and the newly collected strains, from which the degree of homology was extracted. Often in studies, a phylogenetic tree is also constructed. Thus, from 1930's to present (2009), many strains have been collected and have clustered within genetic groups.

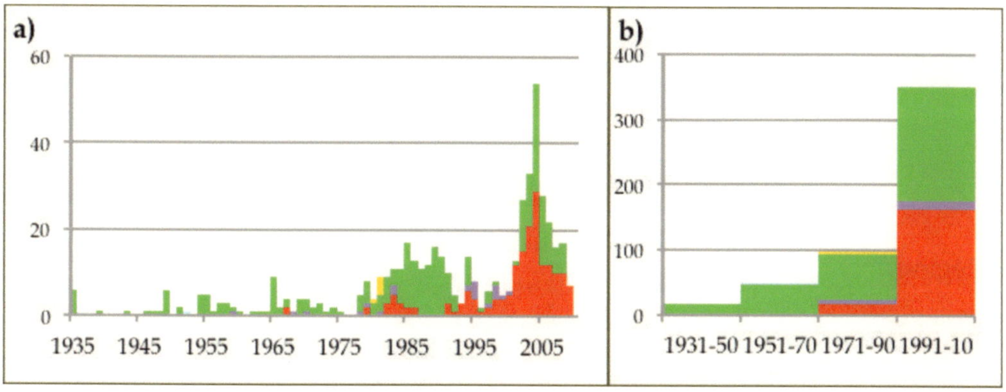

Fig. 4. Number of strains collected and their genotypes: a) from 1935 to 2009; b) during the four 20-years time periods (1931-1950, 1951-1970, 1971-1990 and 1991-2010).
Genotype I in red; Genotype II in purple; Genotype III in green; Genotype IV in gold; Genotype V in light blue (one single strain, 1952)

In figure 4, it appears that until the 80's, no more than 10 strains were collected each year. Then, from 80's to early 90's, a first peak of 17 strains was recorded, in 1985, mainly due to strains from regions 1 and 3. After a 7-years period with relatively constant and low strains collection, another pick was recorded, in 2004. Much higher than the previous one, this peak reached 54 strains, which were collected in region 1 and 2, but above all in region 3 (40 (75.5%) strains, of which 23 (57.5%) originated from South East China). By considering 20-years time periods, the amount of collected strains clearly increased, seemingly in an exponential way.

Spatially, genotypes that have been identified differed between regions and every genotype have not been found in each Asian region yet. As an example, although India-Sri Lanka-Nepal Region (Region 2) has displayed one single genotype (III), strains of the five genotypes have been collected from the Indonesia-Philippines-Malaysia Region (Region 4) (Table 1). In fact, Region 4 is the only one that has been showed to house all the genotype and the only region where genotypes IV and V have been identified.

Moreover, genotypes evolved in time, with genotype III being the predominant genotype until early 1990's, and being progressively replaced by genotype I by then, especially in China, Taiwan, Korea and Japan (i.e. regions 1, 3 and 6) (Fig. 4 and 5).

Contrary to regions 1 and 3 where many strains have been collected (respectively 186 and 240, counting for 85.7% of the 497 strains reported), relatively few strains were found in the remaining four regions (Fig. 5). Thus, region 1 and 3 predominantly contribute to the yearly variation of the number of strains collected. As these two regions comprise the most developed countries with the most efficient epidemiological survey, the variation is expected to reflect the real incidence of JE. Consequently, the figure 5 shows that JEV has intensively circulated in regions 1 and 3 during the last decades.

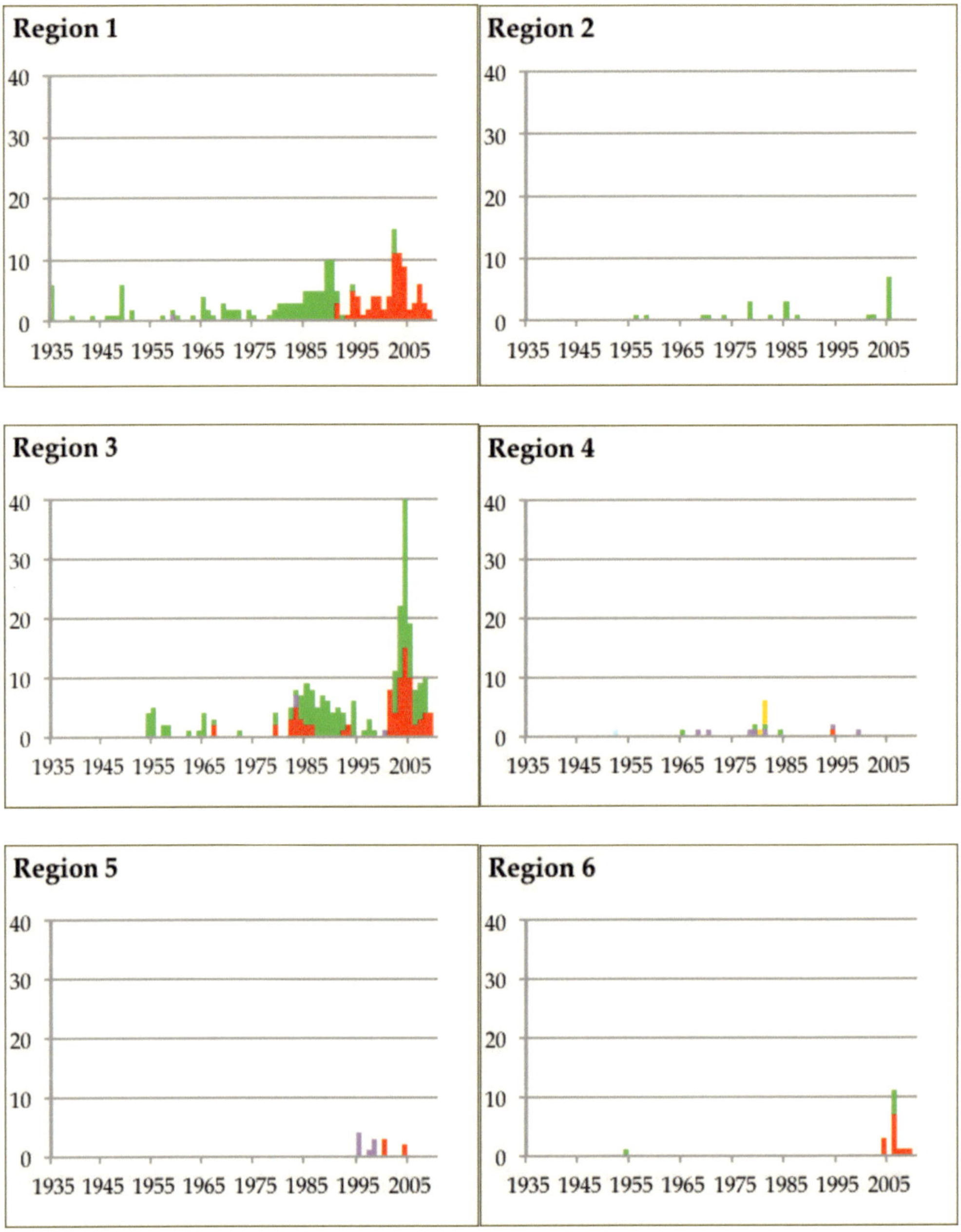

Fig. 5. Temporal evolution of the number of strains collected and their genotype among the fully characterized within the 6 regions. The colour code of the 5 genotypes is the same than in Fig. 4

In region 2 and 4, whereas few strains was collected and isolated, JEV seems to have circulated from early 1950's. Interestingly in region 2, in five instances, each one approximately separated by 5-10 years, a few and lowly variable strains was collected, suggesting a periodic increase of the amount of JEV strains, but quite constant. In region 4, a peak period of circulation was recorded between 1975 and 1985, suggesting that apart from this 10-years period, JEV circulated less actively even if additional strains were still isolated before and after. In region 6, one single strain was isolated before 1955, and after about 50 years without any other strain, several have been collected since 2004. In region 5, the first strain was isolated in 1995. From then, strains have been regularly isolated until 2004.

3.3 Dispersion of the genotypes

The following four figures show how JEV genotypes changed during the four 20-years time periods (Fig. 6a, b, c, d).

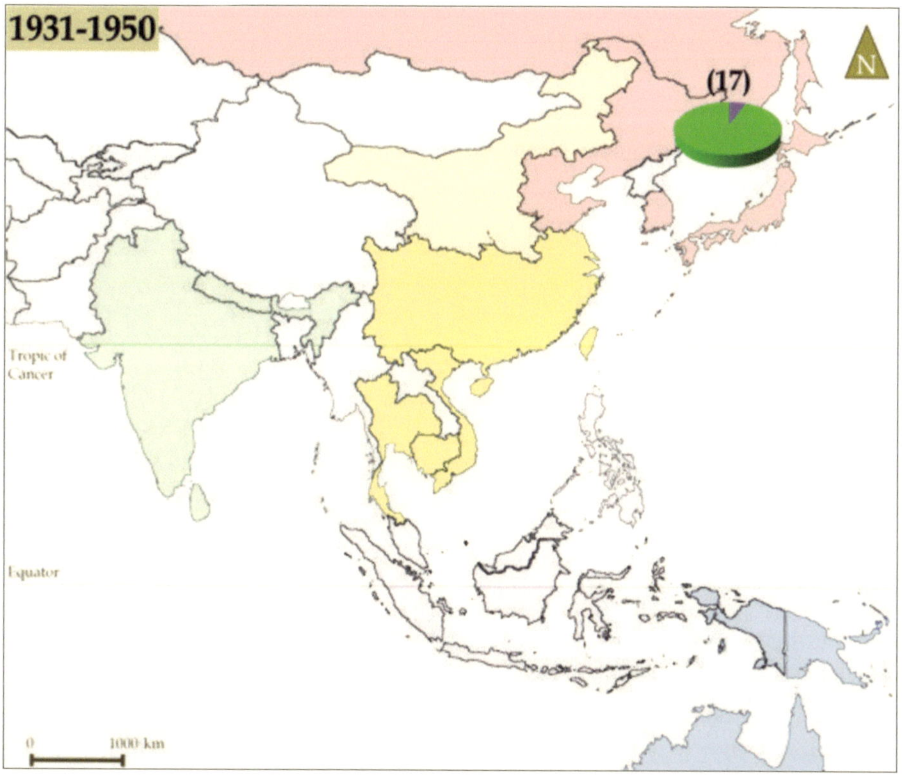

Fig. 6a. Evolution of the proportion of each genotype identified in every region from 1931 to 1950. The total amount of strains collected in every region is in brackets. Regions are coloured as in Fig. 3. Pie charts represent the proportion of each genotype in every region. The colour code used for the genotypes is the same than in Fig. 4 and 5. When no pie chart is presented, no strain was collected in the corresponding region

Between 1931 and 1950 (Fig. 6a), JEV strains were isolated from region 1 only. Among the seventeen strains characterized, about 95% belonged to genotypes III, the remaining ones belonging to genotype II. Then, from early 1950's, strains have been isolated from every areas of Asia, apart from Australasia. On the 47 strains isolated between 1951 and 1970, more than 95% still belonged to genotype III (Fig. 6b). Interestingly, the first, and single, isolation of strain from genotype V was performed in region 4. Rather than illustrating a dispersion of JEV from further north region of Asia towards south-eastern and southern

Asia, our results suggest that from 1931 to 1970, JEV did circulate in the whole continental Asia. Indeed, the proportion of the genotype III did not change within the 40-years period of time (stabilized around 95%), and if considered as control region, the region 1 displayed the same profile: numerous strains from genotype III and a few from genotype II.

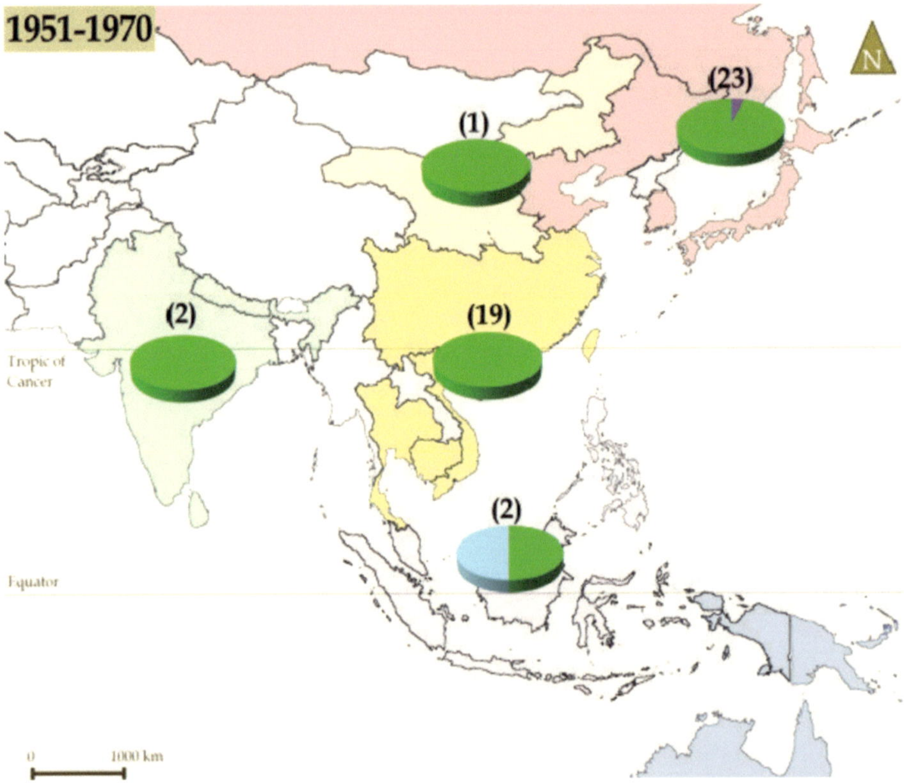

Fig. 6b. Evolution of the proportion of each genotype identified in every region from 1951 to 1970. The legend is the same than if Fig. 6a

Between 1970 and 1990 (Fig 6c), 98 strains were collected, doubling the amount of strains collected between 1951 and 1970. While strains still originated from regions 1, 2, 3 and 4, none was isolated from region 6. Also, for the first time, several strains of genotype IV were collected in region 4. Although genotype II had only been found in the northern region 1 since 1930's, several strains were collected both in region 3 and 4.

More interestingly, proportion of genotype III started to decrease from 95% to 70% between 1971 and 1990, while the new genotype I appeared in region 3 and reached 17%, becoming the second most important JE genotype in Asia. This tendency was then confirmed during the last 20-years time period, between 1990 and 2010 (Fig. 6d), when genotype I reached 46% against 50% for genotype III. However, this change did not occur widely in Asia. Indeed, in region 2, genotype III has ever been the only one that could be identified, and genotype I has seemed to be geographically limited to Eastern areas of Asia and in Australasia. By considering these five eastern regions only, genotype I and III became equally important (50%-50%). Furthermore, temperate areas (regions 1 and 6) were markedly different than tropical areas (regions 3, 4 and 5).

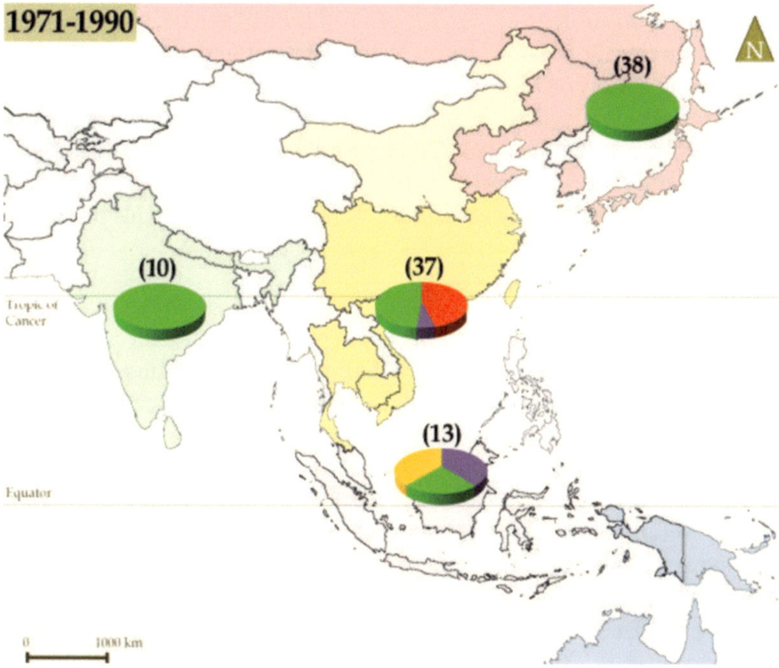

Fig. 6c. Evolution of the proportion of each genotype identified in every region from 1971 to 1990. The legend is the same than if Fig. 6a

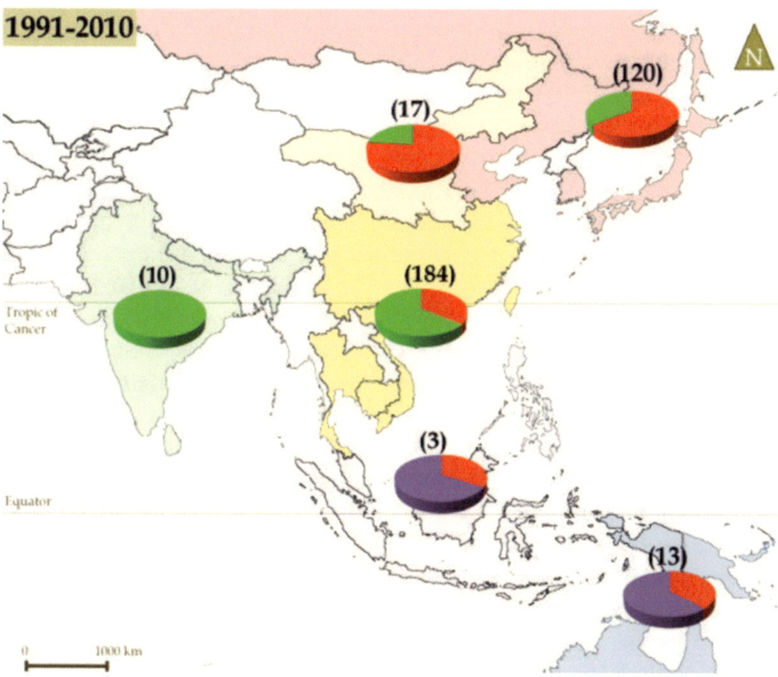

Fig. 6d. Evolution of the proportion of each genotype identified in every region from 1991 to 2010. The legend is the same than if Fig. 6a

Whilst in these three tropical regions, genotypes I, II and III respectively counted for 35.5%, 5.5% and 59%, in temperate regions (1 and 6) genotypes I and III respectively counted for 66% and 34%, making genotype I the most important genotype.
On top of that, for the really first time, JEV strains were obtained from the Australasia region (region 5), firstly in Papua New Guinea and Torres Strait Islands, and secondly in Australia mainland. Genotype II was the first isolated and then genotype I appeared, in lower proportion however (38% against 62% for genotype II during this period).

4. Discussion

More than 500 JEV strains were used to understand the spatio-temporal evolution of JEV genotypes since the disease was detected. Characteristic of strains such as the year of collection and isolation, the exact place it originated from and the genotype it belongs to are not always properly presented in articles. Also, retrieval of the original source of strain isolation very often failed, partially because of the use of more recent references. As a consequent, the scientist who detected a strain for the really first time becomes progressively forgotten. However, the original source of strain sequencing was better conserved. Moreover, a doubt remains on the year. The year of isolation is more often cited in studies (for instance Pyke et al., 2001) while in GenBank database, the year of collection is sometimes given (for instance strains LY5P-09 and YN114, respectively presented in Zhang et al., 2011 and Wang et al., 2010). Even, in other articles, the term year alone is used and serves as an element of description of the history of the strains (for instance Yun et al., 2003). Thus, in our study, we considered the year presented in studies as being the year during which the strains was proven to circulate.
Also, in time, sequencing techniques have improved in the same time that database of sequenced strains enlarged. At that time, more strains were available and molecular and statistical tools allowed reinforcing phylogenetic analysis. However, in some instances, genetic characterization of strains led to different results. As an example, strain B2239, collected in 1984 in Thailand (GenBank accession number U70391) clustered in genotype II (Pyke et al., 2001) and I (Nabeshima et al., 2009). Furthermore, strains JKT6468, collected in 1981 in Indonesia (GenBank accession numbers AY184212, U70407 or L42162) was used in 21 different articles and was suggested to belong to genotype II once (Yang et al., 2004), III once (Yun et al., 2003), IV fifteen times (Huang et al., 2010; Fan et al., 2010). Consequently, we choose to keep the genotype that was the most often and most recently obtained. Finally, we had to eliminate several incomplete strains to our database and used the other to evaluate the spatio-temporal evolution of the genotype over the Asian and Australasian continents.
Since its detection in 1930's, Japanese Encephalitis Virus has continuously circulated in Asia for about seven decades. First isolated in Japan, many JEV strains have been collected since. Despite large vaccination campaigns in developed countries such as Japan, Taiwan or even Thailand, the disease has never been eliminated from any country and human cases still regularly occurs. Furthermore, JE progressively spread in new Asian areas and progressively enlarge its distribution area. Restricted to north-eastern areas of Asia at first, the disease then invaded a majority of the countries of South East Asia, South Asia, East Asia and finally Australasia. Of course, the disease might have not been detected from developing countries in early period because of a lack of health services and epidemiological survey. Especially, the differences in survey effort, virus isolation techniques and public

health services very probably explain why no strains had been characterized before 1950's outside region 1. As evidence, before 1970, most of strains (52.8%) were isolated from human hosts, suggesting that public health services were the first tool used to identify the virus. Thus, in countries where health care was not as well-developed as, for example, in Japan, several human cases may have failed at being diagnosed and virus at being detected. On the contrary, since 1970's, the proportion of strains that have been isolated from mosquitoes and pig has strongly increased, reaching 81.1% while the proportion of strains extracted from humans has fallen to 17.6%. Regarding the serious effects of JE on human health, better attention has been progressively paid to the disease. Thus, this important change of strains sources illustrates the epidemiological survey effort that has been developed in Asia, also confirming that the number of strains collected increased with time partly thanks to improving survey. Therefore, it is more likely that less human cases stayed undetected from 1970's and most of areas where JE outbreaks occurred were recorded.

Even if epidemiological survey improved in time the number of strains that were yearly collected may have not totally reflected the number of strains really circulating until 1970's. However, in a few countries where survey effort has been constantly maintained since the first identification of the JEV, the variation of strains amount is expected to be close to what really happened. Thus, Japan, Korea, India or even Australia can be considered as witness of the temporal evolution of the total amount of JEV strains collected, whereas that does not cover every region. Since it appeared that the increase of collected strains was exponential, the effect of epidemiologic survey effort cannot be easily distinguished from the real increase in JEV circulation. Yet, the examination of the temporal evolution of the amount of strains detected in Japan shows that a few strains were annually present from 1930's to mid-1980's and during 1990's. On the contrary, two peaks of abundance of strains, signs of epidemic manifestations, occurred between mid-1980's and 1992, and then between 2000 and 2009. Moreover, the second peak was higher than the previous one, enforcing the assumption of a general increase of the number of strains circulating. Consequently, JEV most intensively circulated during the last two decades, especially in region 1, 3 and 5, where it appeared for the first time. In region 4 and 6, weaker epidemiologic survey effort were made, and strains, which have been scarce and have temporally scattered there, may have failed at illustrating the real circulation of JEV (see also Solomon et al., 2003). In Central China, drier climate with less developed irrigated agriculture such as rice (Frolking et al., 2001), less important livestock and human population compared to other parts of China do not provide the best conditions for the JEV vectors to breed, and for the JEV to amplify and be transmitted to human. Also, provinces of this area are poorer than coastal provinces. Therefore, until 1990's and the rise of molecular techniques of sequencing, less attention could have been paid to this region for decades, despite an existing risk. In region 2 however, the effort of survey seems to have been maintained since 1970's, and the periodic and constant re-emergence of JEV strains is likely to point out a less intense activity of the virus in South Asia compared the East Asian countries. Also, genotype III is the only one to have ever been found in this region, suggesting that the strains pool little evolutes. Future constant efforts in every country of the Asian region would provide a better insight. As an effective tool, the use of sentinel animals in survey would improve the assessment of the risk of JEV transmission to human. In particular, serological survey on domestic pig herds, which are the main reservoir amplifying hosts of the virus and are widely raised in Asia, would be a means to monitor the JEV activity (Nitatpattana et al., 2011).

However, evidence of recent introduction of the virus was demonstrated. In Australia, intensive surveillance has existed for long. Thus, JEV strains are unlikely to have not been detected before mid-1990's, and the disease has obviously extended its geographical range. The way the virus is introduced is subject to debate. On the first hand, some researchers believe that infected vectors, mostly mosquitoes, may be transported by cyclonic winds. This theory was presented to explain the crossing of the Torres Strait towards Australia mainland (Ritchie & Rochester, 2001) or the several introductions of strains from China towards Japan (Nga et al., 2004). On the other hand, the virus may be transported in long distance by migratory birds, as it has also been suspected to explain the numerous introductions of JEV strains in Japan from China or in northern areas of Asia from the Indochinese peninsula (Nga et al., 2004). Whatever the reason is, these findings show that JE is an emerging-remerging disease which may colonize new areas, whilst trades of goods, as well as transport of people are in constant development and increase the probability of the virus to be introduced in vectors or animals.

In parallel of the increasing of JEV strains and dispersion towards new Asian areas, genotypes changed. After that genotype III remained the major genotype until 1990's, it is very obvious that genotypes I, which emerged in every region of Asia except in South Asia (Nepal, India and Sri Lanka), became the very major genotype in northern temperate regions (i.e. regions 1 and 6 essentially constituted by Japan, South Korea, and North East China, none strain having been isolated from Far East Russia since 1943). Genotype I originated from the Indochinese peninsula in late 1960's and circulated at first in Cambodia, Thailand and South East China by the end of the 1970's, before it enlarged its geographical distribution to further north and southeast areas. Genotype I also indicates a difference of activity between temperate and tropical regions. Indeed, while genotype I invaded tropical Asia (Indochinese peninsula, Philippines, Indonesian-Malaysian region and Australasia) without becoming the main genotype, the major genotype has clearly shifted from genotype III to genotype I in Japan (Ma et al., 2003), South Korea (Yun et al., 2010), North East China (Wang et al., 2007a) and Central China (Wang et al., 2007a), since early 1990's. Furthermore, whereas JEV strains of genotype I were detected, none isolate was obtained from human patients before the second half of the 2000's. Unfortunately, by then, strain has been detected from human, throwing the efficiency of the vaccine used until then into question (Wang et al., 2010). Indeed, existing live or attenuated vaccines used to be derived from genotype III strains (Zhang et al., 2011). Since the infectivity and pathogenecity of JEV genotype I strains may be different to genotype III, the vaccines may become less protective for human, therefore pointing out the need to evaluate them both.

By considering the current map of JEV genotype distribution, it appears that the Indonesia-Malaysia-Philippines region was the source of introduction into Australasia. Also, this region has always been the one where several genotypes cohabited. Eventually, the five genotypes were recognized there. Thus, our data are consistent with the hypothesis of Solomon (2003) suggesting that genotypes IV and V are the most ancestral ones. This region may be the original source of the virus, which spread first towards northern areas, then was detected in Japan, and then spread to other Asian regions. A gradient of dispersion from region 4 to region 3, then to region 6 and 1 further north, and to region 2 further west, and another to region 5 further southeast is indeed probable (Solomon et al. 2006).

5. Conclusion

Although Japanese Encephalitis has been known to recently spread over South Asia since its clinical identification in the late 1870s, followed by the discovery of the etiological agent in the early 1930s, considering the molecular clock, Japanese Encephalitis virus appears to have spread and diversified - as genotypes - across South East Asia more than 200 years ago (Solomon et al., 2003). Actual dispersion of the different JEV genotypes do not present a clear pattern of distribution within the South Asian endemic region; also a temporal and spatial analysis appears to be the most appropriate way to understand the actual distribution of JEV and its significance in term of risk of expansion (emergence) and vaccine strategies.

We provide here some insight for such understanding as for the dynamics of genotype diffusion (i.e.: one genotype rising in a given territory and taking over a previously prevailing genotype). The immunological pressure through vaccination campaign - with a vaccine generated from one single serotype - could drive such actual pattern, while also agricultural practices (ex.: pig farming), changes in the main vector (ex.: *Culex quinquefasciatus*) could theoretically participate to such a distribution. However more study need to be done to identify the fundamentals of genotype emergence within a given territory. Ultimately, taking into account these observations, each JEV genotype dynamic much be considered and understand at a local level with respect to environmental factors of natural and anthropic origins.

6. References

Akiba, T.; Osaka, K.; Tang, S.; Nakayama, M.; Yamamoto, A.; Kurane, I.; Okabe, N. & Umenai, T. (2001). Analysis of Japanese encephalitis epidemic in Western Nepal in 1997. *Epidemiology and Infection*, Vol. 126, No. 1, pp. 81-8

Ali, A.; Igarashi, A.; Paneru, L.R.; Hasebe, F.; Morita, K.; Takagi, M.; Suwonkerd, W.; Tsuda, Y. & Wada, Y. (1995). Characterization of two Japanese encephalitis virus strains isolated In Thailand. *Archives of Virology*, Vol. 140, pp.1557-1575

Bi, P; Tong, C.; Donald, K. Parton, K.A. & Ni, J. (2003). Climate Variability and Transmission of Japanese Encephalitis in Eastern China. *Vector-Borne and Zoonotic Diseases*, Vol. 3, No. 3, pp. 111-115

Chang, G.J.; Hunt, A.R. & Davis, B.A. (2000). A single intramuscular injection of recombinant plasmid DNA induces protective immunity and prevents Japanese encephalitis in mice. *The Journal of Virology*,Vol. 74, No. 9, pp. 4244-52

Chen, W-R.; Tesh, R.B. & Rico-Hesse, R. (1990). Genetic variation of Japanese encephalitis virus in nature. *Journal of General Virology*, Vol. 71, pp. 2915-2922

Cox, C.B. (2001).The biogeographic regions reconsidered. *Journal of Biogeography*, Vol. 28, pp. 511-523

Erlanger, T.E.; Weiss, S.; Keiser, J.; Utzinger, J. & Wiedenmayer, K. (2009). Past, present, and future of Japanese encephalitis. *Emerging Infectious Diseases*, Vol. 15, pp. 1–7

Fan, J-M.; Luo, J.; Chen, L.; Teng, M.; Bu, D.; Wang, F-Y.; Wang, L.; Wang, C-Q. & Zhang, G-P. (2010). Genetic analysis of strains of Japanese Encephalitis Virus isolated from swine in central China. *Virus Genes*, Vol. 40, pp. 357–361

Frolking, S.; Qiu, J.; Boles, S.; Xiao, X.; Liu, J.; Zhuang, Y.; Li, C. & Qin, X. (2002). Combining remote sensing and ground census data to develop new maps of the distribution of rice agriculture in China. *Global Biogeochemical Cycles*, Vol. 16, No. 4, pp. XX-XX 1091

Gao, X.Y.; Nasci, R. & Liang, G.D. (2010). The Neglected Arboviral Infections in Mainland China. *PLoS Neglected Tropical Diseases*, Vol. 4, No. 4, e624

Gao, X.Y.; Wang, H.Y.; Wang, H.Y.; Fu, S.H.; Liu, G.F.; Li, Y.; Li, M.H.; Xu, A.Q. & Liang, G.D. (2009). Molecular characterization of full-length genome of Japanese encephalitis virus (SD08-10) newly isolated in Shandong province. Article in Chinese. *Zhonghua Shi Yan He Lin Chuang Bing Du Xue Za Zhi*, Vol. 23, Issue 4, pp. 242-244

Guirakhoo, F.; Zhang, Z.X.; Chambers, T.J.; Delagrave, S.; Arroyo, J.; Barrett, A.D. & Monath, T.P. (1999). Immunogenicity, genetic stability, and protective efficacy of a recombinant, chimeric yellow fever-Japanese encephalitis virus (ChimeriVax-JE) as a live, attenuated vaccine candidate against Japanese encephalitis. *Virology*,Vol. 257, No. 2, pp. 363-72

Hanna, J.N.; Ritchie, S.A.; Phillips, D.A.; Lee, J.M.; Hills, S.L.; van den Hurk, A.F.; Pyke, A.T.; Johansen, C.A. & Mackenzie, J.S. (1999). Japanese encephalitis in north Queensland, Australia, 1998. *The Medical Journal of Australia*, Vol. 170, pp. 533–536

Hasegawa, H.; Yoshida, M.; Kobayashi, Y. & Fujita, S. (1995). Antigenic analysis of Japanese encephalitis viruses in Asia by using monoclonal antibodies. *Vaccine*, Vol. 13, No. 17, pp. 1713-1721

Huang, J-H. ; Lin, T-H. ; Teng, H-J. ; Su, C-L. ; Tsai, K-H. ; Lu, L-C. ; Lin, C. ; Yang, C-F. ; Chang, S-F. ; Liao, T-L. ; Yu, S-K. ; Cheng, C-H. ; Chang, M-C. ; Hu, H-C. & Shu, P-Y. (2010). Molecular Epidemiology of Japanese Encephalitis Virus, Taiwan. *Emerging Infectious Diseases*, Vol. 16, No. 5, pp. 876-878

Igarashi, A .; Tanaka, M.; Morita, K.; Takasu, T. ; Ahmed, A.; Ahmed, A.; Akram, D.S. & Wagar, M.A. (1994). Detection of West Nile and Japanese encephalitis viral genome sequences in cerebrospinal fluid from acute encephalitis cases in Karachi, Pakistan. *Microbiology and Immunology*,Vol. 38, pp. 827–30

Jan, L-R.; Yueh, Y-Y.; Wu, Y-C. ; Horng, C-B. & Wang, G-R. (2000). Genetic variation of Japanese encephalitis virus in Taiwan. *American Journal of Tropical Medicine and Hygiene*, Vol. 62, No. 4, pp. 446-452

Keiser, J.; Maltese, M.F.; Erlanger, T.E.; Bos, R.; Tanner, M.; Singer, B.H. & Utzinger, J. (2005). Effect of irrigated rice agriculture on Japanese encephalitis, including challenges and opportunities for integrated vector management. *Acta Tropica*, Vol. 95, pp. 40–57

Khan, S.; Hanjra, M.A. & Mu, J. (2009). Water management and crop production for food security in China: A review. *Agricultural water management*, Vol. 96, No. 3, pp. 349-360

Kobayashi, Y; Hasegawa, H.; Oyama, T.; Tamai, T. & Kusaba, T. (1984). Antigenic Analysis of Japanese Encephalitis Virus by Using Monoclonal Antibodies. *Infection and Immunity*, Vol. 44, No. 1, pp. 117-123

Liu, X.; Yua, Y.; Li, M.; Liang, G.; Wang, H.; Ji, L. & Dong, G. (2011). Study on the protective efficacy of SA14-14-2 attenuated Japanese encephalitis against different JE virus isolates circulating in China. *Vaccine, Vol.* 29, pp. 2127–2130

Ma, S.P.; Yoshida, Y.; Makino, Y.; Tadano, M.; Ono, T. & Ogawa, M. (2003). Short report: a major genotype of Japanese encephalitis virus currently circulating in Japan. *American Journal of Tropical Medicine and Hygiene*, Vol. 69, pp. 151-154

Mackenzie, J.S.; Williams, D.T. & Smith, D.W. (2007). Japanese Encephalitis Virus: The Geographic Distribution, Incidence, and Spread of a Virus with a Propensity to Emerge in New Areas, In: *Emerging Viruses in Human Populations*, Edward Tabor, pp. 201-268, Elsevier, ISBN 0-444-52074-0

Mangada, M.N. & Takegami, T. (1999). Molecular characterization of the Japanese encephalitis virus representative immunotype strain JaGAr 01. *Virus Research*, Vol. 59, pp. 101–112

Mohammed, M.A.F.; Galbraith, S.E.; Radford, A.D.; Dove, W.; Takasaki, T.; Kurane, I. & Solomon, T. (2011). Molecular phylogenetic and evolutionary analyses of Muar strain of Japanese encephalitis virus reveal it is the missing fifth genotype. *Infection, Genetics and Evolution*, in press.

Nabeshima, T.; Loan, H.T.K.; Inoue, S.; Sumiyoshi, M.; Haruta, Y.; Nga, P.T.; Huoung, V.T.Q.; del Carmen Parquet, M.; Hasebe, F. & Morita, K. (2009). Evidence of frequent introductions of Japanese encephalitis virus from south-east Asia and continental east Asia to Japan. *Journal of General Virology*, Vol. 90, pp. 827–832

Nam, J.H.; Chae, S.L.; Won, S.Y.; Kim, E.J.; Yoon, K.S.; Kim, B.I.; Jeong, Y.S. & Cho, H.W. (2001). Short report: genetic heterogeneity of Japanese encephalitis virus assessed via analysis of the full-length genome sequence of a Korean isolate. *American Journal of Tropical Medicine and Hygiene*, Vol. 65, pp. 388-392

Nerome, R.; Tajima, S.; Takasaki, T.; Yoshida, T.; Kotaki, A.; Lim, C.K.; Ito, M.; Sugiyama, A.; Yamauchi, A.; Yano, T.; Kameyama, T.; Morishita, I.; Kuwayama, M.; Ogawa, T.; Sahara, K. & Ikegaya, A. (2007). Molecular epidemiological analyses of Japanese encephalitis virus isolates from swine in Japan from 2002 to 2004. *Journal of General Virology*, Vol. 88, pp. 2762-2768

Nga, P.T.; del Carmen Parquet, M.; Cuong, V.D.; Ma, S.P.; Hasebe, F.; Inoue, S.; Makino, Y.; Takagi, M.; Nam, V.S. & Morita, K. (2004). Shift in Japanese encephalitis virus genotype circulating in northern Vietnam: implications for frequent introductions of JEV from Southeast Asia to East Asia. *Journal of General Virology*, Vol. 85, No.6, pp. 1625-1631

Ni, H. & Barrett, A.D.T. (1995). Nucleotide and deduced amino acid sequence of the structural protein genes of Japanese encephalitis viruses from different geographical locations. *Journal of General Virology*, Vol. 76, pp. 401-407

Ni, J. (2001). A biome classification of china based on plant functional types and the BIOME3 model. *Folia Geobotanica*, Vol. 36, pp. 113-129

Nitatpattana, N.; Dubot-Peres, A.; Gouilh, M.A.; Souris, M.; Barbazan, P.; Yoksan, S.; de Lamballerie, X. & Gonzalez, J.P. (2008). Change in Japanese encephalitis virus distribution, Thailand. *Emerging Infectious Diseases*, Vol. 14, No. 11, pp. 1762-1765

Olson, D.M.; Dinerstein, E.; Wikramanayake, E.D.; Burgess, N.D.; Powell, G.V.N; Underwood, E.C.; D'amico, J.A.; Itoua, I.; Strand, H.E.; Morrison, J.C.; Loucks, C.J.; Allnutt, T.F.; Ricketts, T.H.; Kura, Y.; Lamoreux, J.F.; Wettengel, W.W.; Hedao, P. & Kassem, K.R. (2001). Terrestrial Ecoregions of the World: A New Map of Life on Earth. *BioScience*, Vol. 51, No. 11, pp. 933-938

Paranjpe, S. & Banerjee, K. (1996). Phylogenetic analysis of the envelope gene of Japanese encephalitis virus. *Virus Research* 42, 107–117.

Paranjpe, S.; Walimbe, A. &. Banerjee, K. (1997). Statistical analysis of the envelope gene and the prM region of Japanese encephalitis virus evidence suggestive of positive selection. *Journal of Genetics*, Vol. 76, No. 2, pp. 117-131

Pyke, A.T.; Williams, D.T.; Nisbet, D.J.; van den Hurk, A.F.; Taylor, C.T.; Johansen, C.A.; Macdonald, J.; Hall, R.A.; Simmons, R.J.; Mason, R.J.; Lee, J.M.; Ritchie, S.A.; Smith, G.A. & Mackenzie, J.S. (2001). The appearance of a second genotype of Japanese encephalitis virus in the Australasian region. *American Journal of Tropical Medicine and Hygiene*, Vol. 65, pp. 747-753

Richards, E.E.; Masuoka, P.; Brett-Major, D.; Smith, M.; Klein, T.A.; Kim, H.C.; Anyamba, A. & Grieco, J. (2010). The relationship between mosquito abundance and rice field density in the Republic of Korea. *International Journal of Health Geographics*, Vol. 9, p. 32

Rosen, L. (1986). The natural history of Japanese encephalitis virus. *Annual Review of Microbiology*, Vol. 40, pp.395-414

Saito, M.; Taira, K.; Itokazu, K. & Mori, N. (2007). Recent Change of the Antigenicity and Genotype of Japanese Encephalitis Viruses Distributed on Okinawa Island, Japan. *American Journal of Tropical Medicine and Hygiene*, Vol. 77, No. 4, pp. 737-746

Saxena, S.K.; Mishra, N. ; Saxena, R.; Singh, M. & Mathur, A. (2009). Trend of Japanese encephalitis in North India: evidence from thirty-eight acute encephalitis cases and appraisal of niceties. *Journal of Infection in Developing Countries*, Vol. 3, No.7, pp. 517-530

Schuh, A.J.; Tesh, R.B.; Innis, B.L. & Barrett, A.D.T. (2010). Genetic characterization of early isolates of Japanese encephalitis virus: genotype II has been circulating since at least 1951. *Journal of General Virology*, Vol. 91, pp. 95–102

Schuh, A.J.; Tesh, R.B. & Barrett, A.D.T. (2011). Genetic characterization of Japanese encephalitis virus genotype II strains isolated from 1951 to 1978. *Journal of General Virology*, Vol. 92, pp. 516–527

Shimojima, M.; Nagao, Y.; Shimoda, H.; Tamaru, S.; Yamanaka, T.; Matsumura, T. Kondo, T. & Maeda, K. (2011). Full genome sequence and virulence analyses of the recent equine isolate of Japanese encephalitis virus. *Journal of Veterinary Medical Science*, in press

Solomon, T. & Vaughn, D.W. (2002). Pathogenesis and clinical features of Japanese encephalitis and West Nile virus infections. *Current Topics in Microbiology and Immunology*, Vol. 267, pp. 171–194

Solomon, T.; Ni, H.; Beasley, D.W.; Ekkelenkamp, M.; Cardosa, M.J. & Barrett, A.D. (2003). Origin and evolution of Japanese encephalitis virus in Southeast Asia. *Journal of Virology*, Vol. 77, No. 5, pp. 3091-3098

Sumiyoshi H, Mori C, Fuke I, Morita K, Kuhara S, Kondou J, Kikuchi Y, Nagamatu H, Igarashi A.Complete nucleotide sequence of the Japanese encephalitis virus genome RNA. *Virology*. 1987 Dec;161(2):497-510.

Tang, W-F.; Ogawa, M.; Eshita, Y.; Aono, H. & Makino, Y. (2010). Molecular evolution of Japanese encephalitis virus isolates from swine in Oita, Japan during 1980–2009. *Infection, Genetics and Evolution*, Vol. 10, pp. 329–336

Tsuchie, H.; ODA, K.; Vythilingam, I.; Thayan, R.;Vijayamalar, B.; Sinniah, M.; Singh, J.; Wada, T.; Tanaka, H.; Kurimura, T. & Igarashi, D. (1997). Genotypes of Japanese Encephalitis virus isolated in three states in Malaysia. *American Journal of Tropical Medicine and Hygiene*, Vol. 56, No. 2, pp. 153-158

Uchil, P.D. & Satchidanandam, V. (2001). Phylogenetic analysis of Japanese encephalitis virus: envelope gene based analysis reveals a fifth genotype, geographic clustering, and multiple introductions of the virus into the Indian subcontinent. *American Journal of Tropical Medicine and Hygiene*, Vol. 65, pp. 242-251

van den Bergh, G.D.; de Vos, J. & Sondaar, P.Y. (2001). The late Quaternary palaeogeography of mammal evolution in the Indonesian Archipelago. *Palaeogeography, Palaeoclimatology, Plaeoecology*, Vol. 17, pp. 385-408

van den Hurk, A.F.; Montgomery, B.L.; Northill, J.A.; Smith, I.L.; Zborowski, P.; Ritchie, S.A.; Mackenzie, J.S. & Smith, G.A. (2006). Short report: the first isolation of Japanese encephalitis virus from mosquitoes collected from mainland Australia. *American Journal of Tropical Medicine and Hygiene*, Vol. 75, No.1, pp. 21-25

von Economo, C. (1931). Encephalitis lethargica. Its sequelae and treatment. Translated by Newman KO. *London: Oxford University Press*

Vrati, S. (2000). Comparison of the genome sequences and the phylogenetic analyses of the GP78 and the Vellore P20778 isolates of Japanese encephalitis virus from India. *Journal of Biosciences*, Vol. 25, No. 3, pp. 257–262

Wang, H.Y.; Takasaki, T.; Fu, S.H. & Liang, G.D. (2007b). Molecular epidemiological analysis of Japanese encephalitis virus in China. *Journal of General Virololgy*, Vol. 88, No. 3, pp. 885-894

Wang, J-L.; Pan, X-L.; Zhang, H-L.; Fu, S-H.; Wang, H-Y.; Tang, Q.; Wang, L-F. & Liang, G-D. (2009a). Japanese Encephalitis Viruses from Bats in Yunnan, China. *Emerging Infectious Diseases*, Vol. 15, No. 6, pp. 939-942

Wang, L. ; Fu, S. ; Zhang, H. ; Ye, X. ; Yu, D.; Deng, Z.; Yuan, J. ; Zhai, Y. ; Li, M. ; Lv, Z. ; Chen, W. ; Jiang, H. ; Gao, X. ; Cao, Y. ; Wang, H. ; Tang, Q. & Liang, G. (2010). Identification and isolation of Genotype-I Japanese Encephalitis virus from encephalitis patients. *Virology Journal*, Vol. 7, p 345

Wang, L.H.; Fu, S.H.; Wang, H.Y.; Liang, X.F.; Cheng, J.X.; Jiang, H.M.; Cai, G.L.; Li, X.W.; Ze, W.Y.; Lv, X.J.; Wang, H.Q.; Zhang, D.L.; Feng, Y.; Yin, Z.D.; Sun, X.H.; Shui, T.J.; Li, M.H.; Li, Y.X. & Liang, G.D. (2007a). Japanese Encephalitis Outbreak, Yuncheng, China, 2006. *Emerging Infectious Diseases*, Vol. 13, pp. 1123-1124

Wang, W-H. ; Zhang Y-M.; Xu, X-G.; Xing, F-S.; & Tang, Q-H. (2009b) Cloning and Sequence Analysis of the Full-Length Genome of Japanese encephalitis virus Strain SXBJ07 Isolated from Swine. *Agricultural Sciences in China*, Vol. 8, No. 11, pp. 1392-1402

Vaughn, D.W. & Hoke, C.H., Jr. (1992). The epidemiology of Japanese encephalitis: prospects for prevention. *Epidemiological Reviews*, Vol. 14, pp. 197-221

Williams, D.T.; Wang, L.F.; Daniels, P.W. & Mackenzie, J.S. (2000). Molecular characterization of the first Australian isolate of Japanese encephalitis virus, the FU strain. *Journal of General Virology*, Vol. 81, pp. 2471–2480

Xiao, X.; Boles, S.; Frolking, S.; Li, C.; Babu, J.Y.; Salas, W. & Moore B. (2006). Mapping paddy rice agriculture in South and Southeast Asia using multi-temporal MODIS images. *Remote Sensing of Environment*, Vol. 100, pp. 95–113

Yamanaka, T.; Tsujimura, K.; Kondo, T.; Yasuda, W.; Okada, A.; Noda, K.; Okumura, T. & Matsumura T. (2006). Isolation and Genetic Analysis of Japanese Encephalitis Virus from a diseased Horse in Japan. *Journal of Veterinary Medical Science*, Vol. 68, No. 3, pp 293-295

Yang, D.K.; Kim, B.H.; Kweon, C.H.; Kwon, J.H.; Lim, S.I. & Han, H.R. (2004). Biophysical characterization of Japanese encephalitis virus (KV1899) isolated from pigs in Korea. *Journal of Veterinary Science*, Vol. 5, pp. 125-130

Yoshida, Y.; Tabei, Y.; Hasegawa, M.; Nagashima, M. & Morozumi, S. (2005). Genotypic analysis of Japanese encephalitis virus strains isolated from swine in Tokyo, Japan. *Japanese Journal of Infectious Diseases*, Vol. 58, pp. 259–261

Yun, S-I.; Kim, S-Y.; Choi, W-Y.; Nam, J-H.; Ju, Y-R.; Park, K-Y.; Cho, H-W. & Lee, Y-M. (2003). Molecular characterization of the full-length genome of the Japanese encephalitis viral strain K87P39. *Virus Research*, Vol. 96, pp. 129-140

Yun, S-M.; Cho, J.E.; Ju, Y-R.; Kim, S.Y.; Ryou, J.; Han, M.G.; Choi, W-Y. & Jeong, Y.E. (2010). Molecular epidemiology of Japanese encephalitis virus circulating in South Korea, 1983-2005. *Virology Journal*, Vol. 7, p. 127

Zhang, J-S.; Zhao, Q-M.; Zhang, P-H.; Jia, N. & Cao, W-C. (2009). Genomic sequence of a Japanese encephalitis virus isolate from southern China. *Archives of Virology*, Vol. 154, pp. 1177–1180

Zhang, J-S.; Zhao, Q-M.; Guo, X-F.; Zuo, S-Q.; Cheng, J-X.; Jia, N.; Wu, C.; Dai, P-F. & Zhao, J-Y. (2011). Isolation and Genetic Characteristics of Human Genotype 1 Japanese Encephalitis Virus, China, 2009. *PLoS ONE*, Vol. 6, No. 1, e16418

20

Trials for Risk Assessment of Japanese Encephalitis Based on Serologic Surveys of Wild Animals

Mika Saito et al.*
Department of Microbiology and Oncology, Graduate School of Medicine, University of the Ryukyus, Okinawa Japan

1. Introduction

Japanese encephalitis (JE) is a severe and acute encephalitis with a high fatality rate, caused by Japanese encephalitis virus (JEV), a mosquito-borne flavivirus of the genus *Flavivirus*, family *Flaviviridae*. The JEV serogroup of flaviviruses includes West Nile virus, St. Louis encephalitis virus, and Murray Valley encephalitis virus which also cause encephalitis, though with some clinical variation (Mackenzie et al., 2007). JE is a major public health problem in the Asian region, accounting for more than 16,000 reported cases and 5,000 deaths annually. With the near eradication of poliomyelitis, JE is now the leading cause of childhood viral neurological infection and disability in Asia (Halstead and Jacobson, 2003). Approximately half of all survivors suffer from permanent neurological and/or mental impairments due to the invasion and destruction of cortical neurons and Purkinje cells by the virus (Johnson et al., 1985, Monath, 1986).

Historically, severe epidemics of JE had been reported during the summer season in Japan since the 19th Century and more than 1000 cases were reported annually in the 1960s. With the control of epidemics in Japan and Korea due to changes in agricultural and animal husbandry practices, and in part through vaccination, the number of JE cases markedly

* Takashi Ito[2], Yosuke Amano[3], Junji Takara[4], Katsushi Nakata[5], Shoko Tamanaha[5], Yuichi Osa[6], Tomoo Yoshino[7], Manabu Onuma[8], Takashi Kuwana[8], Go Ogura[5], Masayuki Tadano[1], Daiji Endoh[9] and Mitsuhiko Asakawa[7]

[1]*Department of Microbiology and Oncology, Graduate School of Medicine, University of the Ryukyus, Okinawa,*
[2]*Nago Zoological and Botanical Gardens, Okinawa,*
[3]*Nagamine Animal Clinic, Okinawa,*
[4]*Naha Veterinary Hospital, Okinawa,*
[5]*Laboratory of Subtropical Zoology, Faculty of Agriculture, University of the Ryukyus, Okinawa,*
[6]*Wildlife Section, Nature Conservation Department, Hokkaido Institute of Environmental Sciences, Hokkaido,*
[7]*Department of Pathobiology, School of Veterinary Medicine, Rakuno Gakuen University, Hokkaiodo,*
[8]*Biological Resource Laboratory, Laboratory for Intellectual Fundamentals for Environmental Studies, National Institute for Environmental Studies, Ibaraki,*
[9]*Department of Veterinary Radiology, School of Veterinary Medicine, Rakuno Gakuen University, Hokkaido Japan*

decreased, with less than 10 cases reported annually since the early 1990s (Arai et al., 2008). Meanwhile, JE emerged in Thailand, Vietnam and China in the 1980s. Although the incidence has since declined in these countries, recently the disease has emerged in new areas in Pakistan, and Oceania, particularly Papua New Guinea and northern Australia. The incidence of JE is increasing in countries like Bangladesh, Cambodia, India, Indonesia, Laos, Myanmar, North Korea, and Pakistan (Erlanger et al., 2009). Mackenzie et al (2007)

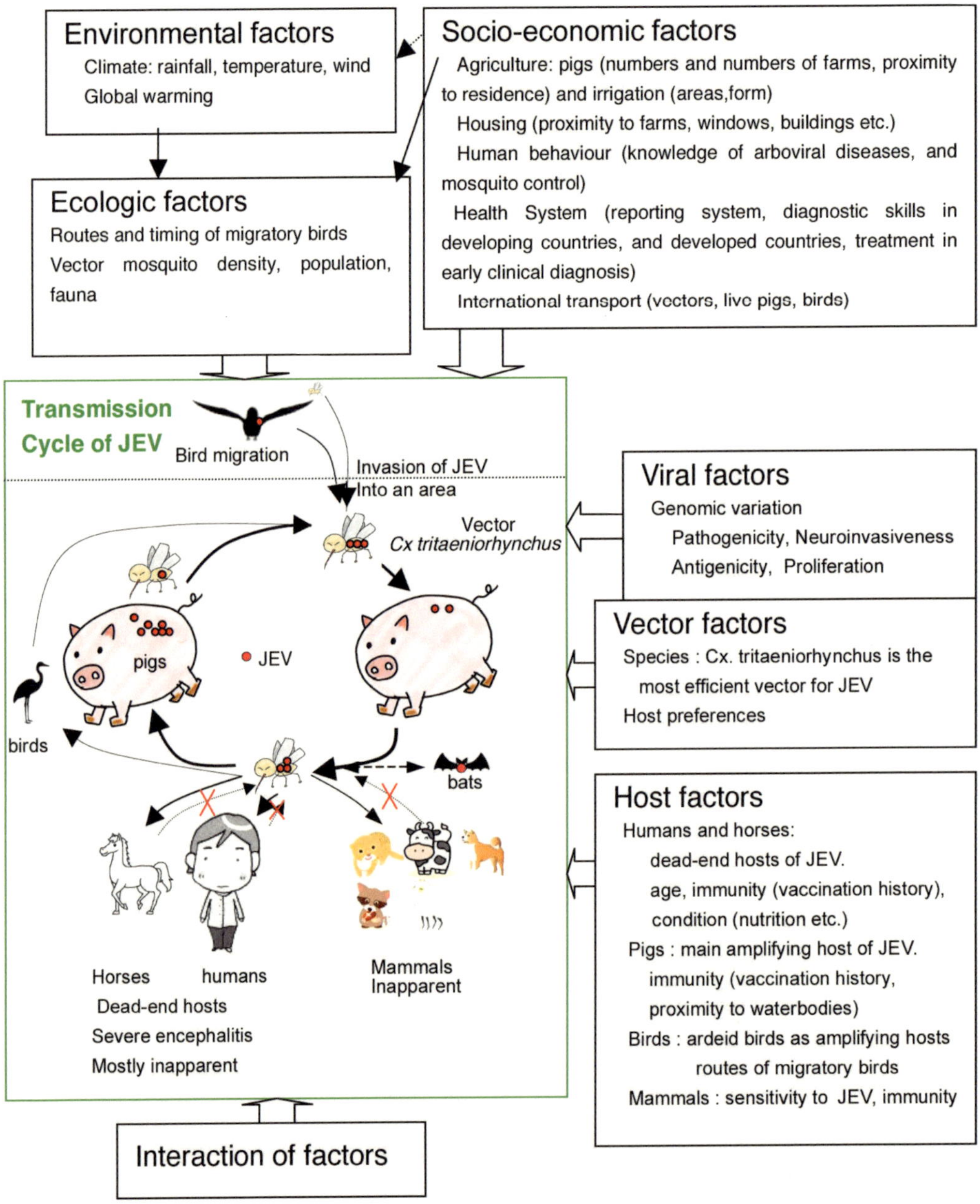

Fig. 1. Transmission cycle of JEV and Risk factors for JE

attributed this phenomenon to the propensity of JEV to spread and colonize new areas. Genetically, five genotypes (genotype 1, 2, 3, 4 and 5) of JEV had been distributed with geographic segregation (Chen et al. 1992. 1994. Uchil and Satchidanandam 2001). The distribution pattern has changed drastically in the last few decades, with a major shift from genotype 3 to genotype 1 in the 1990s in Japan, as well as Vietnam, China, and Korea (Ma et al., 2003, Chung et al. 1996, Nga et al. 2004.) This indicated that an exotic JEV was introduced into these countries and established a transmission cycle.

JEV is maintained in nature by transmission cycles involving *Culex (Cx.) sp.* mosquitoes and amplifying hosts. *Cx. tritaeniorhynchus* is the most efficient vector, and pigs and certain species of birds, particularly *ardeid* birds, are the most effective amplifiers. Humans and horses are incidental, known as dead-end hosts, and most infected mammals do not develop sufficient levels of viremia to infect mosquitoes. As JEV has a wide range of hosts, environmental changes such as global warming, and economic development including irrigation and animal husbandry practices influence its distribution and occurrence.

At present, no specific treatment for JE is available, and the efficacy of ongoing vaccines against various genotypes found in Asia is also controversial. Therefore, surveillance and risk assessment using an interdisciplinary approach are required for the control of JE, and also other flaviviral infections.

Risks of JE infection closely relate to the transmission cycles of JEV, and many factors involved there in. Factors worth considering when assessing risks are described briefly in Figure 1. Risks of JE occurrence in humans relate to both host and viral factors. The ratio of apparent to inapparent JE infections in humans in estimated at 1:200 to 1:1000. The frequency of exposure through infected mosquitoes becomes high in areas where JE is epidemic. Migratory birds, wind-blown vectors, and the transport of vectors and animals would be determinants of the invasion by JEV of new areas.

In this study, a serologic survey of domestic and migratory wild mammals and wild birds was conducted in Hokkaido and Okinawa, Japan, in order to assess risks for JE in humans. The necessity of assessing risks based on serosurveys of wild animals is discussed.

2. Trials for risk assessment of Japanese encephalitis – a serosurvey of wild animals in Japan

2.1 Study design

2.1.1 Study areas

A seroepidemiologic study of wild animals was conducted in Hokkaido, northern Japan, about 850 km from Tokyo, and on Okinawa Island; a small subtropical island, about 2.000 km southwest of Tokyo (Figure 2).

2.1.2 Collection of serum samples from wild mammals

Alien mammals such as the raccoon *Procyon lotor* in Hokkaido and Honshu, and the mongoose *Herpestes auropunctatus* on Okinawa island threaten ecological destruction as predators of endangered species, and government projects to control their population were conducted with the permission of the Ministry of the Environment, Japan. Sera were obtained from 45 raccoons captured in central Hokkaido in 2005, and Mongooses captured in Okinawa between 2001 and 2005 (Saito et al, 2009a). Two serum samples were obtained from injured flying foxes, *Pteropus dasymallus inopinatus* Kuroda, rescued on Okinawa in 2007 and 2008. The isolation of viruses from all serum samples was attempted without success.

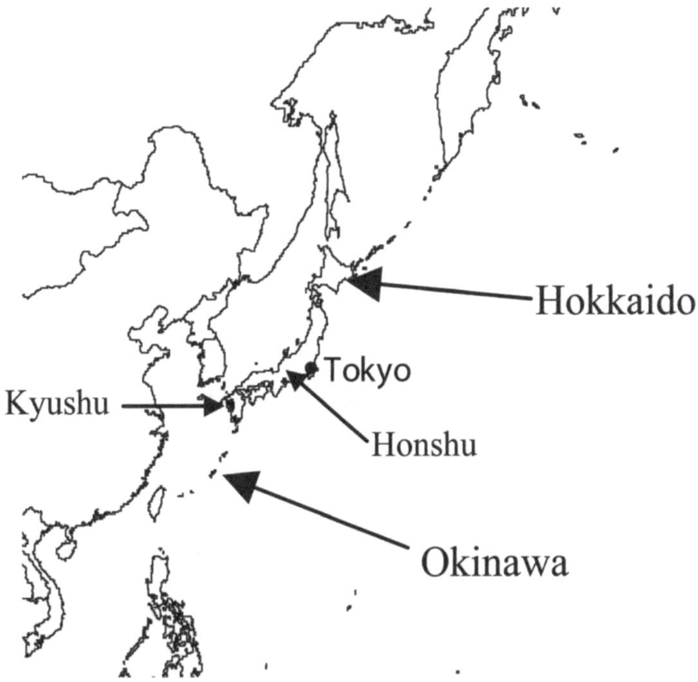

Fig. 2. Location of study areas

2.1.3 Collection of serum samples from wild birds

A total of 50 wild ducks were captured in eastern Hokkaido in 2008, with permission from the Ministry of the Environment, Japan. Eight Spot-billed Ducks (*Anas poecilorhyncha*), 17 Mallards (*A. platyhynchos*), 1 Eurasian Wigeon (*A. penelope*), and 24 Northern Pintails (*A. acuta*) were subjected to a serosurvey. Spot-billed Ducks are recognized as migrant breeders, Mallards as residents breeders or wondering birds, and Eurasian Wigeons and Northern Pintails as winter visitors in Hokkaido.

A total of 72 injured birds, mostly from traffic-related accidents, rescued in animal hospital and zoos as wildlife relief facilities on Okinawa from 2007 to 2009, were subjected to a serosurvey. The order, family, and species of the birds are listed in Table 1. Eleven orders, 17 familiies, and 28 species were collected. Roughly, the birds were classified seasonally, seven individuals (one species) as migrant (summer) breeders, 29 (13 species) as winter vistors, 34 (12 species) as resident breeders, and 2 (2 species) as wondering breeders in Okinawa. Brains, livers, hearts, and spleens were sampled from dead bodies. The isolation of viruses from all samples was attempted without success.

2.1.4 Positive and negative control sera for birds

To conduct the serologic survey of wild birds, negative and positive control sera were used. As maternal antibody levels declined 2 weeks after hatching in chickens, and 3 weeks after hatching in ducks, sera from 10 chicks reared for 2 weeks after hatching in a cage without mosquito bites, and 70 Aigamo juvenile ducks, a cross between wild ducks (*A. platyrhynchos*) and domestic ducks (*A. platyrynchos var. domesticus*), reared for 50 days after hatching in a room until early May, not the breeding season for mosquitoes, 2008, in Hokkaido, were used as negative control. Positive sera for JE were produced in chickens by immunization with an inactivated JE vaccine for animals (Kyoto Biken, Japan) three times weekly, starting from 2 weeks of age, and bleeding the animals 2 weeks after the last immunization. Serum samples from 7 Aigamo ducks infected by West Nile virus (NY-99 strain) were provided and used as reference sera for flavivirus infection (Shirafuji et al., 2009).

Order	Family	species	English name	n (+)*	seasonal
Anseriformes	Anatidae	*Aythya fuligula*	Tufted duck	1 (1)	winter
		Anas poecilorhyncha	Spotbilled duck	1 (0)	residents
Caraciformes	Alcedinidae	*Halcyon coromanda*	Ruddy Kingfisher	7 (0)	summer
Pelecaniformes	Ardeidae	*Bubulcus ibis*	Cattle Egret	2 (2)	winter
		Egretta alba	Great Egret	2 (1)	winter
		Egretta intermedia	Intermediate Egret	3 (0)	winter
		Ardea cinerea	Grey heron	4 (1)	winter
		Egretta sacra	Pacific reef egret	1 (0)	residents
Accipitriformes	Accipitridae	*Butastur indicus*	Grey-faced buzzard	7 (0)	winter
		Accipiter gularis	Japanese sparrow hawk	1 (1)	residents
	Pandionidae	*Pandion haliaetus*	Osprey	1 (0)	winter
Falconiformes	Falconidae	*Falco peregrinus*	Peregrine Falcon	1 (0)	winter
Procellariiformes	Procellariidae	*Puffinus pacificus*	Wedge-tailed shearwater	1 (0)	wondering
Columbiformes	Columbidae	*Streptopelia orientalis*	Eastern turtle dove	5 (2)	residents
		Sphenurus formosae	Whistling Green-pigeon	5 (0)	residents
		Columba livia	Rock dove	1 (0)	residents
Passeriformes	Turdidae	*Turdus pallidus*	Pale Thrush	3 (0)	winter
		Monticola solitarius	Blue Rock Thrush	1 (0)	residents
	Hirundinidae	*Hirundo tahitica*	Pacific swallow	1 (0)	residents
	Corvidae	*Corvus macrorhynchos*	Jungle Crow	3 (0)	residents
Stringiformes	Stringidae	*Ninox scutulata*	Brown hawk owl	11 (2)	residents
		Otus lempiji	Sunda Scops-owl	3 (0)	residents
Charadriiformes	Laroidae	*Larus crassirostris*	Black-tailed gull	2 (0)	winter

Order	Family	species	English name	n (+)*	seasonal
	Charadriidae	*Vanellus vanellus*	Northern lapwing	1 (0)	winter
	Scolopacidae	*Numenius phaeopus*	Whimbrel	1 (0)	winter
	Stercoradriidae	*Stercorarius longicaudus*	Long-tailed jaeger	1 (0)	wondering
Gruiformes	Rallidae	*Gallinula chloropus*	Common Moorhen	1 (0)	residents
		Felica atra	Coot	1 (0)	winter
Total (number of positive)				72 (10)	

* n=number of rescued birds. Values in parenthesis are number of JEV antibody-positive birds

Table 1. The list of injured birds rescued in Okinawa and the number of birds positive for JEV antibodies

	Chicken Negative Control (n=7)	Chicken JE vaccinated (n=4)	Aigamo duck Negative Control (n=70)	Aigamo duck WNV infected (n=7)
$FRNT_{50}$	0 %	100 %	55.7 %	100 %
$FRNT_{90}$	0%	100 %	1.4 %	85.7 %

Table 2. Neutralization antibody titers against JEV Nakayama with different stringencies

2.1.5 Serologic survey

Fifty percent focus reduction neutralization tests ($FRNT_{50}$) were conducted to measure neutralizing antibody titers against JEV strains, Nakayama (prototype strain) and Beijing-1 (laboratory strain), for mammals as described previously (Saito et al., 2009a). Ninety percent focus reduction neutralization tests ($FRNT_{90}$) were employed to measure neutralizing antibody titers against the Nakayama strain for wild birds. The testing was done on BHK-21 cells in 96-well microplates with an immuno-staining method as described previously (Saito et al., 2007).

2.2 Results

2.2.1 Serosurvey of wild mammals

A single sample from 45 raccoons (2.2 %) in Hokkaido had antibody titers of 70 and 40 against the Nakayama and Beijing-1 strains, respectively.

Previously obtained serologic data, showing that 35.4 % (85/240) of mongooses had antibodies for JEV (Saito et al., 2009a), was re-analyzed by GIS on different scales (Figure 4). The analysis on a small scale showed barns, bodies of water and rive paddies to be near the capture points of mongooses with high titers of JE antibody.

Both of the flying foxes captured in Okinawa had antibodies against Nakayama, with titers of 17 and 14, respectively.

2.2.2 Serosurvey of wild birds

To evaluate the reliability of testing, both $FRNT_{50}$ and $FRNT_{90}$ at different stringencies, were conducted on negative and positive control (JE immunized and WNV infected) samples of chickens and Aigamo ducks (Table 2) (Buckley et al, 2003). Non-specific reactions were observed at a high rate (55.7 %) among negative control ducks, by $FRNT_{50}$. Even by $FRNT_{90}$, a single duck showed a non-specific reaction, although the titer was low as 10. Serologic tests using Negative controls of chickens and JE-vaccinated chickens clearly showed all samples to be negative and all to be positive by $FRNT_{50}$ and $FRNT_{90}$. WNV-infected ducks as reference showed positive for JE antibody by both stringencies of test, except a single sample by $FRNT_{90}$. Given the results, FRNT90 against JEV Nakayama was employed for the seroepidemiologic survey of wild birds.

Among 50 serum samples from 4 species of ducks; spot-billed ducks, mallards, northern pintails and Eurasian wigeons, in Hokkaido, only a single sample from spot-billed ducks (2%) recognized as migrant breeders had JE antibodies (Figure 3).

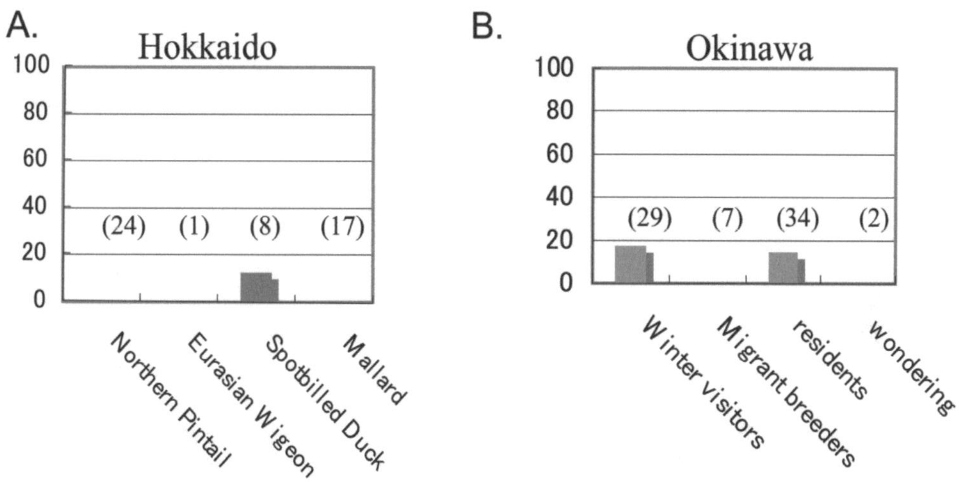

Fig. 3. Antibody-positive rates of ducks captured in Hokkaido (A) and injured birds rescued in Okinawa (B) against the Nakayama strain. Northern Pintails and Eurasian Wigeons are recognized as winter visitors, Spotbilled Ducks as migrant breeders, and Mallards as residents, and partly wonderers. Values in parentheses show numbers of bird species or seasonal groups

A total of 10 (14.2%) sera of wild birds in Okinawa had JE antibodies. Five (2 Cattle Egrets, 1 Grey heron, 1 Great Egret, and 1 Tufted duck) were from 29 winter visitors and 5 (2 Brown hawk owls, 2 Eastern turtle doves, and 1 Japanese sparrow hawk) from 34 resident breeders. Four of the five positive sera in winter visitors were from *ardeid* birds. None of the migrant breeders had antibodies (Table 1 and Figure 3).

3. Discussion

A seroepidemiologic study was conducted on wild mammals and wild birds in Hokkaido and Okinawa, Japan, and risks for JEV infection and JEV invasion were evaluated by knowing local transmission activity and the seroprevalence of migratory species, respectively. JEV activity in Hokkaido is known to be low, as demonstrated by serosurveys of pigs (Infectious Disease Surveillance Center), although focal outbreaks occured in pigs in the 1980s (Takashima et al. 1988). In Okinawa, high JEV transmission rates have been demonstrated by serosurveys of pigs indicating the longest JEV active season in Japan, and the virus has been isolated even in winter (Ura, 1976, Tadano et al. 1994, Infectious Disease Surveillance Center). About 100 JE cases were reported with fluctuations until the mid 1960s. The last reported case was in 1998. Seroconversion in pigs was used for JE surveillance for many years, nationwide in Japan, and thus is generally accepted as reflecting the JEV transmission rate in an area.

We reported a serosurvey of mongooses in Okinawa, valuable for understanding the local transmission activity of JEV in nature. By using mongooses under control projects, it is possible to analyze capture points and antibody titers, enabling estimates of high transmission areas on a small scale (Figure 4A) (Saito et al., 2009a). The environmental condition at the capture point for animals with high antibody titers were suitable for the transmission of JEV, i.e. rive fields and bodies of water for the breeding of vector mosquitoes and barns for pigs as an amplifier of JEV (Figure 4B). However, mongooses mostly inhabit only the Okinawa and Amami islands in Japan. By contrast, raccoons, another alien species is distributed over a wide range in Japan, though not in Okinawa. In this study, a serosurvey of raccoons was conducted in Hokkaido, showing low positive rates with only a single sample having JE antibodies, thus implying low transmission of JEV there. Ohno et al (2009) also conducted a comparative serosurvey of raccoons in Hokkaido and in the Kinki area of western Japan, showing a high prevalence of JEV in western and low prevalence in northern areas. Thus, the animal appears to be a good sentinel for JEV infection. In this study, the suitability of risk assessments with serosurveys of alien animals under control projects, together with fundamental data analysis is indicated.

We also conducted a serosurvey of migratory species. It was reported that flying foxes have a potential role in the transmission cycle and dispersal of JEV (van den Hurk AF et al, 2009). Antibodies against JEV with low titers were observed in both flying foxes caught in Okinawa, a species that can fly short distances within the island or to nearby islands. Flying foxes might play a role in the dispersal of JEV on the island.

Interestingly, in this serosurvey of wild birds, all of the positive ducks collected in Hokkaido, 2008 were Spotbilled ducks, a migrant breeder in Hokkaido, and seemed to have been infected in the south (Saito et al, 2009b). Results from our studies of raccoons and wild ducks showed low transmission rates of JEV in Hokkaido, consistent with those for pigs and other species.

The yearly sero-conversion of JEV in pigs starts in Okinawa, and moves to the north. This phenomenon may be caused by the migration or hibernation of JEV. The migratory flyways of migrant breeders such as the Ruddy Kingfisher correlate with this movement, from south, Australia, to north, Siberia, through Okinawa, and mainland Japan. However, no migrant breeder tested negative for the JEV antibody in this study. Nabeshima et al (2009) described that JEV is frequently introduced into Japan from Southeast Asia and continental east Asia, based on a molecular epidemiologic study and chronological order. Okinawan genotype 1 strains are closely related to strains from other parts of Japan, Korea and China, but different from Australian strains (Saito et al., 2007). Recently genotype 1 with the same subcluster as Kyushu and Shanghai appeared in Taiwan, in 2007, approximately 10 years after their first appearance in China, Korea, and Japan (Huang et al, 2010). Thus, the direction of JEV's introduction seemed to be from north to south. Five winter visitors with antibodies were observed, 2 Cattle Egrets, 1 Grey Heron, 1 Great Egret and 1 Tufted duck. They are thought to have been infected in the north, not in Okinawa, because of seasonal characteristics. *Ardeid* birds, Egrets and Herons are known amplifiers of JEV and involved in JEV invasion (Buescher EL et al, 1959). From the results of this study, together with molecular epidemiologic studies, JEV is suggested to have been introduced into Okinawa from Honshu, and Kyushu, possibly by a winter visitor such as *ardeid* birds. The flyways of most *ardeid* birds remain unknown. Their elucidation and continuous epidemiologic and virologic studies will provide important information for evaluating risks of JEV invasion. Migratory birds are one of the determinants with which to assess invasive viruses like not only JEV, but also flaviviruses with a similar epidemiology.

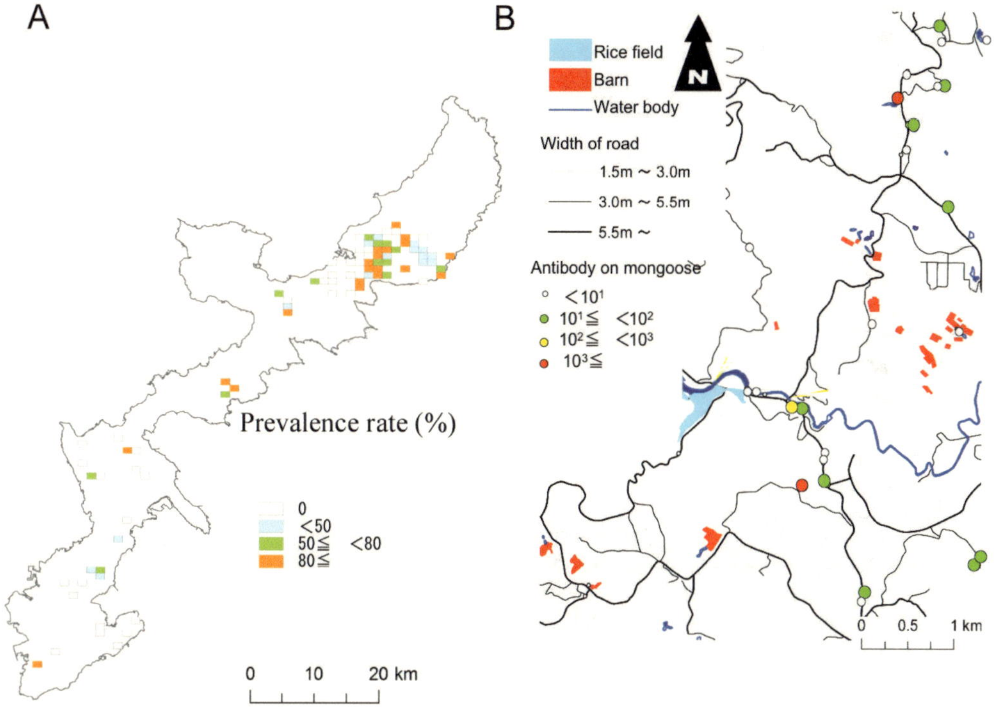

Fig. 4. Map of Okinawa Island used for the GIS analysis using mesh with prevalence rates of JE antibody in mongooses (ref. Saito et al, 2009a) (A). Map of high prevalence areas with the location of farms (B). Dots show capture points and the JE antibody titer

JEV antibodies were detected in 14.3 % (5/35) of resident breeders in Okinawa between 2007 and 2009, a relatively low rate. This however may be due to the inclusion of data from a variety of species and sizes, differing in sensitivity and mosquito preference. In Okinawa, serosurveys of pigs have showed that seroprevalence has gradually decreased since the mid 2000s and was less than 20 % in 2009 and 2010, which indicated that low transmission activity (Infectious Disease Surveillance Center) might correlate with seroprevalence in resident breeders and mongooses.

The Ministry of Health, Labour and Welfare in Japan discontinued the recommendation for JE vaccinations due to adverse events for 5 years from 2005. During this period, no epidemic of JE occurred in Japan, and no cases were reported in Okinawa either. Risk assessments for JE should be strengthened to evaluate the quick and drastic changes in natural transmission that might be occurring in Okinawa with an interdisciplinary approach, including studies of mosquitoes, serosurveys of people, domestic and wild animals, and vaccine evaluation. A reconsideration of JE control is required in step with recent changes.

4. Conclusion

The distribution and occurrence of JE are changing due to environmental influences. Therefore, risk assessment and surveillance are important for controlling JE. Serosurveys of pigs as amplifiers are the predominant means of assessing risks of JEV infection, and also sustainable. Wild mammals such as raccoons and mongooses are valuable sentinels for assessing natural transmission, and strengthen the notion of surveillance using pigs, while control programs for alien mammals provide the opportunity for a detailed geographic analysis of JEV transmission. Virologic and serologic surveys of wild birds, particularly *ardeid* birds as possible amplifiers, and bats should be sustained to assess risks of JEV invasion. Furthermore, they may reveal the mechanisms by which the distribution of JEV is expanding.

5. Acknowledgements

The authors are grateful to Dr. Takashi Nagamine for his cooperation and advice, the staff of the Department of Agriculture, University of the Ryukyus for sampling wild birds, and the staff of Rakuno Gakuen University for sampling raccoons and wild birds in Hokkaido. They also express thanks to Dr. Hiroaki Shirafuji, for providing control sera from Aigamo ducks.

6. Disclosure statements

This study was supported by Grant-in Aid for Exploratory Research (No. 16659121 and No. 19658115) and Scientific Research (No. 20380163 and No. 23510030), from the Ministry of Education, Culture, Sports, Science and Technology of Japan, and by the Global Environment Research Fund of the Ministry of the Environment, Japan, F-3 and F-9.

7. References

Arai S, Matsunaga Y, Takasaki T, Tanaka-Taya K, Taniguchi K, Okabe N, Kurane I, Vaccine Preventable Disease Surveillanve Program of Japan. 2008. Japanese Encephalitis: Surveillance and Elimination Effort in Japan from 1982 to 2004. *Jpn J Infect Dis*. 61, 333-338

Buckley A, Dawson A, Moss SR, Hinsley SA. 2003. Serological evidence of West Nile virus, Usutsu virus and Sindbis virus infection of birds in the UK. *J Gen Virol*, 8, 2807-2817

Buescher EL, Scherer WF, McClure HE, Moyer JT, Rosenberg MZ, Yoshi M, Okada Y. 1959. Ecologic studies of Japanese encephalitis in Japan. IV. Avian Infection. *Am J Trop Med Hyg*, 8, 689-697

Chen WR, Rico-Hesse R. & Tesh RB 1992. A new genotype of Japanese encephalitisvirus from Indonesia. *Am J Trop Med Hyg* 47, 61-69

Chen WT, Tesh RB & Rico-Hesse R. 1990. Genetic variation of Japanese encephalitis virus in nature. *J Gen Virol* 71, 2915-2922

Chung YJ, Nam JH, Ban SJ, and Cho HW. 1996. Antigenic and genetic analysis of Japanese encephalitis viruses isolated from Korea. *Am J Trop Med Hyg*. 55, 91-97.

Erlanger, TE, Weiss S, Keiser J, Utzinger J, and Wiedenmayer, K. 2009, Past, present, and future of Japanese encephalitis. *Emerging Infectious Diseases* 15, 1-7

Halstead SB and Jacobson J, 2003, Japanese encephalitis. *Adv Virus Res* 61, 103-138

Huang JH, Lin TH, Teng HJ, Su CL, Tsai KH, Lu LC, Lin C, Yang CF, Chang SF, Liao TL, Yu SK, Cheng CH, Chang MC, Hu HC, Chu PR. 2010. Molecular Epidemiology of Japanese encephalitis virus, Taiwan. *Emerging Infectious Diseases*, 16, 876-878

Infectious Disease Serveillance Center, http://idsc.nih.go.jp/yosoku/JE/JEmap2009-E.html

Johnson, RT, Burke, DS, Elwell M, Leake CJ, Nisalak A, Hoke CH, and Lorsomrudee, W. 1985. Japanese encephalitis: immunocytochemical studies of viral antigen and inflammatory cells in fatal cases. *Annu. Neurol*. 18, 567-573

Ma SP, Yoshida Y, Nakino Y. Tadano M. Ono T. and Ogawa M. 2003. A major genotype of Japanese encephalitis virus currently circulating in Japan. *Am J Trop Med Hyg* 69, 151-154.

Mackenzie JS, Williams DT, and Smith DW. 2007. *Japanese Encephalitis Virus: The Geographic Distribution, Incidence, and Spread of a Virus with a Propensity to Emerge in New Area.* In *Emerging Virus in Human Population.* pp. 201-268. Edited by T. Tobaor. Elsevir press.

Monath TP. 1986. Pathobiology of the flaviviruses, p.375-440. In Schlesinger, S., and Schlesinger MF. (eds), The Togaviridae and Flaviviridae, Avademic Press, New York.

Nabeshima T, Loan HTK, Inoue S, Sumiyoshi M, Haruta Y, Nga PT, Huoung VTQ, Parquet MC, Hasebe F, Morita, K. 2009. Evidence of frequent introductions of Japanese encephalitis virus from south-east Asia and continental east Asia to Japan. *J Gen Virol*, 90, 827-832

Nga PT, Parquet MC, Cuong VD, Ma SP, Hasebe F, Inoue S, Makino Y, Takagi M, Nam VS and Morita K. 2004. Shift in Japanese encephalitis virus (JEV) genotype circulating in northern Vietnam: implications for frequent introductions of JEV from Southeast Asia to East Asia. *J Gen Virol* 85, 1625-31.

Ohno Y, Sato H, Suzuki K, Yokoyama M, Uni S, Shibasaki T, Sashika M, Inokuma H, Kai K, Maeda K. 2009. Detection of antibodies against Japanese encephalitis virus in raccoons, raccoon dogs and wild boars in Japan. *J Vet Med Sci* 71, 1035-1039

Saito M, Nakata K, Nishijima T, Yamashita, K, Saito A, Ogura G, 2009a, Proposal for Japanese encephalitis surveillance using captured invasive mongooses under an eradication project on Okinawa Island, Japan. *Vector Borne Zoonotic Dis.* 9, 259-266

Saito M, Osa Y, Asakawa M, 2009b, Antibodies to flaviviruses in wild ducks captured in Hokkaido, Japan: Risk assessment of Invasive flaviviruses, *Vector Borne Zoonotic Dis.* 9, 253-258

Saito M, Taira K, Itokazu K, Mori N, 2007, Recent change of the antigenicity and genotype of Japanese encephalitis viruses distribute on Okinawa Island, *Japan. Am J Trop Med Hyg*. 77, 737-746

Shirafuji H, Kanehira K, Kubo M, Shibahara T, Kamio T. 2009, Experimental West Nile virs infection in Aigamo ducks, a cross between wild ducks (Anas platyrhynchos) and domestic ducks (Anas platyrhynchos var. domesticus), *Avian Diseases*, 53, 239-244

Tadano M, Kanemura K, Hasegawa H, Makino Y, Fukunaga T. 1994. Epidemiological and ecological studies of Japanese encephalitis in Okinawa, subtropical area in Japan. I. Investigations on antibody levels to Japanese encephalitis virus in swine sera and vector mosquito in Okinawa, Miyako and Ishigaki islands. *Microbiol Immunol*, 38, 117-122

Takashima I, Watanabe T, Ouchi N, Hashimoto N. 1988. Ecological studies of Japanese encephalitis virus in Hokkaido: interepidemic outbreaks of swine abortion and evidence for the virus to overwinter locally. *J Med Entomol*. 26, 454-458

Uchil PD and Satchidanandam V. 2001. Phylogenetic analysis of Japanese encephalitis virus: envelope gene based analysis reveals a fifth genotype, geographic clustering, and multiple introductions of the virus into the Indian subcontinent. *Am J Trop Med Hyg* 65, 242-51.

Ura M. 1976 Ecology of Japanese encephalitis virus in Okinawa, Japan. I. The investigation on pig and mosquito infection of the virus in Okinawa Island from 1966 to 1976. Tropical medicine 18 151

van den Hurk AF, Smith CS, Field HE, Smith IL, Northill JA, Taylor CT, Jansen CC, Smith GA, Mackenzie JS. 2009. Transmission of Japanese encephalitis virus from the Black Flying Fox, Pteropus alecto, to Culex annulirostris mosquitoes, despite the absence of detectable viremia. *Am J Trop Med Hyg*. 81, 457-462.

21

Prevention and Control of Japanese Encephalitis Viruses: A Challenged Issue

Somsak Pantuwatana[1] and Matti Sallberg[2]
[1]*Burapha University, Bangsaen, Chon Buri,*
[2]*Karolinska Institutet, Stockholm*
[1]*Thailand*
[2]*Sweden*

1. Introduction

Encephalitis caused by Japanese encephalitis virus (JEV) is a leading cause of viral encephalitis of children less than 15 years old in Asia including Thailand. The virus is transmitted to human by several species of culicine mosquitoes including *Culex tritaeniorhynchus, Culex gelidus, and Culex vishnui.* The natural cycle occurs as a zoonotic cycle of which either pigs or birds serve as vertebrate amplifying host and man appears to be accidental hosts. In addition to human disease, JEV produces abortion and neonatal death in pigs and death in horses, which are economically important in the area where Japanese encephalitis occurs. Currently the specific drug for treatment of Japanese encephalitis is not available. The promising strategy for the prevention of this disease is vaccination together with efficient mosquito control, protection of the amplifying hosts, and prevention human from mosquito biting. Thus, the prevention and control of this disease is a challenged issue.

The development of a vaccine that would induce rapid protection in people and animals is currently remained as an important issue. New generation of safe chimeric viruses that are unable to infect mosquitoes is currently ongoing in the development and preclinical studies. This would be a major step toward production of live-attenuated vaccine that is safer for the environment and would minimize the risk for vaccine-born outbreaks as reported in 1970s for TC-83 vaccine. However, additional efficacy trials in nonhuman primates are required to confirm the protective response for some of the candidates and for initiation of potential clinical trials. Some of the recent experimental data indicates that the immune response against Venezuelan Equine Encephalitis virus (VEEV) needed to control the brain infection may differ from the one required to control the peripheral infection. Therefore, vaccines that protect against the natural infection may differ in the future from those that are supposed to protect against high-dose air-borne challenge and may be more attenuated. Our group is also trying to use the most recent pathogenesis data to design a therapeutic vaccine that would reverse already established encephalitis and help clear the virus from the brain.

Plasmid DNA-based vaccination strategies have become an active area of research over the past decade due to their potential to produce safer and cheaper vaccines. These vaccines could be delivered to recipients by intra-muscular (IM) injection or intra-dermal (ID) administration using a gene gun. IM inoculation of plasmid DNA vaccines to mice induces predominantly T helper 1 (Th1) immune responses, while T helper 2 (Th2) type immune responses are generated following the ID delivery. The isotypes of antibodies and the types of cytokines induced by the two methods differ and this could have bearing on the efficacy of the vaccine candidate.

Attempts have been made to construct the plasmid DNA vaccine against JEV by trying to include JEV *e* gene in the plasmid DNA. It has been shown that these plasmids are capable of synthesizing JEV premembrane (prM) and E proteins, which have been evaluated in mice. Both forms of E protein however generated JEV neutralizing antibodies that provided significant protection to mice against lethal JEV challenge.

In pre-clinical studies, after evaluation in rodent models, nonhuman primates are usually the models of choice as they provide a robust system for evaluation of vaccine candidates. The Old World monkeys have predominantly been used in these types of studies with rhesus (*Macaca mulatta*) and cynomolgus (*Macaca fascicularis*) monkeys being most popularly used for evaluation of vaccine candidates against various infectious diseases, including those caused by *Flaviviruses*. It has been shown that the immunogenicity of premembrane-envelop proteins (pMEa and pMEs) delivered intramuscularly (IM) or intradermally (ID) in rhesus monkeys resulted in the DNA immunization induced protective levels of JEV neutralizing antibodies and generated robust memory that led to a rapid and sustained anamnestic response in monkeys sham challenged with mouse brain-grown, formaldehyde inactivated commercial vaccine. Several JEV proteins were evaluated in the DNA vaccine modality for their ability to induce protective immunity in the murine system. These include plasmids could express non-structural protein 1 (NS1), E or prM and E proteins of JEV. It was shown that variable degree of efficacy in murine model systems with plasmids expressing prM and E proteins conferring high degree of protection of mice against lethal JEV challenge, largely due to their ability to induce JEV neutralizing antibodies. Two plasmids could express prM protein along with full-length anchored E or truncated secretory E protein, while both plasmids induced JEV neutralizing antibodies in mice. To achieve this, efforts are underway to further enhance the immunogenicity of JE DNA candidate vaccine.

Another alternative approach for controlling Japanese encephalitis is the reduction in mosquito vector population. It has been shown that the JEV can cause a long-lasting viremic phase in amplifying hosts. The virus can cause infection in pigs with the viremic phase last for 28 days, whereas the viremic phase in infected birds last for 4-5 days with a very high virus titer, about 10^5 pfu/ml in a house sparrow. These long lasting viremia in amplifying hosts provide ample opportunities for the susceptible mosquito vectors to become infected after feeding on them. Therefore, if we can reduce the population of mosquito vectors, the chances are possible to control the epidemic of JEV in the endemic areas. The slow-release formulations of products made from microbial insecticides, i.e., *Bacillus sphaericus*, and *Bacillus thuringiensis* var. *israelensis*, have been used in field trials against certain species of mosquito larvae especially *Culex quiquefasciatus*, with a satisfactory result. However, it is very difficult to apply the aforementioned formulations of microbial insecticides' products in the breeding places of the mosquito vectors, because the mosquito larvae of *Culex* species are filter feeder, which feed on the surface of the water. All larvae of the mosquito vector species are found in polluted water. It has been shown that the effectiveness of microbial insecticides' products is not reached a satisfactory result. Efforts on the development of microbial insecticides for biological control of mosquito vector are underway in parallel with the recent advances in biotechnology

2. Natural cycle of Japanese encephalitis virus

Japanese encephalitis virus (JEV) has long been recognized as a member of viruses, which has been classified in the genus *Flavivirus* of the family *Flaviviridae*. The natural transmission cycles involving avian or swine reservoir hosts, where culicine mosquitoes serve as vectors. The virus has ability to cause fatal infections in horses, and is transmitted to human by several species of culicine mosquitoes including *Culex tritaeniorhynchus, Culex gelidus, and Culex vishnui* in Thailand. In general, the natural cycle occurs as a zoonotic cycle of which either pigs or birds serve as vertebrate amplifying host and man appears to be accidental hosts. In addition to human disease, JEV produces abortion and neonatal death in pigs and death in horses, which are economically important in the area where Japanese encephalitis occurs.

In general, a three-way relationship between virus, host and environment that has evolved over millions of years, is considered as a basic requirement of a given mosquito-borne viruses to occupy a particular ecological niche. A certain virus is confined perhaps to the forests of one continent; it infects one or a small number of species of mosquitoes that habitually feed off one or a few species of vertebrate. Any given species of vertebrate that serves as an efficient host, it must be abundant, must reproduce rapidly, and above all musts maintain a high level of viremia for an adequate period. In its turn, any species of mosquitoes that will serve as an efficient vector, must have a sufficiently low threshold of infection by that virus, must then carry and shed the virus in its salivary secretions for life, but not be adversely affected by it, and must have a distribution, flight range longevity, and biting habits well adapted to the habits and habitats of its principal vertebrate host. Hence the virus flourishes indefinitely in a state of peaceful coexistence with vertebrate and mosquito host in which no one-get hurt. The troubles arise when the virus moves beyond this enzootic cycle.

2.1 Virus properties

It is quite interesting to learn how JEV replicates itself and continually circulates in nature. Japanese encephalitis virus, a 40- to 50-nm-sized enveloped virus, has a single positive-strand RNA genome. The RNA genome contains three structural (capsid, pre-M, and envelope) and seven nonstructural (NS1, NS2A, NS2B, NS3, NS4A, NS4B, and NS5) proteins (Chambers et al., 1999). An inactive vaccine is available against JEV, but multiple doses are required to confer protective immunity and some pathogenic side effects have been reported (Ku et al., 1994). There are no specific effective drugs available to treat Japanese encephalitis virus infections.

Four basic criteria in incriminating the mosquitoes as a vector of JEV have been met by *Culex tritaeniorhynchus* which including, i.e., isolation of JEV from naturally infected mosquitoes, laboratory demonstration of the ability of the mosquitoes to become infected by feeding on a viremic host, laboratory demonstration of the ability of these infected mosquitoes to transmit the virus during blood feeding, and evidence of blood feeding contact between the suspected mosquito vector and suspected vertebrate hosts under natural conditions. All evidences supported these criteria were demonstrated in Thailand (Grossman et al., 1974).

2.2 Virus changes

There are some evidences that the virus itself changes in nature during its replication cycles. In *Flavivirus* transmission, the salivary glands play a major role in establishing the vector status by their ability to produce and maintain a high titer of virus throughout the life of the vector. The replication of virus does not cause a cytopathic change in the salivary glands (Takahashi & Suzuki, 1979). This event is very important for the virus itself to survive in nature. In addition to the ability of JEV that can replicate in various kinds of hosts and vectors, JEV also obtains its envelope from the modification of host cell membrane during the budding process. Thus, it has been postulated that genetic variation of JEV in nature may occur following several replication cycle in different kind of vectors and hosts. This hypothesis has been verified by the comparison of short nucleotide sequences of JEV isolates from various countries, and demonstrated that the similarity of the JEV isolates can be segregated into three groups, i.e., group I in which they were recovered from northern Thailand and Cambodia, group II were those isolates that recovered from southern Thailand, Malaysia, Sarawak and Indonesia, and group III were those isolates that recovered from Japan, China, Taiwan, the Philippines, Sri Lanka, India and Nepal (Chen et al., 1990). This finding provides insight into the evolution, transmission and possibly, pathogenesis of JEV. The possibility of virus changes still exists. Once the virus has been changed, it can lead to new epidemic in an appropriate ecological niche because it can escape from herd immunity, which developed against the previous form of the virus.

Mosquito-borne disease usually occurs when unnatural hosts become involved. When man lives in regions in which a particular mosquito-borne virus is enzootic he is vulnerable to infection and a few of those infected may suffer severe, even lethal, disease. Visitors such as tourists, soldiers, or forest workers are even more vulnerable as, unlike the indigenous population, they will not have acquired immunity from subclinical infection in childhood. In tropical countries where the mosquito vector is plentiful year round, the risk is always present and human disease is endemic. In regions subject to monsoonal rains, epidemics of mosquito-borne diseases may occur toward the end of the wet season due to the abundance of mosquito population. In some temperate countries, and particularly in arid areas, human epidemics of mosquito-borne disease occur following periods of exceptionally heavy rain. A different species of mosquito, with anthropophilic habits, may become involved in transmission of the virus to humans, and may then maintain the virus in a man-mosquito-man cycle without the intervention of the natural vertebrate or invertebrate host.

2.3 Infections and pathogenesis

The infection in man is usually initiated by the viruses are introduced through the skin by the bite of a mosquito vector. The virus is replicated in cytoplasm and maturation with budding process and the mature virions are released into cytoplasmic vesicles. The mature virions gain the envelope by modified the cell membrane of the host with the insertion of specific glycoprotein into the membrane. The mature virions inside cytoplasmic vesicles are easily released from the infected cells. Virions that enter the lymphatic capillaries are carried to the local lymph nodes, which act as filters. As they enter, virions are exposed to the macrophages lining the marginal sinus and are usually engulfed. They may be inactivated and digested and their antigens presented to the underlining lymphoid cells in such a way that the immune response is initiated. However, JEV can multiply in the macrophages which some virions may pass straight through the lymph node and eventually enter the blood stream. Since the macrophage and lymphocytes in the lymph node are constantly circulating in the lymph and blood vascular systems, virus may be passively transported around the body in these cells. The important target organ for JEV is CNS (White & Fenner, 1984).

The degree of severity of the disease in man caused by this virus is rather depended on the degree of neuronal destruction. Case fatality rates average about 10 - 20 % and survivors are often with permanent neurological sequelae such as mental retardation, epilepsy, paralysis, deafness, and blindness (White & Fenner, 1984).

The first know outbreak of JEV in Thailand occurred in 1964 in Phitsanulok Province of northern part of the country. Another outbreak was reported in 1969 in Chiang Mai Province with more than 650 cases and mortality rate of 27 %. Sporadic outbreak occurred in the following year in the same area and spread to adjacent provinces (Sangkawibha et al., 1982). It is of interest that the year 1964 was also a year in which very large JE epidemics occurred in Japan and Korea (Kono & Kim, 1969). Hospital records in Chiang Mai Province reveal that periodic rainy season outbreaks of febrile encephalitis, probably caused by JEV, have occurred in northern Thailand since at least 1962 (Grossman et al., 1973).

Human JEV infections, however, are infrequent events. Incidence rates of clinical JEV infections in Thailand with recurrent JE epidemics have usually been between one and 10, and rarely higher than 30 per 100,000 population per year (Wang, 1964; Chen et al., 1990). The inapparent JEV infections occur more frequently, but, in the relatively sparse data available, infection rates of only about five per cent have been found in the few groups of people (mostly schoolchildren) who have been followed serologically through an epidemic season (Southam, 1956; Scherer et al., 1959a; Wang, 1964).

2.4 Vector capability and transmission of virus

The role of vector in maintaining viruses in nature is very critical and important for the virus. The most extensive epidemiologic studies of JEV have been carried out in northern temperate areas, where mosquitoes are not active in the winter. The virus reappears in the same locality year after year, and consequently considerable effort has been devoted to determining how the virus survives when its vectors are inactive. In fact, JEV had been recovered from adult mosquitoes reared from field-collected larvae and never exposed to JEV in the laboratory (Mitamura et al., 1939). This finding and the reports of transovarial transmission by mosquitoes of La Crosse virus (Watts et al., 1973), and other viruses have led to the experimental studies of transovarial transmission of JEV by mosquitoes. It was shown that such transmission could be demonstrated by *Aedes albopictus* and *Aedes togoi* in 1978 (Rosen et al., 1978). Thus, transovarial transmission may serve as one of alternative ways for JEV survives the winter in the northern temperate zone. But transovarial transmission may not be necessary for JEV in tropical areas where mosquito vectors and amplifying hosts are abundant all year round.

For vector roles of JEV, it has been shown that a small number of closely related species of *Culex* mosquitoes serve as vectors. It is very interesting to note that some species of mosquitoes are not only serving as vectors for the virus transmission, they may also serve as an important tool in epidemiological studies. It is important to appreciate the difficulties involved in this sort of epidemiological detective work. Mosquito-borne viruses are generally so difficult to isolate from man, thus field-collected mosquitoes are the important specimens for virus isolation attempts and in fact most of them are originally discovered in mosquitoes collected from tropical forests or from "sentinel" animals left overnight in mosquito-infested areas. However, only certain species of *Culex* mosquitoes can serve as vectors for JE virus. Several factors may play an important role for species-specific activity in virus transmission. It is believed that gut barrier for virus replication is one factor.

2.5 The relationships between virus and mosquito

The capacity of a vector to transmit high titers of virus is an important factor in the vector potential of the species in addition to the susceptibility of the vector to the virus. In this sense, concentration of JEV as high as $10^{4.2}$ in the saliva of *Culex tritaeniorhynchus* for prolonged incubation periods demonstrate the high vector potential of this mosquito (Takahashi, 1976). It has been shown that when mosquitoes are maintained under autumn or winter conditions virus concentrations of whole mosquitoes are lower than in those exposed to summer conditions, and the virus antigen is restricted to the midgut (Kay et al., 1989).

Culex tritaeniorhynchus is known as the principal vector of JEV in many countries, i.e., Japan (Buescher et al., 1959), Okinawa (Hurlburt & Nibley, 1964), and Thailand (Simasathien et al., 1972). A complete study on vectors of JEV in Thailand was done in Chiang Mai Valley. It was shown that peaks in the population densities of *Culex fuscocephala, Culex gelidus* and *Culex tritaeniorhynchus,* as measured by weekly light-trap collections, occurred during the rainy season (April-October) at the time of human and animal JEV infections. Analysis of mosquito blood meals indicated that, while the three vector species fed on humans and a variety of domestic animals, their most frequent hosts were buffalo and cattle. Feeding activity by the three vector species began after dark and was maintained throughout the night. These mosquitoes were predominantly exophilic, and very few were collected inside houses. All these findings suggest that the three incriminated vector species act principally to maintain a cycle of JEV infection in domestic animal populations that only occasionally involves humans in the Chiang Mai Valley (Gould et al., 1974).

2.6 Man as carrier

Man when bitten by an infected mosquitoes, develops a viremia about the end of the incubation period (usually about 5 to 6 days), be remains infective for other *Culex* mosquitoes biting him during the first 4 or 5 days of illness. The new mosquito after ingesting virus can transmit beginning 8 to 10 or more days later and for as long as it lives. From this we may assume that a person infected with a JEV in Bangkok may fly to Songkhla or other cities or neighboring countries before he is ill, then become ill there and be a source of virus for the local *Culex* mosquitoes, which 10 days later pass it on locally and soon a new epidemic center occurs. From here it is carried up river by boat, or elsewhere by train, car or oxcart to other smaller cities and towns. However, the trouble with all of these assumptions applied of Japanese encephalitides spread is that JEV is known to be present endemically in all of these places for a long time, being carried about originally in this same way before these epidemics of JE started. Something new must have intervened. However, once it is introduced as viremia in a returning traveler, animal or bird, including migrants, for example, or in an infected insect vector accidentally imported by airplane, ship or car, they probably would not become established successfully in the country. Eventually, after the virus is landed in a suitable habitat, they could become established and might even become endemic.

2.7 Vertebrate hosts

Another important factor in natural cycle of JEV is vertebrate host. Japanese encephalitis viruses are believed to be maintained in populations of certain vertebrates, being transmitted among them by mosquitoes and other hematophagous arthropods, with man becoming tangentially infected when entering the environment in which these viruses are circulating.

The presence of antibodies in significant numbers of a particular species of bird or animal suggests that it may be an important natural reservoir or amplifier host (Buescher et al., 1959b). An investigation in Chiang Mai Valley showed that each rainy season enormous numbers of the vector mosquitoes emerged from the flooded rice fields and irrigation ditches of the valley to feed on the numerous buffalo, cattle and pigs present in the rural areas. An analysis of the data suggested that pigs play a major role in the transmission of JEV in the Chiang Mai Valley (Grossman et al., 1974). Other studies also confirm that pigs are important hosts for amplification of virus dissemination in the epidemic region (Buscher & Scherer, 1959) and for maintenance of virus cycling in the endemic region (Simpson et al., 1970).

It was also reported in other studies that many vertebrates were infected (SEATO Med Res Lab, 1969). One experimental infection study demonstrated that adults of a mammal, *Menetes berdmorei*, were susceptible to infection with JEV. Also, one species of rat, *Rattus exulans*, might be infected on occasion (William & Imlarp, 1972).

Birds are considered as important hosts for JEV because Culex mosquitoes are readily fed on birds. It was demonstrated that 20 to 37 per cent of wild Japanese tree sparrows had neutralizing antibodies to JEV. Sparrows free of antibodies were inoculated with 10,000 plaque-forming units of JEV. None of the birds became clinically ill. Virus could be detected in blood plasma during the first three days after inoculation but not thereafter (Yuill, 1969). It has been postulated that a certain species of bird (night heron) as well as migrant bird species might serve as a good vehicle to carry virus from one place to other place in a very long distance during the period of acute viremia (Scherer et al., 1959b). However, migrations of most bird species do not cover great distances such as from tropical to temperate areas in the few days that high titer primary viremia would persist. One may hypothesize transmission of infection to susceptible migrants at intermediate resting areas while in transit. Thus, birds moving in great distance may possibly serve as a source of vector infection.

2.8 Reptile

Beside mammals, it is quite interesting to note that two common species of house gecko lizards, *Hemidactylus frenatus* and *Platyurus platyurus*, are susceptible to JEV infection. It was shown that they developed viremia for six days with the concentration of virus in the blood high enough to be picked up by mosquitoes, *Aedes aegypti* (in the amount of 0.006- 0.06 ml) in which JEV could be detected by suckling mice inoculation and LLC-MK_2 cell culture inoculation (Yuill et al., 1968; Yuill, 1969). It turns out that mosquitoes can be used as successful as needles and syringes for drawing blood from house gecko lizards for viremia determination, despite the fact that the mosquitoes usually draw less blood (0.006 - 0.06 ml) from each gecko than that is obtained with needle and syringe (0.05 to 0.1 ml). This finding is very useful in studying ecology of mosquito-borne viruses. Thus, the virological studies with JEV can be done, at daily intervals for one week when small size house gecko lizards are used as hosts for virus infection. Drawing blood from these very small (3 - 10 g) lizards with a syringe and 27-gauge needle invariably proved fatal.

It has been demonstrated clearly by Grossman and his coworkers (Grossman et al., 1974) that a simple pattern of endemic in Thailand, year-round transmission of JEV between *Culex* mosquitoes and pigs seems sufficient to account for persistence of JEV in Chiang Mai Valley, and the appearance of human encephalitis cases. It was found that the human epidemics which occurred each May through August in the Valley were probably a reflection of a logarithmic increase in vector mosquito populations in April and early May. It coincided with the onset of the seasonal rains and was followed closely by larger numbers of infected mosquitoes as reflected by increased JEV transmission rates in sentinel pigs (Grossman et al., 1974). Human epidemics probably resulted from greater exposure to these infected mosquitoes. The apparent resistance of bovines to infection (Johnsen et al., 1974) the slow rate of turnover in the bovine population, and bovine attractiveness to vector mosquitoes (Gould et al., 1974) indicate that bovines may actually suppress JEV infections, as has been suggested in India (Carey et al., 1969).

Questions have been raised concerning low number of JEV cases during high number of vector population in certain endemic areas. Several factors are used to explain these facts, i.e., blood feeding on non-amplifier species of vertebrates, blood feeding on the immune portion of amplifier populations, inefficient transfer from infected mosquito to susceptible amplifier animal to susceptible mosquito. Not all susceptible amplifier hosts fed upon by infected *Culex tritaeniorhynchus* develop high enough viremia to infect other feeding mosquitoes, and high vector mortality between infectious blood meal and the second post-infection oviposition.

2.9 Ecology of mosquito vector

Concerning the ecology of mosquito vector, some factors of greatest relevance to the abundance of JE vectors include the development of irrigation agriculture, e.g., utilization of rice fields and irrigation waste water by *Culex tritaeniorhynchus*, inadequate disposal of polluted water resulting from burgeoning urbanization and industrialization, e.g. *Culex quinquefasciatus*.

In most areas in which JE in endemic *Culex* mosquitoes are now far more important than *Aedes* species in the transmission of the virus to humans, but species of the latter genus may be significant in the basic ecological cycle of JEV such as vectors to humans in some types of relatively undisturbed natural habitat. For example, although *Culex tritaeniorhynchus* and domestic pigs are now the most important hosts of JEV in Japan from the point of view of human infection, swine have been reared in significant numbers in Japan only since the opening of that country to contact with the outside world in 1853. The southeastern Soviet Union is the one area where the epidemiology of JEV has been studied in a setting not greatly changed by humans. Russian investigators consider three of *Aedes* (*togoi, japonicus,* and *koreicus*) as important vectors of JEV to humans in some types of habitat in this region (Petrischeva et al., 1963).

A small number of closely related species of *Culex* mosquitoes serve as vectors, and many vertebrates are infected. Pigs in particular, are important hosts for amplification of virus dissemination in the epidemic region (Buescher and Scherer, 1959) and for maintenance of virus cycling in the endemic region (Simpson et al., 1970). Although the vectors are much more attracted to pigs than to man, it is presumed that the appearance of viremic pigs each spring in the temperate zone allows a large number of mosquitoes to become infected resulting in virus transmission to humans and encephalitis epidemic.

3. Prevention and control

Because of the shortage of appropriate form of specific treatment for Japanese encephalitis, control of the disease relies mainly on the control of the mosquito vector, on the early identification of cases, and if possible, the isolation of cases from contact with vector mosquitoes. Vaccine against JEV is also available for high-risk group of people such as children in endemic area, military men, physicians and nurses. In addition, vaccine against JEV for pig vaccination is also available which is very useful in terms of reducing the number of susceptible amplifying hosts.

There are three JEV vaccines that currently available for prevention of JEV. They are inactivated vaccine derived from mouse brains; cell culture-derived inactivated vaccine, and cell culture-derived live attenuated vaccines . Formalin-inactivated vaccine (JE-Vax) is the only vaccine currently in used internationally. It is produced from mouse brain tissue and is manufactured by the Research Foundation for Microbial Disease (BIKEN), Osaka, Japan, and also by the Government of Pharmaceutical Organization (GPO), Bangkok, Thailand. The GPO obtains the technical assistance from BIKEN and Japanese government to establish local production of inactivated mouse brain-derived vaccine from Nakayama and Beijing strains of JEV. The GPO has the capacity to produce only 40% of the national vaccine need. All of the rest are imported vaccine. Although it is effective, multiple-dose regimen is needed with the relatively high cost and problems with reactogenicity complicated its use. Inactivated and live-attenuated JE vaccine, prepared from JEV strain SA14-14-2 grown in primary hamster kidney (PHK) cells culture, have been developed and used only in China.

Sporadic cases of viral encephalitis in Thailand have been noted in the northern part before 1969. An epidemic transmission of JE was first recognized in 1969 when an outbreak leading to 685 cases occurred in the Chiang Mai valley. Yearly outbreaks numbering in the thousands of cases and hundreds of deaths recurred in the northern region and JE became a leading cause of mortality and disability in children. Hyperendemic JE transmission has subsequently spread within Thailand, and the adjacent area in Burma (Tsai, 2000). According to the continue public health impact of JE in Thailand, it has led to effort in childhood immunization and vaccine production in 1985.

It was demonstrated by hemagglutination inhibition and neutralization assay that there are definitive antigenic differences among JEV Thai strain and between Thai strains and the standard subtypes, Nakayama and Beijing strains (Ali et al., 1995; Ali & Igarashi, 1997). Most of JEV isolated in Thailand are belonging to genotype I, while some belonging to genotype II, which strains Nakayama and Beijing are belonging to genotype III (Ali & Igarashi, 1997). The monovalent vaccine derived from JEV strain Nakayama or bivalent vaccine consisting of Nakayama and Beijing-1 strains provide 91% protective efficiency in either protocol in Thai children. These currently available vaccines are able to induce high levels of protective immunity against JEV belonging to heterologous genotypes. However, it is possible that vaccines produced from JEV strains isolated in Thailand may induce higher level of protective immunity against the locally circulating strains (Kurane & Takasaki, 2000).

3.1 Vaccine development

The development of a vaccine that would induce rapid protection in people and animals is currently remained as an important issue. New generation of safe chimeric viruses that are unable to infect mosquitoes is currently ongoing in the development and preclinical studies. This would be a major step toward production of live-attenuated vaccine that is safer for the environment and would minimize the risk for vaccine-born outbreaks as reported in 1970s for TC-83 vaccine. It has been proposed that live-attenuated JEV vaccine has several advantages including small dose is required for vaccination, a secretory IgA is produced against certain virus agent and the immune response last longer in recipients. This type of vaccine is an attractive one in vaccine development against several virus agents. An attenuation of virulence of the viruses is one of selected markers used for the development of live-attenuated vaccines.

There is one live-attenuated JE vaccine currently available and being used in China. Live-attenuated JE vaccine derived from SA14-14-2 strain has shown several advantages comparing to inactivated vaccine including lower dose in vaccination, low cost in vaccine production, and induction of long-lasting immune response in immunized children. This attenuated virus has small plaque phenotype. The potential of small plaque size mutants to be used as live-attenuated vaccine strains has been intensively investigated by several investigators. It has been shown that temperature sensitive (ts) mutants of dengue type 4 virus and dengue 2 virus which have small plaque phenotype appeared to be attenuated in mice that may be useful for the development of a recombinant live attenuated vaccine of dengue virus (Blaney et al., 2002, Hanley et al., 2002, Huang et al., 2003). The small plaque mutants of other flaviviruses including West Nile virus (WNV) and tick-borne encephalitis virus (TBE), Murray Valley encephalitis virus (MVE), and JEV that are increase in cells infectivity and increase in affinity of glycosaminoglycan binding, have shown their virulence were attenuated in mouse model (Lee et al., 2004, Lee & Lobigs, 2002, Mandl et al., 2001). In addition, almost all strains of JEV, which are small plaque size variants on BHK-21 cells, except for JaGAr 01, are found to be correlated with the virulence attenuation of the viruses in mice (Kimura et al., 1973). Thus, it is quite interesting to find a small plaque size variant as a short cut to be used for the development of the vaccine.

Live attenuated JE vaccine derived from SA14-14-2 strain has shown several advantages comparing to inactivated vaccine including lower dose in vaccination, low cost in vaccine production, and induction of long-lasting immune response in immunized children. This attenuated virus has small plaque phenotype. The potential of small plaque size mutants to be used as live-attenuated vaccine strains has been intensively investigated by several investigators. It has been shown that temperature sensitive (ts) mutants of dengue type 4 virus and dengue 2 virus which have small plaque phenotype appeared to be attenuated in mice that may be useful for the development of a recombinant live attenuated vaccine of dengue virus (Blaney et al., 2002, Hanley et al., 2002, Huang et al., 2003). The small plaque mutants of other flaviviruses including West Nile virus (WNV) and tick-borne encephalitis virus (TBE), Murray Valley encephalitis virus (MVE), and JEV that are increase in cells infectivity and increase in affinity of glycosaminoglycan binding, have shown their virulence were attenuated in mouse model (Lee et al., 2004, Lee & Lobigs, 2002, Mandl et al., 2001). In addition, almost all strains of JEV, which are small plaque size variants on BHK-21 cells, except for JaGAr 01, are found to be correlated with the virulence attenuation of the viruses in mice (Kimura et al., 1973). Thus, it is quite interesting to find a small plaque size variant to use for the development of the vaccine.

It has been shown that there is a good correlation between small plaque size and attenuation of viruses including several members of flavivirus, i.e., Dengue virus type 2, West Nile virus, Tick-borne encephalitis virus, and Murray Valley encephalitis virus (Tsai, 2000; Blaney et al., 2002; Hanley et al., 2002; Lee et al., 2004; Lee & Lobigs, 2002; Mandl et al., 2001; Huang et al., 2003). The vaccine strain, SA 14-14-2 of JEV, also has a small plaque size and grows quite well in PHK cells. This strain is currently used to produce live attenuated vaccine in China (Tsai, 2000). It has been described that small plaque size phenotype is influenced by the burst size and short incubation. In addition, the sensitivity to interferon and growth conditions of viruses such as the nature of medium and temperature of incubation of infected cells may be involved in the production of small plaque size of the virus. It was documented that the small plaque variants of Sindbis virus were more susceptible to the action of interferon than a large plaque variant (Kimura et al., 1973).

Serial passage the wild type virus in cell culture is a classical method for the selection of the attenuated strain of viruses. Small plaque size phenotype of the virus comparing to their parent strain are used as a marker for the selection of the virulence attenuation. Moreover, amino acid replacement in E protein is one of the markers to determine the phenotypic changes in neuro-virulence of the viruses as shown by several investigators. The most important is that the difference of amino acid changes in E protein of JEV may unique for each strain. However, these markers are useful to determine virulence attenuation for development of live-attenuated vaccine. To further understand the exact molecular mechanism of the small plaque mutants, the complete nucleotide sequence need to be done.

Attempts have been made to select small plaque variants from the local strain of JEV in Thailand. It was demonstrated that the two suspected temperature-sensitive mutants of Japanese encephalitis virus strain KE-093 had an amino acid substitution, lysine for glutamic acid, in envelope protein at residue E-83 in the small plaque variants. The growth patterns and neurovirulence of these two small plaque variants of Japanese encephalitis virus in suckling mice remained the same as that of the parent strain, which suggested that small plaque phenotypes was not always associated with attenuation in vivo (Lorroengsil et al., 2008). In contrast, it has been shown that JEV strain SA 14-14-2, the vaccine strain, could replicate in C6/36 cells better than the parent strain (Bhatt et al., 2000). TBE virus mutant (Oshima C1-1) that was selected by subculturing the parent strain (Oshima 5-10) in BHK-21 cells was replicated better than the parent virus. The TBE virus mutant was attenuated for neuro-invasiveness in mouse model (Goto et al., 2003). This advantage is useful for the production of the live-attenuated vaccine using cell culture techniques. However, one precaution should be aware of is that the possibility of the vaccine strain that are replicating in the body of vaccinated people may serve as a source for the mosquito vector to feed on, and may revert back to the virulent form of the virus again.

3.2 DNA vaccine

The progresses in the development of DNA vaccine in Thailand are in the early phase of the development. Our group is also trying to use the most recent pathogenesis data to design a therapeutic vaccine that would reverse already established encephalitis and help clear the virus from the brain.

Plasmid DNA-based vaccination strategies have become an active area of research over the past decade due to their potential to produce safer and cheaper vaccines. These vaccines could be delivered to recipients by intra-muscular (IM) injection or intra-dermal (ID) administration using a gene gun. IM inoculation of plasmid DNA vaccines to mice induces predominantly T helper 1 (Th1) immune responses, while T helper 2 (Th2) type immune responses are generated following the ID delivery. The isotypes of antibodies and the types of cytokines induced by the two methods differ and this could have bearing on the efficacy of the vaccine candidate.

Attempts have been made to construct the plasmid DNA vaccine against JEV by trying to include JEV *e* gene in the plasmid DNA. It has been shown that these plasmids are capable of synthesizing JEV premembrane (prM) and E proteins, which have been evaluated in mice. Both forms of E protein however generated JEV neutralizing antibodies that provided significant protection to mice against lethal JEV challenge.

The envelope (E) protein of JEV is also the interesting target for vaccine development. Since the E glycoprotein contains antigenic determinants for hemagglutination and neutralization. Mutations in the *E* gene are often responsible for significant alterations in the biological functions of the virus and may affect virulence (Richman et al., 2002). It has been reported that there are the constructed recombinant DNA encoding full-length and sub-fragment E protein (Chen et al., 1999; Kaur & Sachdeva, 2002; Ashok & Rangarajan, 2002), C-terminal part and soluble form of E protein (Chia et al., 2001). These protein products induce neutralizing antibody and protective immunity in mice.

E protein is known as an important protein, which plays roles in virion assembly, receptor binding, membrane fusion, and is a major target for neutralizing antibodies (Chambers et al., 1990). It has been noted that mutations in the E protein are often responsible for significant alterations in the biology of the virus and may affect virulence (Tiroumourougane et al., 2002; Richman et al., 2002; Burke & Monath, 2002; Chambers et al., 1990; Heinz, 2003). Phenotype changes among flaviviruses have also been found to associate with amino acid alteration of E protein. It has been shown that seven amino acids in the virulent parent SA 14 have been substituted in attenuated vaccine clones, SA 14-14-2/PHK and SA 14-14-2/ PDK, when their genomes are compared. Four of them are located in E protein including E-138, E-176, E-315, and E-439. Three amino acids are located in non-structural protein including NS2B-63, NS3-105, and NS4B-106. Several amino acids are also mutated, i.e., glutamic acid to lysine at E-138, isoleucine to valine at E-176, alanine to valine at E-315, lysine to arginine at E-439, glutamic acid to aspartic acid at NS2B-63, alanine to glycine at NS3-105, and isoleucine to valine at NS4B-106 (Ni et al., 1995). The attenuation concerning neuro-invasiveness in mice of the prototype JEV strains, Nakayama-O and an Indian 826309, was observed following six passages in Hela cells. Nine and eight amino acids substitutions were found in M and E protein of the attenuated Nakayama-O and an Indian 826309, respectively. The common one of amino acid substitution of these two attenuated viruses was alanine to valine at E-366 (Cao et al., 1995). It has been proposed that the mutation of the flavivirus strains that have been attenuated by serial passage do not share common genetic mutations that are associated with their phenotypes. However, there is a notable exception that the identical mutation from glutamic acid to lysine occurred at amino acid residue E-138 of the IC47 infectious clone-derived variants from JEV strain JaOArS982 and of the vaccine strain SA 14-14-2 (Kinney and Huang, 2001).

E protein has been noted as the most important antigen in providing of protective immunity against JEV. Among three domains of E protein, neutralizing epitopes of domain III has been described. They were including of residues 308, 310, and 311 of louping ill virus; 384 and 386 of TBE virus; 305 of yellow fever virus; 307, 383-389, and 333-351 of dengue viruses; 306, 331, 333, 373-399, and 387 of JEV (Lin & Wu, 2003). Immunization with 27 amino acid of JEV E protein which is present on Johnson Grass Mosaic virus-like particles able to induce neutralizing antibodies without using adjuvant and protect mice from lethal challenge (Manishia & Vrati, 2003). This peptide, peptide A, contained residues 373 to 399 of JEV E protein was chosen for this study. Moreover, it has been shown by using complementary structural modeling and site-directed mutagenesis of domain III of E protein of JEV in *E. coli* with monoclonal antibody (Mab) E3.3 that serine 331 and aspartic acid 332 have a potential to be neutralizing epitopes (Lin & Wu, 2003). Another peptide, peptide B, contained residues 325 to 333 was also selected.

It has been shown that mouse immunized with virus-like particles (VLPs) presenting amino acid 373 to 399 from JEV E protein on domain III generated JEV neutralizing antibody without using adjuvant, and these mice were protected against a lethal JEV challenge (Manishia & Virati, 2003). It was demonstrated by site-directed mutagenesis that the functional domain at Ser331 and Asp332 on domain III of JEV E protein interacted with neutralizing monoclonal antibody (Mab) E3.3 (Lin & Wu, 2003).

One of interest is the determination of the antigenic determinant of JEV from sub-fragment in domain III region of *e* gene. There is a possibility to insert two selected peptides that have been chopped into small overlapping peptides, synthesized, and linked with hepatitis B core peptide (HBc Ag), which is a B-cell epitope and recognized by mouse MHC. This HBc Ag may help JEV peptides in an activation of antibody response in immunized mice. The peptides, which show neutralizing activity against JEV, may serve as the antigenic epitopes of the virus. This antigenic epitopes will be useful in second-generation vaccine development against the local JEV in the future.

It has been shown that serial passage of virus resulted in cell-adapted mutant that is attenuated in virulence in mice. Some of these mutants have changed in net positive charge of their proteins. They have high affinity for glycosaminoglycans (GAGs), which are highly-sulfate polysaccharides that are present almost ubiquitously on cell surfaces (Goto et al., 2003; Mandl et al., 2001). JEV replication in mice might require other viral or host cell-specific factors which do not present in BHK-21 cells infection. However, the mechanism by which cell-adapted flaviviruses undergo attenuation in vivo is not well understood.

Protection against JEV is mainly antibody dependent. Virus neutralizing antibody alone is sufficient to impart protection. Previous report has been documented that formalin-inactivated JEV vaccine does not induces CTLs but provides protection to vaccinees against JEV (Pan et al., 2001). Therefore, B cell epitopes on JEV E protein are important determinants of protection against virus infection. The whole E protein was not necessary for activating immune response but the small fragments of E protein were sufficient for eliciting the immune response and protect against JEV challenge (Lin & Wu, 2003; Kaur & Sachdeva, 2002; Chia et al., 2001).

As mentioned by previous reports that the whole protein was not necessary for activating immune responses, small protein fragments that contain antigenic epitopes are sufficient for eliciting the desired immune response. Peptide fragments of several pathogens, such as *Brucella abortus*, *Trichinella spiralis* and *Plasmodium yoelii* have potential to be used as vaccines (Moynihan & Howard, 2001). Peptide vaccines are easy to produce, biological stable at high temperature, no infectious agent present in the preparation and safe for human use. A major problem of peptide vaccine is their poor immunogenicity. Synthetic peptide need to be presented with the strong adjuvant or large carrier proteins to elicit good immune responses (Manishia & Virati, 2003). An envelope E gene of Japanese encephalitis virus genotype I, Thai strain KE-093 was successful cloning and heterologous expression in *Escherichia coli* Rosetta 2 strain (Witthajitsomboon et al., 2010). Attempts to develop DNA vaccine are going on by using the cloned *e* gene.

The rodent models have been used to evaluate vaccine candidates in pre-clinical studies, and nonhuman primates are usually the models of choice as they provide a robust system for evaluation of vaccine candidates. The Old World monkeys have predominantly been used in these types of studies with rhesus (*Macaca mulatta*) and cynomolgus (*Macaca fascicularis*) monkeys being most popularly used for evaluation of vaccine candidates against various infectious diseases, including those caused by *Flaviviruses*. It has been shown that the immunogenicity of premembrane-envelop proteins (pMEa and pMEs) delivered intramuscularly (IM) or intradermally (ID) in rhesus monkeys resulted in the DNA immunization induced protective levels of JEV neutralizing antibodies and generated robust memory that led to a rapid and sustained anamnestic response in monkeys sham challenged with mouse brain-grown, formaldehyde inactivated commercial vaccine. Several JEV proteins were evaluated in the DNA vaccine modality for their ability to induce protective immunity in the murine system. These include plasmids could express non-structural protein 1 (NS1), E or prM and E proteins of JEV. It was shown that variable degree of efficacy in murine model systems with plasmids expressing prM and E proteins conferring high degree of protection of mice against lethal JEV challenge, largely due to their ability to induce JEV neutralizing antibodies. Two plasmids could express prM protein along with full-length anchored E or truncated secretory E protein, while both plasmids induced JEV neutralizing antibodies in mice. To achieve this, efforts are underway to further enhance the immunogenicity of JE DNA candidate vaccine.

4. Vector control

4.1 Microbial insecticides

An alternative approach for controlling Japanese encephalitis or any of mosquito-borne viruses is the reduction in mosquito vector population. It has been shown that the JEV can cause a long-lasting viremic phase in amplifying hosts. The virus can cause infection in pigs with the viremic phase last for 28 days, whereas the viremic phase in infected birds last for 4-5 days with a very high virus titer, about 10^5 pfu/ml in a house sparrow(Yuill, 1969). These long lasting viremia in amplifying hosts provide ample opportunities for the susceptible mosquito vectors to become infected after feeding on them. Therefore, one way to block the transmission of the virus can be achieved by reducing the number of mosquito-vector populations. This activity will lead to the reduction of new cases of infected patients in the endemic areas.

The world Health Organization (WHO) has recommended utilization of *Bacillus thuringiensis* var. *israelensis* (Bti) as an agent for biological control of mosquitoes since 1978 (Arata et al., 1978). The recommendation was based on the facts that *Bti* produces proteinaceous parasporal crystals during sporulation. These crystals are composed of multiple proteins ranging from 26 to 135 kilodaltons (kDa) in size with act as a protoxin (135 kDa). The crystals are lethal to larval mosquitoes (Goldberg & Margalit, 1977), and to blackflies (Undeen & Nagel, 1978). No effect is observed on non-target aquatic insects, fish, or frog larvae (Garcia & Goldberg, 1978). It has been shown that several chemicals can persist for a long time in the environment, they are hazardous to humans. Thus, the development of biological controls as an alternative means of mosquito vector control is desired.

4.1.1 *Bacillus thuringiensis* var. *israelensis*

One of the most successful insect pathogens used for insect control is the bacterium *Bacillus thuringiensis* subspecies *israelensis*, which presently is ~ 2% of the total insecticidal market. *Bti* is almost exclusively active against larval stages of different mosquito species, i.e., *Aedes aegypti*, *Culex quinquefascatus*, *Culex gelidus*, and *Culex tritaeniorhynchus* and kills the insect by disruption of the midgut tissue followed by septicemia caused probably not only by *Bacillus thuringiensis* but probably also by other bacterial species (Raymond et al., 2010). The action of *Bacillus thuringiensis* relies mainly on insecticidal toxins that are active during the pathogenic process. In addition, these bacteria also produce an array of virulence factors that contribute to insect killing (Bravo et al., 2005). Upon sporulation, *Bacillus thuringiensis* produces insecticidal crystal inclusions that are formed by a variety of insecticidal proteins called Cry or Cyt toxins. These toxins show a highly selective spectrum of activity killing a narrow range of insect species. The Cry and Cyt toxins belong to a class of bacterial toxins known as pore forming toxins (PFT) that are secreted as water-soluble proteins and subsequent undergo conformational changes in order to insert into the membrane of their hosts. Despite the limited use of *Bacillus thuringiensis* products as spray-able insecticides, Cry toxins have been introduced into transgenic crops providing a more targeted and effective way to control insect pests in agriculture. Concomitantly, this approach has resulted in significant reduction in the use of chemical insecticides in places where this technology has been embraced.

4.1.2 *Bacllus sphaericus*

One promising agent that may be used as microbial insecticides is a spore-forming bacillus, *Bacillus sphaericus*. This bacterium is an aerobic, gram-positive, spore-forming bacillus, which is also widespread in soil and aquatic environments. Some strains produce a toxin which is lethal when ingested by filter-feeding mosquito larvae. Kellen and his colleagues described the isolation of a larvicidal *Bacillus sphaericus* strain K from moribund larvae in the U.S. in 1965 (Kellen et al., 1965). A more pathogenic strain, strain SSII-1, was later isolated by Singer (Singer, 1973) from infected larvae collected in India. Subsequently, more highly toxic strains were isolated from around the world, among which are strain 1593 from Indonesia (Singer & Murphy, 1976), strain 2297 from Sri Lanka (Wickremesinghe & Mendis, 1980), and strain 2362 from Nigeria (Weiser, 1984). The potency and specificity of the *Bacillus sphaericus* toxins make them promising agents for biological control of mosquito pests.

Comparison of the larvicidal toxins from *Bacillus sphaericus* strains SSII-1, 1593 and 2362 revealed several important differences (Myers et al., 1979). *Bacillus sphaericus* yielded better results against larvae of *Culex quinquefasciatus* and *Anopheles minimus* than that of *Aedes aegypti* larvae (Pantuwatana, 1989).

Attempts have been made to produce several formulations of microbial insecticides, *Bacillus sphaericus*, and *Bacillus thuringiensis* var. *israelensis* (*Bti*). Microbial insecticides have been proposed as substitutes for chemicals because they have a narrow and specific spectrum of activities that enable them to kill only certain insect species. But their use is limited since most microbes show a narrow spectrum of activity that enables them to kill only certain insect species. Moreover, they have low environmental persistence and they require precise application practices, since many of these pathogens are specific to young insect larval stages or are sensitive to irradiation.

The slow-release formulations of products made from microbial insecticides, i.e., *Bacillus sphaericus*, and *Bacillus thuringiensis* var. *israelensis,* have been used in field trials against certain species of mosquito larvae especially *Culex quiquefasciatus,* with a satisfactory result. However, it is very difficult to apply the aforementioned formulations of microbial insecticides' products in the breeding places of the mosquito vectors, because the mosquito larvae of *Culex* species are filter feeder, which feed on the surface of the water. All larvae of the mosquito vector species are found in polluted water. It has been shown that the effectiveness of microbial insecticides' products is not reached a satisfactory result. Efforts on the development of microbial insecticides for biological control of mosquito vector are underway in parallel with the recent advances in biotechnology.

5. References

Ali, A., Igarashi, A., Paneru, L. R., Hasebe, F., Morita, K., Takagi, M., Suwonkerd, W., and Tsuda, Y. 1995. Characterization of two Japanese encephalitis virus strains isolated in Thailand. *Arch. Virol.* 140: 1557-1575.

Ali, A., and Igarashi, A. 1997. Antigenic and genetic variations among Japanese encephalitis strains belonging to genotype I. *Microbiol. Immunol.* 41: 241-252.

Arata, A.A., Chapman, H.C., Cupello, J.M., Davidson, E.W., Laird, M., Margalit, J., and Roberts, D.W. 1978. Status of biocontrol in medical entomology. *Nature (London)* 276: 669.

Ashok, M.S., and Rangarajan, P.N. 2002. Protective efficacy of a plasmid DNA encoding Japanese encephalitis virus envelope protein fused to tissue plasminogen activator signal sequences studies in a murine intracerebral virus challenge model. *Vaccine* 20: 1563-1570.

Bhatt, T.R., Crabtree, M.B., Guirakhoo, F., Monath, T.P., and Miller, B.R. 2000. Growth characteristics of the Chimeric Japanese encephalitis virus vaccine candidate, ChemeriVax-JE (YF/JE SA14-14-2), in *Culex tritaeniorhynchus, Aedes albopictus,* and *Aedes aegypti* mosquitoes. *Am. J. Trop. Med. Hyg.* 62: 480-484.

Blaney, J.E., Johnson, D. H., Manipon, G.G., Firestone, C., Hanson, C.T., Murphy, B.R., and Whitehead, S.S. 2002. Genetic basis of attenuation of Dengue virus type 4 small plaque mutants with restricted replication in suckling mice and SCID mice transplanted with human liver cell. *Virology* 300: 125-139.

Bravo, A., Gill, S.S., and Soberón, M. 2005. *Bacillus thuringiensis* mechanisms and use. In: L.I. Gilbert, K. Iatrou and S.S. Gill, Editors, Comprehensive Molecular Insect Science, Elsevier BV (2005) ISBN 0-44-451516-X, pp. 175–206

Buescher, E.L., and Scherer, W.R. 1959. Ecologic studies of Japanese encephalitis virus in Japan. IX. Epidemiologic correlations and conclusions. *Am. J. Trop. Med. Hyg.* 8: 719-722.

Buescher, E.L., Scherer, W.F., Rosenberg, M.Z., Gresser, I., Hardy, J.L., Bullock, H.R. 1959a. Ecologic studies of Japanese encephalitis virus in Japan. II. Mosquito infection. *Am. J. Trop. Med. Hyg.* 8: 651 - 654.

Buescher, E., Scherer, W., Rosenberg, M., and McClure, H.E. 1959b. Immunologic studies of Japanese encephalitis virus in Japan. III. Infection and antibody responses of birds. *J. Immunol.* 83:605-613.

Burke, D.S., & Monath, T.P. 2002. Flaviviruses. In: Knipe DM, Howley PM editors. *Fields Virology* vol.1, 4th ed. ASM Press, Washington DC.

Cao, J.X., Haolin, N., Wills, M.R., Campbell, G.A., Sil, C.B., Ryman, K.D., Kitchen, I., and Barrett, A.D.T. 1995. Passage of Japanese encephalitis virus in HeLa cells results in attenuation of virulence in mice. *J. Gen. Virol.* 76: 2757 -2764.

Carey, D.E., Myers, R.M., Reuben, R., Webb, J.K.G. 1969. Japanese encephalitis in South India. A summary of recent knowledge. *Indian J. Med. Res.* 56: 1340-1352.

Chambers, T.J., Hahn, C.S., Galler, R., and Rice, C.M. 1990. Flavivirus genome organization, expression, and replication. *Annu. Rev. Microbiol.* 44: 649-688.

Chamber, T.J., Nestorowicz, A., Mason, P.W., and Rice, C.M. 1999. Yellow fever/Japanese encephalitis chimeric viruses. Construction and biological properties. *J. Virol.* 73:v3095-3101.

Chen, W.R., Tesh, R.B., and Rico-Hesse, R. 1990. Genetic variation of Japanese encephalitis virus in nature. *J. gen. Virol.* 71: 2915-2922.

Chen, H.W., Pan, C.H., Liau, M.Y., Jou, R., Tsai, C.J., Wu, H.J., Lin, Y.L., and Toa, M.H. 1999. Screening of protective antigen of Japanese encephalitis virus by DNA immunization: a comparative study in conventional viral vaccines. *J. Virol.* 73: 10137-10145.

Chia, S-C., Leung, P.S.C., Liao, C-P., Huang, J-H., and Lee, S.T. 2001. Fragment of Japanese encephalitis virus envelope protein produced in *Escherichia coli* protects mice from virus challenge. *Microb. Pathol.* 31: 9-19.

Garcia, R., and Goldberg, L.J. 1978. University of California Mosquito Control Research. *Annu. Rep.* 1977, p. 29.

Goldberg, L.J., and Margalit, J. 1977. A bacterial spore demonstrating rapid larvicidal activity against *Anopheles serget II, Uranotaenia unquiculata, Culex univitattus, Aedes aegypti*, and *Culex pipiens*. *Mosq. News* 37, 355.

Goto, A., Hayasake, D., Yoshii, K, Mizutani, T., Kariwa, H., and Takashima, I. 2003. A BHI-21 cell culture-adapted tick-borne encephalitis virus mutant is attenuated for neuro-invasiveness. *Vaccine* 21:4043-4051.

Gould, D.J., Edelman, R., Grossman, R.A., Nisalak, A., and Sullivan, M.F. 1974. Study of Japanese encephalitis virus in Chiangmai Valley, Thailand. IV. Vector studies. *Am. J. Epidemiol.* 100: 49-56.

Grossman, R.A., Edelman, R., Willhight, M., Pantuwatana, S., and Udomsakdi, S. 1973. Study of Japanese encephalitis virus in Chiangmai Valley, Thailand. III. Human seroepidemiology and inapparent infections. *Am. J. Epidemiol.* 98: 133 – 149.

Grossman, R.A., Edelman, R., and Gould, D.J. 1974. Study of Japanese encephalitis virus in Chiangmai Valley, Thailand. VI. Summary and conclusions. *Am. J. Epidemiol.* 100: 69-76.

Hanley, K. A., Lee, J. J., Blaney, J. E., Murphy, B. R., and Whitehead, S. S. 2002. Paired charge-to-alanine mutagenesis of Dengue virus type 4 NSS generates mutants with temperature-sensitive, host range, and mouse attenuation phenotypes. *J. Virol.* 76: 525-531.

Hasekawa, T., Takehara, Y., and Takahashi, K. 1975.Natural and experimental infections of Japanese tree sparrows with Japanese encephalitis virus. *Arch. Virol.* 49(4): 373-376.

Heinz FX. 2003. Molecular aspects of TBE virus research. *Vaccine* 21: S/3-S/10.

Huang, C.Y-H., Butrapet, S., Tsuchiya, K. R., Bharmarapravati, N., Gubler, D.J., and Kinney, R.M. 2003. Dengue 2 PDK-53 virus as a chimeric carrier for tetravalent Dengue vaccine development. *J. Virol.* 77: 11436-11447.

Hurlburt, H.S. and Nibly, C.J. 1964. Virus isolations from mosquitoes in Okinawa. *J. Med. Entomol.* 1: 78-82.

Johnsen, D.O., Edelman, R., Grossman, R.A., Maungman, D., Pomsdhit, J., and Gould, D.J.. 1974. Study of Japanese encephalitis virus in Chiangmai Valley, Thailand. V. Animal infections. *Am. J. Epidemiol.* 100: 57-68.

Kaur, R., and Sachdeva, G. 2002. Plasmid DNA immunization against Japanese encephalitis virus: immunogenicity of membrane-anchored and secretory envelope protein. *J. Infect. Dis.* 185: 1-12, 17.

Kay, B.H., Fanning, I.D., and Mottram, P. 1989. Rearing temperature influences flavivirus vector competence of mosquitoes. *Med. Vet. Entomol.* 3(4):415-422.

Kellen WR, Clark TB, Lindegren JE, Ho BC, Rogoff MH and Singer S. *Bacillus sphaericus* Neide as a pathogen of mosquitoes. *J. Invertebr. Pathol.* 7: 442, 1965.

Kimura, T., Iwai, K., and Ueba, N. 1973. Difference in plaque size of Japanese encephalitis virus strains on BHK-21 cells and chick embryo cells. *Biken J.* 16: 57-66.

Kinney, R.M., and Huang, C.Y-H. 2001. Development of new vaccines against Dengue fever and Japanese encephalitis. *Intervirology* 44: 176-197.

Kono, R., and Kim, K.H. 1969. Comparative epidemiological features of Japanese encephalitis in the Repupublic of Korea, China (Taiwan) and Japan. *Bull. Wld. Hlth. Org.* 40; 263-277.

Ku, C.C., King, C.C., Lin, C.Y., Hsu, H.C., Chen, L.Y., Yuch, Y.Y., and Chang, G.J.J. 1994. Homologous and heterologous neutralization antibody responses after immunization with Japanese encephalitis vaccine among Taiwan children. *J. Med. Virol.* 44:122-131.

Kurane, I., and Takasaki, T. 2000. Immunogeneticity and protective efficacy of the current inactivated Japanese encephalitis vaccine against different Japanese encephalitis virus strains. *Vaccine* 18: 33-35.

Lee, E., Hall, R.A., and Lobigs, M. 2004. Common E protein determinans for attenuation of glycosaminoglycan-binding variants of Japanese encephalitis and West Nile virus. *J. Virol.* 78: 8271-8280.

Lee, E., and Lobigs, M. 2002. Mechanism of virulence attenuation of glycosaminoglycan-binding variants of Japanese encephalitis virus and Murray Valley encephalitis virus. *J. Virol.* 76: 4901-4911.

Lin, C.W., and Wu, S-Ch. 2003. A functional determinant on domain III of the Japanese encephalitis virus envelope protein interacted with neutralizing-antibody combining sites. *J. Virol.* 77: 2600-2603.

Lorroengsil, S., Chen, A., Sallberg, M., and Pantuwatana, S. 2008. Genetic differences of E gene of a Thai strain of Japanese encephalitis virus that determine small plaque size phenotype but not neurovirulence in suckling mice. *Southeast Asian J. Trop. Med. Public Health* 39:387-393.

Mandl, C.W., Kroschewski, H., Allison, S.L., Kofler, R., Holzmann, H., Meixner, T., and Heinz, F.X. 2001. Adaptation of tick-born encephalitis virus to BHK-21 cells results in the formation of multiple heparan sulfate binding sites in the envelope protein attenuation in vivo. *J. Virol.* 75: 5627-5637.

Manishia, S., and Vrati, S. 2003. A Japanese encephalitis virus peptide present on Johnson grass mosaic virus-like particles induces virus-neutralizing antibody and protects mice against lethal challenge. *J. Virol.* 77: 3487-3494.

Mitamura, T., Kitaoka, M., Watanabe, S., Hosoi, T., Tenjin, S., Seki, D., Nakahata, K. Jo, K., and Shimizu, T. 1939. Weitere Untersuchungen uber die Ubertragung der japanischen Enzephalitis durch Mucken. *Trans. Soc. Pathol. Jpn.* 29: 92.

Moynihan, J.S., and Howard, C.R. 2001. Recent advances in the development of peptide vaccines for Hepatitis B. *Intervirology* 44: 65-77.

Myers, P., Yousten, A.A., and Davidson, E.W. 1979. Comparative studies of the mosquito-larval toxin of *Bacillus sphaericus* SS II-I and 1593. *Can. J. Microbiol.* 25, 1227.

Ni, H., Chang, G-J J., Xie, H., Trent, D.W., and Barrett A.D.T. 1995. Molecular basis of attenuation of neurovirulence of wild-type Japanese encephalitis virus strain SA 14. *J. Gen. Virol.* 76: 409-413.

Pan, C.H., Chen, H.W., Huang, HW., and Tao, M.H. 2001. Protective mechanisms induced by a Japanese encephalitis virus vaccine. Requirement for antibody but not $CD8^+$ cytotoxic T-cell response. *J. Immunol.* 75:11457-11463.

Pantuwatana, S. The prospect of *Bti* and *B sphaericus* in mosquito control in Thailand. *Israel J. Entomol.* 23: 51-57, 1989.

Raymond, B., Johnston, P.R., Nielsen-LeRoux, C., Lereclus, D., and Crickmore, N. 2010. Bacillus thuringiensis: an impotent pathogen? *Trends Microbiol.* 18: 189–194.

Richman, D.D., Whitley, R.J., and Hayden F.G. 2002. Flaviviruses. In: Monath, T.P., Tsi, T.F., (ed) *Clinical Virology* 2nd ed. ASM Press, Washington D.C.

Rosen, L., Tesh, R.B., Lien, J.C., and Cross, J.H. 1978. Transovarial transmission of Japanese encephalitis virus by mosquitoes. *Science* 199: 909-911.

Sangkawibha, N., Nakornsri, S., Rojanasuphot, S., and Ahandarik, S. 1982. Japanese encephalitis in Thailand. *J. Dept. Med. Sci. (Thailand)* 24: 1-20.

Scherer, W.F., Kitaoka, M., grossberg, S.E., et al. 1959a. Immunology studies of Japanese encephalitis virus in Japan. II. Antibody response following inapparent hunan infection. *J. Immunol.* 83: 594-604.

Scherer, W.F., Moyer, J.T., Izumi, T., Gresser, I., and McCown, J. 1959b. Ecological studies of Japanese encephalitis in Japan. Parts VI. Swine infection. *Am. J. Trop. Med. Hyg.* 8: 644-722.

Simasathien, P., Rohitayotshin, S., Nisalak, A., Singharaj, P., Halstead, S.B., and Russel, P.K. 1972. Recovery of Japanese encephalitis virus from wild caught mosquitoes in Thailand. *Southeast Asian J. Trop. Med. Public Health* 3: 52-54.

Simpson, D.I.H., Bowen, E.T.W., Platt, G.S., Way, H.G., Smith, C.E., Peto, S., Kamath, S., Lim, B.L., and Lim, T.W. 1970. Japanese encephalitis in Sarawak: virus isolation and serology in a Land Dyak village. *Trans. Roy. Soc. Trop. Med. Hyg.* 64: 503-510.

Singer, S. 1973. Insecticidal activity of recent bacterial isolates and their toxins against mosquito larvae. *Nature* 244, 110.

Singer, S., and Murphy, D.J. 1976. New insecticidal strains of *Bacillus sphaericus* useful against *Anopheles albimanus* larvae. *Abstr. 76th Annu. Meet., American Society of Microbiology*, 181).

Sutham, C.M. 1956. Serological studies of encephalitis in Japan. II. Inapparent Infections by Japanese B encephalitis virus. *J. Infeect. Dis.* 99: 163-169.

Takahashi, M. 1976. The effects of environmental and physiological conditions of *Culex tritaeniorhynchus* on the pattern of transmission of Japanese encephalitis virus. *J. Med. Entomol.* 13: 275-284.

Takahashi, M., and Suzuki, K. 1979. Japanese encephalitis in mosquito salivary gland. *Am. J. Trop. Med. Hyg.* 28(1):122-135.

Tiroumourougane, S.V., Raghava, P., and Srinivasan, S. 2002. Japanese viral encephalitis. *Postgrad. Med. J.* 78: 205-215.

Tsai, T. F. 2000. New initiative for the clonal of Japanese encephalitis by vaccination: Minutes of WHO/CVI meeting, Bangkok, Thailand. 13 - 15 October 1998. *Vaccine* 18: 1-25.

Undeen, A.H., and Nagel, W.L. 1978. The effect of *Bacillus thuringiensis* ONR-60A strain (Goldberg) on *Simulium* larvae in the laboratory. *Mosq. News* 38, 524.

Wang, S.P. 1964. Japanese encephalitis in Taiwan: A review of recent studies. *Bull. Wld. Hlth. Org* 30: 297-284.

Watts, D.M., Pantuwatana, S., DeFoliart, G.R., Yuill, T.M., and Thompson, W.H. 1973. Transovarial transmission of La Crosse virus (California Encephalitis group) in the mosquito *Aedes triseriatus. Science* 82: 1140-1141.

Weiser, J. 1984. A mosquito-virulent *Bacillus sphaericus* in adult *Simulium damnosum* from northern Nigeria. *Zentralbl. Microbiol.* 139: 57.

White, D.O., and Fenner, F., 1984, *Medical Virology*, Academic Press, INC. (Orlando, U.S.A., 3rd ed, ch 5).

Wickremesinghe, R.S.B., and Mendis, C.L. 1980. *Bacillus sphaericus* spore from Sri Lanka demonstrating rapid larvicidal activity on *Culex quinquefasciatus. Mosq. News* 40, 387.

Williams, J.E. and Imlarp, S. 1972. Susceptibility of rodents to Japanese encephalitis virus. *Bull. Wld. Hlth. Org.* 46: 854-855.

Witthajitsomboon, N., Chen, A., Lorroengsil, S., Sallberg, M., and Pantuwatana, S. 2010. Cloning and expression of envelope protein of Thai genotype I strain KE-093 of Japanese encephalitis virus. *Southeast Asian J. Trop. Med. Public Health* 41:1359-1367.

Yuill, T.M., Sukhavachana, P., Nisalak, A., and Russel, P.K. 1968. Dengue virus recovery by direct and delayed plaques in LLC-MK_2 cells. *Amer. J. Trop. Med. Hyg.* 17: 441-448.

Yuill, T.M. 1969. Mosquitoes for drawing blood from small reptiles. *Trans. Roy. Soc. Trop. Med. Hyg.* 63(3): 407-408.

22

Systems Thinking: Prevention and Control of Japanese Encephalitis - "The Plague of the Orient"

Kaliyaperumal Karunamoorthi[1,2]
[1]*Unit of Medical Entomology & Vector Control, College of Public Health and Medical Sciences, Jimma University,*
[2]*Research & Development Centre, Bharathiar University, Tamil Nadu*
[1]*Ethiopia*
[2]*India*

1. Introduction

Insect-transmitted diseases impose enormous burden on the world's population in terms of loss of life (millions of death per year) and morbidity. These diseases are also responsible for huge economic losses, both in terms of health-care costs and lost productivity, mostly in countries that can least afford them (Jacobs-Lorena & Anthony, 2002) and, contribute significantly to disease burden, death, poverty, and social debility in the tropical countries (Jang *et al.*, 2002). In particular, developing countries are the foremost sufferer and the major victims of several vector-borne diseases (Karunamoorthi & Sabesan, 2010). More specifically, mosquitoes are the vectors of the dreadful diseases affecting mankind. World Health Organization (WHO) has declared mosquitoes as "the public enemy number one" as they are predominantly responsible for the transmission of various dreadful diseases, such as malaria, filariasis, dengue, yellow fever, and Japanese encephalitis.

1.1 Global public health impact of Japanese encephalitis (JE)

JE is one of the most dreaded mosquito-borne viral encephalitis known to afflict humans and is the leading cause of viral encephalitis (inflammation of the brain) all through the world especially in large parts of Asia with temperate and subtropical or tropical climate (Sabesan *et al.*, 2008). Encephalitis is an infection on the membrane around the brain and spinal cord and is commonly known as **"brain fever"** with high case fatality (Igarashi, 1992a). In Southeast Asia, the incidence of JE appears to be increasing, probably as a result of a steady rise in population density, deforestation, and increasing irrigation of agricultural areas (Igarashi, 1992b).

JE affects predominantly school-age children and is greatly feared because of its high lethality and frequency of permanent neurologic sequelae. Today, approximately 3 billion people are living under the current JE-endemic region (Dutta *et al.*, 2010). The estimated annual incidence and mortality rates are 30,000–50,000 and 10,000, respectively, where as the estimated global burden of JE in 2002 was 709,000 disability-adjusted life years lost (Keiser *et al.*, 2005).

JE outbreaks occur frequently in 14 Asian countries. However, the lack of reporting system and poor diagnostic tools available for JE limits the appropriate estimation of cases as on date. The use of vaccine is restricted to certain situations only, and no standard formulation is available yet (Sabesan, 2003). Nearly half of the survivors suffer from severe neuropshychiatric sequelae (Dutta *et al.*, 2010). In addition, the social prognosis for handicapped survivors of JE is often poor in developing countries.

2. The historical background of Japanese encephalitis virus (JEV)

From the 1870s, recurring epidemics of encephalitis have been reported from the islands of Japan, especially during the summer season, with major outbreaks occurring every 10 years. This summer encephalitis was termed as type B encephalitis, to differentiate from von Economo's encephalitis lethargica. The name type B was later dropped and in 1935 the Nakayama strain of Japanese encephalitis virus (JEV) was isolated from the brain of a fatal case (Solomon *et al.*, 2000). In just six weeks in 1924, there were more than 6000 cases and 3000 deaths (Solomon, 2006). The virus was later classified as a member of the genus Flavivirus (family Flaviviridae) named after the prototype Yellow fever virus (Latin; flavi = yellow). The genus consisted of over 70 other closely related virus species (Dutta *et al.*, 2010).

The mode of transmission by mosquito vector was elucidated only 25 years after the recognition of JEV (Tiroumourougane *et al.*, 2002). The origins of JEV are uncertain, but phylogenetic comparisons with other flaviviruses suggest that it has evolved from an African ancestral virus, perhaps as recently as a few centuries ago (Gould, 2002) and evolved into its present form in the Indonesia–Malaysia region (Solomon *et al.*, 2003a).

3. Epidemiology

Because of its prevalence and mortality JE is a major public health problem in endemic-epidemic regions. Acute encephalitis occurs in about 1 to 20 cases per 1000 infections, leading to death in 25% of the cases and producing serious neurological lesions in 30% (Burke & Leake, 1988). Children and young adults are most susceptible (Solomon, 1997). The peak transmission period is in summer (from May to October), corresponding with the rainy season and the proliferation of mosquitoes (Halstead, 1992). In endemic zones the percentage of JE antibodies among local resident increases with age. However, during an epidemic outbreak in a previously unaffected region both adults and children are equally susceptible (Umenai *et al.*, 1985). JE is primarily found in South East Asian countries (see Fig. 1). Three epidemiological regions can be distinguished as follows (Rhodain, 1996);

- **The endemic region** made up of southern India, southern Vietnam, southern Thailand, the Philippines, Malaysia and Indonesia. In these regions mosquitoes are more often attracted by birds and pigs where human cases are rare.
- **The intermediary subtropical region** which includes northern India, Nepal, North and Central Burma, northern Thailand, northern Vietnam, southern China and Bangladesh. Transmission is permanent and of low intensity; however, it increases to higher levels

during the rainy season (between April and October). Epidemics in contrast, are severe and concentrated among children.

- **The temperate epidemic region**, spanning northern China, Korea, Japan, Taiwan and the southern extremities of Russia. Transmission is variable coupled with environmental temperature. In winter, mosquitoes are inactive but huge epidemics can be seen in summer and autumn. The geographical area of this disease is showing a trend towards expansion. Postulated explanations are migration of birds, certain irrigation projects, animal smuggling and global warming. Development of rice plantations is theoretically foreseeable in other regions (Pakistan, Afghanistan, Nile Valley, Madagascar and Oriental Africa) creating a favorable environment for further vector proliferation (Rhodain, 1996).

3.1 The geographical distribution of JE

At present, the geographical distribution of JE ranges from Japan, maritime Siberia and the Republic of Korea in the North, to most parts of China and the Philippines in the East, Papua New Guinea in the South, and India and Nepal in the West (see Fig. 1) (Broom *et al.*, 2003). JE is now an emerging viral disease having international importance as it is invading the previously non-endemic areas too. From Asia, it has stretched to Papua New Guinea and Torres Strait of northern Australia (Hanna *et al.*, 1996; Mackenzie *et al.*, 1997). Recent outbreaks of JE have been reported southward in Australia, and westward in Pakistan (Solomon *et al.*, 2000). In recent decades, JE has gradually spread to previously non-affected Asian regions. The reasons for this increased geographic distribution are uncertain, but may include population shifts, and changes in agricultural practices, animal husbandry, migratory bird patterns, and movement of vector mosquitoes to wider areas (Halstead & Jacobson, 2003).

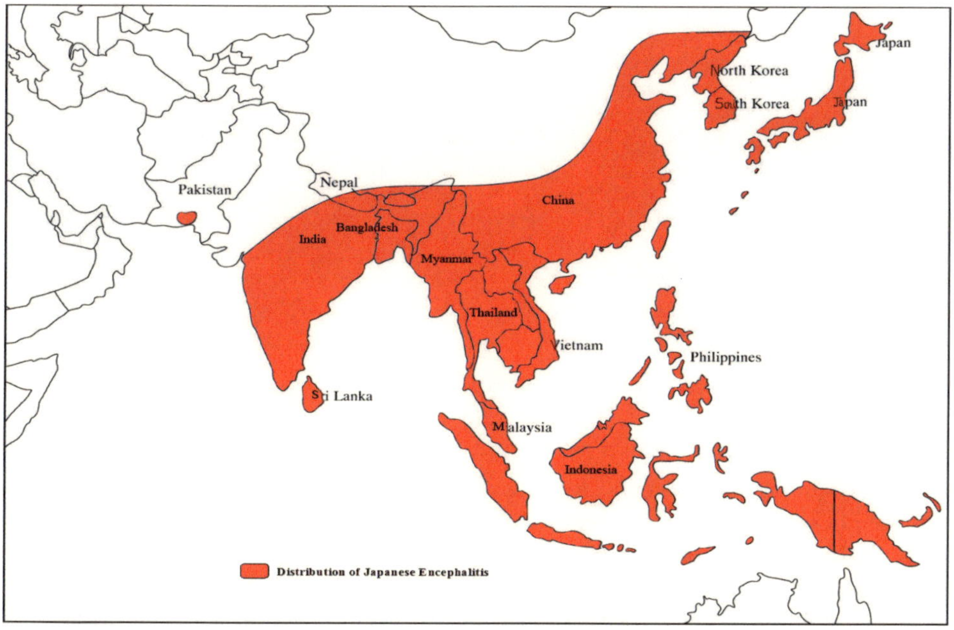

Fig. 1. Map showing the distribution of Japanese Encephalitis

3.2 The causative agent - Japanese encephalitis virus (JEV)

JE virus, is the most common documented cause of viral encephalitis in Asia, and potentially ranks next to the Human Immunodeficiency Virus (HIV) as the most common cause of viral encephalitis in the world (Tsai, 1994). The virus is able to replicate within the salivary glands of the mosquitoes. Mature JE virions remain entrapped in intracellular vacuoles and are later released into the apical cavity of salivary gland cells through the fusion of these vacuoles with the apical plasma membrane. This process is associated with primary re-synthesis of saliva in mosquitoes following blood feeding activity. Another type of shedding involves virus particles, either singly or in mass, being released directly through the apical plasma membrane (Takahashi & Suzuki, 1979).

3.3 Enzootic cycle of JEV

JEV is an arbovirus transmitted in an enzootic cycle involving birds, particularly wading ardeids, such as herons and egrets. Pigs can become infected and act as amplifying hosts. Many mosquito species are potential vectors, but Culex species such as *Culex tritaeniorhynchus* and *C. vishnui,* which breed in rice paddies and other dirty water, are especially important. Humans become infected when they are bitten by infected mosquitoes, but since they have transient and low-level viremia, they are "dead-end" hosts that do not normally transmit virus (Fig. 2).

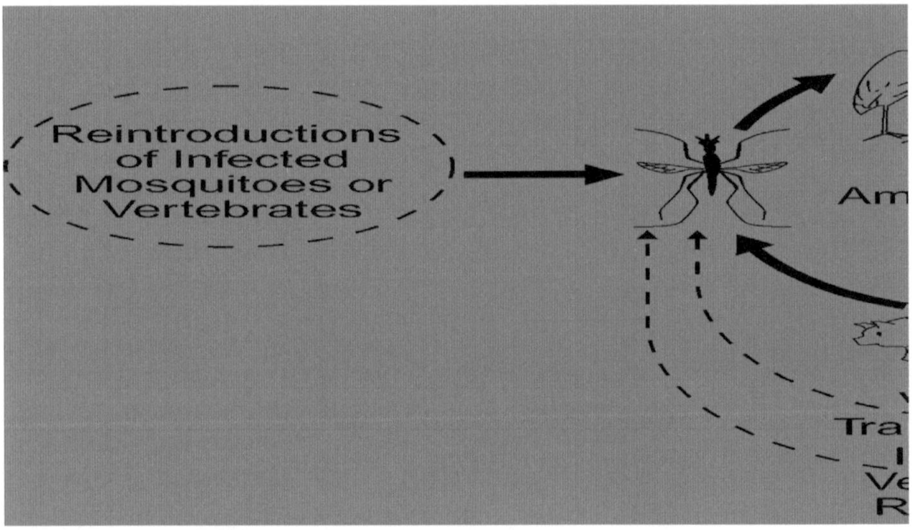

Fig. 2. The transmission cycle of JE

3.3.1 Vector mosquitoes

JE vector mosquitoes are zoophilic, feeding primarily on animal and wild birds and human beings are not considered as a reservoir for viral transmission. It is feeds most often in the outdoors, with the peak biting times after sunset and again after midnight (Fischer *et al.*, 2008). Female mosquitoes get infected after feeding on a viraemic host and can transmit the virus to other hosts after an extrensic incubation period of 9 to 12 days. Man to man transmission has not been documented. The mosquitoes remain infected for life. The average life period of a mosquito is about 21 days and undergoes three gonotrophic cycle (WHO, 2006).

Human infections are mainly transmitted by *Culex tritaeniorrhynchus* Giles, which is the principal vector of JE in India and South East Asian countries (Suman *et al.*, 2008). The female specimens are infective 9–10 days after having taken the viraemic blood meal, having undergone three gonotropic cycles (Gajanana *et al.*, 1997). Other culicine mosquitoes that can transmit JE include *Cx. bitaeniorhyncus, Cx. epidesmus, Cx. fuscocephala, Cx. gelidus, Cx. pseudovishnui, Cx. sitiens, Cx. vishnui* and *Cx. whitmorei* (Sehgal & Dutta, 2003). The JE incidence, however, varies from country to country; the highest occurrence is found in the rice-growing areas of the country. From this, one may surmise an ecological connection with the irrigation facilities and paddy cultivation (Rajagopalan & Work, 1969).

3.3.2 The pig

Mosquitoes pick the virus from the pigs (which are supposed to be the major reservoir of the virus) and transfer it to humans (Singh, 2007). Pigs with high and prolonged viraemias, are often common in endemic countries, and are generally reared in open and unroofed pigpens, which are located near houses (Mishra *et al.*, 1984; Solomon *et al.*, 2000). In different parts of India, 12 to 44 percent of pig population has been found to be positive for JE antibodies particularly in JE endemic areas (WHO, 2006).

3.3.3 The human, cattle and birds

The presence of JE antibodies in the sera of birds belonging to different species have indicated that *Ardeola grayii* (pond heron) and *Bubulcus ibis* (cattle egret) play a definite role in maintenance of JE virus in nature (WHO, 2006). Humans, goats, cattle and horses are considered to be the dead-end hosts (Reuben *et al.*, 1992). For example, in the Thanjavur district, India, an area with extensive rice agriculture, a very low JE incidence has been reported. This has been explained by high cattle to pig ratio (400:1) (Vijayarani & Gajanana, 2000). In rice-growing villages without herons, seroconversion rates in children aged 0–5 and 6–15 years were 0% and 5%, respectively. In ecologically-similar villages with herons, the corresponding rates were 50% and 56%, respectively (Mani *et al.*, 1991).

4. Clinical manifestations

The disease is characterized by a wide range of presentations, as both the symptoms and the clinical course can differ broadly among patients (Solomon, 1997). On average, only 1 in 300 cases produce clinical symptoms (WHO, 1998). The first signs of infection appear after an incubation period between 6 and 14 days. It usually starts with a fever above 38°C, chills, muscle pain and meningitis-type headaches accompanied by vomiting. The initial presentation in children usually begins with gastrointestinal symptoms: nausea, vomiting and abdominal pains similar to those found in an acute abdominal syndrome. These non-specific signs can continue for 2 to 4 days. However, the patient's state deteriorates rapidly. A progressive decline in alertness takes place eventually leading to deepening coma. Convulsions are experienced by 85% of subjects (Kumar *et al.*, 1990).

The meningeal syndrome predominates with painful neck stiffness. Motor paralyses including hemiplegia and tetraplegia may also be present. Signs of extra pyramidal involvement, including tremor, rigidity, and abnormal movements are observed in around 30% of the patients (Kumar *et al.*, 1994). Severe clinical cases are likely to have life-long neurological sequelae. Mostly children and young adults are affected (Solomon *et al.*, 2000; Tsai, 2000; Halstead & Jacobson, 2003). Presence of one clinical case in the community suggests that 300 to 1000 people have been infected (WHO, 2006).

5. Laboratory diagnosis

The diagnosis of JE viral infection should be made within an epidemiological context (Endy & Nisalak, 2002). During epidemic outbreaks, a febrile meningeal syndrome should be considered for JE above any other diagnostic consideration. In endemic regions, other arbo-viruses should be investigated when symptoms of viral encephalitis are present, especially in children (Diagana *et al.*, 2007). Nowadays, confirmation of JE virus infection depends mostly on serologic assays such as IgM antibody detection by enzyme-linked immunosorbent assays (ELISA) (Mathur *et al.*, 1990; Shope & Meegan, 1997).

5.1 Detection/isolation of antigen/virus

- Demonstration of viral antigen in the autopsied brain tissue by the fluorescent antibody test.
- Isolation and identification of the virus from CSF, occasionally from peripheral blood (within 3 to 4 days after onset of symptoms) or autopsied brain tissue.

5.2 Detection of antibody

- The diagnosis of JE is supported by serological tests. The tests include detection of IgM antibodies which appear after the first week of onset of symptoms and are detectable for one to three months after the acute episode.
- IgG antibodies indicate previous infection and are useful for conducting seroepidemiological studies to determine the extent of silent infection and immunity levels in the local population.
- The detection of antibodies to JE virus can be done routinely by Haemagglutination Inhibition Test (HI) test to demonstrate fourfold rise in total antibodies and IgM Capture ELISA test for demonstration of IgM antibodies.
- Confirmation of the diagnosis of JE must be based on multiple criteria including clinical, biological, europhysiologic and cerebral imaging findings (Diagana *et al.*, 2007).

6. Approaches for prevention and control of JE

Environmental degradation, socio-economic decline, rapid population movements, migratory birds' movement and the concomitant effects of global warming are contributing to changing pattern of morbidity and mortality and posing serious challenge to public health. Japanese encephalitis remains as major cause of viral encephalitis in Asia, imposing a significant burden on poor rural families. It is a disease of public health importance due to its epidemic potential and high case fatality rate. Even, if patients survive, complications may lead to lifelong sequelae. Therefore the epidemic form of the disease can be minimized by applying the effective control or prevention measures in order to save the lives especially young children. The strategy for prevention and control of JE includes the following avenues;

1. Surveillance
2. Vector control
3. Personal Protection Interventions
4. Immunization
5. Case management
6. Health education and training
7. Epidemic preparedness and response

6.1 Surveillance

The component of JE surveillance consists of three major areas: (1) Clinical/syndromic surveillance through PHC system for early diagnosis and proper management of JE patients. (2) Vector surveillance in JE prone areas for monitoring vector behaviour and population build up for timely implementation of intervention methods (3) Sero-surveillance to delineate high risk population groups and to monitor JE specific antibodies in sentinel animals or birds as an indication of increasing viral activity (WHO, 2006).

6.2 Vector control intervention strategies

Vector control remains to be the most generally effective measure to prevent/interrupt the disease transmission and is therefore one of the basic technical elements of the vector-borne disease control programme. Currently the following strategies are mainly implemented in order to control the JE vectors and eventually to minimize the disease burden among the rural poor community, despite of their limitations.

6.2.1 Environmental management control strategies

Alternate wet and dry irrigation (AWDI)

Traditionally, flooded rice fields have been the ideal breeding place for several mosquito species, including those that transmit JE. An important feature of this technique involves the alternate wetting and drying of paddy fields, which in turn curtails the life cycle development of the mosquito from larvae and pupae to adult (Keiser *et al.*, 2005). In order to achieve a significant reduction of mosquito larvae, AWDI (also termed intermittent irrigation) has to be applied during the entire cropping season and should cover all rice fields. This method is particularly feasible in places where control of the water supply and drainage is possible, hence where soil and climatic conditions are suitable (Mogi, 1988).

In China, large-scale application of the AWDI technique has been held responsible for significant reductions of rice field breeding vectors and malaria. Growing water shortages in many areas create an incentive to better control of irrigation water. AWDI is also one such strategy (Keiser *et al.*, 2005). A study found that the AWDI has reduced the immature stages of *Cx. tritaeniorhynchus* by 14–91% in rice fields and adult population by 55–70%. The crop yield was examined in two trials and increases between 4 and 13% were observed in AWDI rice fields (Lu-Baulin, 1988). The effect of this method on the incidence of JE has to be investigated (Keiser *et al.*, 2005).

Limitations

- The potential of AWDI is, however, limited in areas where there is a threat of insufficient resources to re-flood the fields and where farmers perceive a risk of reduced yields by letting their fields dry out.

6.2.2 Biological control strategies

Biological control refers to the introduction or manipulation of organisms to suppress vector populations. A wide range of organisms helps to regulate mosquito populations naturally through predation, parasitism and competition (Chandra *et al.*, 2008). Concern about the threat of strong forms of insecticide resistance (Hargreaves *et al.*, 2000) has stimulated renewed interest in alternative control methods including biological control and biopesticides. The best known is the use of *Bacillus thuringiensis* var. *israelensis* (*Bti*) and *B. sphaericus* and, another biocontrol method, the use of larvivorous fish in appropriate water bodies, have been used in mosquito control for over 100 years (Bay, 1967).

6.2.2.1 Larvivorous fish as a biological agent

Recognizing the high larvivorous potential of the fish species *Gambusia` affinis,* it has widely been used to control the immature stages of various vector mosquitoes. Other fish species include *Tilapia* spp., *Poecilia reticulata or Cyprinidae* (Lacey & Lacey, 1990). After stocking rice fields with 1–10 natural predator fish perm^2, larval populations of *Cx. tritaeniorrhynchus* were reduced by 55.2–87.8% (Kim *et al.*, 1994). Larvivorous fish cannot be applied in rice fields, where irregular irrigation is practiced. It should also be noted that predator populations are strongly influenced by the temperature, rice growth, vegetation, use of pesticides or chemical pollutants (Lacey & Lacey, 1990).

In addition, recent research has shown that ovipositing mosquitoes may move to other breeding sites in response to the stocking of rice fields with predatory fish (Angelon & Petranka, 2002). Furthermore, the introduction of exotic predators such as *Gambusia* might displace the native fish populations to reduce their natural value, as being observed in Japanese rice fields (Wada, 1988). Therefore, the compatibility of the chosen fish with local fauna and flora is of high importance (Lacey & Lacey, 1990).

6.2.2.2 Bacteria as biocides

The larvicidal activity of the spore forming bacteria *B. sphaericus* and *B. thuringiensis israelensis* were discovered in 1965 and 1976, respectively (Mittal, 2003). In Tamil Nadu, India, the application of 4.3 kg/ha of a microgel droplet formulation of *B. sphaericus* 1593M resulted in a 44–79% reduction of early instar and 82–100% reduction of late instar culicinae larvae (*Cx. fuscanus, Cx. pseudovishnui* and *Cx. tritaeniorhynchus*) for at least 5 weeks (Sundararaj & Reuben, 1991). Similarly, up to 95–98% of *Cx. tritaeniorhynchus* larvae were reduced in three other field sites evaluating *B. sphaericus or B. thuringiensis* formulations (Balaraman *et al.*, 1983; Rhee *et al.*, 1983; Kramer, 1984). However, the larvicidal activity did not persist in these rice fields beyond a couple of days; in the Republic of Korea the residual effect of *B. thuringiensis* H-14 was found to last only for 24 h (Rhee *et al.*, 1983).

Limitations

- The application of larvicides may not be an appropriate control strategy in terms of cost effectiveness because of the widespread breeding reservoirs of *Cx. tritaeniorrhynchus.*

- Biocides are not only expensive but also their effectiveness can withstand only for a few days. Therefore, it requires frequent and repeated applications at least at the end of every week.
- *In general, biocides are* effective against mosquito larvae but cannot control the pupal stage.

6.2.2.3 Invertebrate predators

Invertebrate predators, i.e. *Coleoptera, Hemiptera* or *Odonata,* though less common than the use of fish, are also known to substantially reduce mosquito larval populations in rice fields. However, they are highly sensitive to temperature, presence of vertebrates, growth of rice and chemical pollutants (Lacey & Lacey, 1990). In India, the presence of notonectids was negatively associated with the larval abundance of *Cx. pseudovishnui, Cx. tritaeniorrhynchus* and *Cx. vishnui* (Sunish & Reuben, 2002).

6.2.2.4 Fungi

Fungi that have been studied extensively for their potential as biological mosquito control agents include *Coelomomyces* spp. and *Lagenidium giganteum.* The former have been investigated with regard to how they impact the development of JE vectors in China (Keiser *et al.,* 2005). Field observations showed a strong effect of the fungus *Coelomomyces indica* on *Cx. tritaeniorhynchus,* as infected larvae were unable to develop into adults (Liu & Hsu, 1982). However, fungi have not been applied for biological control of JE vectors on a large scale so far, as practical problems, for example their production, have yet to be solved (Lacey & Lacey, 1990).

6.2.2.5 Algae

The floating water fern Azolla (Salviniales: Azollaceae) contains a symbiont nitrogen-fixing cyanobacteria, *Anabaena azollae* Strasburger, and is regarded as a source of organic fertilizer for rice cultivation (Lumpkin & Plucknett, 1980). Azolla multiplies rapidly and forms a thick surface mat which has been shown, in laboratory studies, to interfere with oviposition of mosquitoes as well as adult emergence from pupae (Amerasinghe & Kulasooriya, 1986; Rajendran & Reuben, 1988).

In China, the major vectors breeding in rice-fields say, *Cx. tritaeniorhynchus* and *An. sinensis* are found to have significant reductions of larvae in paddy fields where rice was cultivated in association with *Azolla pinnata* (Anonymous, 1986). In Tamil Nadu, India, application of the floating water fern *Azolla microphylla* greatly reduced immature mosquito populations. However, the infestation of the rice field with Azolla was difficult to achieve and 80 percent coverage by *Azolla* was accomplished only 13–14 days after rice transplantation, limiting its wider use as a biological mosquito control agent (Rajendran & Reuben, 1991).

6.2.3 Chemical control strategies

Indoor residual spraying (IRS)

IRS remains to be the most widely used vector control intervention. Its application has been thoroughly standardized and there are clear specifications for suitable equipment and insecticides. As the main effect of IRS is the killing of mosquitoes entering houses and resting on sprayed surfaces, it is not useful for the control of vectors which tend to rest outdoors, although it may be effective against outdoor biting mosquitoes which enter houses for resting after feeding.

IRS is relatively ineffective against the highly exophilic vectors, not only because of the resting habits of the vectors, but also because of the mobility of settlements, which remain unreported and inaccessible. In southern Henan province, China, DDT residual indoor spraying had no effect on the incidence of JE, but it was greatly reduced after the introduction of pyrethroid-impregnated bed nets. Only a small effect on outdoor biting densities of Culex tritaeniorhyncus was found, although the number of mosquitoes resting inside bed nets decreased markedly after the introduction of bed net impregnation (Luo *et al.*, 1994). The recent evidence also shows that IRS is ineffective against JE vectors (Sabesan *et al.*, 2008).

6.3 Personal protection interventions

6.3.1 Insecticide Treated Mosquito Nets (ITMNs)

The insecticidal treatment of nets adds a chemical barrier to the often imperfect physical barrier provided by the net and thus, improves its effectiveness in personal protection. ITMNs are easy to use devices for preventing mosquito -borne diseases such as JE, malaria, etc. The absence of reliable surveillance data, difficulties of vaccine production, and shortages and high costs of the commercial vaccine are thought to restrict the implementation of vaccine programs, especially in low-income countries (WHO, 1998; Monath, 2002). The interventional strategy using ITMNs will have an important epidemiological implication in bringing down the JEV activity in the pig-rearing communities without disturbing their social custom of rearing pigs, which they have been carrying on for ages. As well, this may provide a cost-effective way to reduce JEV transmission and supplement the relatively high cost of vaccines (Dutta et al., 2011).

Limitations

- Majority of the JE vectors have shown the bimodal feeding activity (the peak biting times after sunset and again after midnight) and people often stay outdoors at dusk hours during when ITNs may not be useful to reduce the man-vector contact.
- In addition, the JE vectors feeds most often in the outdoors and therefore, in these above circumstances deployment of ITNs may not be a feasible strategy and therefore, the application of repellents could be a useful alternative intervention measures.

6.3.2 Repellent

Repellents are playing key role in order to reduce the man-vector contact and eventually to reduce the vector-borne diseases (Karunamoorthi & Sabesan, 2010). Protection against insect bites is best achieved by avoiding infested habitats, wearing protective clothing, and applying insect repellent (Curtis, 1992; Fradin, 2001). Although insecticide-treated bed nets protect against mosquitoes and malaria in many parts of the world, people may contract disease in the early evening before they retire to the confines of the net, since exposure to malaria vectors and nuisance mosquitoes starts in the early evening (Maxwell *et al.*, 1998).

Insect repellents are extremely useful to the travelers, who visit for a short-span of time in the JE endemic areas. The main advantage is that the repellents are relatively cheap, highly effective and can be applied as a short-term measure.

Limitations

- Personal protection through mosquito coils and indigenous materials (oils,smokes, etc.) is widely practiced in agricultural communities but is of doubtful effectiveness in terms of protection against transmission, although it often provides some relief from the "nuisance" aspect in situations of high mosquito (including vector) biting densities. Commercial repellents are generally too expensive for poor farmer communities.

6.3.2.1 Plant -based repellents

Plants have been used since ancient times to repel/kill bloodsucking insects in the human history and even now, in many parts of the world people are using plant substances to repel/kill the mosquitoes and other blood-sucking insects (Karunamoorthi *et al.,* 2008). At the moment repellent of plants origin have been receiving massive attention due to their environmental and user friendly nature as they are easily available, accessible and affordable (Karunamoorthi *et al.,* 2009).

6.3.2.2 Plant-based products against JE vector mosquitoes

Petroleum ether (60–80°C) extracts of the leaves of *Vitex negundo* have acted as a promising repellent against *Cx. tritaeniorrhynchus* (Karunamoorthi *et al.,* 2008). Recent study results reveal that the hexane extracts of *A. marmelos* and *A. paniculata* can serve as potential repellent, ovicidal, and oviposition deterrent against Japanese encephalitis vector, *Cx. tritaeniorrhynchus* (Elango *et al.,* 2010). Globally, numerous studies evidently suggest that the traditionally used plant-based insect repellents are promising and could potentially contain many vector-borne diseases in particular JE (Karunamoorthi *et al.,* 2008; 2010).

6.3.2.3 Removal of Pig farming

The removal of the pigs acting as amplification hosts appears to have stopped the circulation of JEV in Singapore. The incidence of reported serological confirmed cases of JEV has been declining since pig farming has been eliminated in the country. The incidence has dropped from 101 cases during 1977–1984 to 15 cases for 1985–1992 (Anonymous, 1994).

Limitations

- This intervention strategy may not be feasible in the resource-poor settings, where majority of the people largely consider pigs as a source of income and desire food.

6.4 Immunization

Immunization provides a reasonable and practical way to control JEs, but the selection of target populations may present a problem in countries where JE outbreaks cannot be clearly defined in terms of places of infection and affected age groups. However, immunization is recommended for protecting populations where JE virus attacks are highly probable. Monitoring of JE activity will help to identify populations at the risk of exposure who can then be given a booster immunization (Umenai *et al.,* 1985).

6.4.1 Types of vaccine

Three types of vaccine against the Japanese encephalitis virus is presently licensed to be produced and administered worldwide. The inactivated mouse-brain derived JE vaccine is available on the international market. Primary hamster kidney (PHK) cell derived inactivated and live attenuated JE vaccines are widely used in China. A comparison between the inactivated mouse-brain derived vaccine and the PHK-derived live-attenuated vaccine shows a similar immunogenicity (84-100% seroconversion after 3 doses vs. 94-100% seroconversion after 2 doses), efficacy (91% with two doses vs. 97% with two doses) and with incidence of minor side effects. The inactivated JE vaccine was associated with rare incidence of severe allergic reactions and neurological complications (Mori & Siegel, 2000).

6.4.2 Dosage and route of administration

Dosage schedules differ for endemic and non-endemic regions. Children in endemic areas may need fewer doses because of previous immunity or subsequent exposures to flaviviruses that boost up antibody levels (ACIP, 1993). In endemic areas, the inactivated Biken vaccine is administered subcutaneously in two 0.5-mL doses between one to four weeks apart. Primary vaccination varies from the age of 18 months in Thailand to 3 years in Japan. Boosters are often given one year after primary vaccination and at intervals of 3 years thereafter (Tsai, 1994). In non-endemic regions, the Advisory Committee on Immunization Practices (ACIP) recommends a three-dose regimen on days 0, 7, and 30 with a booster given after one year and every three years thereafter (ACIP, 1993). Normal administration in China consists of a 0.5-mL dose at years of 1 and 2. A final booster is given in year six (Hennessy *et al.*, 1996).

6.4.3 Pig vaccination

Live attenuated JE vaccine has been developed in Japan primarily for immunization of pigs to prevent still births. In the Republic of Korea live attenuated JE vaccine using baby hamster kidney cells has also been developed and used for the vaccination of pigs (Umenai *et al.*, 1985). Immunization of pigs may be attempted to control JE epidemics because it has been established that these animals, after vaccination with the live vaccine, showed no viraemia on exposure to infected mosquitoes. The immunized pigs must have therefore been unable to "amplify" the virus transmission. However, all investigators engaged in this project pointed out that effective immunization was not easy because of the high turnover in the pig population so that individual pigs might escape being immunized (Umenai *et al.*, 1985). Vaccination of pigs has been used but has not been shown to consistently reduce mosquito and human infections and is not cost-effective in most settings. However, moving pigs away from human habitats also makes sense (Solomon, 2006).

6.4.4 WHO position on JE vaccination

Considering the current existence of safe and effective vaccines at a relatively low cost for wide scale use, the WHO advises the integration of the JE vaccine into the WHO immunization initiative in regions where this disease constitutes a public health risk. Therefore, systematic vaccination campaigns (in the form of 'vaccination days') are needed to allow the progressive integration of JE vaccination into the WHO immunization initiative. Despite a few cases of encephalomyelitis reported in children after having received the Mouse Brain-derived JE Vaccine, the WHO is considering using it in its immunization campaign since the benefits far outweigh the risks. Because of the availability and simplicity of use, the attenuated live vaccine based on the SA 14-14-2 strain offers an interesting alternative (Diagana *et al.*, 2007).

Limitations

- It should be mentioned that JE vaccine is not always available because the cost of commercial vaccines is still too high for use in large-scale vaccination. Work on the development of second generation (genetically engineered) vaccines is in progress.

6.5 Case management

6.5.1 Treatment

At present there are no established antiviral treatments against JE. *Interferon alpha* was the most promising drug in small open-label trials, but it failed to affect the outcome in children with JE (Solomon *et al.*, 2003). Though we are handicapped by the non-availability of a specific drug against JE, mortality and morbidity can be decreased appreciably by control and treatment of factors causing secondary deterioration such as raised intracranial pressure and convulsions. The value of this approach has been documented in traumatic coma (Ghajar & Hariri , 1992).

6.6 Health education

- Simple Information on JE - cause, transmission and prevention of mosquito bites.
- Community action in reducing mosquito breeding places by filling pools, weekly drainage of accumulated water, lowering of water levels in rice fields etc.
- National guidelines for diagnosis, management and prevention of JE - for programme managers and health professionals.

The people of JE-prone areas can be motivated through information, education and communication (IEC) activities/awareness campaigns on the dreadful disease. Using ITMNs for self-protection and protecting pigs from mosquito bites can efficiently check the JEV transmission in the JE prone areas. (Dutta *et al.*, 2011).

6.7 Epidemic preparedness and response

- Immediately notify government authorities by phone, fax or email.
- A team of investigators consisting of clinicians, epidemiologists, entomologists etc. should be immediately sent to the affected site, to take action.
- The team should be provided with proper information on collection of specimens;
  - Stool samples – for isolation of enterovirus
  - Blood or serum on the first three days of the illness – for detection or isolation of virus
  - Paired serum samples at an interval of at least 10 days – for antibody detection.
  - Cerebral Spinal Fluid (CSF) – for virus isolation and antibody tests
  - In case of deaths – tissue samples of brain and liver.

Conclusively, the JE disease control programmes have been focusing on the three major areas; (1) mosquito control, (2) amplifying host (pig) control, and (3) vaccination. However, neither mosquito control nor amplifying host (pig) control has been proven (in India) to be an effective measure to control JE, as they are carried out mostly after the outbreaks. Spraying the entire epidemic prone area is time consuming, expensive, and it is difficult to cover all mosquito habitats. Moreover, it is discouraged on account of environmental pollution. Since the biting activity of JE mosquitoes is at dusk, use of bed nets at night is likely to be ineffective and it shall not be the best solution for JE control. Segregating, slaughtering, or vaccinating pigs is economically not feasible and also difficult in other logistic angles. Since other animals, like birds also act as amplifying hosts just pig elimination shall not override JE (Sabesan *et al.*, 2008).

It seems that there is compelling evidence that human immunization is effective for containing the JE epidemics. Since the epidemic in man appears to follow epizootics which coincide when the vector density shoots up in the anticipated epidemic districts, feasibility of JE vaccination has to be considered as a preventive measure. In such situations, identifying the risk area and determining the target population to be immunized are crucial. Therefore, a routine JE immunization may be initiated in all areas identified for the risk of epidemics (Sabesan *et al.*, 2008).

One cannot affirm with or advocate the universal appropriate JE preventive/control measures. However, selecting the community oriented appropriate control strategy is extremely essential to minimize the mortality and morbidity due to JE. There are a number of effective intervention strategies currently available and therefore, one can select/prefer, the most appropriate intervention based on the local availability, accessibility, and affordability from the following recommendations;

- Changes in agricultural and animal husbandry practices
- Creating awareness by effective health education campaign through electronic media viz., printed pamphlet, news papers, radio and television
- Avoiding the outdoor stay at dusk hours during the main transmission period
- Intermittent irrigation system, if possible.
- Application of repellents during dusk hours in order to reduce the man-vector contact
- Consistent deployment of ITNs
- Immunization to the vulnerable section of the society especially for children (<15 years).
- Rational use of appropriate insecticide in the resting sites of mosquitoes, viz; domestic and peri-domestic areas, cattle sheds, pigsties, chicken coops etc. to suppress the vector density in risky areas prior to transmission (Sabesan et al., 2008).
- Promoting the use of bio-control agents (fishes/'Azolla', etc) and organic fertilizers ('neem' cakes) to reduce the mosquito immatures (Sabesan *et al.*, 2008).
- Monitoring viral activity in vector mosquitoes and reservoir animals in order to supplement with the information on vector abundance to predict the risk of transmission (Sabesan *et al.*, 2008).

7. Acknowledgement

I am greatly indebted to Dr. K. Ilango M.Sc., Ph.D., Scientist, Zoological Survey of India, Chennai, India and Dr. S. Sabesan M.Sc., Ph.D., Scientist, Vector Control Research Center, Ponidcherry, India for their constant encouragement and support. I would like to thank Mrs Melita Prakash for her sincere assistance. My last but not the least heartfelt thanks go to my colleagues of our Department of Environmental Health Science, College of Public Health and Medicine, Jimma University, Jimma, Ethiopia, for their kind support and cooperation.

8. References

Amerasinghe, F.P. & Kulasooriya, S.A. (1986). Azolla vs mosquitoes: some experiments with *Culex quinquefasciatics*. *MIRCEN Journal*, Vol. 2, pp. 355-363.

Angelon, K.A. & Petranka, J.W. (2002). Chemicals of predatory mosquitofish (*Gambusia affinis*) influence selection of oviposition site by *Culex* mosquitoes. *Journal of Chemical Ecology*, Vol. 28, pp. 797–806.

Anonymous. (1986). Azolla study initiated in China. WHO/FAO/UNDP PEEM Newsletter No. 15,3-4.

Anonymous. (1994). Epidemiological News Bulletin 20 (5) (published by the Ministry of the Environment, Singapore).

Balaraman, K., Balasubramanian, M. & Jambulingam, P. (1983). Field trial of *Bacillus thuringiensis* H-14 (VCRC B-17) against Culex and Anopheles larvae. *Indian Journal of Medical Research*, Vol. 77, pp. 38-43.

Bay, E.C. (1967). Mosquito control by fish: A present-day appraisal. WHO Chronicle, Vol. 21, pp. 415-423.

Broom, A.K., Smith, D.W., Hall, R.A., Johansen, C.A. & Mackenzie, J.S. (2003). Arbovirus infections. In: Cook, G., Zumla, A. (Eds.), Manson's Tropical Diseases, 21st ed. Saunders, London, pp. 725–764.

Burke, D.S. & Leake, C.J. (1988). Japanese encephalitis. In: Monath TP, editor. The Arboviroses: Epidemiology and ecology, vol. 3. Boca Raton FL: CRC Press, pp. 63-93.

Centers for Disease Control and Prevention. "Inactivated Japanese encephalitis virus vaccine. Recommendations of the Advisory Committee on Immunization Practices (ACIP)." MMWR. 42: RR1-15, 8 January 1993.

Chandra, G., Bhattacharjee, I., Chatterjee, S.N., & Ghosh A. (2008). Mosquito control by larvivorous fish. *Indian Journal of Medical Research*, Vol. 127, pp. 13-27.

Curtis, C.F. (1992). Personal protection methods against vectors of disease. *Review of Medical and Veterinary Entomology*, Vol. 80, pp. 543–553.

Diagana, M., Preux, P. & Dumas M. (2007) Japanese encephalitis revisited. *Journal of the Neurological Sciences*, Vol. 262, pp. 165-170.

Dutta, K., Rangarajan, P.N., Vrati S., & Anirban Basu, A. (2010) Japanese encephalitis: pathogenesis, prophylactics and therapeutics. *Current Science*, Vol. 98(3), pp. 326-334.

Dutta, P., Khan, S.A., Khan, A.M., Borah, J., Sarmah, C.K. & Mahanta, J. (2011).The Effect of Insecticide-Treated Mosquito Nets (ITMNs) on Japanese Encephalitis Virus Seroconversion in Pigs and Humans. *American Journal of Tropical Medicine and Hygiene*, Vol. 84(3), pp. 466-472.

Elango, G., Rahuman, A.A., Bagavan, A., Kamaraj, C., Zahir, A.A., Rajakumar, G., Marimuthu, S.& Santhoshkumar, T. (2010). Efficacy of botanical extracts against Japanese encephalitis vector, *Culex tritaeniorrhynchus*. *Parasitology Research*, Vol. 106, pp. 481-492.

Endy, T.P. & Nisalak, A. (2002). Japanese encephalitis virus: ecology and epidemiology. In: Mackenzie JS, Barrett ADT, Deubel V, editors. Japanese Encephalitis and West Nile Viruses. Berlin: Springer-Verlag; pp. 12-48.

Fischer, M,, Hills, S., Staples, E., Johnson, B., Yaich, M., & Solomon, T. (2008). Japanese encephalitis prevention and control: advances, challenges, and new initiatives. Scheld WM , Hammer SM , Hughes JM , eds. Emerging Infections 8 . Washington, DC : American Society for Microbiology Press, pp. 93-124 .

Fradin, M.S. (2001). Protection from blood-feeding arthropods. In:Auerbach PS (ed) Wilderness Medicine, 4th edn. Mosby, St.Louis, pp 754–768.

Gajanana, A., Rajendran, R., Samuel, P.P., Thenmozhi, V., Tsai, T.F., Kimura-Kuroda, J. & Reuben, R. (1997). Japanese encephalitis in South Arcot district, Tamil Nadu India: a three-year longitudinal study of vector abundance and infection frequency. *Journal of Medical Entomology*, Vo. 34, pp. 651–659.

Ghajar, J. & Hariri, R.J. (1992). Management of pediatric head injury. *Pediatric Clinics of North America*, Vol. 39, pp. 1093-1012.

Gould, E.A. (2002) Evolution of the Japanese serological group viruses. In Current Topics in Microbiology and Immunology: Japanese Encephalitis and West Nile Virus Infections (eds Mackenzie, J. S., Barrett, A. D. and Deubel, V.), Springer-Verlag, Berlin, pp. 391-404.

Halstead, S.B. & Jacobson, J. (2003). Japanese encephalitis. Advances in Virus Research, Vo. 61, pp. 103-138.

Halstead, S.B. (1992). Arboviroses of the Pacific and Southeast Asia. In: Feigin V, Cherry JD, editors. Textbook of pediatric infectious diseases. 3rd edition. Philadelphia: WB Saunders; pp. 1468–1475.

Hanna, J.N., Ritchie, S.A., Phillips, D.A., Shield, J., Bailey, M.C., Mackenzie, J.S., Poidinger, M., McCall, B.J. & Mills, P.J. (1996). An outbreak of Japanese encephalitis in the Torres Strait Australia. *Medical Journal of Australia*, 1996; 165, 256–260.

Hargreaves, K., Koekemoer, L.L., Brooke, B.D., Hunt, R.H., Mthembu, J. & Coetzee, M. (2000). *Anopheles funestus* resistant to pyrethroid insecticides in South Africa. *Medical and Veterinary Entomology*, Vol. 14, pp. 181-189.

Hennessy, S., Zhengle, L., Tsai, T.F., et al. (1996). "Effectiveness of live-attenuated Japanese encephalitis vaccine (SA14-14-2): a case control study." *Lancet*, Vo. 347, pp. 1583-1586.

Igarashi, A. (1992a). Epidemiology and control of Japanese encephalitis. *World Health Statistics Quarterly*, Vol. 45, pp. 299-304.

Igarashi, A. (1992b). Japanese encephalitis: virus, infection, and control. Kurstak E, ed. Control of Virus Diseases. Second edition. New York: Marcel Dekker, pp. 309-342.

Jacobs-lorena, M., & James, A.A. (2002). Genetic modification of insects of medical importance: past, present and future. Report t of the Scientific Working Group on Insect Vectors and Human Health, TDR/SWG/VEC/03.1 P68-73.

Jang, Y.S., Kim, M.K., Ahn, Y.J., & Lee, H.S. (2002). Larvicidal activity of Brazilian plants against *Aedes aegypti* and *Culex pipiens* pallens (Diptera: Culicidae). *Agricultural Chemistry Biotechnology*, Vol. 45(3), pp. 131-134.

Karunamoorthi, K. & Sabesan, S. (2010). Laboratory evaluation of dimethyl phthalate treated wristbands against three predominant mosquito (Diptera: Culicidae) vectors of disease. *European Review of Medical and Pharmacological Science*, Vol. 14(5), pp. 443-448.

Karunamoorthi, K., Ilango, K. & Endale, A. (2009). Ethnobotanical survey of knowledge and usage custom of traditional insect/mosquito repellent plants among the Ethiopian Oromo ethnic group. *Journal of Ethnopharmacology*, Vol. 125(2), pp. 224-229.

Karunamoorthi, K., Ilango, K. & Murugan, K. (2010) Laboratory evaluation of traditionally used plant-based insect repellent against the malaria vector *Anopheles arabiensis* Patton (Diptera: Culicidae). *Parasitology Research*, Vol. 106(5), pp. 1217-1223.

Karunamoorthi, K., Ramanujam, S. & Rathinasamy, R. (2008). Evaluation of leaf extracts of *Vitex negundo* L. (Family: Verbenaceae) against larvae of *Culex tritaeniorhynchus* and repellent activity on adult vector mosquitoes. *Parasitology Research*, Vol. 103, pp. 545-550.

Keiser, J., Maltese, M.F., Erlanger, T.E., Bos, R., Tanner , M., Singer, B.H. & J¨urg Utzinger, J. (2005). Effect of irrigated rice agriculture on Japanese encephalitis, including challenges and opportunities for integrated vector management. *Acta Tropica*, Vol. 95, pp. 40-57.

Kim, H.C., Kim, M.S. & Yu, H.S. (1994). Biological control of vector mosquitoes by the use of fish predators *Moroco oxycephalus* and *Misgurnus anguillicaudatus* in the laboratory and semi-field rice paddy. *Korean Journal of Entomology*, Vol. 24, pp. 269-284.

Kramer,V. (1984). Evaluation of *Bacillus sphaericus* & *B. thuringiensis* H-14 for mosquito control in rice fields. *Indian Journal of Medical Research*, Vol. 80, pp. 642-648.

Kumar, R., Mathur, A., Kumar, A., Sharma, S., Chakraborty, S. & Chaturvedi, V.C. (1990). Clinical features and prognosis indicators of Japanese encephalitis in children in Lucknow (India). *Indian Journal of Medical Research*, Vol. 91, pp. 321-327.

Kumar, R., Selvan, S.A., Sharma, S., Mathur, A., Misra, P.K., Singh, G.K., et al. (1994). Clinical predictors of Japanese encephalitis. *Neuroepidemiology*, Vol. 13, pp. 97-102.

Lacey, L.A. & Lacey, C.M. (1990). The medical importance of Riceland mosquitoes and their control using alternatives to chemical insecticides. *Journal of American Mosquito Control Association*, Vol. 2 (Suppl.), pp. 1-93.

Liu, S.L. & Hsu,Y.C. (1982). Effect of the fungus *Coelomomyces indica* on the viability of *Culex tritaeniorhynchus* larvae. Kun Chong Xue Bao, Vol. 25, pp. 409-412.

Lu Bao-Lin, (1988). The effect of Azolla on mosquito breeding. *Parasitology Today*, Vol. 4, pp. 328-329.

Lumpkin. T.A. & Plucknett, D.L. (1980). Azolla: botany, physiology and use as a green manure. *Economic Botany*, Vol. 34, pp. 111-153.

Luo, D., Yoa, R., Song, J., Huo, H. & Wang, Z. (1994). The effect of DDT spraying and bed nets impregnated with pyrethroid insecticide on the incidence of Japanese encephalitis virus infection. *Transactions of Royal Society of Tropical Medicine and Hygiene*, Vol. 88(6), pp. 629-631.

Mackenzie, J.S., Poidinger, M., Phillips, D., Johansen, C.A., Hall, R.A., Hanna, J., et al., (1997). Emergence of Japanese encephalitis virus in the Australasian region. In: Saluzzo JF, Dodet B, editor. Factors in the emergence of arboviruses diseases. Paris: Elsevier; pp. 191-201.

Mani, T.R., Rao, C.V., Rajendran, R., Devaputra, M., Prasanna, Y., Hanumaiah, Gajanana, A. & Reuben, R. (1991). Surveillance for Japanese encephalitis in villages near Madurai, Tamil Nadu, India. *Transactions of Royal Society of Tropical Medicine and Hygiene*, Vol. 85, pp. 287-291.

Mathur, A., Kumar, R., Sharma, S., Kulshreshtha, R., Kumar, A. & Chaturvedi, U.C. (1990). Rapid diagnosis of Japanese encephalitis by immunofluorescenct examination of cerebrospinal fluid. *Indian Journal of Medical Research*, Vol. 91, pp. 1-4.

Maxwell, C.A., Wakibara, J., Tho, S. & Curtis, C.F. (1998). Malaria infective biting at different hours of the night. *Medical and Veterinary Entomology*, Vol. 12, pp. 325-327.

Mishra, A.C., Jacob, P.G., Ramanujam, S., Bhat, H.R. & Pavri, K.M. (1983). Mosquito vectors of Japanese encephalitis epidemic in Mandya district (India). *Indian Journal of Medical Research*, Vol. 80, pp. 377-389.

Mittal, P.K. (2003). Biolarvicides in vector control: challenges and prospects. *Journal of Vector Borne Diseases*, Vol. 40, pp. 20-32.

Mogi, M., 1988. Water management in rice cultivation and its relation to mosquito production in Japan. In: Vector Borne Disease Control in Humans Through Rice Agro-ecosystem Management. International Rice Research Institute in collaboration with the WHO/FAO/UNEP Panel of Experts, pp. 101–109.

Monath, T.P. (2002). Japanese encephalitis vaccines: current vaccines and future prospects. *Current Topic on Microbiology and Immunology*, Vol. 267, pp. 105- 138.

Mori, M.C. & Siegel, R. (2000). Live attenuated Japanese encephalitis (SA14-14-2) vaccine: The best alternative? June 3, 2000. http://www.stanford.edu/~siegelr/mori.html. accessed on 9th February 2011.

Rajagopalan, P.K. & Work , T.H. (1969). An Analysis of mosquito collections with special reference to the incidence and prevalence of '*Culex vishnui* Complex' in the Japanese encephalitis infected localities of North Arcot District, Madras State, India, from December 1955 through December 1957. *Indian Journal of Medical Research*, Vol. 57, pp. 1409-1419.

Rajendran, R. & Reuben, R. (1988). Laboratory evaluation of the water fern *Azolla pinnata*, for mosquito control. *Journal of Biological Control*, Vol. 2, pp. 114- 116.

Rajendran, R. & Reuben, R. (1991). Evaluation of the water fern *Azolla microphylla* for mosquito population management in the rice land agro-ecosystem of South India. *Medical and Veterinary Entomology*, Vol. 5, pp. 299-310.

Reuben, R., Thenmozhi, V., Samuel, P.P., Gajanana, A. & Mani, T.R. (1992). Mosquito blood feeding patterns as a factor in the epidemiology of Japanese encephalitis in Southern India. *American Journal of Tropical Medicine and Hygiene*, Vol. 46, pp. 654-663.

Rhee, H.I., Shim, J.C., Kim, C.L. & Lee, W.J. (1983). Small scale field trial with Bacillus thuringiensis israelensis H-14 for control of the vector mosquito (*Culex tritaeniorhynchus*) larvae in rice fields. *Korean Journal of Entomology*, Vol. 13, pp. 39-46.

Rhodain, F. (1996). Données récentes sur l'épidémiologie de l'encéphalite japonaise. *Bulletin of the National Academy of Medicine*, Vol. 180, pp. 1325-1340.

Sabesan, S. (2003). Forecasting mosquito abundance to prevent Japanese encephalitis. *Current Science*, Vol. 84, No. 9, pp. 1172-1173.

Sabesan, S., Konuganti, H.R. & Vanamail, P. (2008). Spatial Delimitation, Forecasting and Control of Japanese Encephalitis: India - A Case Study. *The Open Parasitology Journal*, Vol. 2, pp. 59-63.

Sehgal, A. & Dutta, A.K. (2003). Changing perspectives in Japanese encephalitis in India. *Tropical Doctor*, Vol. 33, pp. 131-134.

Shope, R.E. & Meegan, J.M. (1997). Arboviruses. Evans AS, Kaslow RA, eds. Viral Infections of Humans. Fourth edition. New York: Plenum, 151–183.

Singh, A. (2007). Menace of Japanese encephalitis in rural areas of eastern Uttar Pradesh. *Current Science*, Vol. 93, No. 12, pp 1649.

Solomon, T. (1997). Viral encephalitis in Southeast Asia. *Neurological Infections and Epidemiology*, Vol. 2, pp. 191-199.

Solomon, T. (2006). Control of Japanese encephalitis – within our grasp? *New England Journal of Medicine*, Vol. 355, pp. 869-871.

Solomon, T., Dung, N. M., Kneen, R., Gainsborough, M., Vaughn, D. W. & Khanh, V. T. (2000). Japanese encephalitis. *Journal of Neurology, Neurosurgery and Psych*iatry, Vol. 68, pp. 405-415.

Solomon, T., Dung, N.M., Wills, B., Kneen, R., Gainsborough, M., Diet, T.V., Thuy, T.T., Loan, H.T., Khanh, V.C., Vaughn, D.W., White, N.J. & Farrar, J.J. (2003). Interferon alfa-2a in Japanese encephalitis: a randomised double-blind placebo-controlled trial. *Lancet*, Vol. 361, pp. 821-826.

Solomon, T., Ni, H., Beasley, D.W.C., Ekkelenkamp, M., Cardosa, M.J. & Barrett, A.D. (2003a). Origin and evolution of Japanese Encephalitis Virus in Southeast Asia. *Journal of Virology*, Vol. 5, pp. 3091-3098.

Suman, D.S., Shrivastava, A.R., Parashar, B.D., Pant, S.C., Agrawal, O.P. & Prakash, S. (2008). Scanning electron microscopic studies on egg surface morphology and morphometrics of Culex tritaeniorrhynchus and Culex quinquefasciatus (Diptera: Culicidae). *Parasitology Research*, Vol. 104, pp. 173-176.

Sundararaj, R. & Reuben, R. (1991). Evaluation of a microgel droplet formulation of Bacillus sphaericus 1593M (Biocide-S) for control of mosquito larvae in rice fields in Southern India. *Journal of American Mosquito Control Association*, Vol. 7, pp. 556-559.

Sunish, I.P. & Reuben, R. (2002). Factors influencing the abundance of Japanese encephalitis vectors in ricefields in India-II Biotic. *Medical and Veterinary Entomology*, Vol. 16, pp. 1-9.

Takahashi, M. & Suzuki, K. (1979). Japanese encephalitis virus in mosquito salivary glands. *American Journal of Tropical Medicine and Hygiene*, Vol. 28, pp. 122-135.

Tiroumourougane, S.V., Raghava, P. & Srinivasan, S. (2002). Japanese viral encephalitis. *Postgraduate Medical Journal*, Vol. 78, pp. 205-215.

Tsai, T.F, Yu. (1994). "Japanese encephalitis vaccines." Vaccines.[edited by] Stanley A. Plotkin, Edward A. Mortimer, Jr. Philadelphia : W.B. Saunders Co., 1994.

Tsai, T.F. (2000). New initiatives for the control of Japanese encephalitis by vaccination: minutes of a WHO/CVI meeting, Bangkok, Thailand, 13–15 October 1998. Vaccine 18 (Suppl. 2), 1-25.

Umenai, T., Krzysko, R., Bektimirov, T.A. & Assaad, F.A. (1985). Japanese encephalitis: current worldwide status. *Bulletin of World Health Organizat*ion, Vol. 63(4), pp. 625-631.

Vijayarani, H. & Gajanana, A. (2000). Low rate of Japanese encephalitis infection in rural children in Thanjavur district (Tamil Nadu), an area with extensive paddy cultivation. *Indian Journal of Medical Research*, Vol. 111, pp. 212-214.

Wada, Y. (1988). Strategies for control of Japanese encephalitis in rice production systems in developing countries. In: Vector Borne Disease Control in Humans Through Rice Agroecosystem Management. International Rice Research Institute in collaboration with the WHO/FAO/UNEP Panel of Experts, pp. 153–160.

WHO. (1998). Japanese encephalitis vaccine. WHO position paper. *Weekly Epidemiology Record*, Vol. 73, pp. 337-344.

WHO. (2006). Guidelines for Prevention and Control of Japanese Encephalitis. http://whoindia.healthrepository.org/handle/123456789/187. accessed on 9th February 2011.